A.C. Feller · J. Diebold
Histopathology of Nodal and Extranodal Non-Hodgkin's Lymphomas

Springer
Berlin
Heidelberg
New York
Hong Kong
London
Milan
Paris
Tokyo

Alfred C. Feller · Jacques Diebold

in Collaboration with M. Paulli and A. Le Tourneau

Histopathology of Nodal and Extranodal Non-Hodgkin's Lymphomas

(Based on the WHO Classification)

Third, Completely Revised and Updated Edition

With 307 Figures in 345 Parts

Springer

Prof. Dr. med. Alfred Christian Feller
Universitätsklinikum Schleswig-Holstein, Campus Lübeck
Institut für Pathologie
Ratzeburger Allee 160, 23538 Lübeck

Professor emeritus Jacques Diebold
Hotel-Dieu de Paris
Service Central d'Anatomie et de Cytologie Pathologique
1, place du Parvis Notre Dame, 78181 Paris Cedex 04
Frankreich

ISBN 978-3-642-62224-3 ISBN 978-3-642-18653-0 (eBook)
DOI 10.1007/978-3-642-18653-0

Library of Congress Cataloguing-in-Publication Data
Feller, Alfred C.
Histopathology of nodal and extra-nodal non-Hodgkin's lymphomas/Alfred C. Feller, Jacques Diebold. – 3rd, completely rev. and updated ed.
p.; cm.
Rev. ed. of: Histopathology of non-Hodgkin lymphomas/Karl Lennert. 2nd ed. 1992.
Includes bibliographical references and index.
ISBN 978-3-642-62224-3 (alk. paper)
1. Lymphomas – Histopathology. I. Title: Histopathology of non-Hodgkin lymphomas.
II. Diebold, Jacques. III. Lennert, Karl. Histopathology of non-Hodgkin lymphomas. IV. Title.
[DNLM: 1. Lymphoma, Non-Hodgkin-classification. 2. Lymphoma, Non-Hodgkin – pathology. QZ 350 F318h 2003]
RC280.L9L4613 2003
616.99'446-dc21 2002042885

http://www.springer.de

Originally published by Springer-Verlag Berlin Heidelberg New York in 2004
Softcover reprint of the hardcover 3rd edition 2004

Cover design: E. Kirchner, D-69121 Heidelberg
Typesetting: FotoSatz Pfeifer GmbH, D-82166 Gräfelfing
Printed on acid-free paper 21/3150 – 5 4 3 2 1 0

Preface

Roughly 10 years ago, the second edition of „Histopathology of Non-Hodgkin's Lymphomas“ was published. The book gave an excellent overview of predominantly nodal non-Hodgkin's lymphomas. Since then, advances in the field of immunology and the development of new techniques, including new monoclonal antibodies, have allowed a more precise definition of several lymphoma entities as well as a better understanding of the lymphoid system.

Thus, in addition to the entities described in the updated Kiel Classification, reports of new, especially extranodal entities have appeared in the literature. Of these, the most important is MALT-lymphoma, which is one of the most frequently occurring extranodal lymphomas. In addition, a large number of rare diseases have been identified, some of which seem to be well-defined clinicopathological entities. An increasing number of monoclonal antibodies that react with formalin fixed material, as well as PCR, sequencing techniques, and the detection of chromosomal abnormalities could aid in establishing the relevance of some of these newly described diseases.

Meetings of The European Association of Hematopathology (EAHP) have opened Europe to the United States and have led to closer contact between the EAHP and its American counterpart, the Society for Hematopathology (SH). Based on these joint discussions, a group of well-known hematopathologists from both sides of the Atlantic suggested the Revised European-American Lymphoma Classification (REAL classification), which in many respects was based on the earlier Kiel classification. In turn, this encouraged the WHO to formulate a consensus classification, which was eventually approved by both hematopathological societies and issued in 2001.

Around that time, Prof. Karl Lennert encouraged us to rewrite the second edition of the „Histopathology of Non-Hodgkin's Lymphomas“. Thus, this new edition is completely based on the WHO classification. However, the reader who is familiar with the previous edition and with the Kiel Classification system will recognize that almost all of the nodal lymphoma entities described in the updated Kiel Classification appear in the WHO Classification. For this reason, we feel that the WHO Classification is, in many aspects, based on the Kiel Classification.

In order to stress the importance of distinguishing between nodal and extranodal lymphomas and to clearly differentiate between them, we decided to organize discussions of the lymphoma entities according to the organs in which they primarily occur. Thus, a large chapter is devoted to describing primary nodal lymphomas. Since these lymphomas occur in extranodal sites as well, they are then also discussed in the chapters on the various organs, with cross-references to their extensive description in the chapter on nodal lymphomas, while the organ-specific lymphoma types are described in the respective organ chapters. We think that assigning the distinct lymphoma types to individual chapters makes the book easier to use.

This new edition is intended chiefly for use by pathologists in every-day diagnostics, as was true for the previous edition. Although we have included the latest molecular genetic and cytogenetic results, the information provided is limited, as we feel that, even today, the most important diagnostic principle still lies in the morphology and the immunohistochemistry. Moreover, no attempt was made at providing a complete citation of the literature since an online search quickly renders citations in a printed book out of date.

For diagnostic purposes, we have included a separate chapter that describes in detail the distinct patterns of lymphoma infiltration in the bone marrow. The last chapter of the book provides technical advice, but the reader should be well aware that the information is very incomplete and in some way provisional as new techniques are constantly being developed. However, basic techniques, especially those which are prey to pitfalls arising from the use and interpretation of results of molecular genetics, are discussed.

We would not have been able to write this book without the tremendous work of Karl Lennert, who wrote the first and the second edition. We therefore are most grateful to Prof. Lennert for teaching us over many years and for giving us the possibility to write this third edition.

We are very grateful for the help of many colleagues. We would like to thank Prof. Marco Paulli for writing the chapters on anaplastic large-cell lymphomas and lymphomatoid papulosis. Dr. Agnès Le Tourneau provided us with many photomicrographs. Prof. Philippe Gaulard supported us with the chapter on hepatosplenic NK/T-cell lymphoma, first described by himself. We also want to thank Prof. Hartmut Merz for interesting discussions on many of the topics of this book. Dagmar Schmöe organized the bibliography with great enthusiasm. We are grateful to the many technicians from the institutes in Lübeck and Paris. It would not have been possible to design and write this book without the tremendous help of our secretaries, Catherine Belorgey, Birgit Kalus, Jaqueline Gèron and Silja Klein.

It was a great pleasure to co-operate with Springer-Verlag. First of all, we want to thank Dr. Julia Heidelmann for her continuous stimulation and support in finalizing this book. We also thank Wendy Ran for her excellent copy-editing, and Joachim W. Schmidt for his support during the production process as well as his careful attention to the quality of the illustrations.

Lübeck and Paris, Summer 2003 — Alfred C. Feller, Jaques Diebold

Contents

Chapter 1

History of Lymphoma Classification 1

1.1 Introduction

Before 1970, several purely morphologically oriented description classifications of non-Hodgkin's lymphoma (NHL) were suggested. From that period new classifications based on current immunological concepts [Lukes-Collins classification (Lukes and Collins 1974a,b; Lukes et al. 1978b), Kiel classification (Gérard-Marchant et al. 1974; Lennert et al. 1975; Lennert 1976, 1978)] were proposed. The classification of Dorfman (1974) was a variant of the Rappaport classification. The latter was proposed by Rappaport in 1956 (Mathé et al. 1956), finalized in the Armed Forces Institute of Pathology (AFIP) fascicle "Tumors of the Hematopoietic System" in 1966 (Rappaport 1966), and then revised in 1976 (Nathwani et al. 1976). The classification of the British National Lymphoma Investigation (Bennett et al. 1974), the WHO classification (Mathé et al. 1976), and the classification of the Japanese Lymphoma Study Group (Suchi et al. 1979; see The T- and B-Cell Malignancy Study Group 1981) were independently proposed at about the same time.

In fact, in the United States a dispute developed on the widely used Rappaport classification versus the new immunologically oriented classifications (Kiel and Lukes and Collins Classification). Whereas it was almost impossible to translate from the Rappaport classification into the Kiel classification and vice versa (Krüger et al. 1981), it was relatively easy to translate back and forth between the Lukes-Collins classification and the Kiel classification (Lennert et al. 1983). The Rappaport classification was simple to use and had proved to be prognostically relevant in numerous clinical studies in the 1960s. The difference between nodular and diffuse lymphomas was particularly emphasized. It soon became clear, however, that the Rappaport classification was not consistent with the results of modern immunology, i.e., with new concepts of the lymphoid system. Nevertheless, clinical oncologists and other specialists in the United States insisted on further use of the Rappaport classification because of its simplicity and clinical relevance (clinical studies using the Lukes-Collins or the Kiel classification had not yet been done or were incomplete).

This did not solve the problem, however. Five other classifications had been proposed and were also defended emphatically by their proponents. A compromise agreement was not attained at the meeting at Airlie House in Warrenton, Virginia, USA (in 1975). In view of this situation, a large-scale study was designed, organized, and supported financially by the National Cancer Institute (NCI) of the United States that would permit all authors of the new classifications of NHL, as well as selected pathologists who were not committed to any particular classification, to review in a relatively short time a large number of previously untreated cases at different institutions. The clinical data on 1,153 cases and all histopathological diagnoses according to the six available classifications were recorded at a central facility and subsequently collated for evaluation and discussion. The end result was the presentation of a "*Working Formulation of Non-Hodgkin's Lymphoma for Clinical Usage*" on January 11, 1980 in Palo Alto, California, USA (The Non-Hodgkin's Lymphoma Classification Project 1982).

The Working Formulation (WF) was not a new classification of malignant lymphomas (MLs), but rather a terminological compromise for the definition of entities with different natural histories, prognoses, and responses to therapy. The WF clearly incorporated concepts and terms that derived from the classifications proposed by Lukes and Collins, Dorfman, and the British National Lymphoma Investigation and, to a certain extent, the Rappaport classification. In the WF, the three terms "low grade", "intermediate grade", and "high grade" are defined clinically, and not morphologically, which was justly pointed out by Musshoff (1987). The WF includes ten different categories within the three grades. The Kiel classification recognizes the two groups, low- and high-grade malignant lymphoma, adhering a morphological principle (which leads, nonetheless, to similar prognostic consequences). The low-grade malignant neoplasms are made up essentially of "–cytes" with, in some instances, a minority population of "-blasts", whereas the high-grade malignant neoplasms consist mostly, or exclusively of, "-blasts". The classification is based on morphology, and not on the results of clinical treatment. It defines biological entities.

1.2 The Kiel Classification

The old, simple classification (Lennert 1967, 1969), used in Germany until the introduction of the Kiel classification, differed from the classification recommended by Rappaport (1966), which was widely accepted in Western countries because of its apparent clinical relevance. Since neither the old German classification nor Rappaport's classification were compatible with the knowledge gained from modern research in immunology, it was clearly necessary to apply the results of this research to neoplasms of lymphocytes and their variants. This required taking three steps: (1) the various cell types of lymphoid tissue (and lymphoid neoplasms) had to be defined by hematological and cytochemical methods; (2) the immunological characteristics ("markers") of the morphologically identified cells had to be determined; and (3) lymphoma cells had to be morphologically and immunologically matched with their normal counterparts. These investigations led to a new understanding of ML. By taking the criteria of general pathology and hematology and the clinical behavior of ML into consideration, it was possible to propose a new classification. The so-called Kiel classification (Gérard-Marchant et al. 1974; Lennert et al. 1975; Lennert 1976) is based on that proposition (Fig. 1.1) (Table 1.1).

Lukes and Collins (1974a, b; 1975a, b; Collins et al. 1976; Lukes et al. 1978a) followed a similar course. First, they used the shape of the nuclei to characterize lymphoid cells. They distinguished follicular center cells (FCC) with cleaved nuclei from those with noncleaved nuclei, and lymphoid cells with convoluted nuclei. At the same time, their diagnostic labels indicated whether a lymphoma is composed of B cells, T cells, or "undefined" cells. In contrast, the main terms used in the Kiel classification were originally morphological ones; "B" and "T" were found only in the names

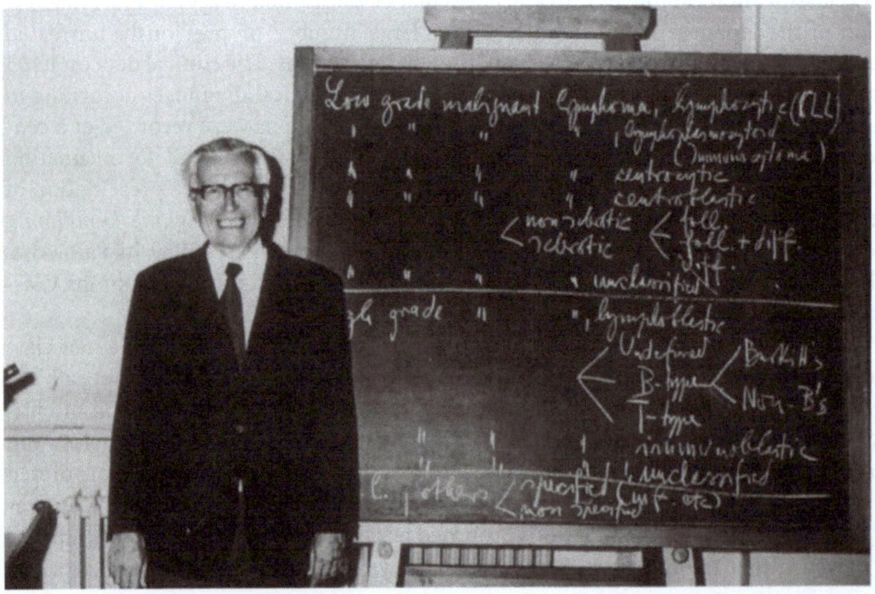

Fig. 1.1. Karl Lennert in Kiel, in 1974, standing in front of a blackboard with the first version of the Kiel classification

Table 1.1. Kiel classification of non-Hodgkin's lymphomas (originally published in 1974; modification of the version published in 1978)

Low-grade malignant lymphomas
Lymphocytic
B-CLL
T-CLL
Hairy cell leukemia
Mycosis fungoides and Sézary's syndrome
T-zone lymphoma
Lymphoplasmacytic/-cytoid (immunocytoma)
Plasmacytic
Centrocytic
Centroblastic-centrocytic
Follicular-diffuse
Diffuse
Sclerosis
High-grade malignant lymphomas
Centroblastic
Lymphoblastic
Burkitt type
Convoluted-cell type
Unclassified
Immunoblastic

of some of the subtypes. The main terms for many B-cell lymphomas indicated that they were derived from the B-cell system (e.g. immunocytoma, plasmacytoma and all germinal center cell tumors), even without the "B" prefix.

Other guiding principles of the Kiel classification were:

1. The cellular composition is of primary importance. This distinguished the Kiel classification from *most* former classifications, whose first criterion had been the growth pattern of the lymphoma (diffuse or nodular).
2. A distinction is made between low-grade and high-grade ML. Low-grade MLs consist of "–cytes", but may also contain a certain number of "–blasts"; high-grade MLs consist of "–blasts" predominately or completely, in other words, low-grade MLs are usually composed of *small cells* that are sometimes interspersed with large cells. High-grade MLs are composed predominately of medium-sized to *large cells.*
3. Since practically all types of ML may be associated with a leukemic blood picture, and since it is often impossible to predict this histologically, leukemias and "solid" lymphomas have been placed together in the Kiel classification.
4. Because paraproteinemia (e.g. macroglobulinemia) is a facultative phenomenon in Ig-producing lymphomas, the disease is defined by its underlying morphological characteristics alone (e.g. immunocytoma).

At this time, about 12% (Lennert et al. 1975) of lymphomas still could not be classified. For the first time, increasingly detailed immunohistochemical definitions of the various lymphoma types were included (Stein et al. 1984). Also molecular genetic methods (O'Connor et al. 1985; Griesser et al. 1986, 1987, 1989; Tkachuk et al. 1988) had been applied, as well as re-embedding of biopsy specimens in synthetics (Hui et al. 1988) in order to achieve a description of the cytological details as exact and as reproducible as possible, especially in cases of T-cell lymphoma and high-grade malignant B-cell lymphoma. As a result a re-evaluation of the existing, "tried and true" Kiel classification became necessary. In particular, it had become possible to classify the relatively rare T-cell lymphomas and to add new entities that were previously not, or not definitely, considered to be NHL (e.g. lymphoepithelioid lymphoma, AILD/LgX type). Moreover, large cell anaplastic lymphoma (LCAL), which had been identified with the monoclonal antibody Ki-1 (CD30), was included. Finally, the B-cell lymphomas of high-grade malignancy that were difficult to distinguish morphologically from one another were reclassified.

In 1988, the European Lymphoma Club decided to introduce an *updated Kiel classification*, with separate columns for B-cell and T-cell types (Table 1.2). The B-cell lymphoma column differed in only two respects from the previous Kiel classification. First, LCAL has been added. Second, Burkitt's lymphoma had been separated from the lymphoblastic lymphomas. The separation into low-grade and high-grade ML had been kept in the updated classification, even though the greater morphological variability of T-cell lymphomas made it difficult to draw strict lines. As there were a number of parallels in morphology and signs of function between the B-cell and T-cell lymphomas, these parallels were taken into account by placing corresponding B-cell and T-cell lymphomas opposite each other, with the goal of making it easier to remember the classification.

By moving lymphoblastic lymphoma to the end of the table and separating it with a broken line, the special status of these lymphomas, which represented neo-

Table 1.2. Updated Kiel classification of non-Hodgkin's lymphomas (1988, modified in 1992)

B	T
Low-grade malignant lymphomas	
Lymphocytic	Lymphocytic
Chronic lymphocytic leukemia	Chronic lymphocytic leukemia
Prolymphocytic leukemia	Prolymphocytic leukemia
Hairy-cell leukemia	Small-cell, cerebriform
	Mycosis fungoides, Sézary's syndrome
Lymphoplasmacytic/-cytoid (immunocytoma)	Lymphoepithelioid (Lennert's lymphoma)
Plasmacytic	Angioimmunoblastic (AILD, LgX)
Centroblastic-centrocytic	T-zone lymphoma
Follicular ± diffuse	
Diffuse	
Centrocytic (mantle cell)	Pleomorphic, small-cell (HTLV-1 ±)
Monocytoid, including marginal zone cell	
High-grade malignant lymphomas	
Centroblastic	Pleomorphic, medium-sized and large cell (HTLV-1 ±)
Immunoblastic	Immunoblastic (HTLV-1 ±)
Burkitt's lymphoma	
Large cell anaplastic (Ki-1+)	Large cell anaplastic (Ki-1+)
Lymphoblastic	Lymphoblastic
Rare types	**Rare types**

plasms of precursor cells, was pointed out. All other lymphoma types were thought to be derived from peripheral lymphocytes and their activation or proliferation forms.

A category called "rare types" was added. In the B-cell series it originally contained monocytoid B-cell lymphoma and large-cell sclerosing B-cell lymphoma of the mediastinum. After publication of the updated Kiel classification, however, it was realized that monocytoid B-cell lymphoma is not as rare as it appeared to be at first; hence, it was included as the last category in the group of low-grade malignant B-cell lymphomas. Two other types were added to the "rare types" category, microvillous, large cell lymphoma and high-grade malignant B-cell lymphomas with a high content of T cells.

When the updated Kiel classification was first made public (Meeting of the European Association for Haematopathology in Geneva, March 1988), it was criticized for leaving out polymorphic immunocytoma. The reasons for not including this subtype were as follows:

1. Subgroups of the lymphoma types were excluded wherever possible in order to maintain clarity. This was done with other entities as well, such as centroblastic-centrocytic lymphoma and centroblastic lymphoma.
2. Polymorphic immunocytoma is diagnosed more often than it actually occurs. Including it in the classification would just further this tendency.

The Kiel Classification did not imply that all ML were classifiable. In most "unclassified" cases, however, the reason for the imprecise diagnosis is shortcomings in biopsy excision or processing techniques. A principle idea was that even poorly prepared slides usually allow the pathologist to say whether it is a case of low-grade or high-grade ML. This should give the clinician at least one criterion on which to base treatment.

The updated Kiel classification of nodal lymphomas, including lymphoblastic lymphomas, reflects the current limits of classification that can be reached with the morphological and immunohistochemical methods available at that time. It was stated that further studies may result in minor variations or reveal rare special types. It was thought to be unlikely, however, that any of the basic entities of the classification will have to undergo significant changes.

If a change should actually become necessary, Lennert and Feller (1992) stated that this would result only from systematic application of new methods such as those of classic and molecular cytogenetics. It was also indicated that it would certainly be necessary to expand the Kiel classification if it was to include all the extranodal lymphomas, especially those of the mucosa-associated lymphoid tissue (MALT). Finally, it was stated that it might be more sensible to ascertain whether different systems of organs develop different types of lymphomas, which would necessitate separate classifications.

1.3 The REAL Classification Proposal

In 1994, a publication appeared, presenting what was then regarded as a new classification, by a group of pathologists called the International Lymphoma Study Group (ILSG) (Harris et al. 1994). This group was founded after the retirement of Professor Karl Lennert in 1989, which resulted in the end of the European Lymphoma Club. The members of the ILSG are hematopathologists from all over the world, mostly from North America and Europe. The successive meetings during the 1980s of the American Society of Hematopathology and of the European Association for Hematopathology allowed these pathologists to meet, get to know each other, and to cooperate. They chose the ambitious acronym REAL (Revised European American Lymphoma) as the name of their classification.

The REAL classification represents a kind of revisited and expanded Kiel classification, using many of the entities defined in the up-dated Kiel classification and adding what was missing, i.e., some extranodal lymphomas, particularly the MALT lymphoma first described by P. Isaacson and D. Wright (1984), as well as new entities. Like the Kiel classification, this classification stressed the importance of morphology and immunohistochemistry. The authors also included cytogenetics and molecular biology, as significant advances had been made in both fields during the 1980s and early 1990s. For European hematopathologists, the REAL classification was regarded as an expanded Kiel classification. But for the USA, the REAL had the effect of a Trojan Horse, allowing the up-dated Kiel classification to penetrate the protected world of hematology and hematopathology.

1.4 The WHO Classification

In 1995, Dr. L.H. Sobin, who was responsible for the WHO classification of neoplasias, proposed to Dr. Elaine Jaffe, one of the member of the ILSG, to publish a "blue book" on the classification of neoplasias arising from hematopoietic cells. To reach the highest rate of consensus, it was decided that this WHO classification should be organized by both the American and the European Societies of Hematopathology. A steering committee was subsequently organized comprising presidents and past presidents of both societies. The steering committee organized ten groups, each with a chairperson. Each chairperson was asked to invite two to six pathologists and hematologists to work together in the group. Each group was instructed to work on one type of hematopoietic or lymphatic neoplasia, to propose a classification comprising all entities, and to describe precisely all the characteristics of the entities. Different general meetings allowed the ten groups to discuss the results achieved so far. Preview publications were prepared in order to acquire a list of entities to be included in the future classification (Jaffe et al. 1998, 1999; Harris et al. 1999). A joint meeting of pathologists, cytologists, hematologists and clinicians in Airlie, Washington DC, was held in 1997. This meeting allowed the proposed classification to be presented to clinicians, who then had the opportunity to modify it.

After this meeting, 3 years were necessary to finish the manuscript. A last meeting was organized in Lyon (France), at the International Agency for Research on Cancer (IARC) in 2000, to discuss the final points and to choose the figures. The book was then published in the new series organized by the IARC in Lyon, under the direction of Dr. Kleihues, and has been available since the end of 2001 (Table 1.3) (Jaffe et al. 2001).

Table 1.3. WHO classification of Hodgkin's, non-Hodgkin's lymphomas and lymphoproliferations

- **B-cell neoplasms**
  - Precursor B-cell neoplasms
    - Precursor B lymphoblastic leukemia/lymphoma
  - Mature B-cell neoplasms
    - Chronic lymphocytic leukemia/small lymphocytic lymphoma
    - B-cell prolymphocytic leukemia
    - Lymphoplasmacytic lymphoma
    - Splenic marginal zone lymphoma
    - Hairy cell leukemia
    - Plasma cell myeloma
    - Solitary plasmacytoma of bone
    - Extraosseous plasmacytoma
    - Extranodal marginal zone B-cell lymphoma of mucosa-associated lymphoid tissue (MALT-lymphoma)
    - Nodal marginal zone B-cell lymphoma
    - Follicular lymphoma
    - Mantle cell lymphoma
    - Diffuse large-B-cell lymphoma
    - Mediastinal (thymic) large B-cell lymphoma
    - Intravascular large-B-cell lymphoma
    - Primary effusion lymphoma
    - Burkitt lymphoma/leukemia
  - B-cell proliferations of uncertain malignant potential
    - Lymphomatoid granulomatosis
    - Post-transplant lymphoproliferative disorder, polymorphic
- **T-cell and NK-cell neoplasms**
  - Precursor T-cell neoplasms
    - Precursor T-lymphoblastic leukemia/ lymphoma
    - Blastic NK-cell lymphoma
  - Mature T-cell and NK-cell neoplasms
    - T-cell prolymphocytic leukemia
    - T-cell large granular lymphocytic leukemia
    - Aggressive NK-cell leukemia
    - Adult T-cell leukemia/lymphoma
    - Extranodal NK-/T-cell lymphoma, nasal type
    - Enteropathy-type T-cell lymphoma
    - Hepatosplenic T-cell lymphoma
    - Subcutaneous panniculitis-like T-cell lymphoma
    - Mycosis fungoides
    - Sezary's syndrome
    - Primary cutaneous anaplastic large-cell lymphoma
    - Peripheral T-cell lymphoma, unspecified
    - Angioimmunoblastic T-cell lymphoma
    - Anaplastic large-cell lymphoma
  - T-cell proliferation of uncertain malignant potential
    - Lymphomatoid papulosis
  - Hodgkin's lymphoma
    - Nodular-lymphocyte-predominant Hodgkin lymphoma
    - Classical Hodgkin lymphoma
      - Nodular sclerosis classical Hodgkin's lymphoma
      - Lymphocyte-rich classical Hodgkin's lymphoma
      - Mixed cellularity classical Hodgkin's lymphoma
      - Lymphocyte-depleted classical Hodgkin's lymphoma

References

Bennett MH, Farrer-Brown G, Henry K, Jelliffe AM (1974) Classification of non-Hodgkin's lymphomas (letter to the editor). Lancet ii:405–406

Collins RD, Leech JH, Waldron JA, Flexner JM, Glick AD (1976) Diagnosis of hematopoietic, mononuclear, and lymphoid cell neoplasms. In: Rose NR, Friedman H (eds) Manual of clinical immunology. American Society for Microbiology, Washington, pp 718–733

Dorfman RF (1974) Histopathology of malignant lymphomas. Clin Hematol 3:39–76

Gérard-Marchant R, Hamlin I, Lennert K, Rilke F, Stansfeld AG, van Unnik JAM (1974) Classification of non-Hodgkin's lymphomas (letter to the editor). Lancet ii:406–440

Griesser H, Feller A, Lennert K, Minden M, Mak TW (1986) Rearrangement of the β-chain of the T-cell antigen receptor and immunoglobulin genes in lymphoproliferative disorders. J Clin Invest 78:1179–1184

Griesser H, Feller AC, Mak TW, Lennert K (1987) Clonal rearrangements of T-cell receptor and immunoglobulin genes and immunophenotypic antigen expression in different subclasses of Hodgkin's disease. Int J Cancer 40:157–160

Griesser H, Tkachuk D. Reis MD, Mak TW (1989) Gene rearrangements and translocations in lymphoproliferative diseases. Blood 73:1402–1415

Harris NL, Jaffe ES, Stein H, Banks PM, Chan JKC, Cleary ML, Delsol G, De Wolf-Peeters C, Falini B, Gatter KC, Grogan TM, Issacson PG, Knowles KM, Mason DY, Müller-Hermelink HK, Pileri SA, Piris MA, Ralfkiaer E, Warnke RA (1994) A Revised European-American classification of Lymphoid neoplasms: a proposal from the International Lymphoma Study Group. Blood 84:1361–1392

Harris NL, Jaffe ES, Diebold J, Flandrin G, Müller-Hermelink HK, Vardiman J, Liser TA, Bloomfield CD (1999) World Health Organization classification of neoplastic diseases of the hematopoietic and lymphoid tissues: report of the clinical advisory committee meeting. Airlie House, Virginia, November 1997. J Clin Oncol 17:3835–3849

Hui PK, Feller AC, Lennert K (1988) High-grade non-Hodgkin's lymphoma of B-cell type. I. Histopathology. Histopathology 12:127–143

Isaacson P, Wright DH (1984) Extranodal malignant lymphoma arising from mucosa-associated lymphoid tissue. Cancer 53:2515–2524

Jaffe ES, Harris NL, Diebold J, Müller-Hermelink HK (1998) World Health Organization classification of lymphomas: a work in progress. Ann Oncol 9:S25–S30

Jaffe ES, Harris NL, Diebold J, Müller-Hermelink HK (1999) World Health Organization classification of neoplastic diseases of the hematopoietic and lymphoid tissues. Am J Clin Pathol 111 [Suppl 1]:8–12

Jaffe ES, Harris NL, Stein H, Vardiman JW (eds) (2001) World Health Organization Classification of Tumours. Pathology and Genetics of Tumours of the Haematopoietic and Lymphoid Tissues. IARC, Lyon

Krüger GRF, Grisar T, Lennert K, Schwarze E-W, Brittinger G (Kiel Lymphoma Study Group) (1981) Histopathological correlation of the Kiel with the original Rappaport classification of malignant non-Hodgkin lymphomas. Blut 43:167–181

Lennert K (1967) Classification of malignant lymphomas (European concept). In: Rüttimann A (ed) Progress in lymphology. Thieme, Stuttgart, pp 103–109

Lennert K (1969) Pathologisch-anatomische Klassifikation der malignen Lymphome. Strahlentherapie [Sonderbd] 69:1–7

Lennert K (1976) Klassifikation und Morphologie der Non-Hodgkin-Lymphome. In: Löffler H (ed) Maligne Lymphome und monoklonale Gammopathien. Lehmanns, Munich, pp 145–166 (Hämatologie und Bluttransfu-sion, vol 18)

Lennert K, in collaboration with Mohri N, Stein H, Kaiserling E, Müller-Hermelink HK (1978) Malignant lymphomas other than Hodgkin's disease. Springer, Berlin Heidelberg New York (Handbuch der speziellen pathologischen Anatomie und Histologie, vol l, part 3B)

Lennert K, Feller AC (eds) (1992) Histopathology of Non-Hodgkin's lymphomas. Springer, Berlin Heidelberg New York

Lennert K, Mohri N, Stein H, Kaiserling E (1975) The histopathology of malignant lymphoma. Br J Haematol 31 [Suppl]:193 203

Lennert K, Collins RD, Lukes RJ (1983) Concordance of the Kiel and Lukes-Collins classifications of non-Hodgkin's lymphomas. Histopathology 7:549–559

Lukes RJ, Collins RD (1974a) A functional approach to the classification of malignant lymphoma. Rec Res Cancer Res 46:18–30

Lukes RJ, Collins RD (1974b) Immunologic characterization of human malignant lymphomas. Cancer 34:1488–1503

Lukes RJ, Collins RD (1975a) New approaches to the classification of the lymphomata. Br J Cancer 31 [Suppl II]:1–28

Lukes RJ, Collins RD (1975) A functional classification of malignant lymphomas. In: Rebuck JW, Berard CW, Abell MR (eds) The reticuloendothelial system (Monographs in pathology, no 16) Williams and Wilkins, Baltimore, pp 213–242

Lukes RJ, Parker JW, Taylor CR, Tindle BH, Gramer AD, Lincoln TL (1978a) Immunologic approach to non-Hodgkin lymphomas and related leukemias. Analysis of the results of multiparameter studies of 425 cases. Semin Hematol 15:322–351

Lukes RJ, Taylor CR, Parker JW. Lincoln TL, Pattengale PK, Tindle BH (1978b) A morphologic and immunologic surface marker study of 299 cases of non-Hodgkin lymphomas and related leukemias. Am J Pathol 90:461–486

Mathé G, Rappaport H, O'Conor GT, Torloni H (1976) Histological and cytological typing of neoplastic diseases of haematopoietic and lymphoid tissues World Health Organization, Geneva. (International histological classification of tumors no 14)

Musshoff K (1987) Maligne Systemerkrankungen. In: Scherer E (ed) Strahlentherapie – Radiologische Onkologie, 3rd edn. Springer, Berlin Heidelberg New York, pp 1080–1332

Nathwani BN, Kim H, Rappaport H (1976) Malignant lymphoma, lymphoblastic. Cancer 38:964–998

O'Connor NTJ, Wainscoat JS, Weatherall DJ, Gatter KC, Feller AC, Isaacson P, Jones D, Lennert K, Pallesen G, Ramsey A, Stein H, Wright DH, Mason DY (1985) Rearrangement of the T-cell-receptor ß-chain gene in the diagnosis of lymphoproliferative disorders. Lancet i: 1295–1297

Rappaport H (1966) Tumors of the hematopoietic System. Atlas of tumor pathology, sect 3, fasc 8. Armed Forces Institute of Pathology, Washington

Stein H, Lennert K, Feller AC, Mason DY (l984) Immunohistological analysis of human lymphoma: correlation of histological and immunological categories. Adv Cancer Res 42:67–147

Suchi T, Tajima K, Nanba K, Wakasa H, Mikata A, Kikuchi M, Mori S, Watanabe S, Mohri N, Shamoto M, Harigaya K, Itagai T, Matsuda M, Kirino Y, Takagi K, Fukunaga S (1979) Some problems on the histopathological diagnosis of non-Hodgkin's malignant lymphoma. A proposal of a new type. Acta Pathol Jpn 29: 755–776

The Non-Hodgkin's Lymphoma Pathology Classification Project (1982) National Cancer Institute sponsored study of classifications of non-Hodgkin's lymphomas. Summary and description of a Working Formulation for clinical usage. Cancer 49:2112–2135

The T- and B-cell Malignancy Study Group (1981) Statistical analysis of immunologic, clinical and histopathologic data on lymphoid malignancies in Japan. Jpn J Clin Oncol 11:15–38

Tkachuk DC, Griesser H, Takihara Y, Champagne E, Minden M, Feller AC, Lennert K, Mak TW (1988) Rearrangement of T-cell data locus in lymphoproliferative disorders. Blood 72:353–357

Further Reading

Aisenberg AC (2000) Historical review of lymphomas. Br J Haematol 109:466–476

Armitage JO (1999) Goals of a lymphoma classification for the oncologist. In: Mason DY, Harris NL (eds) Human lymphoma: clinical implications of the REAL classification. Springer, London, chap 3

Armitage JO, Weisenburger DD (1998) New approach to classifying non-Hodgkin's lymphomas: clinical features of the major histologic subtypes. J Clin Oncol 16:2780–2795

Harris NL (1997) Principles of the Revised European-American Lymphoma classification (from the International Lymphoma Study Group). Ann Oncol 8 [Suppl 2]:11–16

Harris NL (1999) Introduction and rationale for the REAL classification. In: Mason DY, Harris NL (eds) Human lymphoma: clinical implications of the REAL classification. Springer, Berlin Heidelberg New York, chap 1

Isaacson PG (2000) The current status of lymphoma classification. Br J Haematol 109:258–266

Mason DY, Gatter KC (1995) Not another lymphoma classification. Br J Haematol 90:493–497

Stein H (1999) Lymphocyte differentiation. In: Mason DY, Harris NL (eds) Human lymphoma: clinical implications of the REAL classification. Springer, Berlin Heidelberg New York, chap 2

The Non-Hodgkin's Lymphoma Classification Project (1997) A clinical evaluation of the International Lymphoma Study Group Classification of Non-Hodgkins lymphoma. Blood 89:3909–3918

2 Current Status of Lymphoma Classification

2.1 Introduction

An increasing understanding of the immune system as well as the detection of defined chromosomal abnormalities has opened new perspectives for the development of a lymphoma classification system. The Kiel classification was the first, together with that of Lukes and Collins, to recognize and incorporate this knowledge. Still, the use of the Working Formulation in the USA and of the Kiel Classification in Europe has made it difficult to compare results, as the two classification systems differ in their approaches.

Whereas the Kiel classification comprises mostly well-defined clinicopathological entities on a morphologically defined basis, the WF is mostly descriptive, taking neither knowledge of modern immunology nor of cellular origin into account.

To overcome this dilemma, which also made comparisons of lymphoma trials between Europe and the US impossible, a group of 19 hematopathologists from Europe and the USA organized the International Lymphoma Study Group (ILSG), which finally proposed the REAL classification (Harris et al. 1994).

Subsequently, in 1995, Dr. Sobin, of the WHO, proposed to continue and to extend this work with the goal of implementing an international classification; this resulted in 2001 in the WHO classification (see Chap. 1.4).

Also in 1995, Drs. Armitage and Weisenburger, from Nebraska University, Omaha, USA, organized another study (Armitage and Weisenburger 1998). They asked hemato-oncologists of ten institutions in eight countries to each provide up to 200 consecutive cases of previously untreated malignant lymphomas that were representative of the geographic region. These cases were collected between January 1, 1988 and December 31, 1990, at the following study sites: Omaha (Nebraska), Vancouver (Canada), Cape Town (South Africa), London (United Kingdom), Locarno (Switzerland), Lyon (France), Würzburg/Göttingen (Germany), Hong Kong (China).

A group of five expert hematopathologists was invited to visit all ten centers and study the cases so that a consensus diagnosis using the WF, the up-dated Kiel classification, and the REAL classification could be reached. Statisticians were employed to organize the review. The study was organized as follows:

- At each participating institution, the diagnostic slides were reviewed and classified independently by each pathologist using the three classifications mentioned above.
- Routine slides were used from the case files.
- Each pathologist had to propose a first diagnosis based on morphology with only limited clinical data (age and localization), a second diagnosis including immunohistochemistry, and a third after presentation of all clinical data.
- At the end of each day, cases without consensus were discussed after the slides had been viewed with a multiheaded microscope in order to reach a consensus.
- At the end of the visit to each institution, each pathologist re-reviewed 20% of the cases for which a consensus diagnosis had been reached. The cases were randomly selected by the statisticians, without knowledge of the initial interpretation.
- The overall survival of all cases was measured from primary diagnosis until death. Estimates of failure-free survival and overall survival distribution were calculated using the method of Kaplan and Meier.

The results were based on 1,378 cases out of the initial 1,403 cases (The Non-Hodgkin's lymphoma Classification Project 1997).

The five most important results were:

1. For the majority of the cases, a high rate of agreement with a consensus diagnosis between pathologists was achieved for 85–94% of the different entities.
2. Problems were found in Burkitt's lymphoma, which had the lowest rate of agreement for both the first diagnosis and the consensus. The same was true for grading follicular lymphoma. T-cell lymphomas could only be diagnosed by including immunohistochemistry. The additional clinical data were of very limited diagnostic help (Table 2.1).
3. Pathologist agreement upon re-review of 20% of the cases was also good. The overall (intra-observer) agreement reached a mean value of 85% (ranging from 82 to 89% for the five hematopathologists).
4. Using overall and failure-free survival for each type of lymphoma, the various lymphoma types could be divided into four broad groups for prognostic purposes. The 5-year survival was greater than 70% in the first group, was 50–70% for the second group, between 30 and 49% for the third group, and less than 30% for the fourth group.
5. Only the up-dated Kiel and the REAL classifications allowed these four different groups to be correlated with survival.

Finally, these results, presented at the second Airlie meeting in 1997, confirmed that an international classification based on the up-dated Kiel and the REAL classifications would show more or less identical results. Based on the four different types of survival, clinicians accepted that terms like low-, intermediate-, and high-grade should no longer be used. Each lymphoma entity should instead be given a precise diagnosis using the WHO classification scheme, and survival estimated according to the survival curves defined in this study.

Beyond the entities identified in the Kiel classification, a number of new, especially extranodal, lymphoma entities have been recognized during the 10 years since the last edition of this book. Although many of these new entities are rare diseases, they are well-defined clinicopathological entities, such as subcutaneous panniculitis like T-cell lymphoma, and thus have to be described separately. Moreover, some of these entities have a quite distinct morphology, e.g., hepatosplenic T-cell lymphoma, or a characteristic immunophenotype, e.g., natural killer (NK)/T-cell lymphomas. It also became clear that some clinicopathological entities may show a variable morphology and have thus to be defined by their primary localization and their immunophenotype, such as the enteropathy-type T-cell lymphoma and the extranodal NK/T-cell lymphoma, nasal type. Beyond that, the increasing knowledge of the lymphocyte development facilitates a better and more detailed understanding and definition of lymphocytes subsets. This understanding made it possible to define the cell of origin for some lymphoma types (Fig. 2.1 and 2.2).

Thus today, the definition of a clinicopathological lymphoma entity is given not only by morphology but

Table 2.1. Expert pathologist agreement with the consensus diagnosis (from the Non-Hodgkin's Lymphoma Classification Project 1997; Nathwani et al. 1999). *CLL* Chronic lymphocytic leukemia

Consensus diagnosis	Diagnosis 1[a] (%)	Diagnosis 2[b] (%)	Diagnosis 3[c] (%)
Follicular, any grade	93	94	94
Follicular, grade 1	72	73	73
Follicular, grade 2	61	61	61
Follicular, grade 3	60	61	61
Marginal zone B-cell, MALT	84	86	86
Small lymphocytic (CLL)	84	87	87
Lymphoplasmacytoid	53	56	56
High-grade B-cell, Burkitt-like	47	53	53
Primary mediastinal large-B-cell	51	58	85
Marginal zone B-cell, nodal	55	63	63
Mantle cell	77	87	87
Diffuse large-B-cell	73	87	87
Precursor T-lymphoblastic	52	87	89
Anaplastic large-T-/null-cell	46	85	85
Peripheral T-cell, all types	41	86	86

[a] Diagnosis 1 based only on histology, [b] Diagnosis 2 based on histology and immunophenotype, [c] Diagnosis 3 based on histology, immunophenotype and clinical data

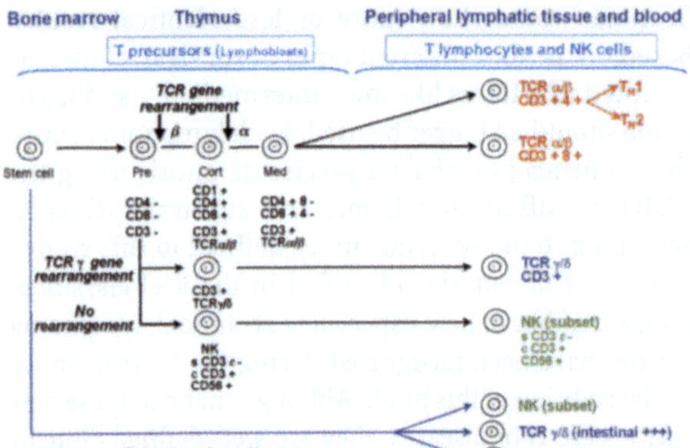

Fig. 2.1

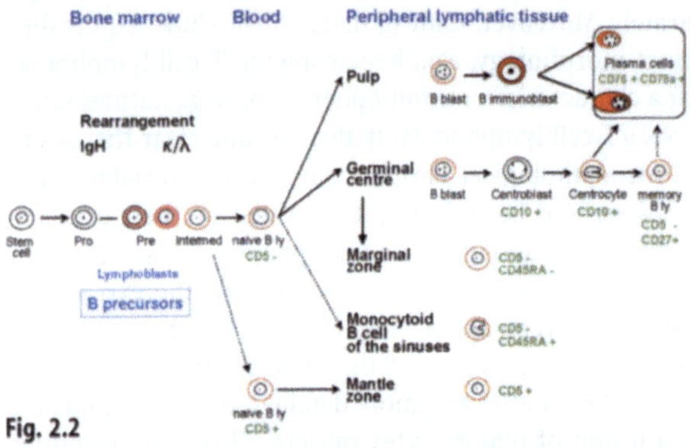

Fig. 2.2

also considers immunophenotypic and genetic aberrations, as well as clinical data and lymphocyte development.

Nevertheless, it is interesting that most of the newly described entities were primarily recognized by morphology and subsequently more precisely defined by additional techniques or clinical data. A prominent example is the important and frequent entity of MALT lymphoma.

Among B-cell neoplasms, almost all entities of the Kiel classification were included into the WHO classification. The MALT concept was added as was the splenic marginal zone lymphoma, which had been mostly described in the Kiel classification as splenic immunocytoma. Some rare entities have been added, like intravascular large B-cell lymphoma and primary effusion lymphoma. Finally, centroblastic and immunoblastic as well as rare types such as T-cell/histiocyte-rich and anaplastic B cell lymphoma have been fused within the term diffuse large B-cell lymphoma.

Among T-cell lymphomas- a number of rare extranodal lymphomas- mostly of NK/T-cell phenotype- have been added including extranodal NK/T-cell lymphoma, nasal type; enteropathy-type T-cell lymphoma; hepatosplenic T-cell lymphoma; and subcutaneous panniculitis-like T-cell lymphoma. The pleomorphic T-cell lymphomas of the Kiel classification have been fused under the term "peripheral T-cell lymphoma, unspecified" including the rare types T-zone lymphoma and Lennert's lymphoma.

Despite the world-wide agreement documented in the WHO classification, it has become clear that some problems remain. These are listed below.

2.2 Small- and Large-Cell Versus Low- and High-Grade

The description of low- and high-grade lymphomas in the Kiel classification is based on the size and the morphology of the nuclei of a lymphoma. This system was first proposed by K. Lennert in the initial Kiel classification (Gérard-Marchant et al. 1974). Using this approach as a prognostic means of categorization, it was only correct for the natural history of a lymphoma in the absence of treatment. Thus, it was indicated in the Kiel classification that these terms are only for practical use, to roughly assign categories describing small cells or "cytes" as low-grade and blasts or large cells as high-grade.

In Europe, these terms were accepted especially for those cases which could not be sub-classified and which could then be treated according to low- or high-grade protocols. Of course, these terms did not attempt to give prognostic information, as today it is possible to achieve complete remission for some large-cell (high-grade) lymphomas. By contrast, small B-cell lymphomas (low-grade) have a long evolution but complete remission is only very rarely achieved by treatment and the disease is mostly responsible for the death of the patient. Another small B cell lymphoma, mantle cell lymphoma, has an even more aggressive evolution and is hardly influenced by treatment.

For all these reasons, the terms small- and large-cell lymphoma or low- and high-grade give no indication in terms of prognosis. Nonetheless, these terms may be useful in the B-cell lineage, although they only cover a part of the NHLs.

As mentioned above, in the past, if a definite classification of an individual lymphoma was not possible, for various reasons, the terms low- and high-grade lymphoma were helpful in forming a clinical decision regarding treatment strategy. In such cases, a lymphoma could be classified as either small-cell (cytic) or blastic, the latter term covering, in addition to the diffuse large B-cell lymphoma, also Burkitt lymphomas and lymphoblastic lymphomas.

The situation among T-cell lymphomas is even more complicated. Most NK/T-cell lymphomas have a more or less similar, aggressive evolution with a poor prognosis whatever the histological type is. Exceptions are the anaplastic large-cell lymphomas (ALCL) of T, which show mostly a rather good prognosis, if it is ALK positive as well as the rare T-large-granular-lymphocytes (T-LGLs) and most cutaneous T-cell lymphomas. In all of these NK/T-cell lymphomas, clinical information should be taken into account since the clinical appearance might be typical, as in angioimmunoblastic T-cell lymphoma, or the clinical appearance might influence the diagnosis, as in exceptional cases of panniculitis-like T-cell lymphomas, which can be localized and indolent in their clinical behavior.

We think that it is still justified in cases which do not allow for a subclassification to use the terms low- and high-grade or small-cell (cytic) or large-cell (blastic) to enable a clinical decision for treatment.

2.3 Primary Versus Secondary Lymphoma

About 10 – 20 % of small-cell (so-called low-grade) lymphomas may transform during their clinical course into a large-cell or blastic lymphoma. This phenomenon is, for example, well-known from small lymphocytic lymphomas/B-cell chronic lymphocytic leukemia (CLL), which may transform into a blastic lymphoma also known as Richter's syndrome. Mostly, such transformations occur after a longer period (8 – 10 years after primary diagnosis) of the primary small-cell lymphoma. Other lymphoma types like follicular lymphomas may also show a transformation at the time of their primary manifestation either at the same location or elsewhere.

Both types of transformed lymphomas are secondary blastic or large-cell lymphomas which either occurred subsequently or simultaneously. It has been shown that this is of major prognostic importance. The transformation of a lymphocytic lymphoma after many years worsens the prognosis significantly. The simultaneous occurrence of a small- and large-cell or blastic component is of importance for therapeutic strategies as the small-cell component may not be eradicated by a therapeutic protocol for large-cell lymphomas.

Although this phenomenon is not detailed in the WHO classification, we believe that such observations are of major clinical importance and should thus be detailed in the report (primary versus secondary, simultaneously or subsequently).

2.4 Definition of Immunocytoma and Its Border with Marginal Zone B-Cell Lymphoma

Immunocytoma is a term which has been proposed to describe lymphoproliferations of immunoglobulin-secreting cells. Improved immunohistochemistry was mandatory in the Kiel classification in order to recognize this type of lymphoma. This term is no longer used in the WHO classification. Lymphoplasmacytoid and lymphoplasmacytic immunocytoma are now classified as two different diseases. One represents a peculiar type of B-cell chronic lymphocytic leukemia (B-CLL), in which the small lymphocytes exhibit a plasmacytoid differentiation (lymphoplasmacytoid immunocytoma). The second (lymphoplasmacytic immunocytoma) is designated as lymphoplasmacytic lymphoma in the WHO classification. Thus, it has to be kept in mind that in the WHO classification cases of lymphocytic lymphoma/B-CLL may clinically present as macroglobulinemia Waldenström.

Moreover, the border between such immunoglobulin-secreting lymphocytic lymphoma and lymphoplasmacytic lymphoma (immunocytoma), on the one hand, and some marginal zone (MZ) lymphomas with a plasmacytic component occurring as primary splenic or nodal MZ lymphoma or, more rarely, as MALT lymphoma, on the other hand, is not sharp. In the past, most cases of MZL have been called immunocytoma. Lymphoplasmacytic lymphoma has been regarded as the histopathologic background of macroglobulinemia Waldenström. However, about 50 % of primary splenic and probably nodal MZ lymphomas are associated with the presence of a serum M component, sometimes more than 3 g/dl, which is the definition of Waldenström's macroglobulinemia (van Huyen et al. 2000). Even patients with MALT lymphoma may present with such a high serum M component (van Huyen et al. 2000). Thus today we don't know whether lymphoplasmacytic lymphoma (immunocytoma) and MZ lymphoma represent more or less the same disease or whether different lymphoma entities may be responsible for a Waldenström's macroglobulinemia. More detailed studies are needed to understand these diseases and their borders with each other.

2.5 Indistinct Border Between Nodal Marginal Zone B-Cell Lymphoma and Follicular Lymphoma with Marginal Zone Differentiation

Nathwani et al. (1999) have shown that about 10% of follicular lymphomas show a more or less marked marginal zone differentiation. This kind of differentiation could be so pronounced that it is almost impossible on purely morphological grounds to differentiate this type of follicular lymphoma from a primary marginal zone lymphoma with follicular colonization. As both may show a clonal plasma cell component, immunohistochemistry is of limited help. The detection of the translocation t(14;18) on the molecular level can be decisive.

2.6 Grading of Follicular Lymphoma

In contrast to the Kiel classification, the WHO classification proposed a complicated grading system for follicular lymphoma, although the clinical relevance is not clear and the results of grading are not reproducible. First, stratification based on the number of blasts present in the neoplastic follicles is not reproducible. This is obvious, as it is impossible for individual cells to clearly distinguish between centroblasts and anaplastic centrocytes or even small blasts, which are found in the blastic variant of mantle cell lymphoma. Moreover, multilobulated cells are not taken into account. Finally, it is not possible in daily practice to definitively count and to correlate the results to the diameter of the field of view. The reproducibility using this system was around 50% among different experienced hematopathologists; thus it is clear that this system has no value.

We recommend estimating the number of blasts (only clearly recognizable centroblasts and multilobulated cells should be counted) and adapting the result to the grading system. In our opinion, it is of major importance to distinguish between diffusely distribulated blasts and solid sheets. The latter (corresponding to grade 3b) indicates a transformation into a diffuse large B-cell lymphoma, which should be noted in the report.

2.7 Distinction Between Diffuse Large B-Cell Lymphoma and Burkitt's Lymphoma: Reproducibility and Value of Subclassification

In individual cases, the distinction of Burkitt's lymphoma and its variants from diffuse large B-cell lymphoma (DLBCL) cannot reproducibly be done. If these two groups cannot be clearly distinguished from each other, it is even more difficult to distinguish variants of Burkitt's lymphoma. We therefore recommend to indicate whether a specific case belongs to the group of Burkitt's lymphoma. In this lymphoma type immunohistochemistry is mandatory (see Chap. 4.2.3).

The subclassification of DLBCL is still a matter of debate. In the past, it was said that a morphological subclassification is not reproducible, although different investigators could even demonstrate the clinical value of such. Furthermore, new data from DNA-array profiling has underlined the clinical value of subclassification. It is clear that morphology alone is limited although able to distinguish between subtypes. The minimal prerequisite is a reliable technique. Routine slides such as those used in different trials are not enough to achieve reproducibility.

2.8 Problems in Reproducibly Recognizing Anaplastic Large-Cell Lymphoma and Lymphoblastic Lymphoma on Purely Morphological Grounds

Although ALCL and lymphoblastic lymphomas are well-defined clinicopathological entities, it is surprising that major difficulties exist to reproducibly diagnose them only on the basis of morphology. The primary consensus for these diagnoses in the NHL classification project was 46% and 52%, respectively. Thus, in both cases immunohistochemistry is necessary if one of the above-mentioned diagnosis is included in the differential diagnosis.

2.9 Is Peripheral T-Cell Lymphoma, Unspecified, a Distinct Clinicopathological Entity or a Catchall Term?

The classification of peripheral T-cell lymphomas is still artificial. About 50% of all T-cell lymphomas fall into the category "peripheral T-cell lymphoma, unspecified". At least the pathologist should describe the specific findings of growth pattern and cytology (T zone, pleomorphism), although we know that today this is of limited clinical value and we do not always define clinicopathological entities. Nevertheless, the morphological findings, together with new biological findings, will certainly allow for better definitions in the future.

2.10 Neither the WHO nor the EORTC Classification of Cutaneous Lymphoma Covers Today's Knowledge

Concerning the classification of cutaneous lymphomas, neither the WHO nor the European Organization for Research and Treatment of Cancer (EORTC) classification is completely satisfactory. The EORTC classification gives a better clinical correlation; however, a number of new entities are not included. The WHO classification tried to include the major entities; but it seems difficult to completely include them into the current classification system. Especially the clinical behavior of many nodal and extranodal lymphomas differs, and the same is true for some biological parameters. In this book we have tried to fuse the EORTC and WHO classifications in order to cover all major entities. Although not definitive, we have tried to propose a separate list for cutaneous lymphomas.

New studies based on immunohistochemistry, molecular biology, and cytogenetics in close correlation with clinical data are needed to define more precisely all the different entities.

References

Armitage JO, Weisenburger DD (for the Non-Hodgkin's Lymphoma Classification Project) (1998) New approach to classifying non-Hodgkin's lymphoma: clinical features of the major histologic subtypes. J Clin Oncol 16:2780–2795

Gérard-Marchant R, Hamlin I, Lennert K, Rilke F, Stansfeld AG, van Unnik JAM (1974) Classification of non-Hodgkin's lymphomas (letter to the editor). Lancet ii:406–440

Harris NL, Jaffe ES, Stein H, Banks PM, Chan JKC, Cleary ML, Delsol G, De Wolf-Peeters C, Falini B, Gatter KC, Grogan TM, Issacson PG, Knowles KM, Mason DY, Müller-Hermelink HK, Pileri SA, Piris MA, Ralfkiaer E, Warnke RA (1994) A revised European-American classification of lymphoid neoplasms: a proposal from the International Lymphoma Study Group. Blood 84:1361–1392

Nathwani BN, Anderson JR, Armitage JO, Cavalli F, Diebold J, Drachenberger MR, Harris NL, MacLennan KA, Müller-Hermelink HK, Ullrich FA, Weisenburger DD (1999) Clinical significance of follicular lymphoma with monocytoid B cells. Non-Hodgkin's Lymphoma Classification Project. Hum Pathol 30:263–268

The Non-Hodgkin's Lymphoma Classification Project (1997) A clinical evaluation of the International Lymphoma Study Group Classification of non-Hodgkin's lymphoma. Blood 89:3909–3918

Van Huyen JP, Molina T, Delmer A, Audouin J, Le Tourneau A, Zittoun R, Bernadou A, Diebold J (2000) Splenic marginal differentiation with or without plasmacytic differentiation. Am J Surg Pathol 24:1581–1592

3 Epidemiology

3.1 Introduction

Already during the early 1970s, an increase in the incidence rates of lymphoma was recognized, only part of which was due to the increase in lymphomas associated with HIV infection. The increase was reported to be more marked than for all other cancer types, except melanoma of the skin and lung cancer in women (Devesa and Fears 1992), and was greater for extranodal than for nodal lymphomas.

The incidence of non-Hodgkin's lymphomas (NHLS) for white men in the USA was 6.9/100,000 per year during the period 1947–1950 compared to 17.4/100,000 during the years 1984–1988 (Hartge and Devesa 1992). Recently, Birch et al. (2002) described the same tendency for the age group between 15 and 24 years old.

Part of this 152% increase in the occurrence of lymphomas can be explained by the recognition of new entities, earlier misdiagnoses, HIV and other immunosuppressive conditions, the increased use of immunosuppressive drugs, and occupation-related disease. Nonetheless, subtracting these causes still leaves an estimated 80% increase in the incidence rate for white males (Hartge and Devesa, 1992). Thus, unknown etiological factors must play an important role. The increase incidence rate of lymphoma is in contrast to the declining incidence of Hodgkin's disease (Hartge et al. 1994).

Recent data of the American Cancer Society also indicate an increase in the total number of cases of malignant lymphomas, with an incidence for males and females of 10.06 and 5.54/100,000, in respectively, in the years between 1990 and 1992 (Newton et al. 1997).

In a recent collaborative study on lymphoma incidence, based on data from eight lymphoma registries from seven European countries, the same tendency was found with an overall annual increase in the incidence of NHLs of 4.2% (Cartwright et al. 1999).

During the last several decades, most values for incidences and frequencies reflected those of nodal lymphomas. Only during the last 10–15 years has it become clear that extranodal lymphomas are, in part, clinicopathological entities and thus have their own biology.

The frequency values, especially those for nodal lymphomas reported by different countries or continents, indicate that there are considerable differences in the incidence rate which are due not only to actual differences but also to variations in practice. In Germany, for example, biopsies are often performed in cases of acute and chronic lymphoid leukemia, whereas in other countries such cases are frequently diagnosed based on blood and bone marrow smears alone.

The incidence rate for all NHLs combined varies from a low of 2/100,000 per year in Thailand to about 10/100,000 per year in whites in the USA. Within Europe, differences can also be observed; for example, the incidence is roughly two-fold lower in Slovakia (4/100,000) than in the Netherlands (8/100,000) (Newton et al. 1997).

The percentage of all NHLs of extranodal origin is between 25% and 35% in most countries, with the stomach, the skin, the small intestine and the tonsils being the most common extranodal sites of involvement. The age-incidence curve of each site is similar to that of nodal lymphomas (Newton et al. 1997).

A study carried out in Denmark, using the REAL classification, compared the number of cases before 1986 and those collected between 1986 and 1992, and found an increase of 21.2% over 6 years, or an average annual increase in incidence of 3.5% (Brincker et al. 2000). There was an increased incidence of diffuse large-B-cell lymphoma (DLBCL) between the two

Table 3.1. Distribution of NHL cases by the consensus diagnosis (NHLCP, 1998). *CLL* Chronic lymphocytic leukemia

Consensus diagnosis	Number of cases	Percent of total cases
Diffuse large-B-cell	422	30.6
Follicular	304	22.1
Marginal zone B-cell, MALT	105	7.6
Peripheral T-cell	96	7.0
Small B-lymphocytic (CLL)	93	6.7
Mantle cell	83	6.0
Primary mediastinal large-B-cell	33	2.4
Anaplastic large T/null-cell	33	2.4
High grade B-cell, Burkitt's-like	29	2.1
Marginal zone B-cell, nodal	25	1.8
Precursor T-lymphoblastic	23	1.7
Lymphoplasmacytoid	16	1.2
All other types	84	~8

cohorts of patients from 39.2 to 47.4%, corresponding to a change in incidence of +43.1% compared to 2.5% for all other subtypes combined. In this study, 24.6% of the patients presented with only primary extranodal disease, while a further 26.8% presented with both nodal and extranodal disease. Thus, 51.4% of patients had extranodal manifestations.

The Non Hodgkin Lymphoma Classification Project (NHLCP) (Anderson at al. 1998) (Table 3.1) found that the distribution of subtypes varied considerably in eight different geographical regions from all over the world; for example, follicular lymphomas varied from 8 to 33% and DLBCL from 25 to 36%.

The Lymphoma Study Group of Japanese Pathologists (2000) reviewed 3,194 lymphomas, comparing these data to those from a HTLV1-endemic area (Kyushu Island) and reclassifying the lymphomas according to the WHO classification. The results were the following:

Hodgkin's lymphoma is an extremely rare disease in Japan (4.4%). T-cell lymphomas are, in general, much more frequent than in all other countries all over the world, predominately due to the HTLV1-endemic areas. In endemic areas, the frequency of T-cell lymphomas increases up to 40% (between 10 and 15% in Europe and the USA). Follicular lymphomas are rare (6.7–11%) compared to the incidence in Europe (20.4%), the USA (35%) and in India (12.6%) (Naresh et al. 2000; Lymphoma Study Group of Japan 2000; Ohshima et al. 2002). According to the NHLCP, a greater percentage of follicular lymphoma is seen in North America, London and Cape Town (31% versus 14% at other geographical sites (Anderson et al. 1998) (Table 3.2).

Table 3.2a. Incidence of malignant lymphoma entities between November 1994 and October 1996, Japan (Lymphoma Study Group of Japanese Pathologists 2000)

Non-Hodgkin's lymphoma	94.71%
B-cell neoplasms	68.53%
NK/T-cell neoplasms	24.92%
B/NK/T-cell, undefined cases	1.25%
Hodgkin's lymphoma	4.41%
Malignant lymphoma, unclassifiable	0.56%
Histiocytic/dendritic neoplasms	0.31%

Table 3.2b. Incidence of malignant B-cell lymphoma entities between November 1994 and October 1996, Japan (Lymphoma Study Group of Japanese Pathologists (2000)

B-cell neoplasms	Percent
Precursor B-lymphoblastic leukemia/lymphoma	3.4
B-cell chronic lymphocytic leukemia/small lymphocytic lymphoma	2.0
B-cell prolymphocytic leukemia	
Lymphoplasmacytic lymphoma	1.0
Mantle cell lymphoma	4.1
Follicular lymphoma	9.8
Marginal zone B-cell lymphoma of MALT	12.3
Nodal marginal zone B-cell lymphoma	1.5
Splenic marginal zone B-cell lymphoma	<1
Hairy cell leukemia	<1
Plasma cell myeloma	13.3
Diffuse large-B-cell lymphoma	48.7
Burkitt's lymphoma	2.1
Unclassifiable	2.1

Table 3.2c. Incidence of malignant NK/T-cell lymphoma entities between November 1994 and October 1996, Japan (Lymphoma Study Group of Japanese Pathologists (2000)

NK/T-cell neoplasms	Percent
Precursor T-lymphoblastic leukemia/lymphoma	6.9
T-cell prolymphocytic leukemia	<1
T-cell granular lymphocytic leukemia	<1
Indolent NK/large-cell granular lymphocyte disorder	<1
Aggressive NK-cell leukemia	<1
Nasal-type NK/T-cell lymphoma	10.4
Mycosis fungoides/Sézary syndrome	4.6
Angioimmunoblastic T-cell lymphoma	9.7
Peripheral T-cell lymphoma, unspecified	26.8
Adult T-cell lymphoma/leukemia	29.9
Anaplastic large-cell lymphoma	6.2
Primary cutaneous CD30-positive lymphoproliferative disorder	<1
Subcutaneous panniculitis-like T-cell lymphoma	<1
Enteropathy-type intestinal T-cell lymphoma	<1
Hepatosplenic gamma/delta T-cell lymphoma	<1
Unclassifiable	1.8

3.2 Statistical Data of the Kiel Lymphoma Registry

At the time of analysis (1983) of the Kiel Lymphoma Registry, the collection, which consisted predominately of nodal lymphomas, contained 78% B-cell lymphomas and 17% T-cell lymphomas. If all the unclassified cases were added to the T-cell lymphomas there would be 22%. Hence the actual frequency of T-cell lymphomas would be at most 20%. In the United States, Lukes et al. (1987a, b) found 21% T-cell lymphomas. In Japan (Suchi 1987) the proportion of HTLV-1-negative T-cell lymphomas is about one-third of all NHLs.

The most frequent types of nodal lymphomas in the Kiel collection were follicular lymphomas (centroblastic-centrocytic lymphoma) (20.4%), centroblastic lymphoma (13.7%), immunocytoma, including some extranodal marginal zone lymphomas(12.3%) (lymphoplasmacytoid and lymphoplasmacytic combined), and B-cell chronic lymphocytic leukemia (B-CLL) (11.1%). The most frequent type of T-cell lymphoma was angioimmunoblastic lymphadenopathy with dysproteinemia (AILD) (lymphogranulomatosis X-type) (angioimmunoblastic T-cell lymphoma) (3.6%).

3.2.1 Age and Sex Distribution

Small-B-cell lymphomas generally do not occur before the age of 20 years and show a peak incidence in the seventh decade. The only exception is follicular lymphoma, which shows a peak in the sixth decade. In adults, almost all types of malignant lymphoma show a slight or moderate male predominance. Only follicular lymphoma exhibits a slight female predominance (male-to-female ratio of 1:1.2).

3.2.2 Malignant Lymphoma of Childhood

In children, an annual incidence of 0.9 NHLs/100,000 was observed, with a male to female ratio of 4.1:1.0 (Samuelsson et al. 1999). Some types of blastic B-cell malignant lymphoma (lymphoblastic and Burkitt's lymphoma) are found more frequently in the first two decades of life than in adulthood. Anaplastic large-cell lymphoma is also observed more often in children and adolescents than in adults (Bucsky et al. 1988, 1989, 1990; Dura and Gladkowska-Dura 1981; Müller-Weihrich et al. 1984, 1985).

Between 1983 and 1987, in Kiel a total of 448 malignant lymphomas were diagnosed in children under the age of 15 years; 56% were Hodgkin's lymphomas and 44% were NHLs. The latter included only 6.6% low-grade malignant lymphomas (Table 3.3), most of which were of the pleomorphic, small-cell T-cell type (peripheral T-cell lymphoma, unspecified) (5.1%). Only one case of immunocytoma and two cases of follicular lymphoma (making up a total of 1.5% low-grade malignant B-cell lymphomas) were found in children age 13 and 14 years. Of the blastic/large cell malignant lymphomas, the lymphoblastic type was diagnosed most frequently (45.9%), but these cases included a considerable number of acute lymphoblastic leukemias (ALLs). The second most frequent type was Burkitt's lymphoma (24.5%), followed by anaplastic large-cell lymphoma (12.2%), centroblastic lymphoma and immunoblastic lymphoma (totaling 5.1%).

Table 3.3. Non-Hodgkin's lymphomas diagnosed from lymph node biopsies at the Lymph Node Registry in Kiel in 1983 (n=1,284). Repeated biopsies and extranodal lymphomas are not included. *CLL* Chronic lymphocytic leukemia, *PLL* prolymphocytic leukemia, *HCL* hairy cell leukemia

B-cell	%	T-cell	%
Small cell (54.4%)			
Lymphocytic		Lymphocytic	
CLL, PLL	11.1	CLL, PLL	0.8
HCL	–		
Immunocytoma	12.3	Mycosis fungoides and Sézary's syndrome	0.9
Plasmacytic	<0.5	Angioimmunoblastic	3.6
Follicular	20.4	Peripheral T, unspecified	7.3
Mantle cell	5.4		
Nodal marginal zone	0.5		
Secondary DLBCL	3.0		
Unclassified	1.2		
Large-cell/blastic malignant lymphomas (23.4%)			
Centroblastic	13.7	Anaplastic large-cell	1.3
Immunoblastic	4.3	Lymphoblastic	3.2
Burkitt's lymphoma	2.6		
Anaplastic large cell	0.1		
Lymphoblastic	0.9		
Unclassified	1.9		
Total	**77.9**[a]		**17.1**[a]

[a] 5% could not definitely be classified as B- or T-cell lymphoma

Table 3.4. Non-Hodgkin's lymphomas diagnosed on lymph node biopsies from children (0-14 years old) at the Lymph Node Registry in Kiel from 1983 through 1987

	n	%
Low-grade malignant lymphomas	13	6.6
Lymphoplasmacytic	1	1.5
Follicular lymphoma	2	
T-cell lymphoma, unspecified	10	5.1
High-grade malignant lymphomas	171	87.2
Centroblastic	5	5.1
Immunoblastic	5	
Burkitt's lymphoma	48	24.5
Anaplastic large cell	24	12.2
Lymphoblastic (including ALL)	89	45.9
Unclassified	12	6.1
Total	196	

In 6.1 % of the cases it was not possible to make a definitive diagnosis, usually due to technical reasons.

It is not possible to calculate the ratio of B-cell lymphomas to T-cell lymphomas in childhood on the basis of the available data, because not all cases were examined immunohistochemically. An immunohistochemical analysis would be absolutely necessary for immunoblastic, lymphoblastic and large-cell anaplastic lymphomas since they cannot be classified reliably as being of the B-cell or T-cell type by morphology alone. Hence, we can make only a rough estimate by extrapolation on the basis of immunologically analyzed cases of other series. The results are listed in Table 3.4, showing that, in childhood, almost *half of the cases of NHL are of the T-cell type*. In adults the percentage of T-cell lymphomas is much lower (see Chap. 3.1).

References

Anderson JR, Armitage JO, Weisenburger DD (1998) Epidemiology of the non-Hodgkin's lymphomas: distributions of the major subtypes differ by geographic locations. Non-Hodgkin's Lymphoma Classification Project. Ann Oncol 9:717-20

Birch JM, Alston RD, Kelsey AM, Quinn MJ, Babb P, McNally RJ (2002) Classification and incidence of cancers in adolescents and young adults in England 1979-1997. Br J Cancer 87:1267-74

Brincker H, Pedersen NT, Bendix-Hansen K, Johansen P (2000) Non-Hodgkin's lymphoma subtypes over time in an unselected population of 646 patients: a study of clinico-pathological data and incidence based on a review using the REAL-classification. Leuk Lymphoma 39:531–41

Bucsky P, Schwarze E-W, Reiter A, Feickert H-J, Odenwald E, Müller-Weihrich S, Riehm H (1988) Heterogeneity of childhood non-Hodgkin's lymphomas: The BFM experience. Presentation at the 20th Meeting of the International Society of Pediatric Oncology, Trondheim, August 22–26

Bucsky P, Feller AC, Beck JD, Gadner H, Heitger A, Ludwig W-D, Reiter A, Riehm H (1989) Zur Frage der Definition der malignen Histiozytose und des großzelligen anaplastischen (Ki-1) Lymphoms im Kindesalter. Klin Pädiatr 201:233–236

Bucsky P, Feller AC, Reiter A, Beck J, Bertram U, Eschenbach C, Gerein V, Lakomek M, Stollmann B, Tausch W, Urban C, Riehm H (1990) Low grade malignant non-Hodgkin's lymphomas and peripheral pleomorphic T-cell lymphomas in childhood – a BFM Study Group report. Klin Pädiatr 202:258–261

Cartwright R, Brincker H, Carli PM, Clayden D, Coebergh JW, Jack A, McNally R, Morgan G, de Sanjose S, Tumino R, Vornanen M (1999) The rise in incidence of lymphomas in Europe 1985-1992. Eur J Cancer 35:627–33

Devesa SS, Fears T (1992) Non-Hodgkin's lymphoma time trends: United States and international data. Cancer Res 52(19 Suppl):5432s–5440s

Dura WT, Gladkowska-Dura MJ (1981) Non-Hodgkin's lymphoma in the first two decades. Morphology and immunocytochemical study. Virchows Arch [A] 390:23-62

Hartge P, Devesa SS, Fraumeni JF Jr. (1994) Hodgkin's and non-Hodgkin's lymphomas. Cancer Surv 19-20:423–53

Hartge P, Devesa SS (1992) Quantification of the impact of known risk factors on time trends in non-Hodgkin's lymphoma incidence. Cancer Res 52(19 Suppl):5566s–5569s

Lukes RJ, Parker JW, Taylor CR, Tindle BH, Gramer AD. Lincoln TL (1978 a) Immunologic approach to non-Hodgkin lymphomas and related leukemias. Analysis of the results of multiparameter studies of 425 cases. Semin Hematol 15:322-351

Lukes RJ, Taylor CR, Parker JW. Lincoln TL, Pattengale PK, Tindle BH (1978b) A morphologic and immunologic surface marker study of 299 cases of non-Hodgkin lymphomas and related leukemias. Am J Pathol 90:461-486

Lymphoma Study Group of Japanese Pathologists (2000) The world health organization classification of malignant lymphomas in Japan: incidence of recently recognized entities. Pathol Int 50:696-702

Müller-Weihrich S. Beck J, Henze G, Jobke A, Kornhuber B, Lampert F, Ludwig R, Prindull G, Schellong G, Spaar HJ, Stollmann B, Treuner J, Wahlen W, Weinel P, Riehm H (1984) BFM-Studie 1981/83 zur Behandlung hochmaligner Non-Hodgkin-Lymphome bei Kindern: Ergebnisse einer nach histologisch-immunologischem Typ und Ausbreitungsstadium stratifizierten Therapie. Klin Pädiatr 196:135 142

Müller-Weihrich S, Henze G, Odenwald E, Riehm H (1985) BFM trials for childhood non-Hodgkin's lymphomas. In: Cavalli F, Bonadonna G, Rozencweig M (eds) Malignant lymphomas and Hodgkin's disease: experimental and therapeutic advances. Proc 2nd Int Conf Malignant Lymphomas. Lugano 1984. Nijhoff, Boston, pp 633-642

Naresh KN, Srinivas V, Soman CS (2000) Distribution of various subtypes of non-Hodgkin's lymphoma in India: a study of 2773 lymphomas using R.E.A.L. and WHO Classifications. Ann Oncol 11 Suppl 1:63-7

Newton R, Ferlay J, Beral V, Devesa SS (1997) The epidemiology of non-Hodgkin's lymphoma: Comparison of nodal and extra-nodal sites. Int. J. Cancer 72:923–930

Ohshima K, Suzumiya J, Kikuchi M (2002) The World Organization classification of malignant lymphoma: incidence and clinical prognosis in HTLV-1-endemic area of Fukuoka. Pathol Int 52:1–12

Samuelsson BO, Ridell B, Rockert L, Gustafsson G, Marky I (1999) Non-Hodgkin lymphoma in children: a 20-year population-based epidemiologic study in Western Sweden. J Pediatr Hematol Oncol 21:103-10

Suchi T, Lennert K, Tu LY, Kikuchi M, Sato E, Stansfeld AG, Feller AC (1987) Histopathology and immunohistochemistry of peripheral T cell lymphomas: a proposal for their classification. J Clin Pathol 40:995-1015

Chapter 4

Nodal B-Cell Lymphoma

4.1 Precursor B-Cell Lymphoblastic Leukemia[1]/ Lymphoblastic Lymphoma[2] (ICD-O: 9835/3[1]; 9728/3[2])

About 80% of lymphoblastic (LB) lymphomas/acute lymphoblastic leukemia are of B-cell origin, 20% of T-cell origin. The distinction between lymphoma and leukemia is arbitrary. A leukemic blood picture and/or a bone marrow involvement of more than 20% leads clinically to the term acute lymphoblastic leukemia, whereas a predominant nodal involvement leads to the term lymphoblastic lymphoma (Bernard et al. 1981). The different manifestations seem to be more related to different age groups and type of precursor cell development than to other biologically relevant phenomena. The prognosis of the T-cell type seems to be a bit less favorable than the B-cell type.

Synonyms

- Kiel: Lymphoblastic lymphoma of B-cell type
- REAL: Precursor B-lymphoblastic leukemia/lymphoma
- WHO: Precursor B-lymphoblastic leukemia/lymphoma

Definition

B-lymphoblastic lymphoma/leukemia is derived from committed precursor cells of peripheral B-lymphocytes. The neoplasm consist chiefly of medium-sized "blast cells" with scanty, more or less basophilic cytoplasm. The nucleus of these cells shows fine chromatin and is usually round, but sometimes gyrate or "convoluted". The infiltrate is diffuse and appears quite monotonous. Primary-tissue-based lymphoblastic lymphoma and a leukemic acute lymphoblastic leukemia can not be distinguished by morphology. Cytogenetics should be included into the final differentiation as the extent of polyploidy is of prognostic importance.

Morphology

The lymph node is infiltrated by a very monotonous-looking population of medium-sized lymphoblasts (9–11 µm; see Fig. 4.1). The nuclei are round, oval, and in some cells indented or gyrate ("convoluted") (Fig. 4.2). They have very fine chromatin and one to three small or medium-sized, slightly basophilic nucleoli. The cytoplasm is scanty and stains grayish-blue or blue with Giemsa. Mitotic figures are plentiful (approximately 10/high-power field). Occasionally, there is a starry-sky cellular pattern, but it is not very pronounced. The trabeculae and capsule, especially in the leukemic variant, are sometimes heavily infiltrated, but still clearly distinguishable from the sinuses.

Cytology. In imprints or smears, the nuclei show only little variation in their shape and size, thus appearing quite monotonous. In a few cases the cells show slightly larger and more variable nuclei (Fig. 4.3). Whereas the more monotonous-appearing lymphoblasts correspond to the L1 morphology of the FAB classification, the latter group have a L2 morphology. The slightly to moderately basophilic, scanty cytoplasm of lymphoblasts is easier to recognize in imprints.

Immunohistochemistry

CD79α is the earliest detectable cytoplasmic antigen in the B-cell lineage. All B-lymphoblastic lymphomas express the B-cell-associated antigen CD19; they coexpress HLA-DR and usually terminal deoxynucleotide transferase (TdT) (Bollum 1979; Kung et al. 1978). Approximately 90% simultaneously show CD22. Usu-

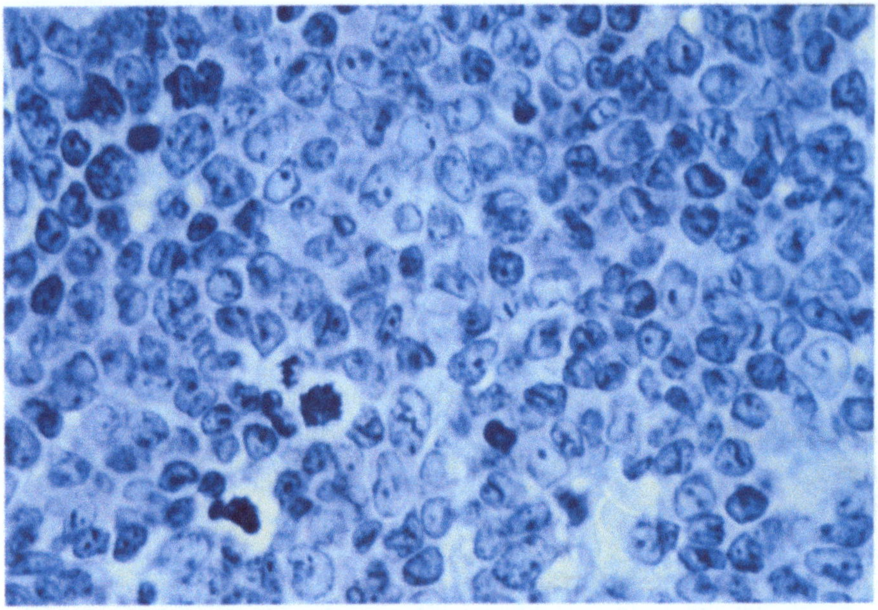

Fig. 4.1. Precursor B-lymphoblastic lymphoma (Giemsa stain). Small to medium-sized tumor cells with a narrow cytoplasmic rim. The nuclei are round or oval

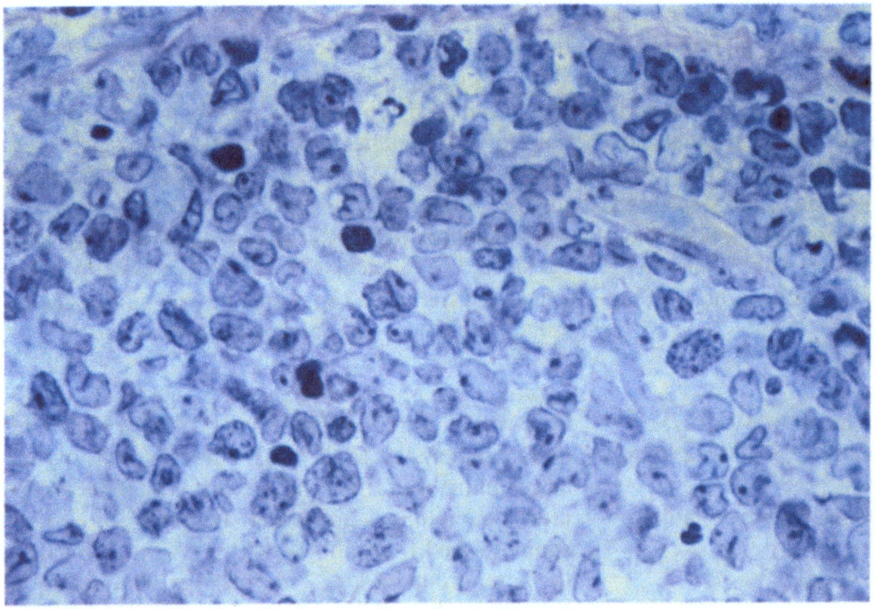

Fig. 4.2. Precursor B-lymphoblastic lymphoma with irregular-shaped nuclei with strong indentations and a light chromatin pattern (Giemsa stain)

ally, in the absence of CD22, surface immunoglobulin s (sIg) is also not detectable. Similar to CD22, CD20 is found in more than 90% of cases. About 80% of the lymphoblastic lymphomas of B type express common acute lymphoblastic leukemia (ALL) antigen (CD10). The proportion of proliferating cells lies between 60 and 80%. Follicular dendritic cells (FDC) cannot be detected.

The earliest detectable B-cell phenotype is thus a coexpression of HLA-DR, CD79α, CD34, and TdT. Following the line of phenotypic B-cell differentiation CD19 and next CD10 are subsequently expressed. This is followed by cytoplasmic IgM expression without light-chain. These steps of differentiation can be designated as progenitor B-cell, pre-pre-B-cell, pre-B-cell and immature B-cell. Most cells in the B-cell lineage are

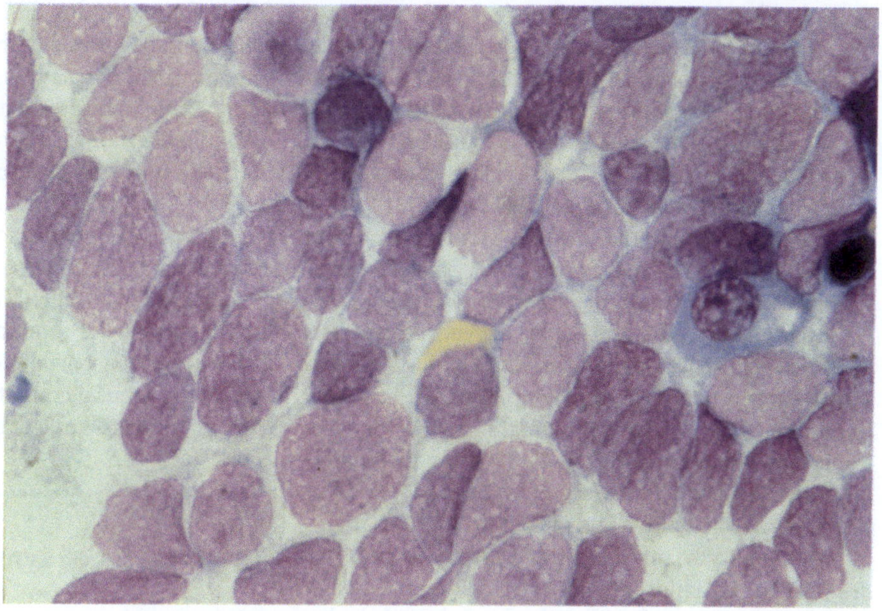

Fig. 4.3. Touch-imprint of precursor B-lymphoblastic lymphoma. The tumor cells have round to oval nuclei and medium-sized nucleoli with only slightly basophilic cytoplasm (Pappenheim stain)

of pre-B and pre-pre-B-cell phenotype (Weiss et al. 1986). The expression or leak of antigens such as CD34, CD13, CD33, and CD10 may have particular prognostic impact (Kersey et al. 1982; Hoelzer et al. 1984; Vannier et al. 1989; Sobol et al. 1987; Thomas et al. 1995; Uckun et al. 1997).

It is noteworthy that about 50% of leukemia/lymphoma (B-LBs) coexpress myeloid antigens. This finding is more frequent in pediatric cases than in adults (Khalidi et al. 1999).

Genetic Features

About 70% of B-LBs have their Ig heavy-chain genes rearranged, in the remaining cases both heavy- and light-chain, indicating a more mature immunophenotype (Korsmeyer et al. 1983). Moreover, there is a high number of cases in which there is cross-lineage rearrangement, or so-called lineage promiscuity. Using probes for T-cell receptor (TCR)-γ, a rearrangement can be found in around 50–60% of B-LBs (Felix et al. 1987; Greenberg et al. 1986; Chen et al. 1987; Pelicci et al. 1985; Greaves et al. 1986). Using TCR-β probes the percentage is somewhat lower (Tawa et al. 1987).

The extent of polyploidy is of major prognostic importance in B-LB/B-ALL. One group has hyperdiploid chromosomes, which have to be divided into those with >50 or <51 chromosomes. The former group has the most favorable prognosis among all, since these cells derive from precursor B-LB (Look et al. 1985; Williams et al. 1982). The latter group has a less favorable prognosis (Raimondi 1993; Pui 1995).

A frequent and prognostically unfavorable translocation is t(9;22), which translocates the abl oncogene into the bcr gene on chromosome 22, resulting in the Philadelphia translocation (Suryanarayan et al. 1991). The translocation t(1;19) occurs in about 20% of precursor B-ALL and also has unfavorable prognostic impact (Crist et al. 1990). Other translocations involve chromosomes 11q23, 12p or abnormalities on 9q. The translocation t(12;21)(p13;q22) has been shown to be the most frequent translocation in childhood ALL of B type (up to 30%) (Amor et al. 1998).

Diagnosis and Differential Diagnosis

The diagnosis of lymphoblastic lymphoma (without subtyping) is simple. The monotonous appearance of the medium-sized blast cells provides the decisive clue even at a low magnification. It is not possible to distinguish between T and B types by morphology alone, however. An immunological examination is indispensable.

The differential diagnosis must include not only *T-lymphoblastic lymphoma/leukemia* (see Chap. 5.1), but also *acute myeloid leukemia, myelomonocytic leukemia and mantle cell lymphoma* (see Chap. 4.2.1.7).

Acute myeloid or myelomonocytic leukemia infiltrates lymph nodes fairly frequently, which therefore may be submitted for histological examination. These types of leukemia may also show medium-sized blast cells that can hardly be distinguished from lymphoblasts. In acute myeloid leukemia, the blast cells are occasionally somewhat more basophilic and larger than those of lymphoblastic lymphoma. If a monocytic component occurs, the nuclei show an irregular, occasionally bean-shaped configuration. In the differential diagnosis silver impregnation is helpful. Fibers are more numerous and thicker in acute myeloid and myelomonocytic leukemia than in lymphoblastic lymphoma or ALL. Sections stained with silver impregnation reveal the most important feature, a considerable increase in capillaries, which is more pronounced in myelomonocytic leukemia than in acute myeloid leukemia.

Cytochemically, myelocytes and promyelocytes that are positive for chloroacetate esterase can usually be found in paraffin sections from both myelogenic leukemias. These cells often lie together in groups, especially in the sinuses and connective tissue of the node. In imprints, the same cells can be found easily with the aid of the chloroacetate-esterase or peroxidase reaction. Immunohistochemically, staining for CD34, CD15, CD33, CD68 and lysozyme are decisive.

T-lymphoblastic leukemia/lymphoma is excluded by immunohistochemistry(see Chap. 5.1). The same is true for rare *NK/T-cell neoplasms*, some of which have a lymphoblastic appearance. These neoplasias occur predominately in adults. (see Chap. 5).

Occurrence

On the whole, lymphoblastic lymphoma/leukemia is a rare disease, making up roughly 2,5% of all non-Hodgkin's lymphomas (NHLs). However, among children this disease constitutes about 40–50% of all childhood NHLs (Kjeldsberg et al. 1983; Neth et al. 2000). The median age is below 40 years among adults (Zinzani et al. 1996), with some clinicians describing a second age peak around 70 years (Nathwani et al. 1981b). Among children, the median age is variable mostly due to the exclusion or inclusion of B-ALL (see Burkitt's lymphoma, Chap. 4.2.3). A median age of around 6 years (Neth et al. 2000) has been reported, while an earlier study found that 50% of patients were older than 10 years (Kjeldsberg et al. 1983). There is a clear male predominance within all age groups.

Clinical Presentation and Prognosis

Most patients present primarily with signs of bone marrow insufficiency and/or lymph-node enlargement. About half of the patients have advanced stage III or IV disease. Some patients have been reported to primarily present with lytic bone lesion, at times simulating Ewing sarcoma (Ozdemirli et al. 1998). About 80% of children with pre-B and pre-pre-B types of ALL and lymphoblastic lymphoma had an 5 year event-free survival (Reiter et al. 1999; Neth et al. 2000). In adults, the overall survival is around 50% (Hoelzer et al. 1996). There is a strong correlation between distinct chromosomal abnormalities and the prognosis of lymphoblastic lymphoma (Okuda et al. 1996).

4.2 Peripheral B-Cell Lymphoma

4.2.1 Small-B-Cell Lymphoma

We have chosen this term to summarize those lymphomas which in the Kiel classification have been called *low grade B-cell lymphomas* and to contrast this group with the group of *large-B-cell or blastic lymphomas*. This section thus includes lymphocytic lymphomas, e.g. B-cell chronic lymphocytic leukemia (CLL), hairy cell leukemia and immunocytoma as well as marginal zone lymphomas, and lymphomas of germinal center origin, e.g. follicular lymphomas and mantle cell lymphomas. As mentioned above, these lymphomas had been summarized in the Kiel classification as *low grade B-cell lymphomas*, defining the grade by the cytology of a dominating -cytic or non-blastic cell population. This latter term has been deleted in the WHO classification; however, it might still be helpful for clinical purposes if a subclassification within the group of small-B-cell lymphomas is not possible. The same is true for the term *lymphocytic lymphoma*, which thus includes B-cell chronic lymphocytic leukemia (B-CLL), small lymphocytic lymphoma (SLL), immunocytoma, and hairy cell leukemia.

4.2.1.1 Chronic Lymphocytic Leukemia[1]/Small Lymphocytic Lymphoma[2] (ICD-O: 9823/3[1]; 9670/3[2])

Lymphocytic lymphomas comprise B-CLL/SLL as well as the lymphoplasmacytoid immunocytoma of the Kiel classification. Moreover B-cell prolymphocytic leukemia (B-PLL) is also included.

Both terms (B-CLL/SLL) are used for these same disease. Cases of pure tissue involvement without leukemia are designated as SLL. Although the lymphoplasma*cytoid* immunocytoma is now included into this category, a separate description is given below as a number of such cases, for example, have a monoclonal gammopathy or present as Waldenström disease (Pangalis et al. 1999) and thus should not be confused with B-CLL/SLL. This type of clinical sign is of importance for the clinical behavior and prognosis of the disease.

Synonyms

- Kiel: Chronic lymphocytic leukemia of B-cell type (B-CLL) and lymphoplasmacytoid lymphoma (immunocytoma)
- REAL: B-cell chronic lymphocytic leukemia
- WHO: Chronic lymphocytic leukemia/small lymphocytic lymphoma

Definition

B-CLL/SLL is a neoplasm of mature B-lymphocytes. Histologically, small lymphocytes predominate, but there are *always* at least a few large blast cells and some prolymphocytes as well as lymphoplasmacytoid cells. Mostly these cells form pseudofollicles as proliferation centers. The lymphoplasmacytoid immunocytoma has now been included into this category by the WHO (see below).

As a rule, the blood picture is leukemic, lymph nodes and bone marrow are almost always infiltrated. If a leukemic phase is missing, this neoplasm is designated as SLL although there is overlap.

By mutational analysis, cases of B-CLL/SLL characterized by a pre- and with a post-germinal-center genotype have been identified, indicating a possible origin from either mantle zone cells or peripheral blood lymphocytes which might be of prognostic value.

Morphology

The lymph-node architecture is completely effaced, and sinuses cannot be recognized with H and E or Giemsa stains. The infiltration usually spreads into the tissue surrounding the node. When this happens, the fibers in the capsule usually remain intact, and only a small or moderate number of lymphocytes are found in the capsule, which is thus expanded. Residual lymphoid tissue is rarely seen; it is recognizable from the presence of lymphocytes that are smaller than the leukemic lymphocytes and show a more intense nuclear staining, thus these areas appear slightly darker. Remnants of germinal centers are also seldom. There are a small to moderate number of mostly fine reticulin fibers in a diffuse arrangement.

Cytologically, small lymphocytes with a usually round nucleus, coarse chromatin, and scanty, pale-staining cytoplasm predominate. Occasionally the nuclei are somewhat pleomorphic and hence suggestive of small centrocytes. Among the small lymphocytes are somewhat larger lymphoid cells ("prolymphocytes") with less dense chromatin and more abundant, pale-staining cytoplasm. Finally, one *always* finds at least a few large-cells with a usually oval nucleus containing a large, often solitary, central nucleolus. These cells have a moderate amount of cytoplasm that stains grayish blue with Giemsa, i.e. shows weaker staining than the cytoplasm of immunoblasts. Thus, these cells are called "paraimmunoblasts" (Fig. 4.4). Mitotic activity is low; mitotic figures are found only in paraimmunoblasts and prolymphocytes.

Only a small number of macrophages and "reticulum cells" are seen, eosinophils are absent. In occasional cases, there are a few typical plasma cells, sometimes with plasmablasts; they are found especially near vessels, the capsule, or trabeculae. Immunohistochemical staining reveals that the light-chains in the plasma cells have a polyclonal Ig pattern; hence the cells can be interpreted as reactive plasma cells and not as components of CLL. Giant cells of the Reed-Sternberg type are seldom seen (Fig. 4.5). Cases in which Hodgkin cells are more numerous have been described as composite lymphomas. However it has been shown that both lymphoma parts have an identical Ig heavy-chain gene rearrangement pattern (Weisenberg et al. 1995) (see Differential Diagnosis).

The histological impression of B-CLL varies with the number of prolymphocytes and paraimmunoblasts. (1) When there is only a small number of prolymphocytes and paraimmunoblasts, they cannot be recognized as such at a low magnification. Hence the growth pattern appears diffuse ("diffuse subtype",

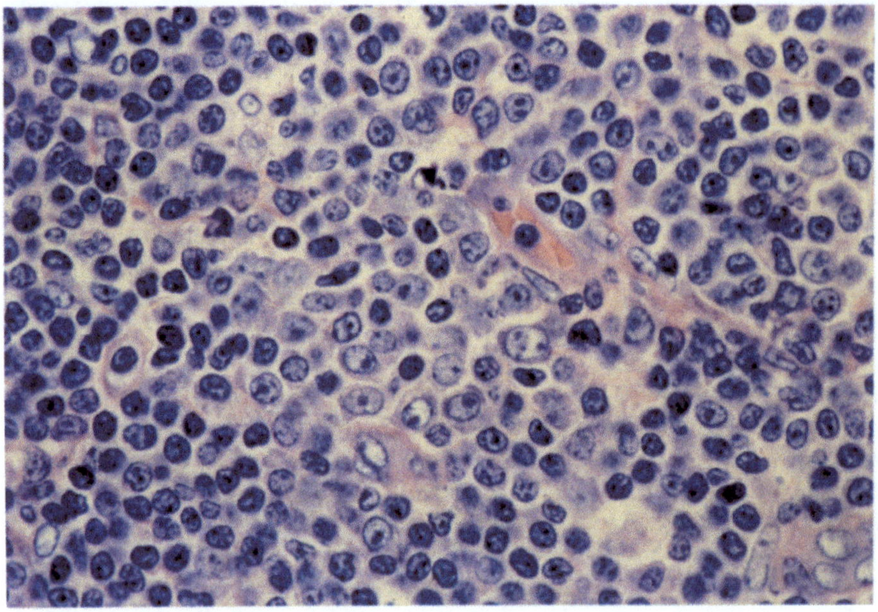

Fig. 4.4. Chronic lymphocytic leukemia of B-cell type. In the center, a pseudofollicular structure with prolymphocytes and paraimmunoblasts is surrounded by small lymphocytes (Giemsa stain)

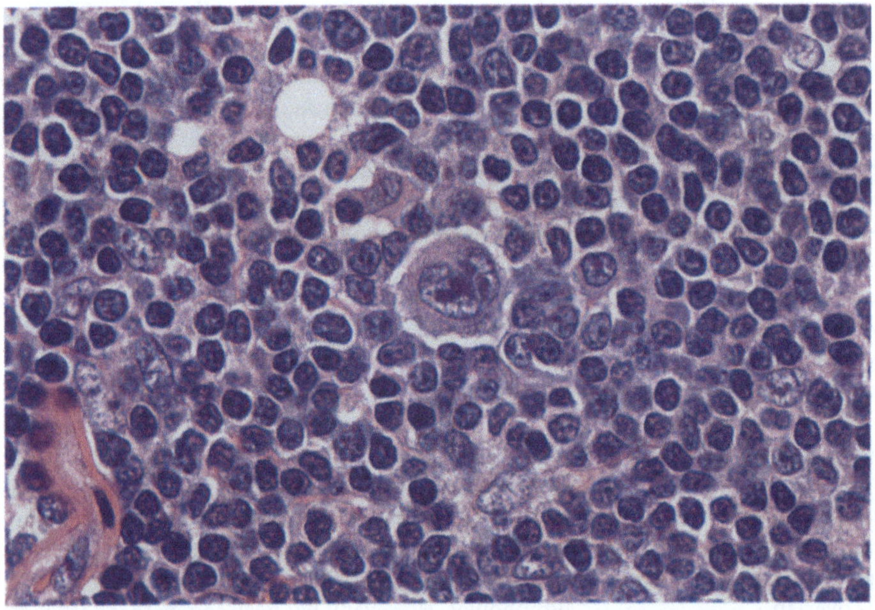

Fig. 4.5. Chronic lymphocytic leukemia of B-cell-type with a classical Hodgkin cell (Giemsa stain)

constituting about 7% of our cases). (2) When there are moderate numbers of prolymphocytes and paraimmunoblasts, they are seen in clusters (proliferation centers), which are evident as light foci in Giemsa-stained slides at a low magnification ("pseudofollicular subtype", accounting for about 85% of our cases of B-CLL; Fig. 4.6). (3) Finally, prolymphocytes (and occasional or quite numerous paraimmunoblasts) may infiltrate large areas of the lymph node (Fig. 4.7); these areas are clearly demarcated from the rest of the CLL infiltration ("tumor-forming subtype", constituting about 8% of the biopsy cases). (4) Some patients have a more prominent lymphoplasmacytoid differentiation with monoclonal cytoplasmic immunoglobulin (cIg) in the plasmacytoid cells. Such cases have been included by the WHO into the group of lymphocytic lymphomas.

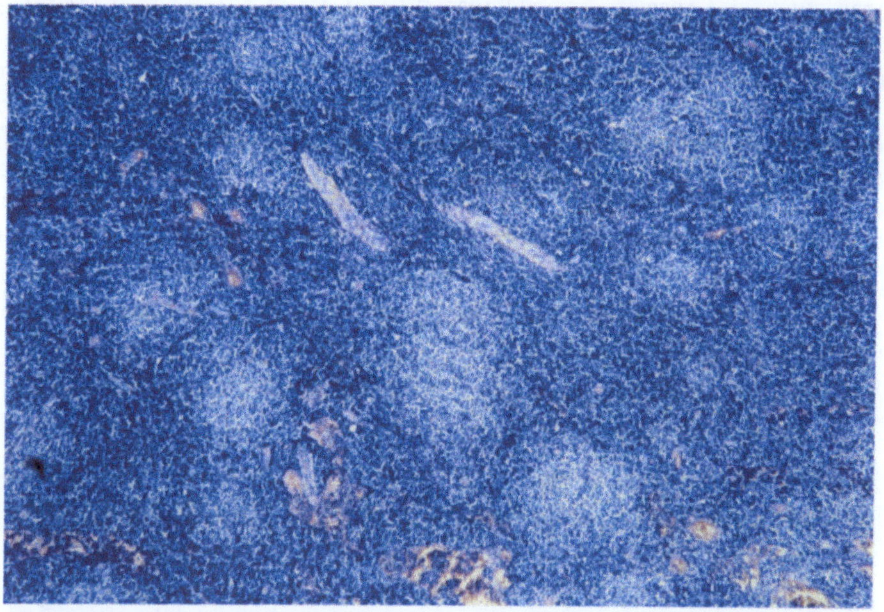

Fig. 4.6. Chronic lymphocytic leukemia of B-cell-type with a typical pseudofollicular pattern. The pseudofollicles appear as light areas (Giemsa stain)

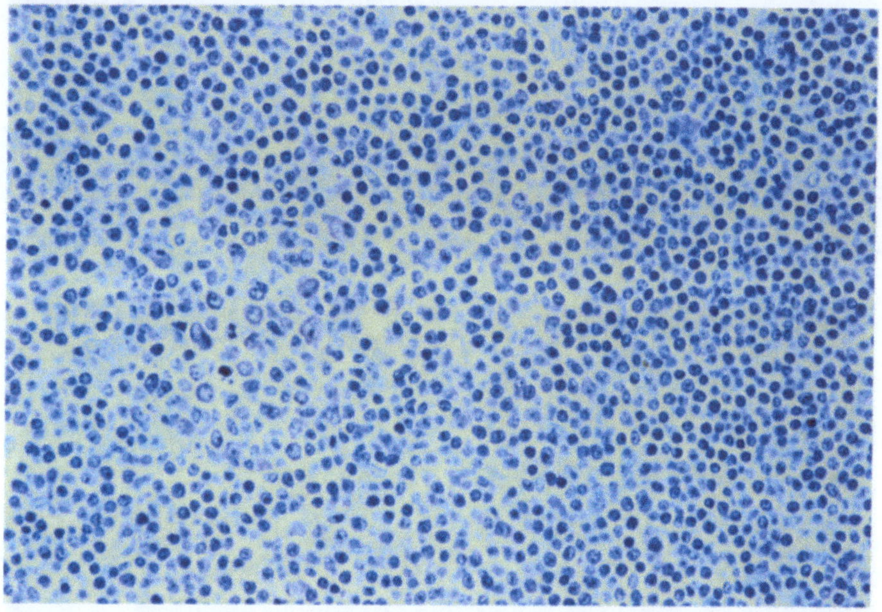

Fig. 4.7. Chronic lymphocytic leukemia of B-cell-type. On the *left* side, the lighter area has a high number of prolymphocytes and some paraimmunoblasts in a tumor-forming B-cell chronic lymphocytic leukemia (B-CLL) (Giemsa stain)

We still prefer to describe this as a special variant (see below).

In 5–10% of lymphocytic lymphomas there may be a predominately interfollicular or perifollicular/marginal zone growth pattern. In these cases the same pseudofollicles are found as in the diffuse type. These pseudofollicles can be either perifollicular or diffuse interfollicular. The two patterns may be linked to the mutational status of the neoplastic cells, which seems to influence the response to therapy (Hamblin et al. 1999; Damle et al. 1999) Mutated variable heavy (V_H)-chain genes were found more frequently in perifollicular proliferation centers (Bahler et al. 2000), whose phenotype is typical of lymphocytic lymphomas but which may be morphologically misinterpreted as mantle cell or marginal zone lymphomas (Ben-Ezra et al.

1989; Ellison et al. 1989; Nguyen et al. 1995; Gupta et al. 2000). A reasonable number of such cases may be lymphoplasmacytoid immunocytomas.

Development into Lymphoma of Higher-Grade Malignancy – Diffuse Large B-Cell. In about 15% of the cases of B-CLL, the cells terminally develop a tumor-like macroscopic appearance. Histologically, this corresponds in about 12% of cases to the "tumor-forming subtype", which can often be recognized in the blood from an increase in the number of prolymphocytes. Such cases have been described as "transition into prolymphocytic leukemia" (York et al. 1984; Stark et al. 1986), but this must not be confused with the primary prolymphocytic leukemia of Galton (Galton et al. 1974). (see Chap.4.2.1.1.1 and 6.10.1.5). Some tumor-

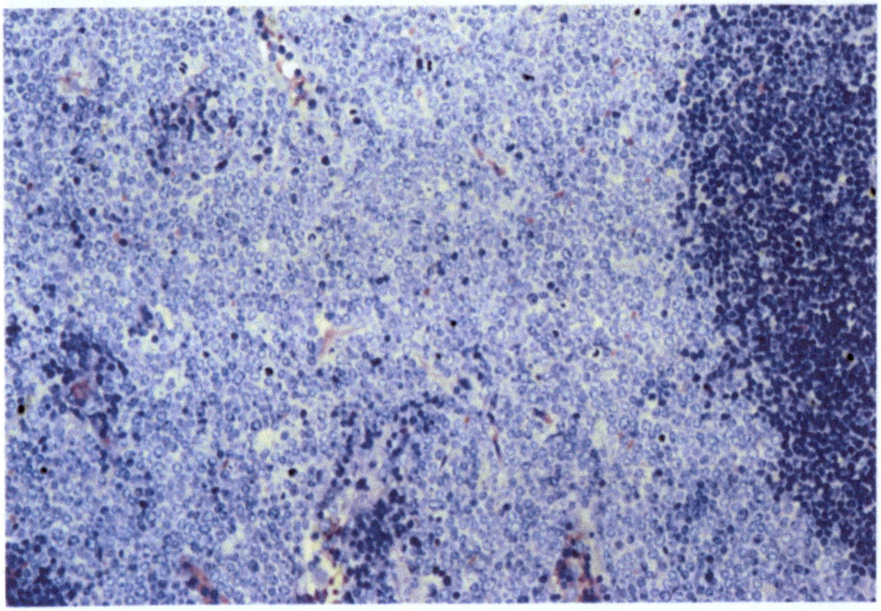

Fig. 4.8. Chronic lymphocytic leukemia of B-cell-type with transformation into a diffuse large-B-cell lymphoma. Note the light area which is sharply demarcated from the remnants of the lymphocytic lymphoma (Giemsa stain)

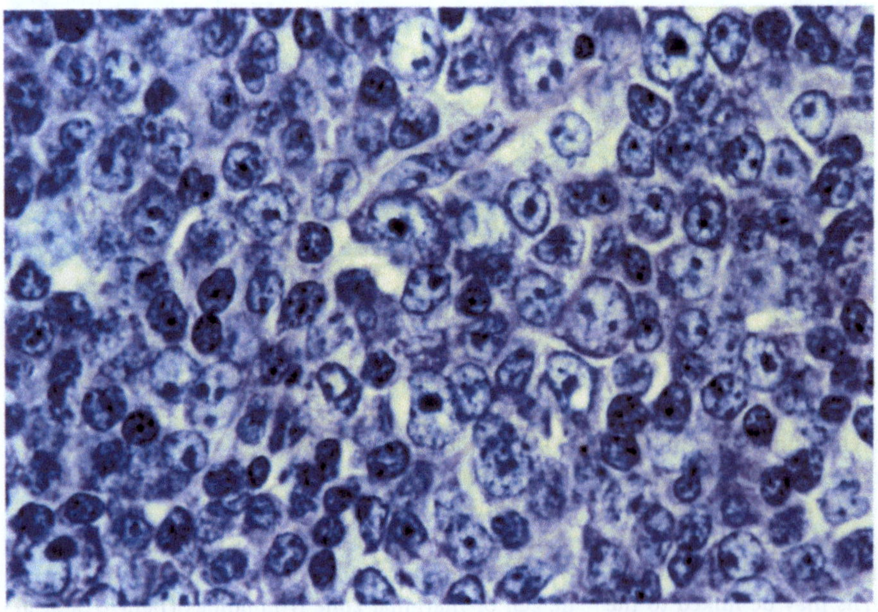

Fig. 4.9. High-power view of so-called Richter's syndrome with immunoblasts and centroblasts (Giemsa stain)

forming subtypes with a high content of prolymphocytes also contain numerous paraimmunoblasts; such cases correspond to the paraimmunoblastic variant described by Pugh et al. (1988). Approximately 4% of B-CLL cases in which there is a terminal tumor-like appearance show a diffuse large-cell lymphoma, either immunoblastic or centroblastic lymphoma (so-called Richter syndrome; Figs. 4.8, 4.9). In contrast, a terminal lymphoblastic phase is evidently rare in CLL. Figure 4.10 shows a case that was interpreted as the blastic phase of B-CLL. The "blasts" contained a large amount of cytoplasmic IgM and were CD23-negative (Fig. 4.11); instead, the cells looked more like prolymphocytes than immunoblasts.

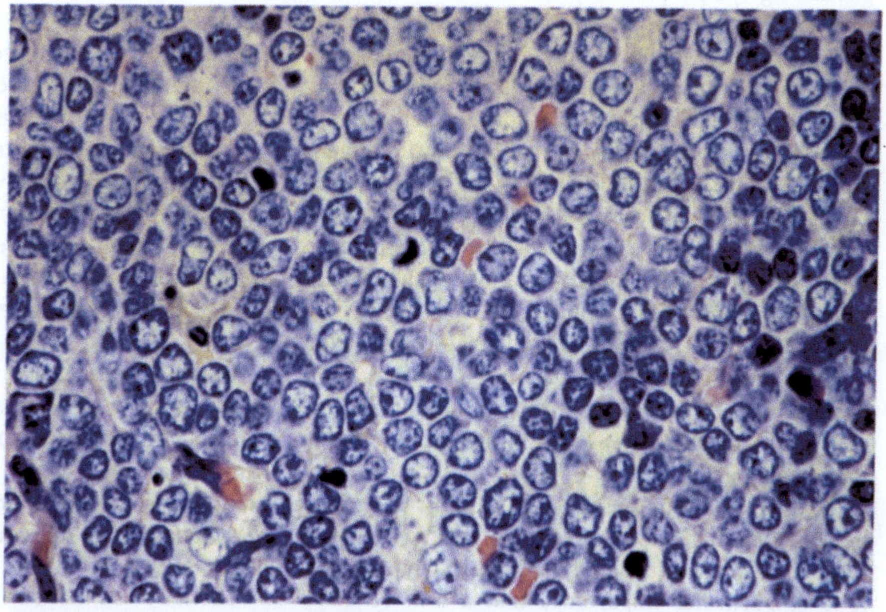

Fig. 4.10. High-power view of a blastic phase of a B-CLL. The cells are mostly paraimmunoblasts (Giemsa stain)

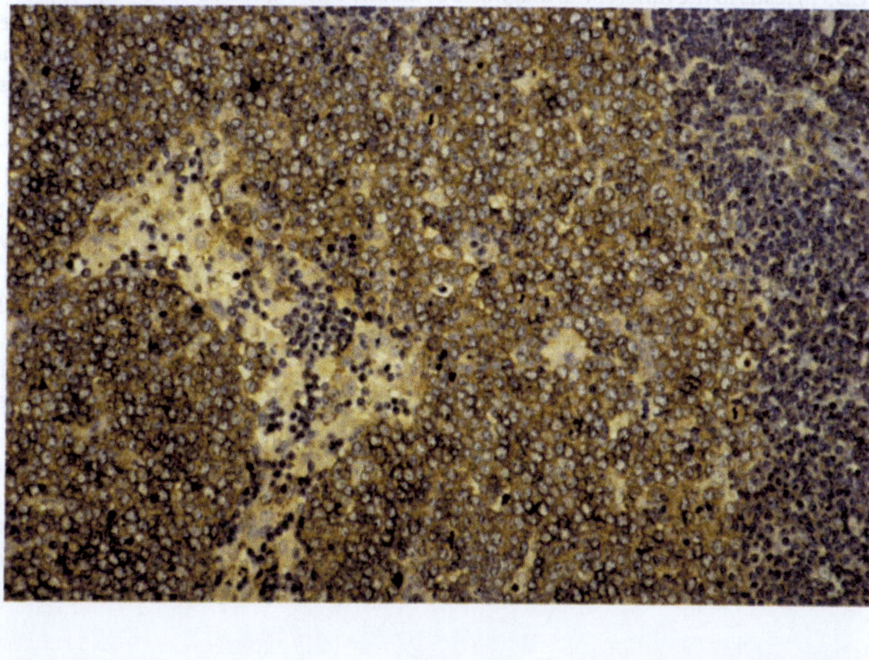

Fig. 4.11. Immunohistochemical staining of the same tumor as in Fig. 4.8; with strong surface and intracytoplasmic IgM expression in a transformed B-CLL (immunoperoxidase stain)

Immunohistochemistry

B-CLL-lymphocytes bear sIg of the IgM type, often together with IgD, and light-chains of either κ or λ type. Approximately 20% of cells lack expression of IgD, and occasionally cells lack IgM as well. IgG on the surface of tumor cells almost always also reveals intracytoplasmic IgG-positive lymphoplasmacytoid cells. This finding is not consistent with a diagnosis of B-CLL; rather, such cases can be diagnosed as a variant of lymphocytic lymphoma, e.g. lymphoplasmacytoid immunocytoma (see Chap. 4.2.1.2). In paraffin sections, monotypic cIg either is not seen or is found in only a few lymphoid cells. Paraimmunoblasts, however, may show moderate cIg reactivity, especially in the tumor-forming subtype (see Fig. 4.11). B-CLL/SLL cells express the B-cell antigens CD19, CD22, CD20, and CD79α. CD5 and CD23 usually show a characteristic coexpression (Kumar et al. 1996; Singh and Wright 1997; Tworek et al. 1998; Watson et al. 2000). The expression of CD20 is mostly low in these cases. The proportion of proliferating cells (Ki-67+) is usually about 5%. The pseudofollicular proliferation centers show a higher percentage of positive cells. Complement receptors (CD35) are not a constant finding. The T-cell content is low (<10%). Residual FDC are found only rarely.

In about 3–5% of the cases, CD5 and/or CD23 may be absent. Partial CD23 expression may indicate a partial transformation into a diffuse large-cell lymphoma. It is of particular importance that a lack of CD23 (CD5+) leads to the differential diagnosis of mantle cell lymphoma. The cells have to be stained for cyclin D1, which is expressed in about 80% of mantle cell lymphomas but is negative in lymphocytic lymphomas (de Leon et al. 1998).

Whether CD5-B-CLL is biologically identical to CD5+ B-CLL is not yet clear (Huang et al. 1999). It has been reported that they differ in their adhesion molecule profile (Finn et al. 2001).

Individual cases of B-CLL have been described in which there is coexpression of CD5 and CD10; however, the significance of this finding is not yet known (Barekman et al. 2001).

Genetic Features

In about 50–70% of B-CLL/SLL patients, chromosomal abnormalities can be identified by classical cytogenetic analysis (Offit et al. 1991). By molecular genetic studies (FISH) the frequency is somewhat higher – up to 80% (Döhner et al. 1999). Frequent, although not specific and probably secondary abnormalities are trisomy 12 as well as primary structural abnormalities of chromosomes 13q14, 14q32 and 11q22–23 (Raghoebier et al. 1992; Stilgenbauer et al. 1993; Döhner et al. 1997). In 13q14, new candidate genes for leukemogenesis have recently been described (Mabuchi et al. 2001; Migliazza et al. 2001). Structural abnormalities of chromosome 17p seem to be associated with disease progression (Callet-Bauchu et al. 1999); deletions of 11q have also been found to indicate a poor prognosis (Döhner et al. 1997). Patients with deletions of 11q have also been shown to have a more rapid disease progression (Döhner et al. 1997).

Recently it was reported that cells with trisomy 12 have a minimal level of mutations whereas cells with 13q14 abnormalities show significant levels (Oscier et al. 1997). Moreover this mutation status seems to be associated with a different prognosis, with low or unmutated genes associated with a more aggressive form of B-CLL (Hamblin et al. 1999; Damle et al. 1999).

Differential Diagnosis

Immunocytoma. This type of lymphoma shows monoclonal cIg in lymphoplasmacytoid and/or plasma cells with at least one cell per high-power field or in large groups of cells. There are often periodic-acid-Schiff (PAS)-positive globular inclusions in the nuclei of neoplastic cells.

The above mentioned cIg expression has to be distinguished from cIg expression in prolymphocytes and paraimmunoblasts in pseudofollicles, which is also found in B-CLL. Lymphoplasmacytic lymphoma (immunocytoma) is almost always negative for CD23 and CD5.

Marginal Zone B-Cell Lymphoma. Some cases have a predominant monocytoid differentiation and are thus morphologically similar to SLL. There may also be plasmacytoid or plasmacytic differentiation; however, the immunophenotype is distinct with positivity for CD5 and CD23 in SLL and lymphoplasmacytoid immunocytoma. Moreover, the growth pattern within the sinuses or perifollicular may be of help in distinguishing between these diseases and marginal zone B-cell lymphoma. A primary extranodal occurrence speaks very much in favor of the latter. It has not yet been clarified whether rare cases of *primary extranodal small-B-cell lymphomas* in the gastrointestinal tract or spleen with positivity for CD5 and/or CD23 belong to the group of SLL or marginal zone B-cell lymphoma.

Mantle Cell Lymphoma. There are no blast cells in the infiltrate. Some mantle cell lymphomas show remnants of germinal centers which can make it difficult to distinguish them from neoplastic blasts of a lymphocytic lymphoma. In such cases, cyclin D1 staining is imperative. The reticulin fibers are thick and more abundant in mantle cell lymphoma.

T-Cell Lymphocytic/Prolymphocytic Leukemia. T-cell regions are infiltrated, and there is a marked increase in the number of epithelioid venules. A pseudofollicular pattern is not seen. T-immunoblasts are extremely rare.

Sézary's Syndrome. T-cell regions are infiltrated, and a marked increase in the number of epithelioid venules is seen. Nuclei of lymphocytes are pleomorphic. Interdigitating cells are increased in number. There may be giant cells of the mycosis fungoides type.

Hairy Cell Leukemia. B-cell regions and connective tissue (trabeculae, capsule) are infiltrated. The lymph node is usually only partially involved. Nuclei are often reniform. Blast cells and mitotic figures are absent.

Lymphocyte-Predominant Hodgkin's Lymphoma. This type of lymphoma contains Reed-Sternberg cells of the L and H type. It often shows infiltration by clusters of epithelioid cells. The growth pattern is frequently nodular ("nodular paragranuloma") and can best be seen by silver impregnation.

Diffuse Lymphoid Hyperplasia. The sinuses are clearly demarcated, often dilated and filled with lymphoid cells.

Occurrence

At the present time, cases of B-CLL account for about 11 % of the NHL lymph-node biopsy material assessed by pathologists in Germany. Outside Germany, lymph-node biopsies are seldom performed on patients with CLL, because blood and marrow examinations are considered to be sufficient for a diagnosis. The International Non-Hodgkin's Lymphoma Classification project gives a percentages of 6.7 % for B-CLL and 1.2 % for lymphoplasmacytoid immunocytoma, although only lymphoplasmacytic immunocytoma is included within the International Lymphoma Study Group (ILSG) provisional entities. Thus, a frequency of around 7–8 % can be assumed (The Non Hodgkin's Lymphoma Classification Project 1997).

B-CLL is usually a disease of late adult life and shows a peak occurrence in the seventh decade. B-CLL does normally not occur before the age of 20, and it is rare before the age of 30. The male-to-female ratio is 1.47 : 1.

Clinical Presentation, Evolution, and Prognosis

Patients with CLL/SLL usually present with an absolute lymphocytosis and/or asymptomatic lymphadenopathy. At diagnosis, the disease presents in more than 70 % of patients at an advanced clinical stage. The bone marrow is also infiltrated in at least 70 % of the cases. Constitutional symptoms are found in about 10 % (Coiffier et al. 1999). The duration of survival of patients with B-CLL is relatively long, but depends on the stage of the disease at the time of diagnosis. According to Rai et al. (1975) and Binet (French Cooperative Group on Chronic Lymphocytic Leukemia 1986), the stage of the disease is determined by criteria other than those used for other types of NHL. The pseudofollicular subtype shows the most favorable prognosis, while the prognosis for patients with the other subtypes is significantly worse (Brittinger et al. 1984).

Clinical stage, β2-microglobulin levels, B symptoms, and percentage of abnormal karyotypes have been described to be of prognostic significance (Rai et al. 1975; Keating 1999; Montserrat et al. 1986).

Recently it has been shown that the mutational status of the neoplastic cells is useful in predicting the therapeutic response (Hamblin et al. 1999; Damle et al. 1999).

4.2.1.1.1 Variant: B-Cell Prolymphocytic Leukemia (ICD-O: 9833/3)

Galton et al. (1974) distinguished a special type of leukemia from typical B-CLL: the lymphocytes are larger and have a large, prominent nucleolus (Fig. 4.12). The patients must have more than 55 % prolymphocytes in the blood or bone marrow according to the definition of the FAB group, which is now also accepted for the WHO classification. In typical cases, patients have marked splenomegaly and high blood cell counts. Initially, the lymph nodes are only slightly infiltrated, but later they may be massively infiltrated by prolymphocytes. The prolymphocytes are quite monotonous looking, significantly larger than B-CLL-lymphocytes,

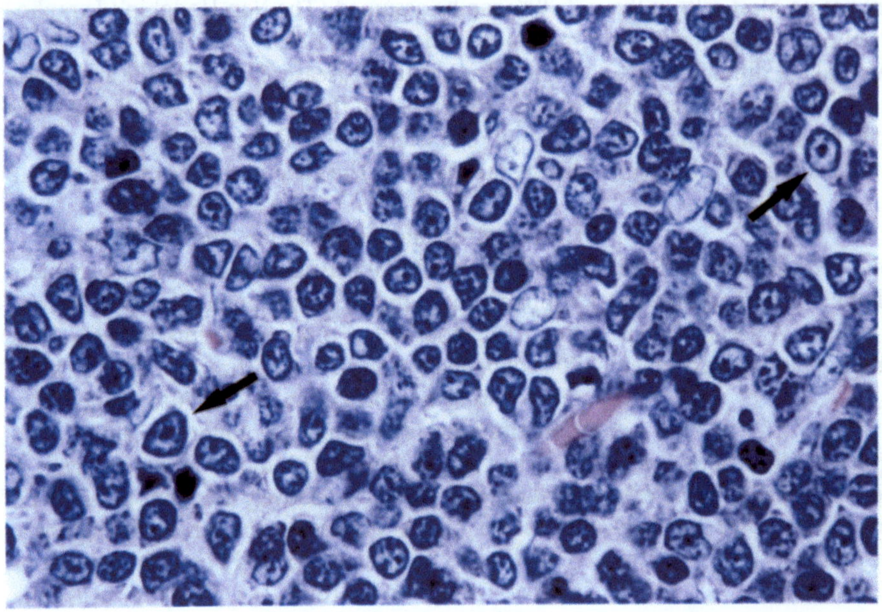

Fig. 4.12. B-prolymphocytic leukemia (B-PLL) with homogeneous sheets of prolymphocytes and only very few paraimmunoblasts (→) (Giemsa stain)

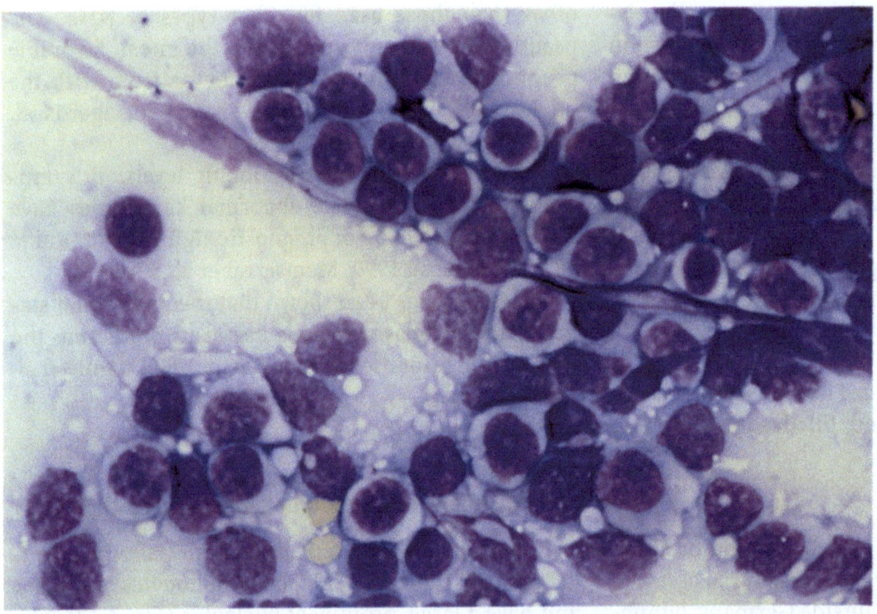

Fig. 4.13. Touch-imprint of a B-cell prolymphocytic leukemia (B-PLL) with round nuclei, prominent nucleoli and a broad cytoplasmic rim (Pappenheim stain)

and show more abundant, weakly basophilic cytoplasm (Fig. 4.13). The nucleus is mostly round, but may show marked nuclear indentations. Proliferation centers are not present. The large paraimmunoblasts seen in B-CLL do not occur in this type of leukemia, but occasionally there may be a somewhat larger, basophilic cell with a larger nucleolus.

A second group of B-PLLs which is morphologically identical but without pronounced splenomegaly and lower leukocyte counts at the time of primary diagnosis has a more favorable prognosis (Shvidel et al. 1999).

By definition, transformed CLL is excluded. However, on purely morphological grounds this can not always be differentiated in lymph-node sections. As this difference is of prognostic importance the clinical history has to be taken into account.

The lymphoma types to be considered in a differential diagnosis are mantle cell lymphoma and lymphoblastic lymphoma, especially those cases with t(11;14) which have been described as morphologically typical PLL. Most probably, such cases have to be designated as mantle cell lymphomas.

The immunophenotypic profile of B-PLL is very similar to that of B-CLL/SLL. B-PLL shows more intensive sIg staining, CD5 is mostly absent, and CD23 is almost always absent. The number of cells expressing the proliferation-associated antigen (Ki-67+) is significantly larger than in B-CLL.

Deletions of 11q23 and 13q14 are frequently described in primary B-PLL (Lens et al. 2000) as well as abnormalities on chromosome 7 (Schlette et al. 2001).

4.2.1.1.2
Variant: Lymphoplasmacytoid Lymphoma (Immunocytoma) (ICD-O: 9823/3)

Synonyms

- Kiel: Lymphoplasmacytoid immunocytoma
- REAL: B-cell chronic lymphocytic leukemia/small lymphocytic lymphoma
- WHO: B-cell chronic lymphocytic leukemia/small lymphocytic lymphoma

Definition

Immunocytoma is a monoclonal neoplasm of B-lymphocytes and is thus morphologically very similar to B-CLL/SLL. In addition to lymphocytes, however, the lymphoplasmacytoid immunocytoma always contains some lymphoplasmacytoid cells that express monoclonal cIg, as shown immunohistochemically; the lymphocytes show sIg staining.

Cases of immunocytoma are often simply classified as "malignant lymphoma lymphocytic". The reasons for this are in part technical: In H and E-stained slides, plasmacytoid differentiation can be recognized only when it is pronounced; hence it is often necessary to apply special stains or immunohistochemical analysis to make the correct diagnosis. The WHO included the lymphoplasmacytoid type into the group of small lymphocytic lymphomas. We think that this type at least should be described as a separate variant of lymphocytic lymphomas as there may be a marked lymphoplasmacytoid differentiation, and about 20–30% of such cases are accompanied clinically by a monoclonal gammopathy (Waldenström's macroglobulinemia)

Morphology

As in B-CLL/SLL, small lymphocytes predominate markedly in immunocytoma, making up more than 50%, and usually more than 90% of the tumor cells. In

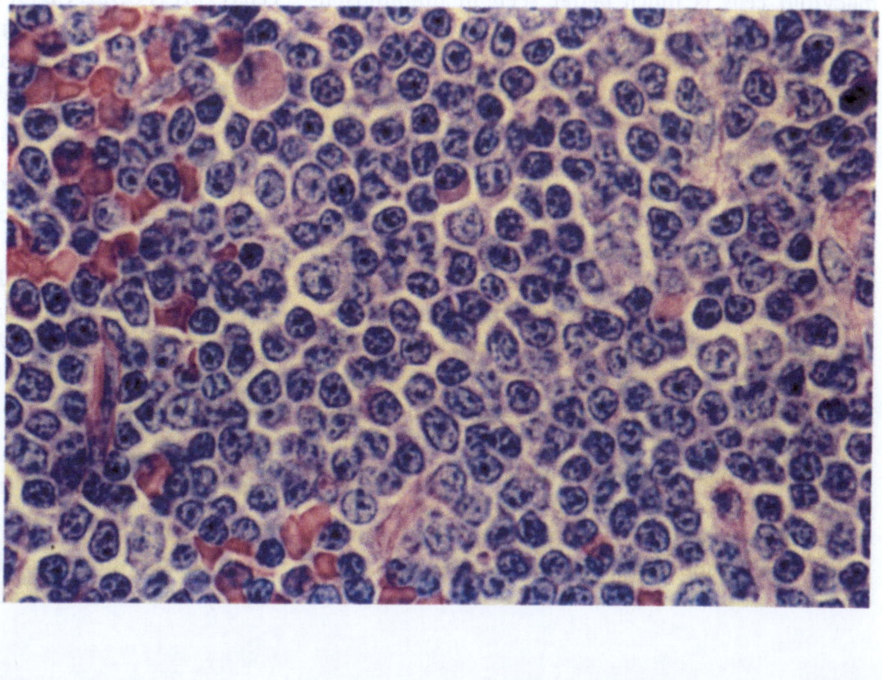

Fig. 4.14. Lymphocytic lymphoma of B-cell-type, variant lymphoplasmocytoid lymphoma (immunocytoma) with a large number of small lymphocytes and prolymphocytes and some plasmacytoid cells (Giemsa stain)

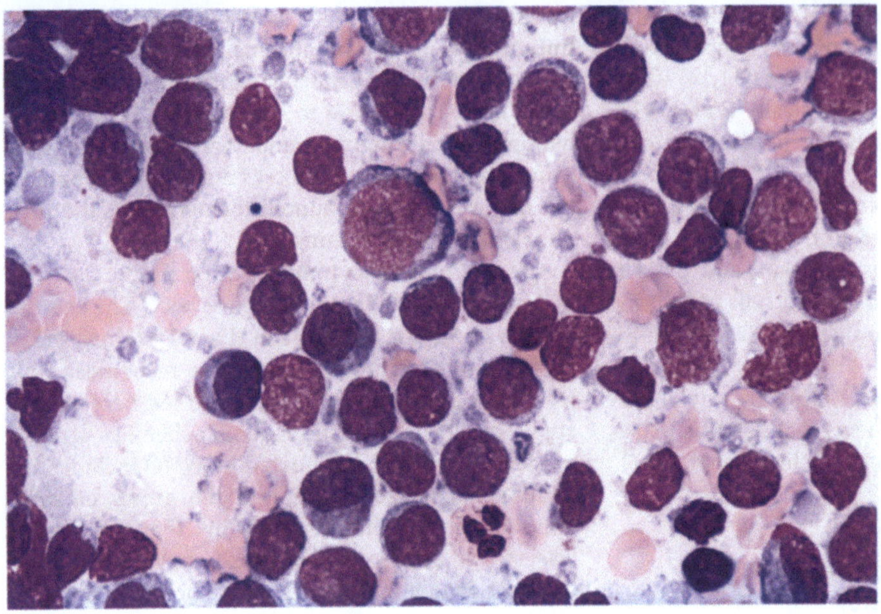

Fig. 4.15. Touch-imprint of a lymphocytic lymphoma, variant lymphoplasmocytoid immunocytoma, with a large number of lymphoplasmocytoid cells and a single blast (Pappenheim stain)

contrast to B-CLL/SLL, however, there is also a number of lymphoplasmacytoid cells, i.e. cells with a more abundant, basophilic cytoplasm and a somewhat eccentric nucleus (Fig. 4.14). These plasmacytoid cells do not have prominent Golgi bodies. Their cytoplasm is less basophilic and less abundant than that of plasma cells of the lymphoplasmacytic immunocytoma (Fig. 4.15). Frequently, the number of monoclonal plasmacytoid cells is much better seen in immunostainings, since these cells can easily be overlooked by conventional Giemsa stain (Fig. 4.16a, b).

Furthermore, there are always a few immunoblasts. In some cases there are a larger number of immunoblasts, and there may be very large proliferation centers, as in tumor-forming B-CLL. Nevertheless, lymphocytes are still the predominant cells. Sometimes a pseudofollicular pattern is found, although less frequently than in B-CLL/SLL.

A significant increase of mast cells is found in one-third of lymphoplasmacytoid immunocytoma. Hemosiderosis is not seen.

In the diagnosis of immunocytoma the most valuable histological feature is the presence of globular PAS-positive inclusions (Dutcher bodies) in the *nucleus* of lymphoplasmacytoid cells (Fig. 4.17).

Some immunocytomas show groups of epithelioid cells (see lymphoplasmacytic immunocytoma).

Immunohistochemistry

The immunophenotype is almost identical to that of B-CLL/SLL. In contrast to B-CLL cells, lymphoplasmacytoid cells also contain cIg of the same isotype as the small lymphocytes. The most frequent heavy-chain class is IgM. Approximately 70 % of the cases both IgM and IgD are present. IgG can be demonstrated in about 10 % of cases. IgA and IgE are rarely found. The tumor cells express CD22, CD19, and CD20. In at least 90 % of the cases of lymphoplasmacytoid subtype the cells express CD5 and CD23. In individual cases one or the other antigen may be lacking. The proportion of proliferating cells (Ki-67+) is, on the average, somewhat larger in immunocytoma than in B-CLL. Small remnants of networks of FDC can be detected in about half of the cases (see Harris and Bhan 1985; Hall et al. 1987).

Genetic Features (see B-CLL)

It has been described that the translocation t(9;14)(p13;q32) as well as del(7)(q32) are more frequently associated with plasmacytoid differentiation (Offit et al. 1992, 1995).

Diagnosis and Differential Diagnosis (see B-CLL and lymphoplasmacytic immunocytoma)

Occurrence

The age distribution of immunocytoma is approximately the same as that of B-CLL, except for the occa-

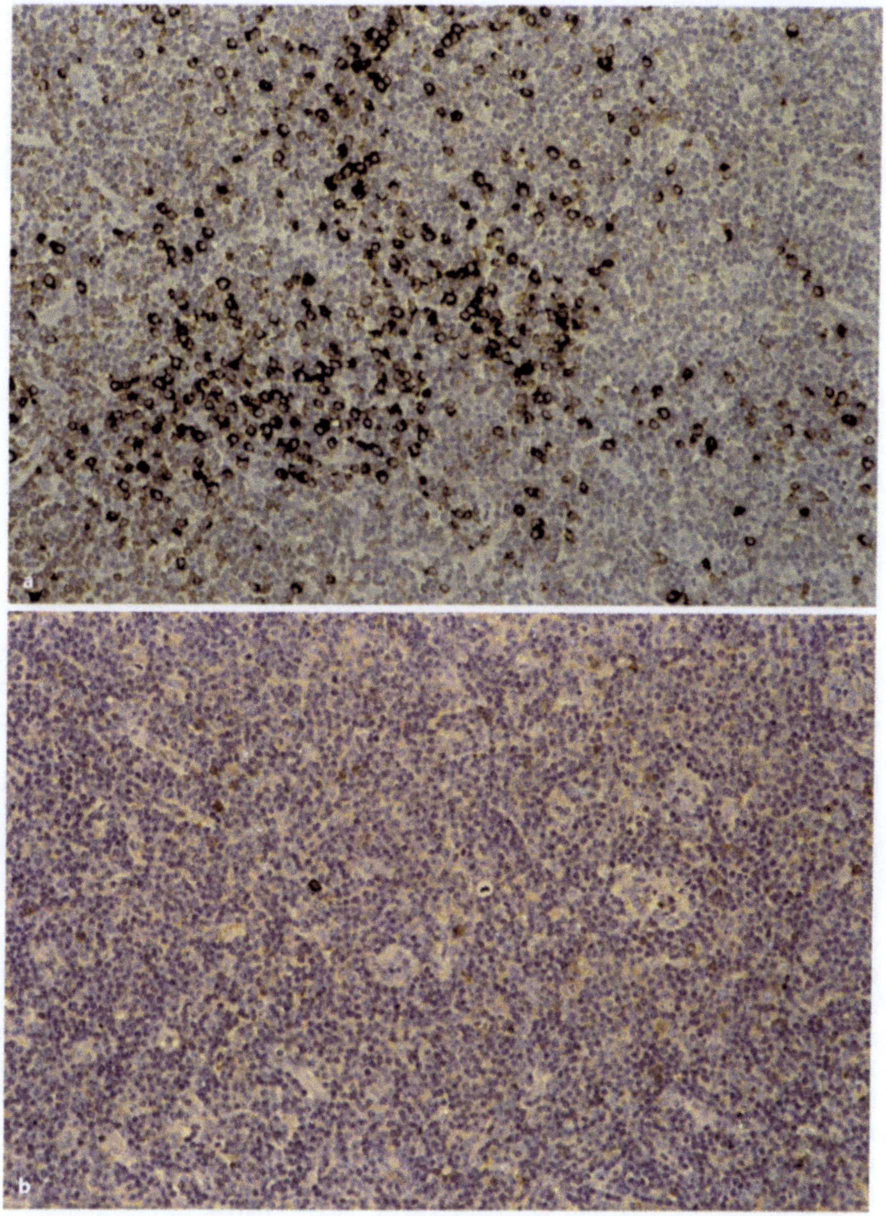

Fig. 4.16 a, b. Lymphocytic lymphoma, variant lymphoplasmocytoid immunocytoma, immunostained for light chain κ (**a**) and λ (**b**). Note the cytoplasmic positivity for κ in **a** (immunoperoxidase stain)

sional case of immunocytoma in childhood. The youngest patient was 13 years old. The male-to-female ratio is about 1.1 : 1.

Clinical Presentation and Prognosis

In general, lymphoplasmacytoid immunocytoma is similar to B-CLL. In most patients, lymphadenopathy develops slowly and affects many regions. In some patients, however, an excessively enlarged spleen is the first sign of disease (Heinz et al. 1979).

Immunocytoma may develop primarily at an extranodal site and occasionally does not involve lymph nodes at all. However, today most of such extranodal cases are recognized as marginal zone B-cell lymphomas.

The blood serum of about 10–20% of patients shows a monoclonal increase in the Ig level, usually

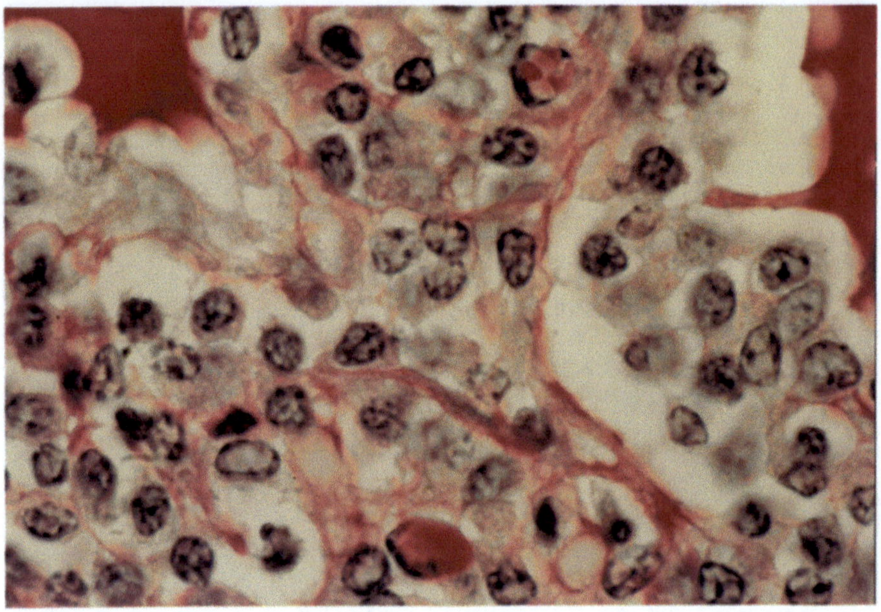

Fig. 4.17. Lymphocytic lymphoma, variant lymphoplasmocytoid immunocytoma, with two cells containing PAS-positive nuclear inclusions (Dutcher bodies)

IgM, sometimes IgG, rarely IgA or IgE. In a few cases either light-chains or heavy-chains alone are present. About 60% of patients have lymphocytosis (>4,109 lymphocytes/l), which looks very much like B-CLL, but is sometimes striking owing to the presence of basophilic lymphoplasmacytoid cells.

On the whole, the overall survival rate is somewhat lower than in B-CLL (Andriko et al. 2001; Papamichael et al. 1999). A study done by the Kiel Lymphoma Study Group (Heinz et al. 1979) did not reveal any significant differences between the two subtypes, i.e. lymphoplasmacytoid and lymphoplasmacytic immunocytoma. Kuse et al. (1983), however, reported a poorer prognosis for "polymorphic" immunocytoma. According to Kimby and Mellstedt (1991), the prognosis for immunocytoma patients with a leukemic blood picture is more favorable than the prognosis for patients with a leukemic immunocytoma.

Thirty to 40 years ago, a number of cases of chronic lymphocytic leukemia containing "atypical azurophilic crystals" were described. These crystals are needle-like inclusions that can be found in the cytoplasm of peripheral blood or bone marrow smears, mostly described in B-CLL and in some cases of Waldenström's disease. Some of these crystals have a slightly beaded appearance (Lagios et al. 1974). As they do not normally stain with Giemsa, they impose a delineated rectangular negative image in the cytoplasm. This rectangular configuration allows a clear distinction from the needle-like azurophilic crystals of Auer bodies. The crystalline inclusions in B-CLL stain positive for immunoglobulin light- and heavy-chain. Thus these crystals seem to be atypical protein precipitates (De Man et al. 1962). We therefore think that these inclusions are predominately found in lymphoblastic lymphomas or the variant of B-CLL (lymphoplasmacytoid immunocytoma) that is in part equivalent to Waldenström's macroglobulinemia.

Interestingly, during the last 30 years there have been no further reports in the literature on the occurrence of this phenomenon. However, it may be that that the inclusions are partly overlooked since they are not found in sections and are not Wright-Giemsa-stained in smears.

4.2.1.2
Lymphoplasmacytic Lymphoma – Partially Corresponding to Macroglobulinemia Waldenström (ICD-O: 9671/3)

Lymphoplasmacytic lymphoma (lymphoplasmacytic immunocytoma) is distinguished from lymphoplasmacytoid immunocytoma by the WHO classification as it is thought to be a distinct clinicopathological entity. Lymphoplasmacytoid immunocytoma cannot be clearly distinguished from lymphocytic lymphomas in all cases and is thus included under lymphocytic lymphomas. Although some immunohistochemical and cytogenetic data favor this view, the clinical data available today indicate mostly a mixture of both types.

The WHO includes Waldenström's disease into this category and uses the terms synonymously. We find this arbitrary as it is clear that Waldenström's disease (WD) is a clinical term and is clinically defined. It was described in 1948 (review Waldenström 1958) as a malignancy of lymphoplasmacytoid cells with immunoglobulin secretion distinguished from that of plasmacytic myeloma.

A serum M component is present with an excess of 3 g/dl. Today, this symptom, primarily thought to be specific for immunocytoma, may also occur associated with other lymphoma types such as B-CLL, multiple myeloma, splenic, and nodal marginal zone B-cell lymphoma (see Chap. 4.2.1.5)and even rare cases of follicular lymphoma (Groves et al. 1998). We therefore do not use the terms WD and lymphoplasmacytic immunocytoma as synonyms.

Synonyms

- Kiel: Lymphoplasmacytic lymphoma (immunocytoma)
- REAL: Lymphoplasmacytoid lymphoma/immunocytoma
- WHO: Lymphoplasmacytic lymphoma/Waldenström macroglobulinemia

Definition

Lymphoplasmacytic lymphoma (immunocytoma) (lymphoplasmacytic lymphoma) is a monoclonal neoplasm of B-lymphocytes and is thus similar to B-CLL. In addition to lymphocytes, however, lymphoplasmacytic lymphoma contains some lymphoplasmacytoid cells and *monoclonal plasma cells.* The lymphocytes show sIg expression, while both the lymphoplasmacytoid cells *and* plasma cells (including precursor cells) contain cytoplasmic Ig of the same type.

The lymphoplasmacytic immunocytoma is almost always CD5- and CD23-negative; it is less often leukemic and more often paraproteinemic than lymphoplasmacytoid immunocytoma.

Morphology

As in B-CLL and lymphoplasmacytoid immunocytoma small lymphocytes predominate markedly. They make up usually more than 90% of the tumor cells. In contrast to B-CLL, however, there is also a number of lymphoplasmacytoid cells and plasma cells, i.e. cells with more abundant, basophilic cytoplasm. In addition, there are always a few immunoblasts (Fig. 4.18).

The *lymphoplasmacytic lymphoma* to some extent corresponds to Waldenström's macroglobulinemia as described in the earlier literature. However, other types of B-cell lymphoma may have the same clinical picture with a marked plasmacytic differentiation (see below).

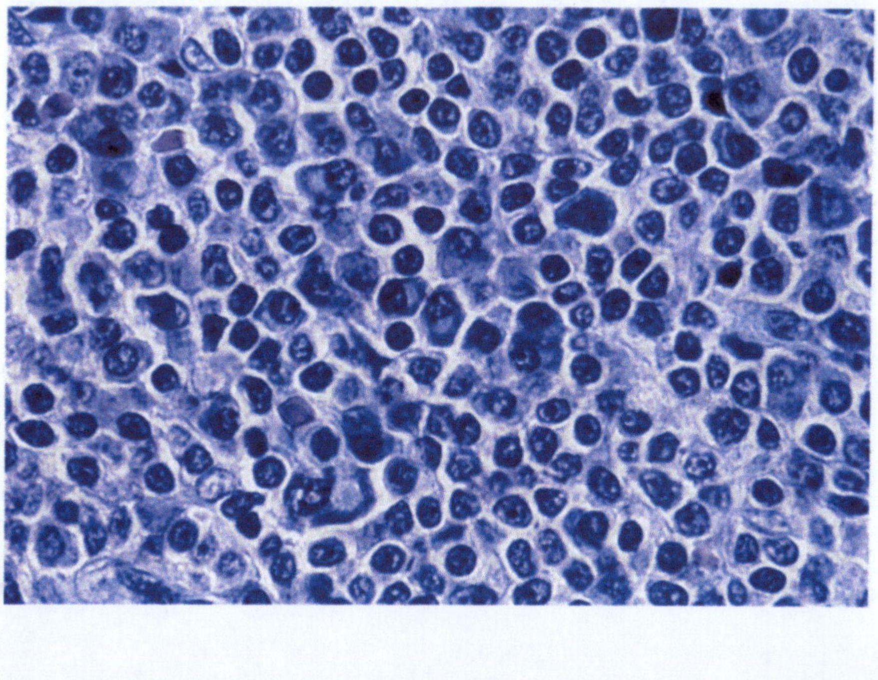

Fig. 4.18. Lymphoplasmocytic lymphoma with small lymphocytes and a large number of plasmacytoid cells and plasma cells, only some of which have prominent nucleoli. Most of the plasma cells are inconspicuous (Giemsa stain)

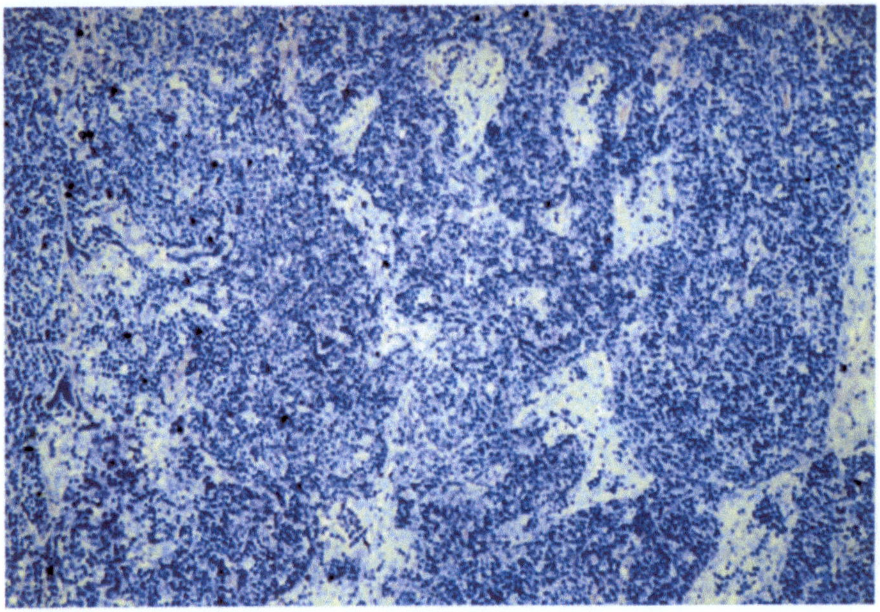

Fig. 4.19. Lymphoplasmocytic lymphoma with dilated sinuses and an increased number of mast cells (Giemsa stain)

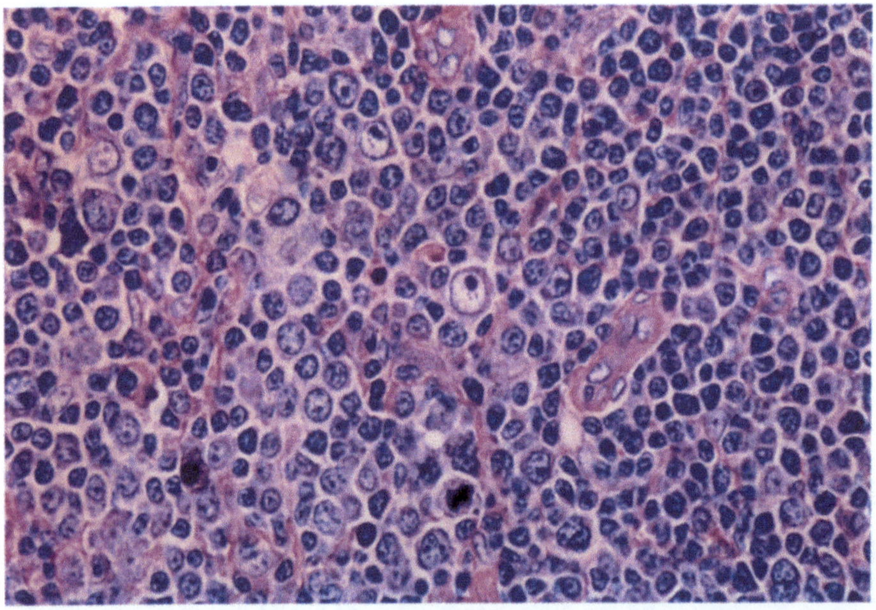

Fig. 4.20. Lymphoplasmocytic lymphoma with an increased number of blasts. Such tumors were described as polymorphic immunocytoma in the old Kiel classification (Giemsa stain)

The numbers of immunoblasts and mitotic figures are low. Proliferation centers like those seen in the pseudofollicular subtype of B-CLL are hardly found in lymphoplasmacytic lymphoma. An increase in the number of mast cells is observed in about two-thirds of the cases. The lymph node sinuses are usually dilated; occasionally they show cavernous dilatation (Fig. 4.19), hemosiderosis is often evident, especially in the sinuses. Other cases show prominent hyperplastic follicles, some cases showed a diffuse effacement of the lymph node structure (Andriko et al. 2001). These two latter types of growth patterns may be associated with an infiltrate of epithelioid cells which then may mimic a lymphoepithelioid T-cell lymphoma (Lennert's lymphoma).

In the past, we have classified lymphomas with higher numbers of immunoblasts as the *polymorphic*

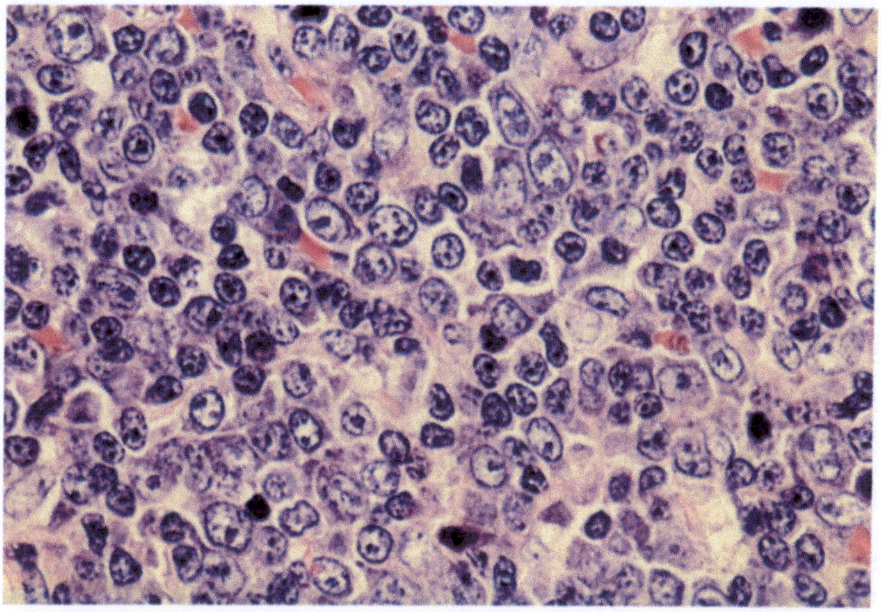

Fig. 4.21. Lymphoplasmocytic lymphoma with transformation into a diffuse large-B-cell lymphoma. These tumors were previously described as polymorphic immunocytomas (compare Fig. 4.20) (Giemsa stain)

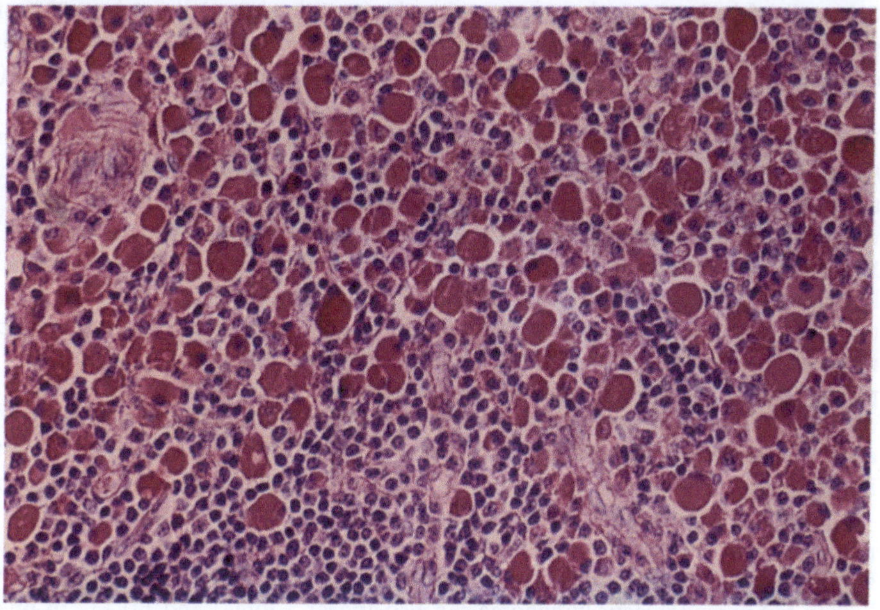

Fig. 4.22. Lymphoplasmocytic lymphoma with PAS-positive globules in the cytoplasm

subtype of immunocytoma. This category is now considered to be superfluous. When we diagnose a case of immunocytoma of the lymphoplasmacytic type, we can determine whether there is a large number of immunoblasts, which is a sign of a higher proliferation rate (Figs. 4.20, 4.21). By making a diagnosis of this sort, one can avoid the danger of overdiagnosing immunocytoma of the polymorphic type. Over the years, the polymorphic immunocytoma category has become a collection box for many different lesions with a high content of plasma cells and immunoblasts, e.g. immunoblastic lymphoma with plasmacytic differentiation, immunocytoma transforming into immunoblastic lymphoma, T-cell lymphomas with a high content of plasma cells, Hodgkin's lymphoma, and infectious mononucleosis. By avoiding the term "polymorphic immunocytoma" it is possible to classify a case of immunocytoma with a high content of blast cells within either the lymphoplasmacytoid category or the lymphoplasmacytic category, which are evidently different in nature.

Similar to lymphoplasmacytoid immunocytoma, one of the most valuable histological feature is the presence of globular PAS-positive inclusions (Dutcher bodies) in the *nucleus* of lymphoplasmacytoid cells and plasma cells (Fig. 4.22). PAS-positive inclusions in the cytoplasm are not as significant, because they also occur in B-CLL. Intranuclear PAS-positive inclusions are found in only one-quarter of cases. Besides globular inclusions, crystalline deposits are rarely seen in plasma cells, whereas diffuse PAS positivity is found more often. Paraproteins are rarely seen in the form of amorphous masses between the tumor cells. In such cases one sometimes finds foreign-body giant cells attempting to remove the deposits. The paraproteins seldom induce amyloidosis (Newland et al. 1986; usually λ subtype). Giant cells of the Reed-Sternberg type are found in occasional cases, especially when there is a high content of epithelioid cells.

Transformation to Diffuse Large-B-Cell Lymphoma /Borderline Cases. The borderline between immunocytoma and *immunoblastic lymphoma* is not distinct when the number of immunoblasts is very high (see Fig. 4.21). When may one speak of an immunoblastic lymphoma, and when is the neoplasm still immunocytoma? The presence of *large accumulations* of immunoblasts is an indication of a diffuse large-B-cell lymphoma (DLBCL) (mostly immunoblastic) (transformation). A high content of lymphocytes evenly spread about the section is inconsistent with a diagnosis of immunoblastic lymphoma.

About 4–15% of immunocytomas show transformation into a DLBCL (Papamichael et al. 1999). In some instances, this may already be evident in the first biopsy, but immunoblastic lymphoma can also appear after immunocytoma has existed for a variable period of time. When immunoblastic lymphoma has developed, one finds a "pure" proliferation of immunoblasts, replacing part, or all, of the immunocytoma.

A high content of diffusely distributed B-lymphocytes within a diffuse large-B-cell lymphoma-immunoblastic may be an indication of a secondary nature of the large-cell lymphoma having developed from an immunocytoma. Secondary development of centroblastic lymphoma is rarely observed.

Immunocytoma often develops in patients with autoimmune diseases, especially Sjögren's syndrome. Today, most of these cases are regarded as marginal zone B-cell lymphomas with a plasmacytic component.

Immunohistochemistry

The lymphocytes express monoclonal sIg. The plasmacytoid cells and the plasma cells must show a monoclonal cytoplasmic Ig expression. The tumor cells express CD20. In contrast to B-CLL/SLL and lymphoplasmacytoid immunocytoma, lymphoplasmacytic lymphoma is almost always negative for CD5 and CD23. Exceptions have been observed. Similar to lymphoplasmacytoid immunocytoma the proportion of proliferating cells (Ki-67+) is, on the average, somewhat larger than in B-CLL. A diffuse admixture of T-cells (both CD4-positive and CD8-positive) is a regular finding in immunocytoma. Remnants of FDC are found with or without germinal center cells in about 50% of the cases of lymphoplasmacytic lymphoma, whereas they are rarely seen in the lymphoplasmacytoid subtype (similar to B-CLL). The presence of FDC and complete, polytypic germinal centers is reminiscent of findings in marginal zone B-cell lymphoma (see Chap. 4.2.1.5).

Genetic Features

A translocation t(9;14) and rearranged Pax5 have been reported in about 30–50% of the cases. The translocation may lead to aberrant protein expression (Iida et al. 1996; Ohno et al. 2000).

Diagnosis and Differential Diagnosis

The diagnosis is based on the demonstration of monoclonal plasma cells among the *predominating* small lymphocytes.

The most frequent problem is the distinction between lymphoplasmacytic lymphoma (immunocytoma) and B-CLL. In one-quarter of such cases it is possible to make this distinction by looking at the PAS reaction: PAS-positive nuclear inclusions in the lymphoplasmacytoid cells or plasma cells are an indication of immunocytoma. In the remainder, the immunohistochemical detection of monoclonal plasma cells is decisive. Moreover, lymphoplasmacytic lymphoma is negative for CD5 and CD23. Other histological or cytological criteria are of limited value and should be supplemented with one of the two reliable criteria.

Some cases of immunocytoma with a perifollicular growth have to be differentiated from *nodal marginal zone B-cell lymphoma*. The cytology of the latter entity is different, with monocytoid and or centrocyte-like cells; however, also such tumors may exhibit a marked plasmacytic differentiation (see below).

Other diseases to be considered in the differential diagnosis of immunocytoma have been described in the section on B-CLL (see Chap. 4.2.1.1).

Lymphomas with Plasmacytic/Plasmacytoid Differentiation. A number of so-called small-B-cell lymphomas may be accompanied by a marked plasmacytic differentiation, e.g. nodal marginal zone B-cell lymphoma, follicular lymphoma grades I and II, and mantle cell lymphoma.

Occurrence

When lymph node biopsies are often performed in cases of B-CLL, as is true in Germany, the number of reported cases of immunocytoma is also higher. In Europe, about 12% of NHL are immunocytomas. In the United States, immunocytoma appears to be less common (approx. 5% of the NHL), but this may be due to differences in the definition.

The age distribution of immunocytoma is approximately the same as that of B-CLL, except for the occasional case of immunocytoma in childhood. The youngest patient in the Kiel collection was 13 years old. The male-to-female ratio is about 1.1:1.

Clinical Presentation and Prognosis

In most patients, lymphadenopathy develops slowly and affects many regions. The blood serum of at least one-third of patients shows a monoclonal increase in the Ig level, usually IgM, sometimes IgG, rarely IgA or IgE. A few tumors exhibit light-chains or heavy-chains alone. About 60% of patients have lymphocytosis ($>4\times10^9$ lymphocytes/l), which looks very much like B-CLL, but is sometimes striking owing to the presence of basophilic lymphoplasmacytoid cells. Coombs-positive hemolytic anemia was reported in 13.5% of patients (Heinz et al. 1979), whereas it is rarely, if at all, seen in patients with B-CLL.

On the whole, the overall survival rate is somewhat lower than that of B-CLL. A study done by the Kiel Lymphoma Study Group (Heinz et al. 1979) did not reveal any significant differences between the two subtypes. According to Kimby and Mellstedt (1991), the prognosis for immunocytoma patients without a leukemic blood picture is more favorable than the prognosis for those with a leukemic immunocytoma.

4.2.1.3 Hairy Cell Leukemia (ICD-O: 9940/3)

Synonyms

- Kiel: Hairy cell leukemia
- REAL: Hairy cell leukemia
- WHO: Hairy cell leukemia

Definition

Hairy cell leukemia (HCL) is a neoplasm of small lymphoid cells that often reveal hair-like surface projections in blood smears (especially in unfixed slides), thus the term "hairy cells". While they are a special type of B-lymphocyte, an equivalent cell has not yet been found in normal or reactive lymphoid tissue.

Morphology

The primary infiltration of lymph nodes by HCL is very rare. There is a slight increase in lymph node infiltrates over the time of the disease. Abdominal lymphadenopathy is reported in up to 20–30% of patients, again depending on the duration of the disease (Mercieca et al. 1994). HCL primarily infiltrates spleen and bone marrow (see Chaps. 6.10.11 and 9.3.1.7).

Lymph nodes show infiltration by monomorphic lymphocytoid cells that are somewhat larger than lymphocytes (Figs. 4.23, 4.24). The nuclei of the tumor cells are somewhat irregular and often reniform; they lie farther apart from each other than do the nuclei of CLL cells and thus have a somewhat clear cell appearance. Blast cells or mitotic figures are not seen in HCL. The infiltration begins in B-regions and connective tissue, with cells infiltrating the trabeculae. A marginal zone pattern of the infiltrate can be observed (Piris et al. 1998). The sinuses are dilated and filled with erythrocytes (Fig. 4.25).

The hair-like projections of "hairy cells" can be recognized most easily with acid-phosphatase staining. Hairy cells show a granular acid-phosphatase reaction which is tartrate-resistant in a variable number of cells in almost all cases.

In blood smears, a hairy cell variant can be recognized in that the cells have more prominent vesicular nucleoli and a more basophilic cytoplasm, thus resembling somewhat B-PLL (see Chap. 6.10.11). Tartrate-resistant acid-phosphatase staining can be helpful.

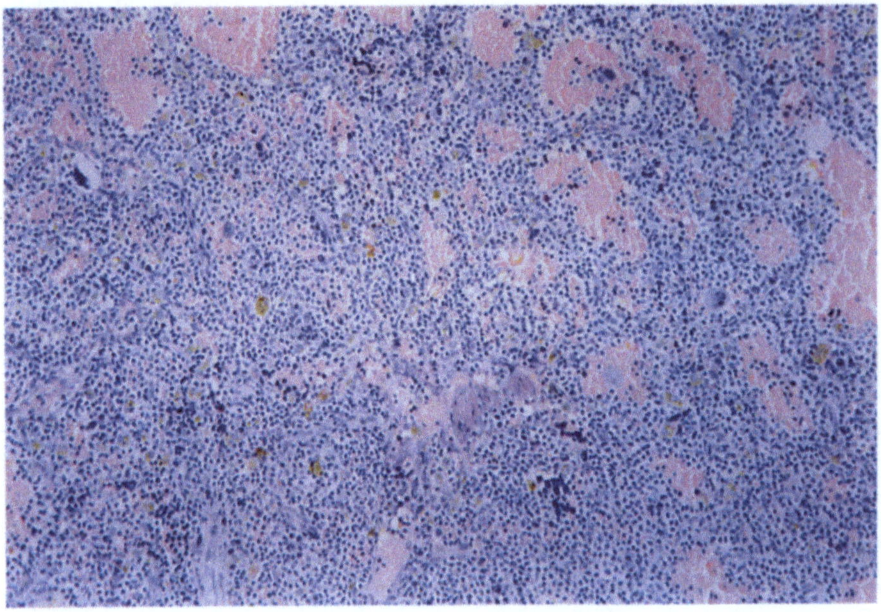

Fig. 4.23. Diffuse lymph node infiltrate by hairy cell leukemia (Giemsa stain)

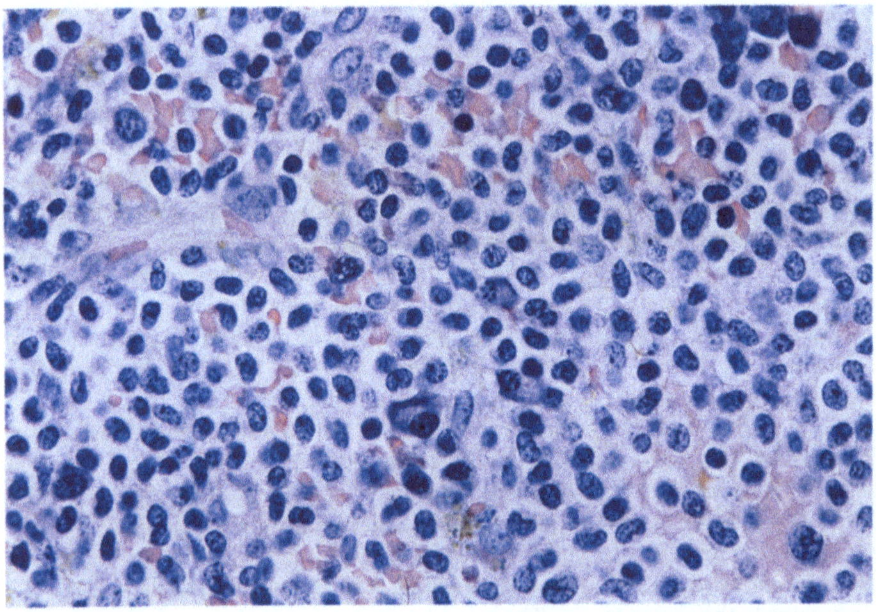

Fig. 4.24. Lymph node infiltrate of a hairy cell leukemia. The infiltrate appears monotonous, featuring cells with small nuclei and a light zone (cytoplasm) surrounding the nuclei resulting in a clear-cell-like appearance (Giemsa stain)

Individual cases with a blastic transformation have been described (Nazeer et al. 1997).

Immunohistochemistry

Hairy cells always express sIg as well as CD20. A special feature of hairy cells is their expression of CD103 (also staining intraepithelial T-lymphocytes) as well as myelomonocytic antigen CD11c and CD25 (Robbins et al. 1993). Some 5–20% of HCL are reported to express CD23, CD10 and on rare occasions CD5 (Aljurf et al. 1994; Dunphy et al. 1999; Miranda et al. 2000; Usha et al. 2000). Recently, it has been described that about 60% of the tumors coexpress cyclin-D1.The number of Ki-67-positive cells is smaller (<5%) than in all other types of malignant lymphoma (ML).

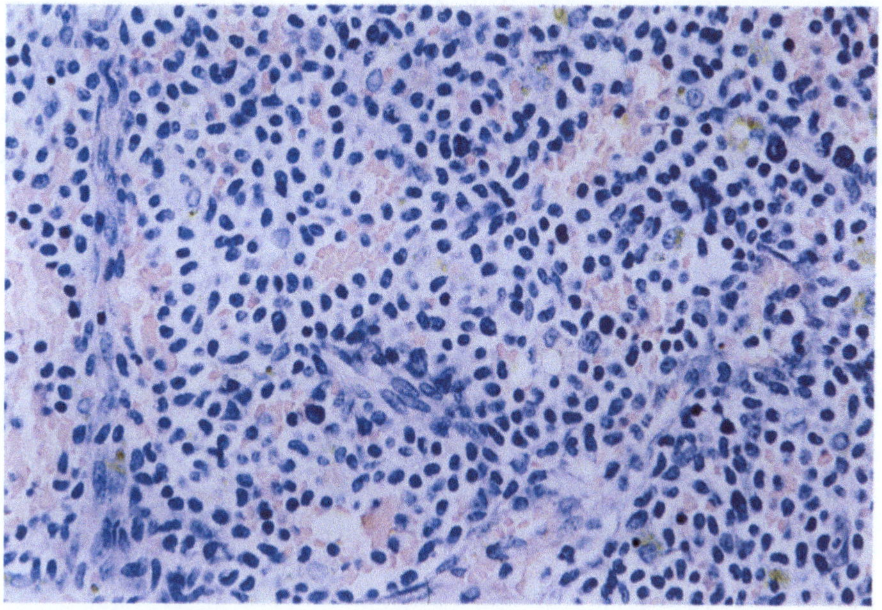

Fig. 4.25 Lymph node infiltrate of a hairy cell leukemia. Note the dilated sinuses filled with erythrocytes (Giemsa stain)

Occurrence

See the chapter on the spleen (Chap. 6.10.11).

Clinical Presentation and Prognosis

HCL is a markedly chronic disease. The paramount signs are splenomegaly and pancytopenia. Lymphadenopathy does not appear until late in the course of the disease and is not pronounced. In the bone marrow there is a massive increase in the number of fibers and infiltration by small lymphoid cells; the latter eventually replacing the whole of the normal marrow. Substantial enlargement of mediastinal and retroperitoneal lymph nodes has been reported (Vardiman and Golomb 1984; Malik et al. 1989). The peripheral blood

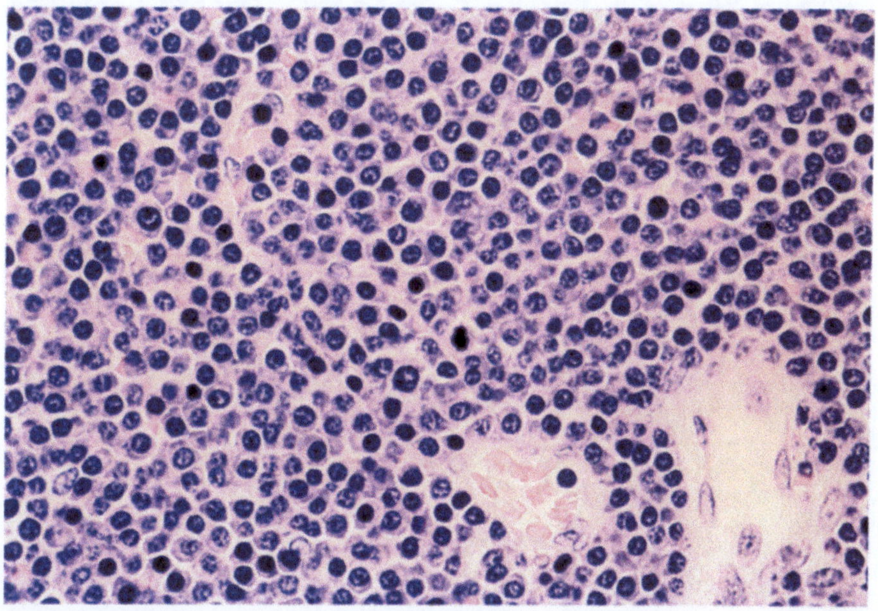

Fig. 4.26. Lymph node infiltrate of a primary nodal plasmacytoma with mostly mature, only slightly polymorphic plasma cells

contains a small to moderate number of hairy cells. There is a relatively high incidence of infections with *Mycobacterium kansasii* (Rice et al. 1982) and of secondary malignant tumors (Jacobs et al. 1985) in patients with HCL (Kampmeier et al. 1994).

4.2.1.4
Plasmacytoma (ICD-O: 9734/3)

Synonyms
- Kiel: Plasmacytic lymphoma (plasmacytoma)
- REAL: Plasmacytoma/plasma cell myeloma
- WHO: Plasmacytoma

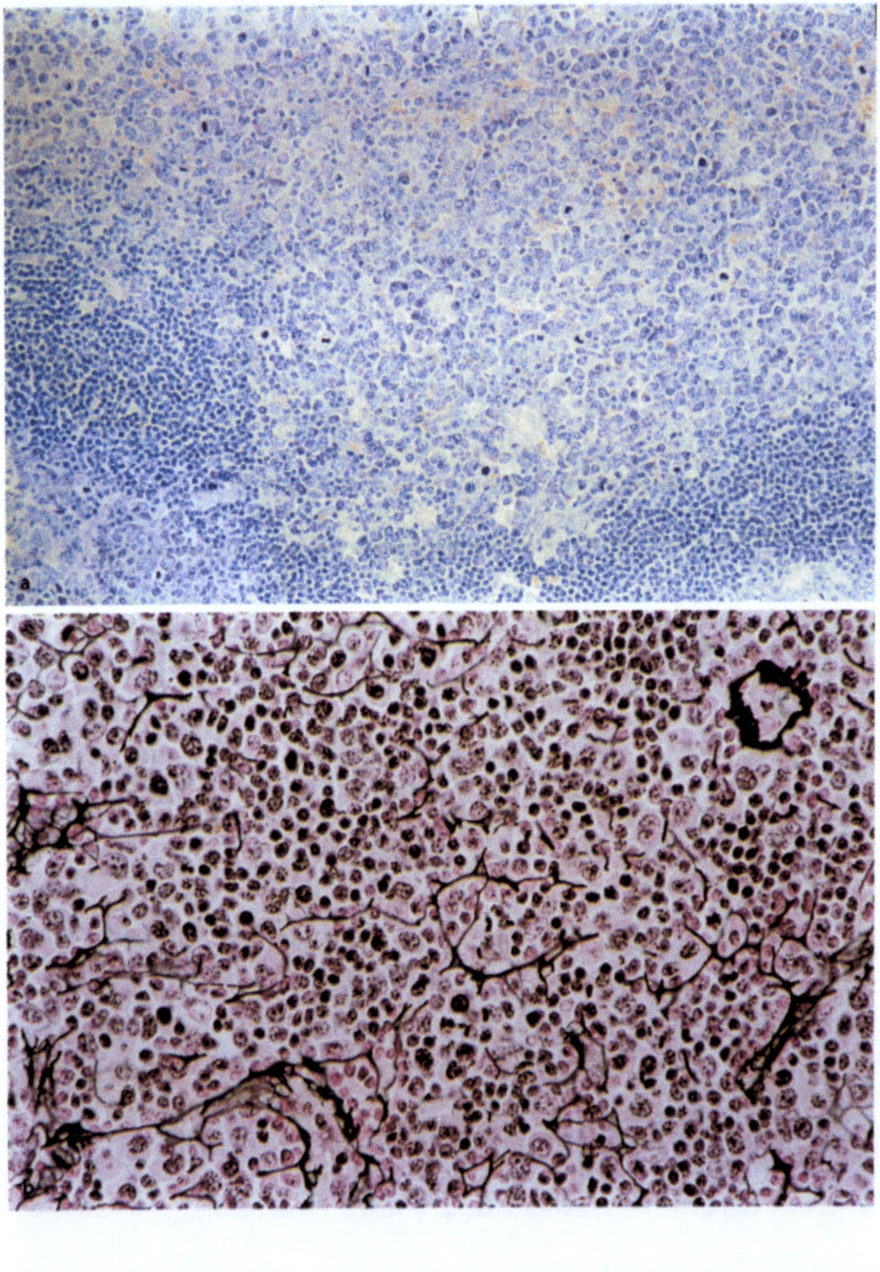

Fig. 4.27a,b. Nodal plasmacytoma (**a**) with interfollicular spreading of neoplastic plasma cells in Giemsa stain. (**b**) Alveolar-like pattern of argyrophilic fibers (Gomori stain)

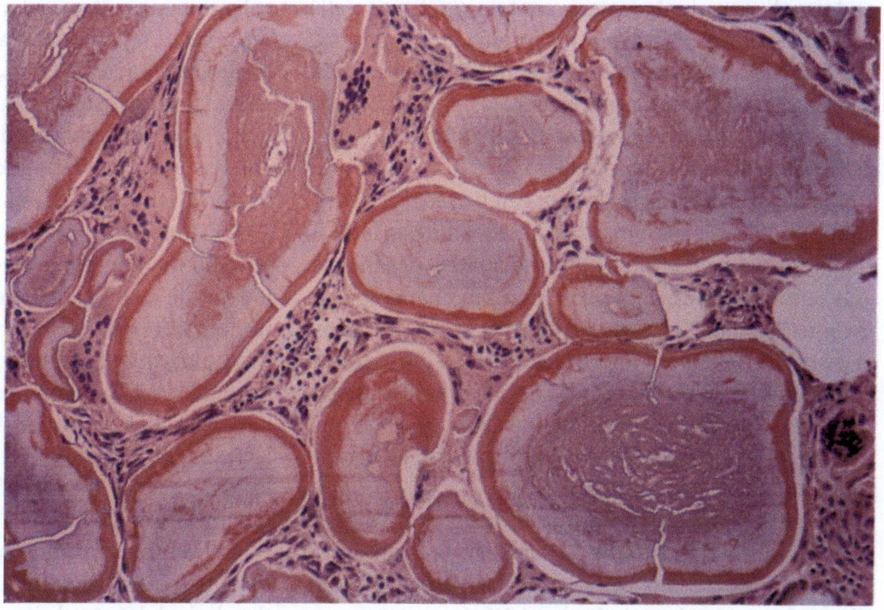

Fig. 4.28. Lymph node plasmocytoma with marked amyloidosis (H and E stain)

In this group we include only the "extramedullary" plasmacytomas, i.e. those that develop primarily in lymphoid tissue (lymph nodes and tonsils; Wiltshaw 1971).

The tumor consists exclusively of well-differentiated ("reticular") plasma cells (Figs. 4.26). Immunoblasts, plasmablasts, and lymphocytes are rare. The reticulin fibers are thick and produce an alveolar pattern (Fig. 4.27a, b). Occasionally, amyloid deposits can be demonstrated in the tumor tissue or vessel walls (Fig. 4.28). Pseudo-angiomatous structures are occasionally evident . In such cases bleeding into the tumor causes the formation of vessel-like lacunae that are not lined with endothelial cells.

The immunophenotype is given in detail in Chap. 6.14.1.3..

Histologically, the main characteristics of lymph node plasmacytoma are the "monotony" and predominance of small cells. Although the plasma cells may show a certain degree of pleomorphism, with giant or multinucleate forms, there are no large basophilic cells with large nucleoli. The nuclear structure of the giant cells is the same as that of the mature plasma cells. This uniformity distinguishes plasmacytoma from most cases of *reactive plasmacytosis*, in which one can recognize all maturational stages of plasmacytopoiesis (immunoblasts, plasmablasts, proplasmacytes, and plasma cells).

Compared to lymph node metastasis of *myeloma*, primary lymph node plasmacytoma usually consists of smaller cells and shows a higher degree of differentiation. One of the reasons for this difference is probably that myeloma usually spreads to lymph nodes late in the course of the disease and after the cells have become anaplastic. The infiltrate is mostly interfollicular (Fig. 4.27a).

In contrast, *plasma cell leukemia* shows a small-cell picture like that of lymph node plasmacytoma (Isobe et al. 1979), but there is a greater tendency to infiltration of the capsule and surrounding tissue in plasma cell leukemia. It should not be difficult to diagnose plasma cell leukemia, however, because of the obvious changes in the blood picture.

In contrast to *immunocytoma*, plasmacytoma does not contain lymphocytes. When we find a small-B-cell component in a tumor otherwise composed of plasma cells, we diagnose immunocytoma or marginal zone B-cell lymphoma with marked plasmacellular differentiation, even if the lymphocytes are confined to small areas.

Angiofollicular Hyperplasia (Castleman's Disease) with a high content of plasma cells. This condition may simulate plasmacytoma, especially when the plasma cells are monotypic. Histologically, the follicles exhibit regressive changes, with perivascular hyaline deposits and small germinal centers containing fewer cells; these are not features of plasmacytoma. Some patients show generalized lymphadenopathy ("multicentric angiofollicular lymph node hyperplasia"; Leibetseder and Thurner 1973; Diebold et al. 1980; Frizzera et al. 1983; Weisenburger et al. 1985).

A similar histological picture can be seen in a clinicopathological syndrome that has been described in the literature as POEMS (polyneuropathy, organomegaly, endocrinopathy, M proteins, skin changes) syndrome (Takatsuki et al. 1976; Gaba et al. 1978; Kojima et al. 1983; Takatsuki and Sanada 1983). This condition is characterized by polyneuropathic and endocrinological symptoms and a usually monoclonal increase in plasma cells in lymph nodes and bone marrow.

Primary lymph node plasmacytoma is a rare disease (<0.6% of the NHLs in the Kiel collection from 1988). Most patients are between the ages of 30 and 70 years. The male-to-female ratio is about 2.6:1.

Clinically involved lymph nodes are mostly cervical; axillary lymph nodes are also involved quite often, whereas lymph nodes in other regions are rarely affected. In general, paraproteinemia is not found in early stages (because of the low tumor cell mass). The possibility of myeloma has to be excluded.

Lymph node plasmacytoma shows a much more favorable prognosis than does myeloma, because it is generally recognized at an earlier stage and the tumor can often be completely removed by surgery.

4.2.1.5
Nodal Marginal Zone B-Cell Lymphoma (ICD-O: 9699/3)

In 1958 and 1961, Lennert described a "benign immature sinus histiocytosis and monocytoid cells". From 1982 to 1984, the cells were primarily considered to be histiocytes and were then finally identified as a special variant of B-cells. The reactive lesion was thus called monocytoid B-cell reaction. Lennert and coworkers observed "monocytoid B-cells" in myoepithelial sialadenitis and especially in the immunocytoma that may subsequently develop in the salivary gland. Schmid et al. 1982; Sheibani et al. 1988; Cousar et al. 1987; Piris et al. 1988; Ng and Chan 1987 described a number of cases of lymphoma that they considered to be derived from monocytoid B-cells. During 1990 and 1992, the relation between marginal zone B-cell lymphoma (MZBCL)and MALT lymphomas, on the one hand, and MZBCL and splenic marginal zone lymphomas, on the other, was recognized (Nathwani et al. 1992).

Between 1982 and 1992, 28 cases of B-cell lymphoma in lymph nodes in which a considerable portion of the lymphoma was composed of large collections of small and medium-sized monocytoid B-cells were observed by the Kiel group (Cogliatti et al. 1990; Nizze et al. 1991). Nine of the patients also showed an extranodal lymphoma of similar histology that was diagnosed as low-grade malignant B-cell lymphoma of MALT; the tumors were located in the stomach (four patients), salivary gland (two patients), thyroid gland (one patient), nasopharynx (one patient) and hypopharynx (one patient). These extranodal tumors contained large collections of monocytoid B-cells in addition to the lesions that are typical of low-grade malignant B-cell lymphoma of MALT.

Although nodal and extranodal MZBCL share many morphological and immunophenotypic similarities, the clinical data made it reasonable to establish two different categories.

Synonyms

- Kiel: Monocytoid B-cell lymphoma
- REAL: Marginal zone B-cell lymphoma
- WHO: Nodal marginal zone B-cell lymphoma

Definition

This indolent small-B-cell lymphoma originates from the nodal marginal zone or sinusoidal B-cells. It mainly spreads within confluent sinuses and only rarely shows a perifollicular (naked follicles) or marginal zone growth pattern. The cells are mostly small or medium-sized with abundant cytoplasm. A secondary lymph node involvement by an extranodal marginal zone or MALT lymphoma has to be excluded.

The monocytoid B-cell reaction represents the normal counterpart of this lymphoma.

Morphology

In most cases, monocytoid B-cell lymphoma can be suspected at a low magnification. One sees compact, sharply demarcated plaques or less sharply delineated, peritrabecular and subcapsular collections of medium-sized cells that look relatively pale. The infiltrations are located in the sinuses or around, chiefly the intermediate and marginal ones (Figs. 4.29a, b, 4.30, 4.31). In-between, numerous or few follicles or naked germinal centers are visible in more than 80% of the cases.

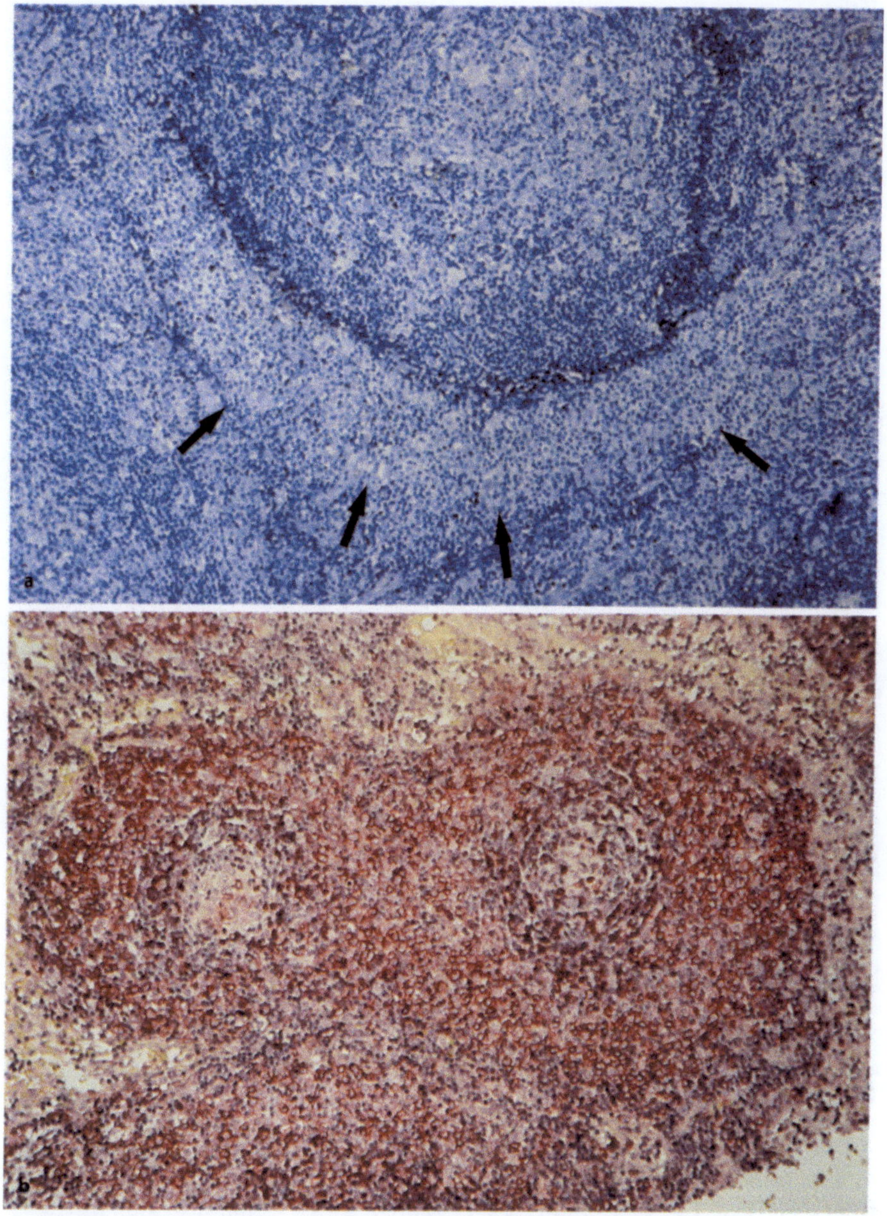

Fig. 4.29. a Primary nodal marginal zone lymphoma with a perifollicular infiltrate (Giemsa stain). **b** Immunohistochemical staining of KiB3 (CD45RA) with detection of the perifollicular infiltrate of a nodal marginal zone B-cell lymphoma. In the center, positively stained remnants of follicles are seen (alkaline phosphatase stain)

The tumor cells stand out clearly against the other lymph node structures, whose cells have darker nuclei (Fig. 4.32a, b). The nuclei of the pale cells lie relatively far apart from one another, which indicates that the cytoplasm is relatively abundant. The monocytoid B-cells have medium-sized, round or occasionally somewhat indented or cleaved nuclei with moderately coarse chromatin and small, usually solitary nucleoli. Sometimes the nuclei are more irregular than those of reactive monocytoid B-cells. The cytoplasm is abundant and stains gray with Giemsa (Fig. 4.33). With CD20 staining it looks cohesive. In some of the cases typical large (cIg+) immunoblasts are interspersed among the monocytoid B-cells. Small numbers of neutrophil granulocytes are often found. Mitotic figures are quite numerous.

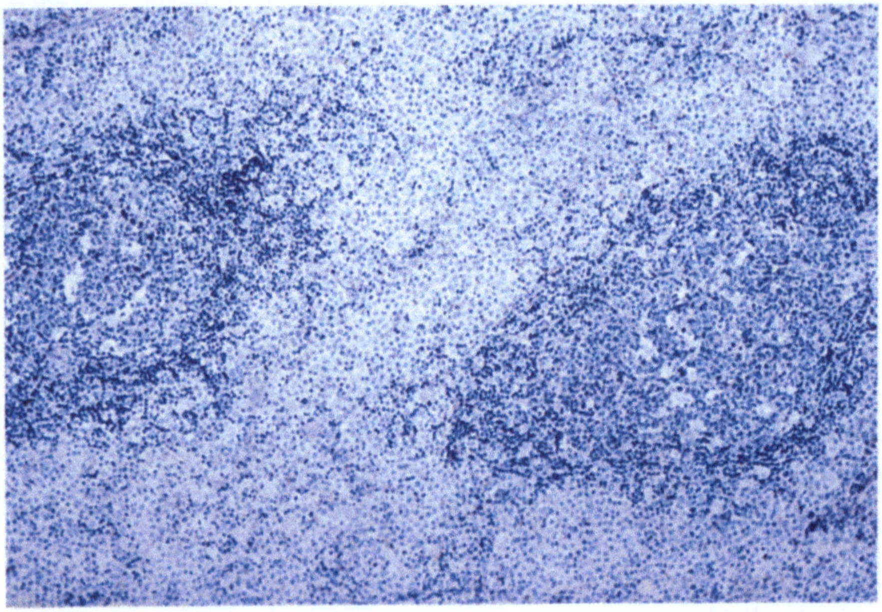

Fig. 4.30. A peri- and interfollicular infiltrate of quite monotoneous looking monocytoid B-cells in a primary nodal marginal zone B-cell lymphoma (Giemsa stain)

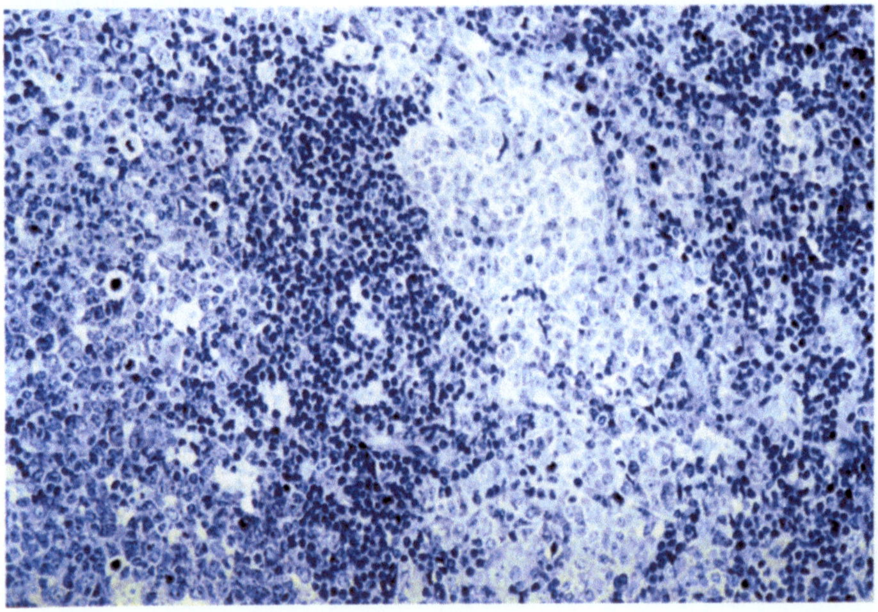

Fig. 4.31. Intrasinusoidal infiltrate of a nodal marginal zone B-cell lymphoma that is well demarcated from the follicular mantle (Giemsa stain)

The monocytoid B-cells can be readily recognized in imprints (Fig. 4.32b). They are medium-sized, and their (bean-shaped) nuclei resemble those of monocytes in shape more often than they do in sections. The chromatin is darker than that of monocytes. Nucleoli usually cannot be recognized. The cytoplasm is a rich grayish blue, and sometimes it was highly vacuolated (on electron microscopy the vacuoles proved to be fat). The PAS reaction is often finely or coarsely granular; sometimes it is diffusely positive (glycogen).

Remnants of lymphoid tissue (pulp) are not always recognizable between the follicular structures and the collections of monocytoid B-cells. Usually, large areas are infiltrated by somewhat larger (B) lymphocytes and

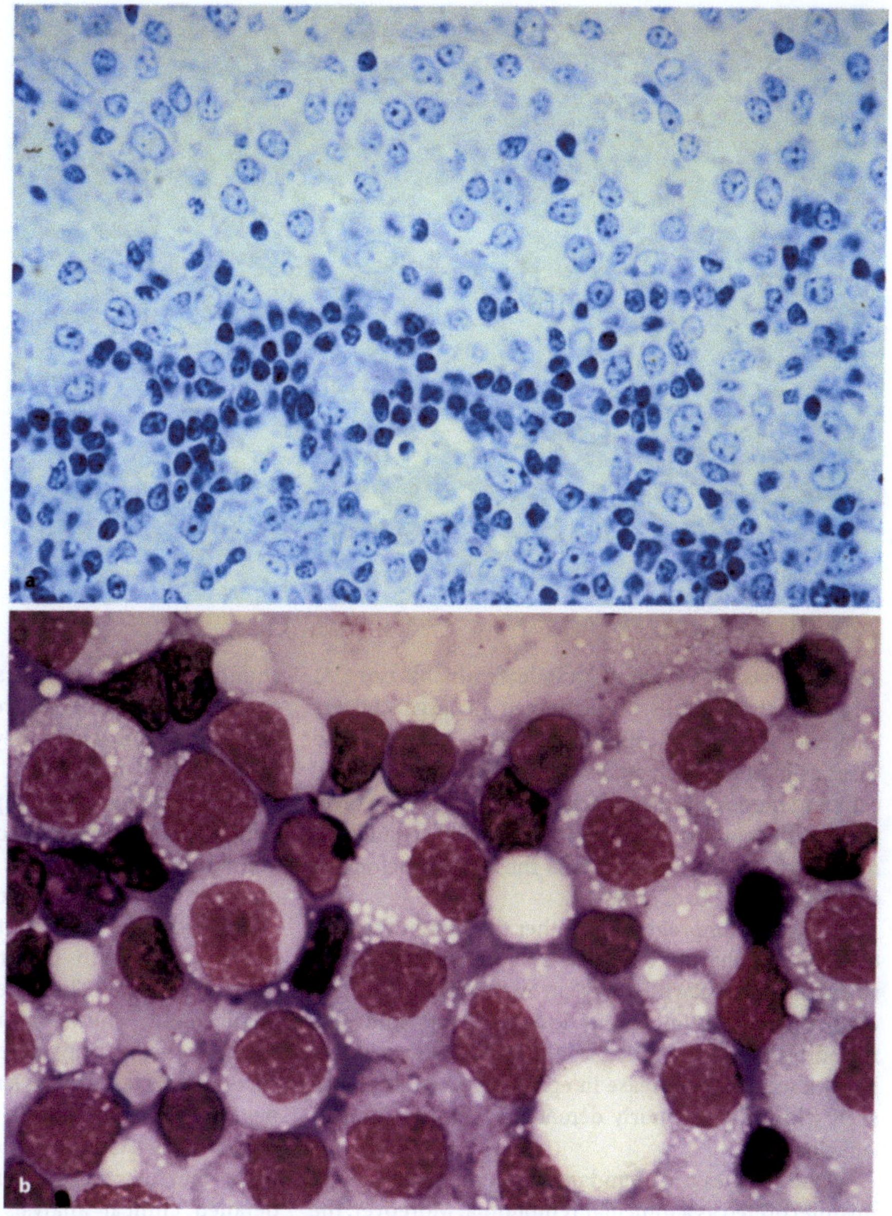

Fig. 4.32. High-power view of infiltrate in Fig. 4.31. The cells have medium sized nuclei and inconspicuous nucleoli. The cytoplasm is not clearly demarcated and stains lightly. **a** Giemsa stain, **b** Pappenheim stain. Touch imprint of a nodal marginal zone B-cell lymphoma. The cells have a broad vacuolated cytoplasm

a variable number of plasma cells. The latter can be so abundant that one gets the impression of a plasmacytoma, especially as the cells may present as demarcated sheets or clusters (Davis et al. 1992). Occasionally even Russell bodies can be found. In other areas, a more lymphocytic infiltrate like that in immunocytoma can be observed. Some of these areas are circumscribed, others extensive. The sheets are CD5-negative, making a distinction from lymphocytic lymphoma possible (see Differential Diagnosis).

In some cases a considerable number of epithelioid cells can be found thus raising suspicion of an immunocytoma. Careful reading of the slides, however, most often demonstrates some foci of monocytoid B-cells, substantiating the diagnosis of marginal zone B-cell lymphoma. At times the monocytoid B-cells appear to

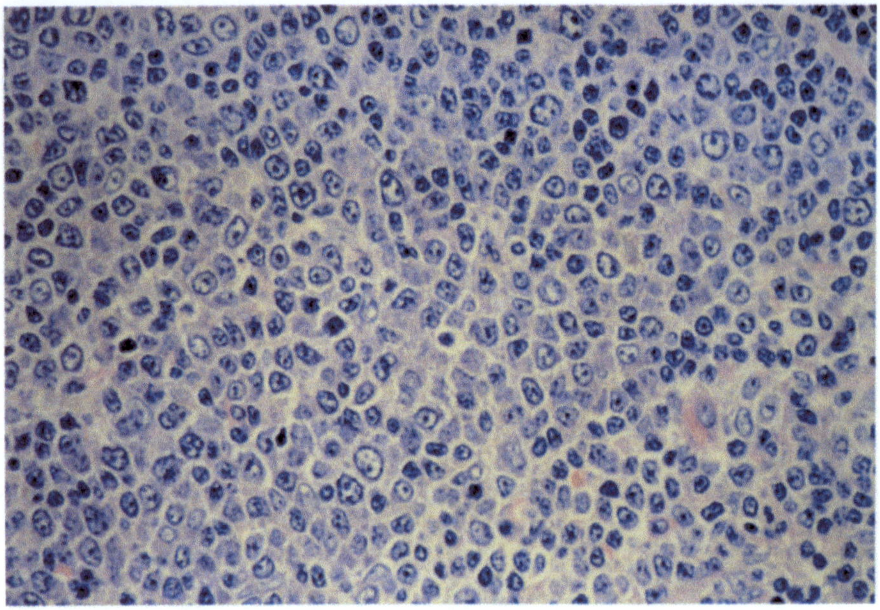

Fig. 4.33. Diffuse infiltrate of a nodal marginal zone B-cell lymphoma; monocytoid B-cells are intermingled with blasts and lymphoplasmacytoid cells (Giemsa stain)

lie in thin-walled vessels of an indeterminable type. At other times, the cells are arranged in large clusters enclosed by a wall of collagenous fibers. In all of these cases as in infiltrates with a high content of epithelioid cells and monocytoid B-cell clusters, there was involvement of the parotid gland by myoepithelial sialadenitis or merely sicca syndrome; thus these cases belong to the group of MZBCL of MALT.

With silver impregnation, either the monocytoid B-cell foci are sharply bounded by a dense network of fibers, or only a few fibers occur with about equal frequency in the monocytoid B-cell clusters and surrounding pulp. A remarkable, and still incomprehensible finding is the increase in epithelioid venules often seen within large, poorly demarcated monocytoid B-cell clusters.

If the follicles are abundant, the lymphoma can be misinterpreted as a follicular lymphoma. Moreover, the reactive follicles are frequently infiltrated (colonized) by neoplastic monocytoid B-cells (see Differential Diagnosis).

In addition to the typical lesion of MZBCL consisting of medium-sized cells that primarily infiltrate the sinuses, we have observed a second variant which we have described as the "small cell variant of monocytoid B-cell lymphoma" (Nizze et al. 1991). It consists of smaller cells that usually show round or only slightly indented (centrocyte-like) nuclei. The cytoplasm is less abundant and also non-basophilic (see Fig. 2c in Nizze et al. 1991). The cells are frequently located in the marginal zone, from where they invade and massively infiltrate the lymphoid tissue (see Fig. 1b in Nizze et al. 1991). A plasmacytic component has not been found. This variant is more frequently associated with an extranodal localization in the MALT system and thus does not belong to the primary nodal MZBCL.

Recently, two different types of nodal MZBCL with respect to growth pattern and immunophenotype were described. The splenic type (without splenic involvement) shows a predominately perifollicular pattern with IgD positivity, whereas the other group shows a perivascular or sinusoidal pattern and is IgD negative. The patients in the first group were diagnosed in early stages I and II. These patients had no bone marrow involvement. In the latter group, a detailed clinical analysis showed that 44% of the patients had an additional extranodal involvement (Campo et al. 1999a).

Evolution and Transformation. Individual cases of transformed nodal MZBCL are described (Fig. 4.34a, b); however, a consensus definition of a transformation does not exist. In the cases we observed, transformation into a diffuse large-cell lymphoma of the B-cell series (polymorphic centroblastic lymphoma in one case, unclassified in the other) took place. The overall

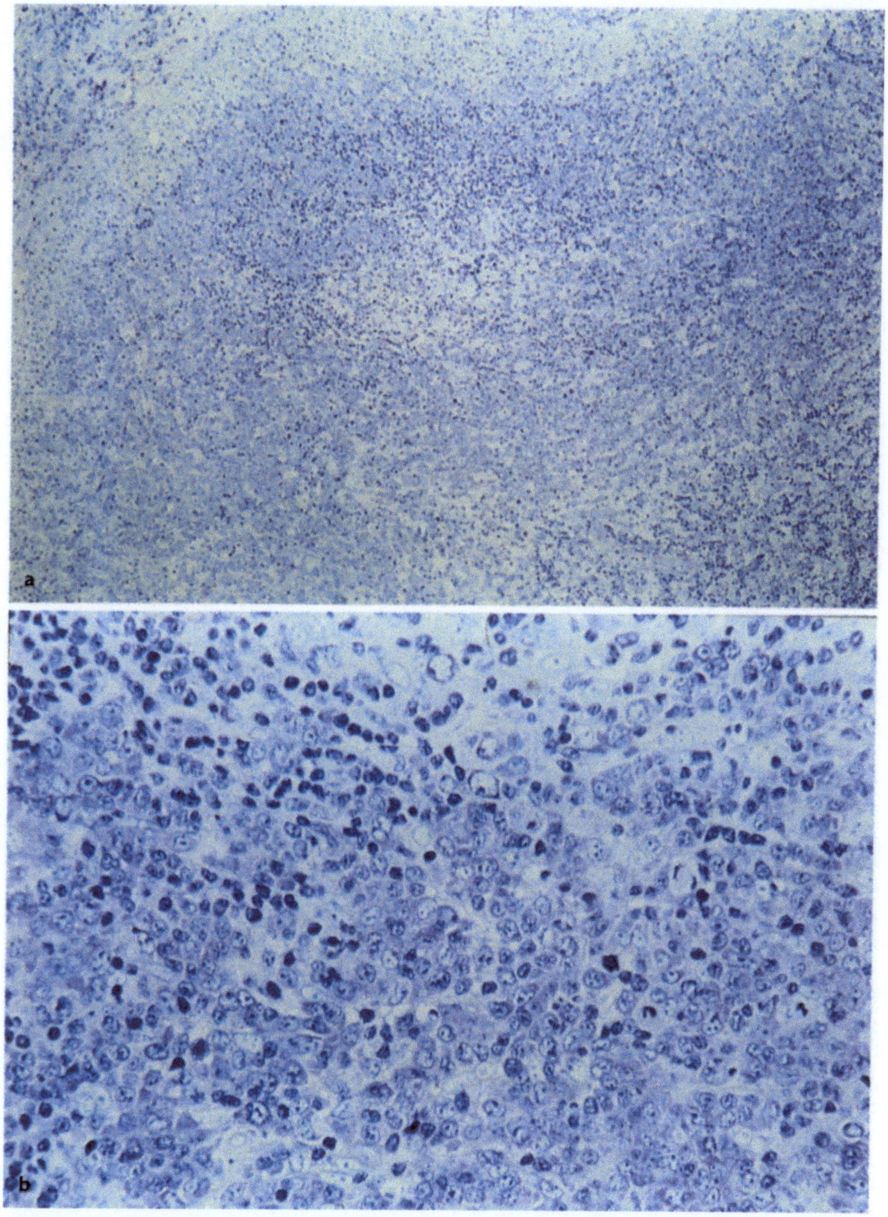

Fig. 4.34 a, b. Blastic variant (diffuse large-B-cell lymphoma) of a marginal zone B-cell lymphoma in Giemsa stain. **a** Low and **b** high-power view

frequency of transformation from the cases studied by the ILSG is 20% (five out of 25).

Finally, we observed individual cases which morphologically fulfilled the criteria of a primary blastic large-cell lymphoma with sinusoidal and perifollicular spreading. We thus think that rare cases of a primary diffuse large B-cell variant of nodal MZBCL do exist.

Immunohistochemistry

cIg can be demonstrated in about half the cases of monocytoid B-cell lymphoma. The tumor cells are interspersed with plasma cells that belong to the same cell clone. IgM is found in two-thirds of the cases, IgG in one-third. A varying number (20–60%) of monocytoid B-cells show monoclonal Ig, chiefly IgM, on their surface. Antigens CD19, CD20, CD22, and Ki-B3 (relat-

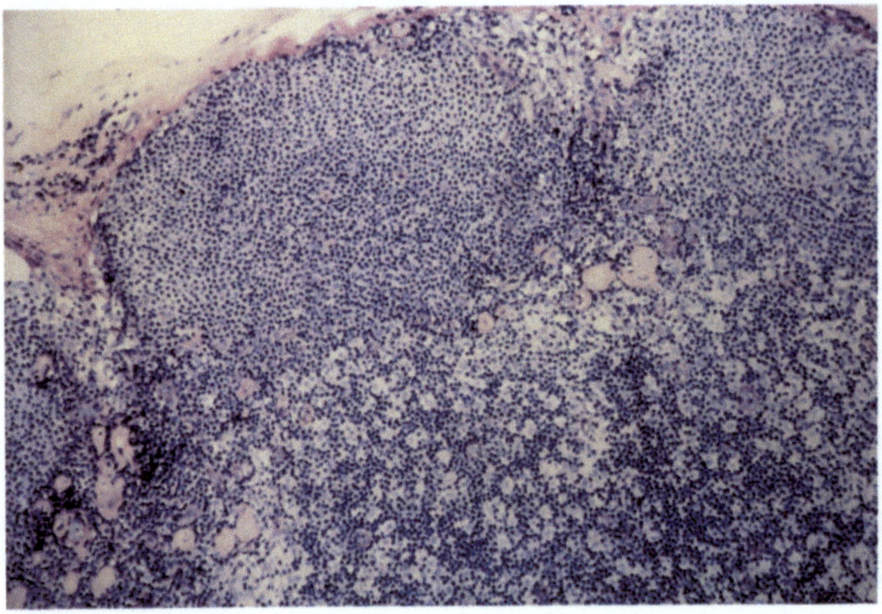

Fig. 4.35. Reactive lymph node with hyperplasia of the marginal zone appearing as an outer rim surrounding the follicle (Giemsa stain)

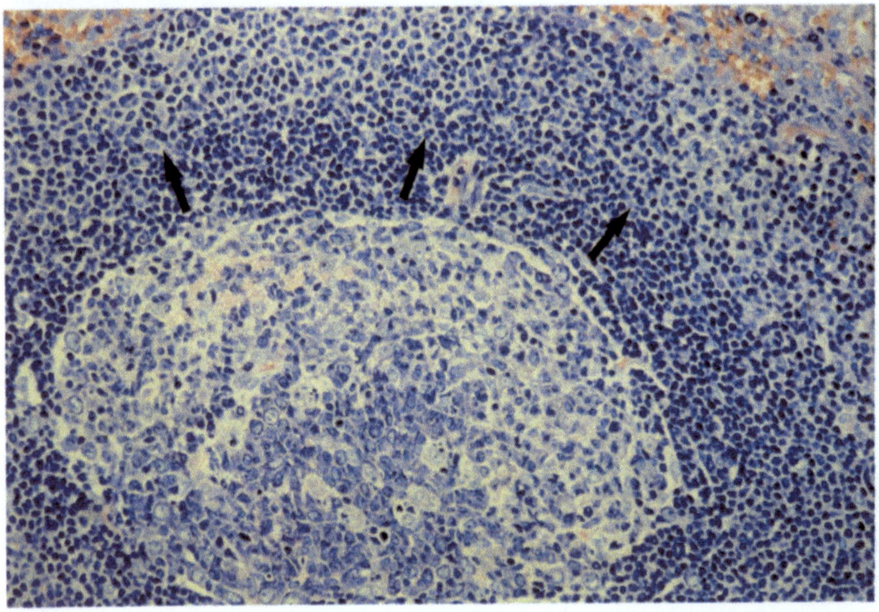

Fig. 4.36. A reactive marginal zone is located above the follicular mantle appearing as a light zone (→) (Giemsa stain)

ed to CD45RA) are expressed constantly and CDw75 (LN1) weakly. The macrophage antibody Ki-M1p (Radzun et al. 1991) has proved to be particularly useful. It can be applied to paraffin sections for identifying both macrophages (strong, diffuse reaction) and monocytoid B-cells (paranuclear granular reactivity). However, positivity is also found in a broad spectrum of other B-cell lymphomas.

CD5, CD10, CD23and CD25 are regularly negative. bcl-2 is expressed weakly in the majority of cases, about 80% (Lai et al. 1998), whereas it is negative on reactive monocytoid B-cells.

The reactive follicles are typically negative for bcl-2. If follicular colonization takes place, however, the follicles become positive for bcl-2 and may thus give the impression of a follicular lymphoma.

Genetic Features

The chromosomal abnormalities for marginal zone B-cell lymphomas of different sites such as nodal, MALT, and splenic are nearly identical and found in about 90% of the cases. Most frequently, a complete or partial trisomy 3 (60%) is detected followed by trisomy 7, 12 and 18 (30–40%) and structural abnormalities in 1q21 or 1q34 (60%) (Dierlamm et al. 1996; Brynes et al. 1996).

The most frequent gains found by comparative genomic hybridization were material from chromosomes 3, 18,X, and 1.

Mutation analysis of the Ig variable regions showed evidence of antigen selection in the sense that marginal zone lymphomas involve clonal expansions of postgerminal center memory cells (Miranda et al. 1999). However, these data are controversial. Other groups found signs for antigen selection only in a small percentage of the different nodal and extranodal marginal zone lymphomas and thus argued for different subsets of marginal zone B-cells from which the differently localized marginal zone B-cell lymphomas arise (Tierens et al. 1998).

Diagnosis and Differential Diagnosis

Diagnosis. The pathologist can often decide in favor of a monocytoid B-cell lymphoma when examining a slide at a low magnification, which reveals that the sinuses are infiltrated by medium-sized cells. These infiltrates stand out clearly against the rest of the lymph node, which shows follicular hyperplasia and usually infiltration of the pulp resembling immunocytoma.

When the tumor infiltration has progressed and the lymph node architecture has been completely effaced, it is difficult to make a diagnosis. The lymphoma types listed below (see Differential Diagnosis) have to be considered.

The *differential diagnosis* comprises the following entities: follicular hyperplasia with monocytoid B-cell reaction, follicular lymphoma with marginal zone differentiation, mantle cell lymphoma, extranodal marginal zone lymphoma, especially of MALT, and small cell lymphocytic lymphoma, especially immunocytoma.

Monocytoid B-cell lymphoma is usually distinguishable from inflammatory lesions showing a pronounced *monocytoid B-cell reaction* combined with marked follicular hyperplasia (toxoplasmosis, infectious mononucleosis, AIDS, purulent inflammation of tissue drained by a node). In such cases immunohistochemistry quickly substantiates the diagnosis, depending on the monoclonality or polyclonality of the sinusoidal B-cells. Moreover, reactive monocytoid B-cells are usually bcl-2-negative whereas the neoplastic counterpart is mostly weakly positive.

A normal marginal zone is hardly seen in reactive lymph nodes. Sometimes it can be observed around primary follicles as a small light zone around the upper part of the follicular mantle. It is mor prominant in mesenteric lymph nodes (Figs. 4.35–4.37).

Follicular lymphoma with marginal zone differentiation is sometimes impossible to distinguish from marginal zone lymphoma with follicular colonization, as the follicles become positive for bcl-2 when colonized. In such cases, a molecular analysis for the detection or exclusion of the translocation t(14;18) – specific for follicular lymphoma – can be decisive.

Mantle cell lymphoma sometimes shows a nodular growth pattern and completely replaces the follicular mantle. The growth pattern is similar to the perifollicular growth around naked germinal centers, such as found in MZBCL. Mantle cell lymphoma does not contain blast cells or plasma cells of the same clone. Immunohistochemical staining for cyclin D1 is helpful for detecting mantle cell lymphoma.

The distinction between nodal and *extranodal marginal zone lymphomas* is clinically important. It has to be kept in mind that it is not possible to distinguish a secondary involvement of a lymph node by an extranodal MZBCL from a primary one by morphology or immunohistochemistry. Thus, it is necessary to include the clinical data into the final diagnosis. It should be especially determined whether there is a Sjögren's syndrome or lymphoma involvement of the MALT system.

Finally, cases of *small lymphocytic lymphoma* – B-CLL or immunocytoma – may show some similarity with monocytoid B-cell lymphoma, especially as in individual cases the lymphocytic component may dominate. Such nodal infiltrates are mostly associated with an extranodal involvement. Moreover, small clusters of monocytoid B-cells must be carefully searched for. The lymphocytic infiltrate in MZBCL is CD5-negative but positive in immunocytoma.

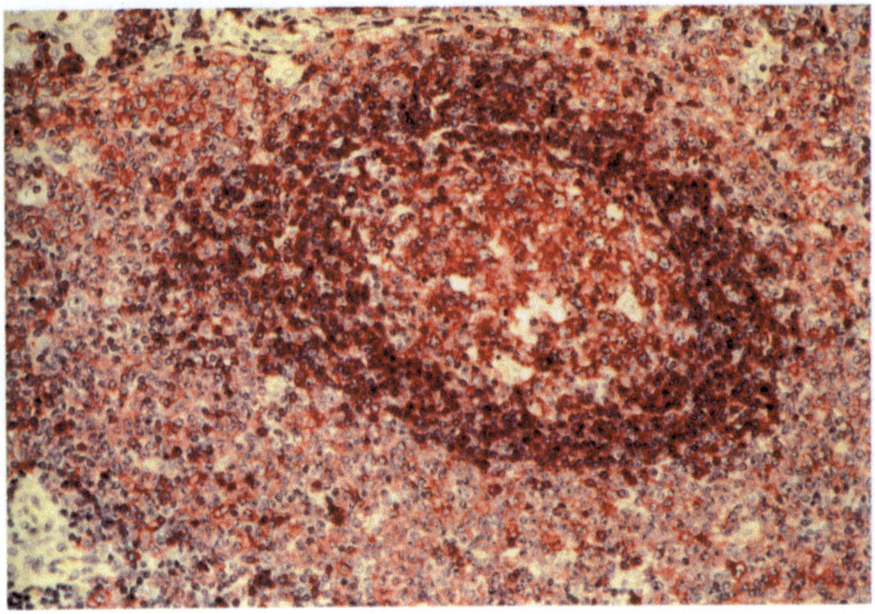

Fig. 4.37. Staining for KiB3 (CD45 RA) with reactive positive marginal zone cells surrounding a reactive follicle (alkaline phosphatase stain)

Occurrence

Monocytoid B-cell lymphoma is rare. In the primary series of the Kiel lymph node registry series it accounted for about 0.2%–0.3% of the NHLs. However, the real frequency seems to be slightly higher as we might have included some immunocytomas, cases in which the monocytoid B-cells made up a smaller percentage. The frequency in the cases studied by the ILSG is 1.8% (25 out of 1,378 cases). The age curve shows a peak around 60 years. The youngest patient was 30 years old, the oldest was 87. The different studies show either a slight female predominance or an equal distribution among both sexes.

Clinical Presentation and Prognosis

Monocytoid B-cell lymphoma of the lymph node chiefly occurs in the cervical lymph nodes (80%). Occasionally, axillary or inguinal nodes are primarily involved. In earlier studies the majority of patients were described as having stage I or stage II disease. However, the new data, clearly separating nodal and extranodal MZBCL (especially associated Sjögren's syndrome), demonstrate that nodal MZBCL mostly presents with an advanced stage III or IV (Mollejo et al. 1994; Nathwani et al. 1992, 1999b). According to the clinical reports, a relatively small percentage of the patients show B symptoms (about 15%). A leukemic blood picture is rare. Other leukemic cases have been described by Carbone et al. (1989) and Traweek et al. (1989). In the blood of one patient, not only were there monocytoid B-cells but also some lymphoplasmacytoid forms were found. In another patient, monoclonal gammopathy (IgG) was documented clinically.

Bone marrow infiltration is found in about 30% of the patients. More than half of the patients have an International Prognostic Index (IPI) score between 0 and 1.

The Kiel group was able to evaluate the clinical course of 18 patients with nodal monocytoid B-cell lymphoma (Cogliatti et al. 1990). Patients in early stages (I and II) were treated mainly with radiotherapy (involved/extended field radiation), patients in later stages (III and IV) mostly with chemotherapy (COP, CHOP, ABVD, Knospe, COP-BLAM). Patients with extranodal primary lymphoma were usually subjected to local postoperative irradiation following resection. Complete remission, lasting from 1–78 months (mean: 28 months), was achieved in 15 patients. Over an average observation period of 34 months (the maximum was more than 6.5 years) six patients remained free of recurrence (30%). In more than half the patients there was a relapse after a mean remission period of 20 months (range: 1–55 months). Five patients (28%) died after 3–54 months (mean: 24 months), in each case from causes related to the lymphoma.

The study of Nathwani et al. (1999b) showed an overall 5-year survival of 56 %, and a 5-year failure-free survival of 28 %. Thus, it is clear that this lymphoma type is only curable at the early stages of disease.

4.2.1.6 Follicular Lymphoma (ICD-O: 9690/3)

Synonyms

- Kiel: Centroblastic-centrocytic and (in part) centroblastic follicular
- REAL: Follicular lymphoma (grade I–III)
- WHO: Follicular lymphoma (grade 1 – 3)

Definition

Follicular lymphomas are neoplasms of germinal centers and thus consist of all their elements, i.e. centroblasts, centrocytes, FDC and macrophages. Centrocytes mostly predominate. The tumors show a follicular, sometimes a follicular and diffuse growth pattern. Exceptional cases are completely diffuse. Depending on the number of blasts, the WHO suggests distinguishing three histological grades:

- Grade 1: 0 – 5 blasts/high-power field
- Grade 2: 6 – 15 blasts/high-power field
- Grade 3: > 15 blasts/high-power field

Grade 3 is subdivided into 3a and 3b (detailed below).

bcl-2 expression is found in almost all grade 1 and 2 lymphomas (centroblastic-centrocytic) and in about 75 % of grade 3 lymphomas. The normal counterpart are germinal center B-cells.

Morphology

Follicular lymphoma is characterized by its cellular composition and its growth pattern.

The WHO classification proposes to use a grading system with grades 1 – 3, subdividing grade 3 into a and b (definition is given below).

About 90 % of the cases belong to follicular lymphoma grades 1 and 2 (grade I and II – REAL, centroblastic-centrocytic – Kiel), only 10 % are follicular (in part) large-cell lymphomas designated as grade 3 (grade III – REAL, in part centroblastic follicular – Kiel). Although follicular lymphoma is characterized by its follicular growth pattern (Fig. 4.38), it may contain diffuse areas (Figs. 4.39, 4.40).

Follicular lymphomas grade 1 (0 – 5 % blasts/high-power field) are most frequently of the purely follicular type (about 50 – 70 %), followed by the follicular and diffuse variant (25 – 40 %) and, finally, the rare diffuse variant (< 5 %). (Molenaar et al. (1984) studied 424 cases in our collection and found only 0.9 % with a diffuse growth pattern!) Besides the growth pattern, the presence of sclerosis should be noted. Sclerosis is seen least often in the purely follicular variant (17 %) and

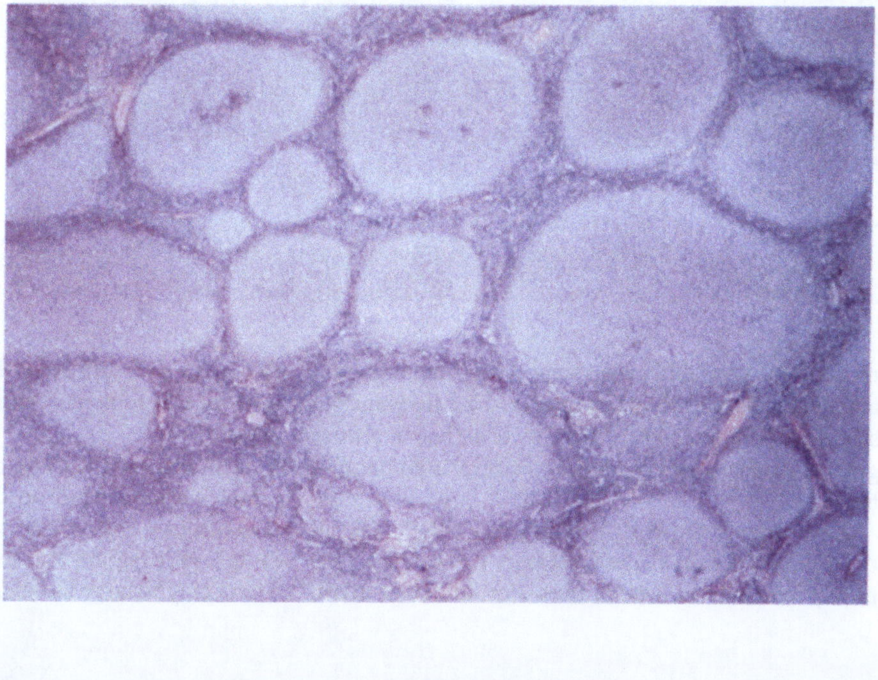

Fig. 4.38. Lymph node section from a follicular lymphoma (Giemsa stain)

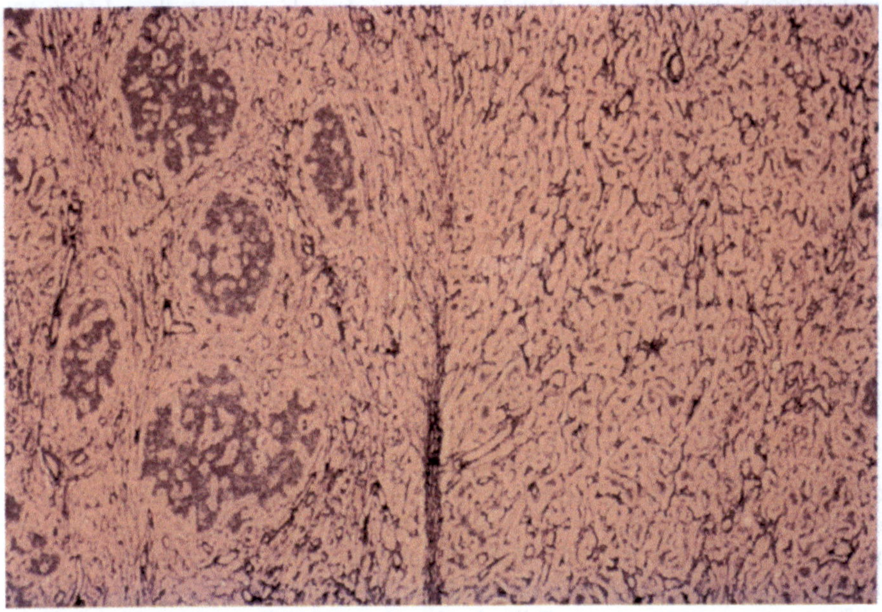

Fig. 4.39. Silver impregnation of a follicular lymphoma. On the *left*, neoplastic follicles can be seen; on the *right*, a diffuse growth pattern is visible

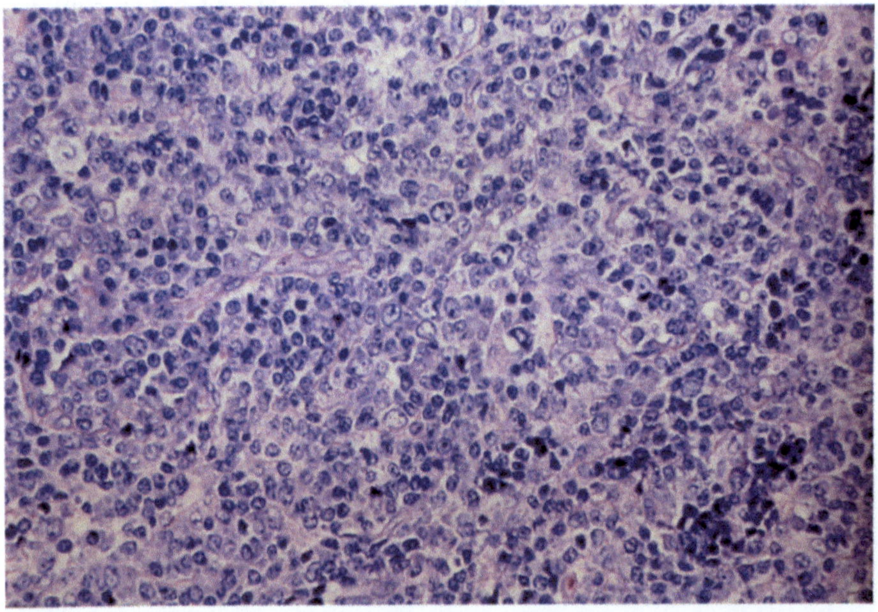

Fig. 4.40. Giemsa staining of a follicular lymphoma with a diffuse growth pattern. Among the centrocytes and lymphocytes, blasts (centroblasts) are dispersed throughout the infiltrate

most often in the diffuse variant (100%); the follicular and diffuse variant shows an intermediate frequency of sclerosis (approx. 65%). This means that a diffuse growth pattern and a tendency to sclerosis go hand in hand.

According to the WHO classification, the extent of the diffuse areas should be described. The lymphoma is purely follicular with more than 75% follicular areas, follicular and diffuse with 25–75% follicular areas, and focally follicular with less than 25% follicular areas.

Sclerosis, which often affects only one side of the lymph node, appears to begin near the capsule and sometimes within it, and to spread first into the outer lymph node regions and surrounding tissue (Fig. 4.41). There may be large bundles of fibers and a pronounced tendency to hyalinization in these regions. If the sclerosis progresses, then large areas of the lymph node may be replaced by hyaline fibrous tissue (this has been called "nodular sclerotic lymphosarcoma" by Bennett and Millett 1969). In such cases the tumor develops a certain resemblance to the nodular sclerosis type of Hodgkin's lymphoma.

Formation of follicles is seen in the lymph node cortex and medulla. The lymph node architecture thus appears to be effaced. Between the neoplastic follicles, however, there are variable-sized T regions containing small lymphocytes, epithelioid venules and some reticulin fibers. These regions occasionally show a large number of plasma cells that are of the

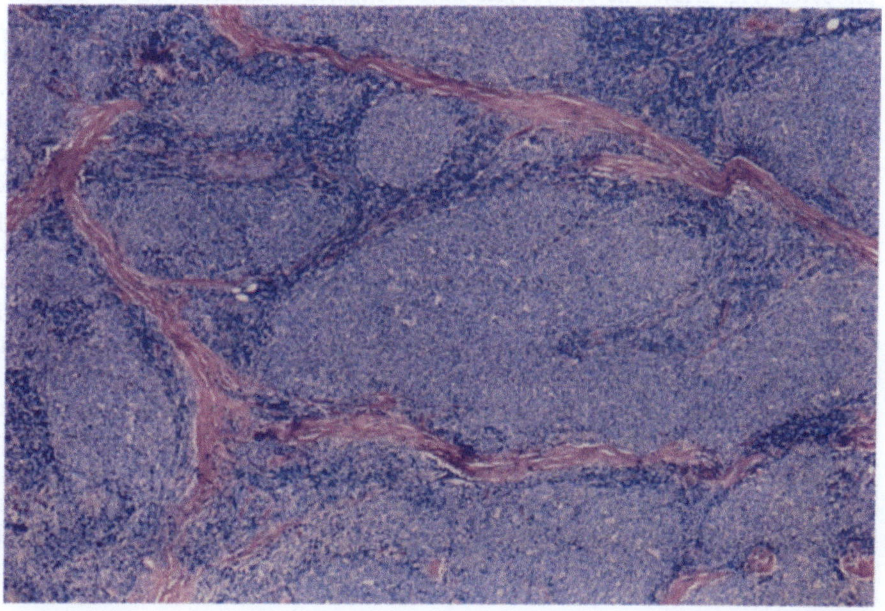

Fig. 4.41. A typical follicular growth pattern in a follicular lymphoma grade 1: there is minimal sclerosis, mostly between the neoplastic follicles (Giemsa stain)

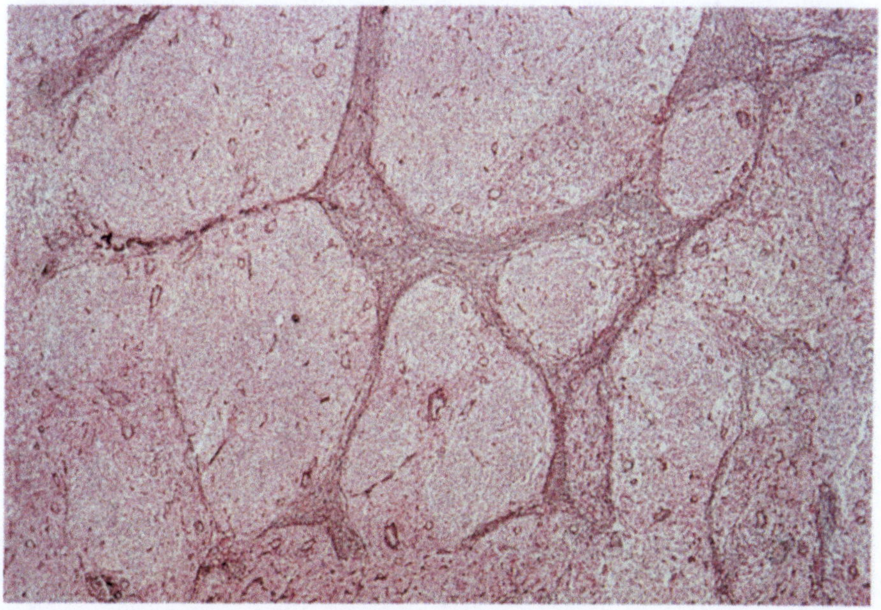

Fig. 4 42. Follicular lymphoma grade 1 with silver impregnation. Note the paucity of fibers in the neoplastic follicles (Gomori silver impregnation)

same Ig light-chain as the neoplastic germinal center cells. Paraproteinemia is often seen in such cases (see Alberti and Neiman 1984; Mann 1985; Frizzera et al. 1986). The follicles contain only a small number of fibers or are often almost completely devoid of fibers (Fig. 4.42).

The neoplastic follicles consist chiefly of small or medium-sized centrocytes, but they always contain centroblasts, FDC and macrophages as well as T-lymphocytes (Fig. 4.43). The centrocytes have elongated indented nuclei with a dispersed chromatin pattern and small inconspicuous nucleoli. The cytoplasmic rim is usually not visible. From these characteristic small to medium-sized cells, there is a continuous spectrum to more anaplastic cells with a lighter chromatin pattern, making the differentiation from medium-sized blasts difficult or even impossible (see below: grading). The centroblasts are medium-sized or large cells and have a scanty, basophilic cytoplasm in Giemsa stain. The nuclei are round or oval with multiple, medium-sized, often marginal nucleoli and have a vesicular chromatin pattern (Fig. 4.44). In some instances, centroblasts are evident in only some of the follicles. Occasionally, the follicles also may contain immunoblasts. Van der Putte et al. (1984) pointed out the presence of germinal center cells with lobulate (multilobulated) nuclei (Fig. 4.45).

The neoplastic follicles differ from reactive follicles in the uniform, dense arrangement of the cells without compartmentalization into light and dark zones and by the absence of starry-sky macrophages. Neoplastic follicles may contain some basophilic giant cells of an uncharacteristic morphology.

Kjeldsberg and Kim (1981) described polykaryocytes resembling Warthin-Finkeldey giant cells. These cells, or at least most of them, probably represent multinucleate FDC. Occasionally, one finds epithelioid cell clusters or even epithelioid cell granulomas ("tubercles") without evidence of tuberculosis or sarcoidosis (Kim and Dorfman 1974).

In both the neoplastic follicles and the interfollicular tissue, there are occasionally deposits of a PAS-positive substance in centrocyte-like or plasma-cell-like cells. The PAS-positive deposits are often globular and may lead to a signet-ring-cell-like deformation of the cells. The term "signet-ring-cell lymphoma" has been applied to tumors showing substantial numbers of such cells. Sometimes the PAS-positive substance is stored in clumps and larger, amorphous aggregates in the neoplastic germinal centers (Chittal et al. 1987). The deposits are sometimes phagocytosed by macrophages.

A diagnostically important, although infrequent, lesion especially in follicular lymphoma grades 1 and 2

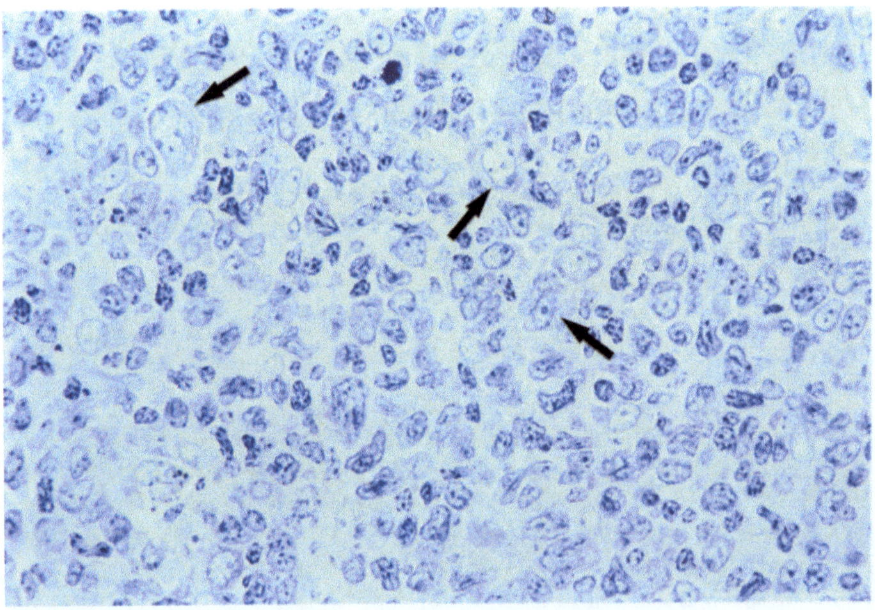

Fig. 4.43. Typical follicular grade 1 lymphoma. Typical blasts are marked (→) (Giemsa stain)

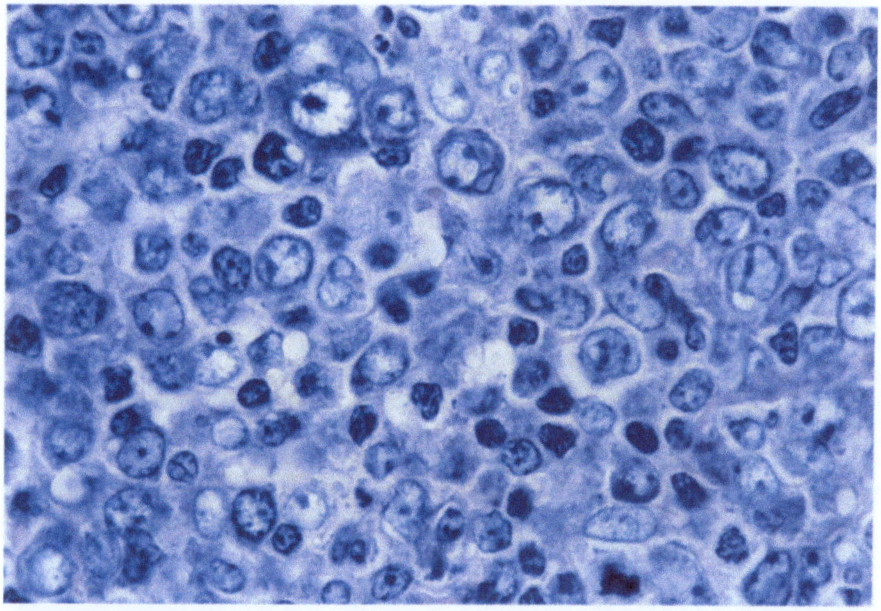

Fig. 4.44. A typical follicular lymphoma grade 3a, with several typical centroblasts intermingled with medium-sized and small centrocytes (Giemsa stain)

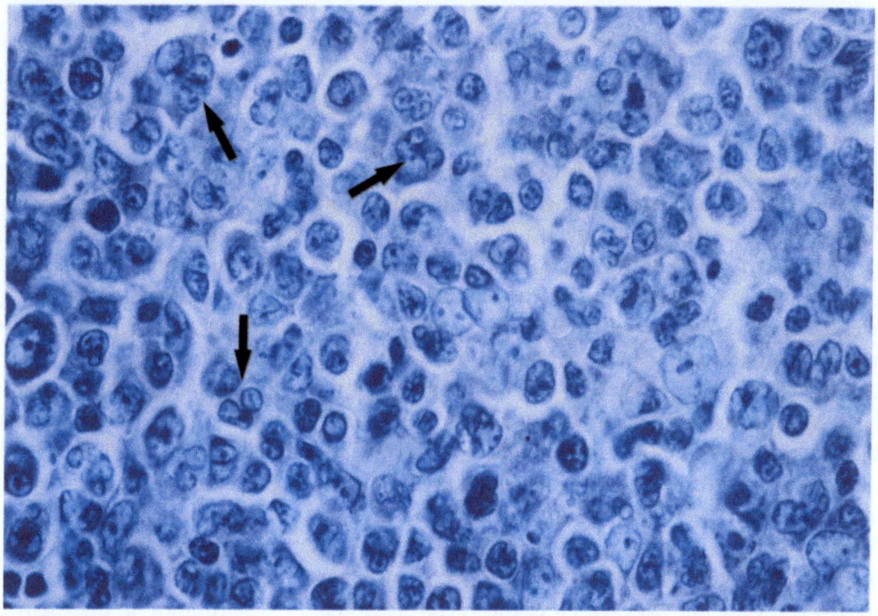

Fig. 4.45. Follicular lymphoma grade 3a. There is a large number of blasts many of which show multilobulated nuclei (→) (Giemsa stain)

is total necrosis of infiltrated lymph nodes. It is found almost exclusively in this type of ML. In such cases it is easy to diagnose the lymphoma on sections stained by silver impregnation.

When purely follicular lymphoma grades 1 - 3a start to show a diffuse growth pattern, the neoplastic follicles appear to be split into pieces and permeated with numerous reticulin fibers and lymphocytes. The diffuse areas consist chiefly of a mixture of centrocytes, lymphocytes and a few centroblasts. One must make a clear distinction between this picture and the development of diffuse *secondary centroblastic* lymphoma (diffuse large-cell - centroblastic).

Follicular lymphoma grade 2 is identical to grade 1

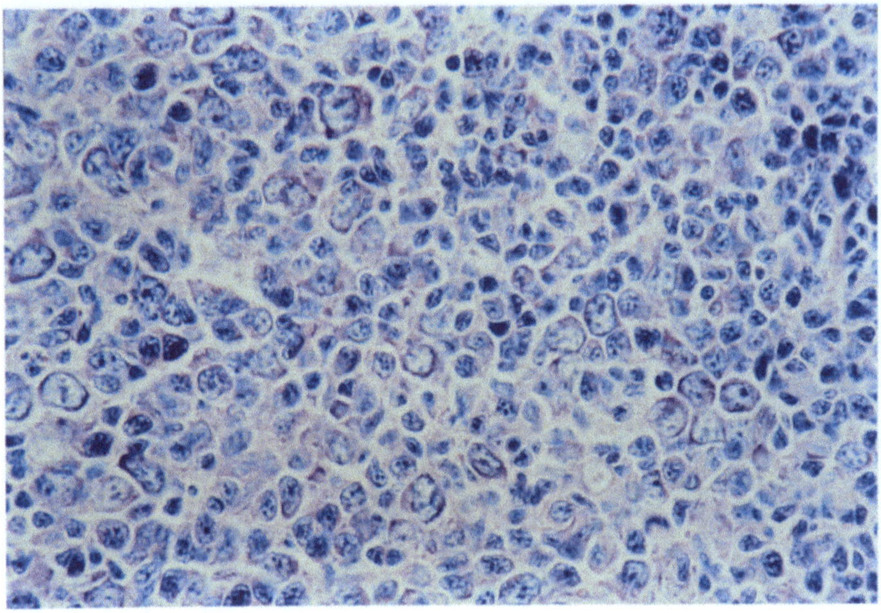

Fig. 4.46. Follicular lymphoma grade 2 (Giemsa stain)

except the number of blasts which lies between 6 and 15/high-power field (Fig. 4.46).

Follicular lymphoma grade 3 shows an identical growth pattern, mostly indistinguishable from grades 1 and 2 under low power. Diffuse areas may indicate a transformation to a diffuse centroblastic lymphoma (diffuse large B-cell lymphoma).

Overall, the number of centroblasts is variable within this lymphoma type, ranging from tumors with only single blasts (grade 1) within a whole section to follicular lymphomas which predominately or even completely consist of blasts (grade 3b). Whereas in the Kiel classification tumors with a higher number of blasts were designated as centroblastic-centrocytic and described to be transformed when clusters or cohesive sheets of blasts were found, other classifications preferred a grading system counting cells or blasts. It is well-excepted that counting the number of blasts is hardly reproducible. Nevertheless, the WHO classification proposed a grading system counting the number of centroblasts per high-power field. One major reason for the non-reproducibility lies in the lack of a proper consensus regarding which cells should be designated as blasts. Adapted to the proposal of Mann and Berard (1983), counting the number of centroblasts in a certain number of high-power fields, the WHO included three grades indicating that grades 1 and 2 are closely related and should be distinguished from grade 3:

- Grade 1 = 0 – 5 centroblasts/high-power field
- Grade 2 = 6 – 15 centroblasts/high-power field
- Grade 3 = > 15 centroblasts/high-power field

At least 10 high-power fields should be counted.

Grades 1 and 2 are almost equivalent to the centroblastic-centrocytic lymphoma in the Kiel classification.

Moreover, the WHO classification proposes to distinguish two subtypes of grade 3. Grade 3a comprises tumors in which the centroblasts (more than 15/high-power field) are dispersed and separated by centrocytes (Fig. 4.47). This type most probably corresponds to a low grade centroblastic-centrocytic lymphoma with high content of blasts in the Kiel classification. Grade 3b comprises tumors in which centroblasts are present as clusters or cohesive sheets corresponding to the high-grade follicular centroblastic lymphoma in the updated Kiel classification (Fig. 4.48).

Although a one-institution study postulated the clinical relevance of grading follicular lymphomas, it seems doubtful that this system will be applicable for multicenter studies. Clinical studies have so far failed to show significant differences for the overall survival of patients with these three subtypes. The interobserver reproducibility within the ILSG was around 50 % differentiating grades 1 – 3 according to the REAL classification. For the significance of prognostic parameters compare Clinical Presentation and Prognosis (p. 65 f).

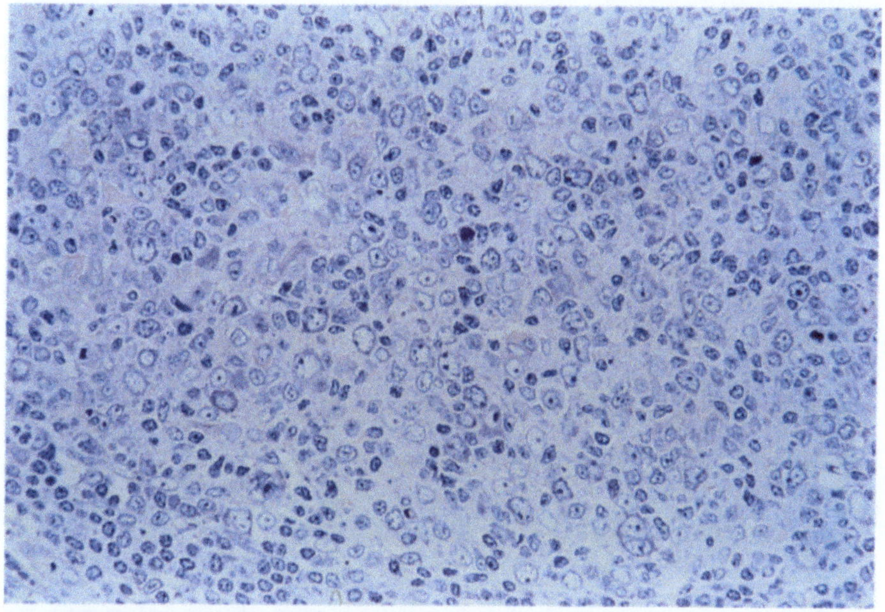

Fig. 4.47. Follicular lymphoma grade IIIa. Note the numerous large blasts intermingled with centrocytes

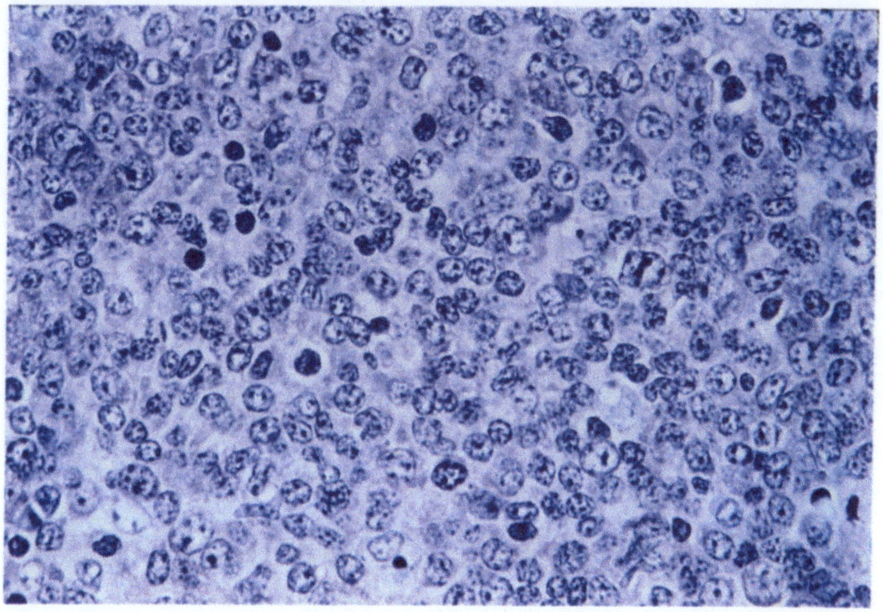

Fig. 4.48. Follicular lymphoma grade IIIb (Giemsa stain)

4.2.1.6.1 Morphological Variants of Follicular Lymphoma: Follicular Lymphoma with Marginal Zone Differentiation

About 5–9% of follicular lymphomas exhibit signs of monocytoid B-cell differentiation ranging from small clusters of monocytoid B-cells to large bands spreading in a sinusoidal and/or perifollicular/marginal zone pattern (Fig. 4.49a, b).

Morphologically, this kind of differentiation can be recognized either by this growth pattern and/or by the cytology of the neoplastic cells. Monocytoid B cells have a more abundant, pale cytoplasm and slightly irregular sometimes round or monocytoid nuclei with

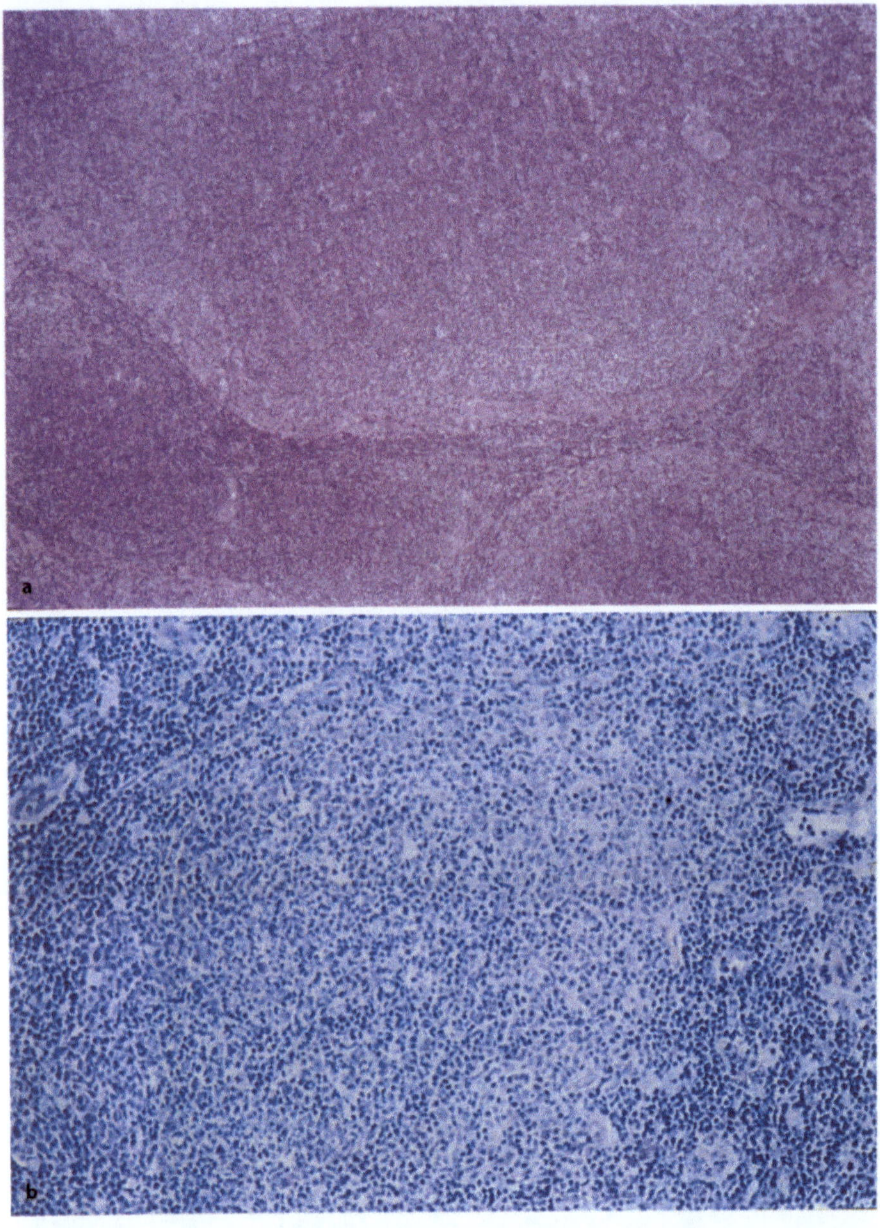

Fig. 4.49 ab. Follicular lymphoma with marginal zone differentiation. The marginal zone is a light area in the paratrabecular sinuses (**a**) and surrounding the germinal center of the neoplastic follicle (**b**) (Giemsa stain)

a light chromatin pattern. These cells can also be found as small clusters within the follicles.

These observations lead to two major issues:

1. The marginal zone differentiation can be abundant, making the differential diagnosis between primary marginal zone lymphoma and a follicular lymphoma with marginal zone differentiation difficult or even impossible. The immunophenotype is of no help as marginal zone lymphoma and marginal zone differentiation in follicular lymphoma have the same phenotype: CD20+, CD5–, CD10–. It can be helpful to detect the translocation t(14;18) on a molecular level, which then indicates a primary follicular lymphoma.
2. It has been described that a partial marginal zone differentiation of follicular lymphomas significantly influences the overall and failure-free survival.

Patients with prominent perifollicular marginal zone differentiation (more than 5%) have a worse prognosis than patients with a pure follicular differentiation (Nathwani et al. 1999a).

4.2.1.6.2
Cytological Variants of Follicular Lymphoma

1. Signet-ring-cell lymphoma (see Weiss et al. 1985 for review). A few cases of follicular lymphoma show globular or diffuse, PAS-positive deposits in numerous centrocytes, lymphoplasmacytoid cells and plasma cells. These deposits represent IgM. Occasionally, they cause displacement and indentation of the nuclei (Lennert 1978; Van den Tweel et al. 1978); this gives the vague impression of signet-ring cells. Hence such tumors have been called signet-ring-cell lymphoma (Kim et al. 1978).
   The term "signet-ring-cell lymphoma" is also applied to another morphological picture, in which vacuoles of various sizes fill the cytoplasm and push the nucleus to the periphery (Fig. 4.50) (Kim et al. 1978; see Weiss et al. 1985 for review). The picture is otherwise that of follicular lymphoma with a follicular or follicular and diffuse growth pattern. In our cases, the vacuoles were PAS-negative or showed, at most, a very weak PAS reaction. The tumors were usually IgG-positive lymphomas (Weiss et al. 1985). The large vacuoles have been interpreted as giant multivesicular bodies, although they are lysozyme-negative (Harris et al. 1981).
   Stansfeld (1985) suggested that the term "signet-ring-cell lymphoma" should be used only for the second type of tumor with large cytoplasmic vacuoles, because only this type is confined to *one* cytologically defined entity, i.e. follicular lymphoma. In contrast, PAS-positive Ig deposits occur in cytologically different lymphoma types, e.g. immunocytoma and follicular lymphoma. The term "signet-ring-cell lymphoma" is superfluous, and even confusing, in such cases. Signet-ring-cell lymphoma of T-cell type (Weiss et al. 1985) has rarely been observed.
2. Follicular lymphoma with a high content of cells containing lobulated nuclei (see Fig. 4.45). Van der Putte et al. (1984) described two cases of follicular centroblastic-centrocytic lymphoma and one case of follicular and diffuse centroblastic-centrocytic lymphoma in which numerous germinal center cells showed "multilobulate" nuclei. The nuclear lobation was seen in centroblasts, centrocytes and lymphoplasmacytoid cells in the neoplastic germinal centers. Subsequently, the investigators looked in reactive germinal centers for cells with multilobate nuclei and actually found them in five of 40 cases.
3. Follicular plasmacytoma. Schmid et al. (1985) described a case of follicular lymphoma in which the neoplastic follicles consisted predominantly of

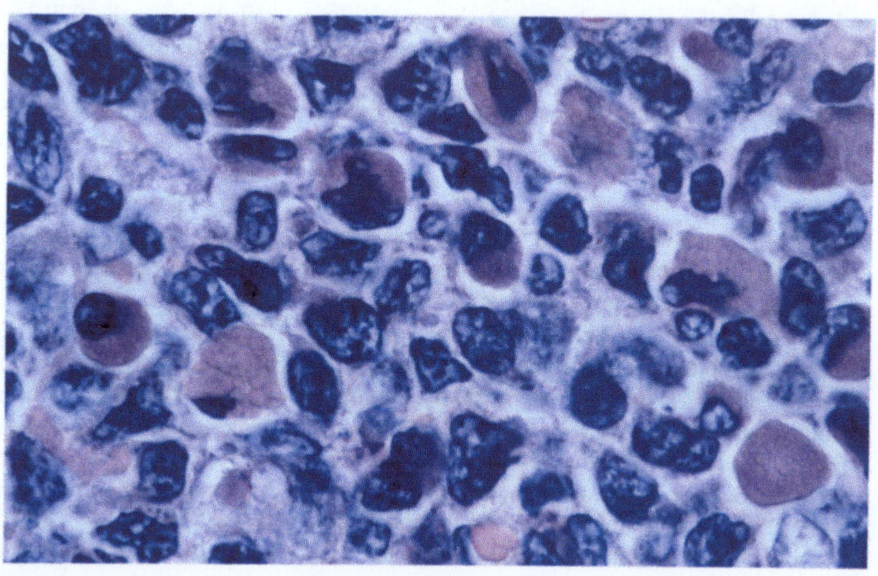

Fig. 4.50. "Signet-ring" follicular lymphoma grade 1. Note the PAS-positive deposits Giemsa-stained red to orange in the cytoplasm of centrocytes and plasma cells in a neoplastic germinal center

typical plasma cells. Some of the follicles, however, contained centroblasts and centrocytes. Hence the tumor was considered to be a special variant of centroblastic-centrocytic lymphoma.

4. Follicular lymphoma with a floral pattern. Osborne and Butler (1987) were the first to report this so-called floral pattern, which is thought to represent florid, progressive, transformed germinal centers. Today it is clear that these cases represent follicular lymphoma which derive in part from atypical lymphocytes that irregularly invade and invaginate the germinal center leading to a floral appearance. These follicles are surrounded by a prominent follicular mantle (Goates et al. 1994). In some cases, coexpression of CD5 on the neoplastic cells is described (Tiesinga et al. 2000).

4.2.1.6.3 Evolution and Transformation

Follicular lymphoma evolves in 30–40% of patients into a large-cell ML (secondary centroblastic lymphoma), which is more frequently than any other type of B-cell lymphoma of small-cell malignancy. In the autopsy collection of the lymph node registry in Kiel (1974–1989), this development was found in 40% of the cases of centroblastic-centrocytic lymphoma, mostly equivalent to follicular lymphoma grades 1–3a; in the other 60% of cases, the follicular lymphoma diagnosed on a lymph node biopsy was still evident at autopsy. The transformed tumor is made up of medium-sized or large cells of only *one* type and shows a *diffuse* growth pattern – large-B-cell lymphoma-centroblastic.

Rare cases of follicular large-cell lymphoma (follicular lymphoma grade 3b) transforming into a Burkitt's lymphoma have been described (Sham et al. 1989).

Borderline Cases. Follicular grade 3b lymphoma is used equivalently to the term follicular large-cell lymphoma and is defined by the number of blasts (> 15/high-power field) as well as the existence of clusters or sheets of blasts. In our opinion, a lymphoma *transforming* into a *secondary large-cell centroblastic lymphoma* must be distinguished from a *primary follicular large-cell centroblastic lymphoma.* For the detection of a transformation into a large-cell lymphoma, not only the number of blasts is decisive but also the presence of circumscribed areas or clusters of centroblasts and the existence of follicular lymphoma grade 1 to grade 3a (see p. 53 and 58).

Thus we believe that different categories of follicular lymphoma do exist:

- *Primary* follicular lymphoma grades 1, 2, 3 a and b
- Follicular lymphoma grade 1 to grade 3a transforming into a *secondary* diffuse or – less frequently – into a follicular large-cell lymphoma
- *Primary follicular centroblastic* lymphoma, only in part identical to grade 3b

Immunohistochemistry

The phenotype of follicular lymphoma tends to reflect the phenotype of its normal counterpart, i.e. germinal center cells. The tumor cells bear sIg, mostly IgM and IgD; at least 30% of cases show IgG. The cells are also characterized by the constant expression of CD22, CD19, CD20, CD79α and CD10. The expression of CD10 is usually more pronounced in neoplastic follicles than in reactive ones (Almasri et al. 1998). The lymphoma cells are negative for CD5 and CD43, which is helpful in the distinction from nodular growing mantle cell lymphoma. The interfollicular areas contain CD20-positive B-cells that belong to the same cell clone as those in the follicles. However, the phenotype is slightly different concerning activation antigens. Whereas the neoplastic follicles are positive for CD10 and CD95, these antigens are down-regulated or even completely negative in the interfollicular infiltrate (Dogan et al. 1998). The presence of CD10-positive cells between the follicles is a valuable criteria for the diagnosis of a follicular lymphoma. In areas of follicular growth, there is generally a preserved network of FDC, which appears to be less dense than that seen in reactive follicles. The FDC stain positive for CD35, CD21 and CD23. Almost all nodal follicular lymphomas grade 1 (97%) and 2 (83%) are positive for bcl-2 protein, the percentage in grade 3 is about 75% (Lai et al. 1998), whereas reactive germinal centers are negative (Pezella et al. 1990). When the growth pattern becomes more diffuse, CD10 may disappear and be replaced by the expression of CD23. The network of FDC is also much thinner in areas with a diffuse growth pattern. Rare cases of the diffuse subtype show no such network at all. The number of T-cells may be high, reaching as much as 40–60% even within the follicular structures. The staining for T-cells has to be carefully evaluated and compared to bcl-2 staining when the differential diagnosis is between follicular lymphoma and follicular hyperplasia, as reactive T-cells are bcl-2-positive and may thus mimic positive germinal center B-cells. The reactive T-cells predominately express CD4 and less frequently CD8. The number of CD57-positive cells is equivalent to the number found in reactive follicles.

The number of Ki-67- (Mib-1)-positive cells varies from case to case (range: 10–80%; mean: approx. 35%). In general, the percentages of Ki-67-positive cells increases with increasing grade; however, it does not parallel the grading system in all cases. This is in part due to the fact that remnants of reactive germinal center cells may still exist within the neoplastic follicle. Moreover, tumors with an increased number of more anaplastic centrocytes which do not have all features of blasts and which are graded as grade 1 or 2 may show extremely high Ki-67 indices, up to 80%. The biology and the clinical relevance of this observation is not yet understood. The proliferation index in the infiltrated interfollicular areas is significantly lower than in the neoplastic follicles.

p53, which is involved in the regulation of bcl-2, is found with increasing frequency from grade 1 to grade 3, underlining that the expression of p53 indicates a progression or even a transformation of the lymphoma (Cooper and Haffajee 1997).

Genetic Features

The characterizing chromosomal translocation in follicular lymphoma is t(14;18), which transposes the bcl-2 gene next to the heavy-chain gene on chromosome 14. This event leads to the expression of the bcl-2 protein in neoplastic follicular center cells. The translocation is detected in 65–95% of the patients with follicular lymphomas. The range of positivity mostly depends on the different detection techniques used. Most of the t(14;18) translocations in follicular lymphomas grades 1 and 2 can be detected by classical cytogenetics, fluorescence in situ hybridization (FISH) or comparative genomic hybridization (CGH) (up to 95%). Most grade 3 follicular lymphomas are also positive; however, the actual frequency of this translocation in grade 3 lymphomas has not yet been estimated.

Beside this characteristic translocation, other, mostly secondary chromosomal events have been described. They are predominately found in progressing or transforming follicular lymphomas although they are not specific for follicular lymphomas. Among these are a large number of trisomies (3, 5, 7, 19, 21, X). Deletions were found especially on 6q. A gain of chromosome 7 was described in 30% of grade 1 and 2 with increasing frequency in grade 3 and in transformed diffuse large-cell lymphomas (Bernell et al. 1998). Other abnormalities are found on chromosomes 1p, 3qs and 10q. Recently, Ott et al (2002) described the t(14;18) in 73% of grade 3a and 13% of grade 3b. By contrast, a chromosomal break in 3q27 was predominately found in grade 3b (44%), and rarely in grade 3a (18%).

Mutations in p53 have also been found. This is interpreted as a secondary event and may also indicate transformation into a diffuse large-cell centroblastic lymphoma.

Differential Diagnosis

It is most important, although sometimes difficult, to distinguish *follicular* lymphoma grades 1–3a (centroblastic-centrocytic lymphoma) from *follicular lymphoid hyperplasia*. The distinction can usually be made on the basis of the morphological criteria given in Table 4.1 (reviews: Rappaport et al. 1956; Nathwani et al. 1981a; Mann 1985). Important information is already provided by a low-power view. Follicular lymphoma shows relatively poorly defined germinal centers without, or with only a narrow lymphocyte mantle and without a zonal arrangement. In contrast, the germinal centers in follicular hyperplasia are more clearly defined and often have a distinct mantle zone; they also show a zonal arrangement, with a lower, dense zone containing numerous blast cells (basophilic in Giemsa stain!) and an upper, less dense zone containing numerous centrocytes (non-basophilic!). Cytologically, neoplastic germinal centers in grade 1 and 2 lymphomas as a rule contain many more centrocytes than do reactive germinal centers. In addition, mitotic activity is generally much lower in neoplastic germinal centers than in reactive ones. Starry-sky cells (macrophages with "tingible bodies") are not seen in follicular lymphoma unless the tumor is transforming into centroblastic lymphoma, whereas such cells are often found in reactive germinal centers.

Of the criteria listed in Table 4.1, the following are particularly important. An admixture of other types of "inflammatory" cells (especially large groups of well-differentiated, polyclonal plasma cells) and a sinusoidal B-cell reaction occur only in follicular lymphoid hyperplasia. However, a marginal zone differentiation

Histological features	Follicular lymphoma	Follicular lymphoid hyperplasia
Lymph node architecture	Effaced	Largely preserved
Sinus catarrh	–	Sometimes +
Germinal centers		
Outline	Ill-defined	Distinct
Size and shape	Relatively uniform	Variable
Lymphocyte mantle	Absent or narrow	Usually well-developed
Zonal architecture	Never	Often
In perinodal tissue	Often	Very rarely
Mitotic figures	Often only a few	Often very many
Protein precipitates	Almost never found	Frequently found
Cytology of follicles		
Centrocytes	Large number	Relatively small number
Centroblasts	Often small number	Often very large number
Starry-sky cells	None	Often abundant
Interfollicular tissue	Monotonous; small cells	Sometimes polymorphic
Cytology of the interfollicular tissue (besides lymphocytes)		
Plasma cells	Sometimes (monotypic)	Often (polytypic)
Immunoblasts	–	Sometimes
Neutrophil granulocytes	–	Occasionally
Eosinophils	Occasionally	Occasionally
Mast cells	Occasionally	Occasionally

Table 4.1. Differential diagnosis of follicular lymphoma and follicular lymphoid hyperplasia

is sometimes seen partly surrounding the neoplastic follicles. Grade 1 and 2 lymphomas tend to spread also outside the capsule, which is unusual in follicular hyperplasia. Very large germinal centers containing numerous centroblasts and starry-sky cells are also typical of lymphoid hyperplasia, especially in children and in early stages of HIV infection. However, early infiltrates of primary follicular large-cell lymphoma (follicular centroblastic) have to be differentiated from such florid follicular hyperplasia. Since follicular lymphoma very rarely occurs in patients younger than 20 years of age, the patient's age is another important criterion.

An immunohistochemical analysis is the most reliable way to distinguish between reactive and neoplastic germinal centers in paraffin sections from ambiguous cases. To detect light-chain restriction is mostly problematic in paraffin sections of follicular lymphoma. Reactive germinal centers contain κ- and λ-chains, whereas neoplastic germinal centers contain light-chains of only *one* type. When light-chain staining does not allow a clear distinction between follicular lymphoma and follicular hyperplasia, the use of bcl-2 antibody is helpful. However, one has to consider that individual cases of follicular lymphoma can be negative (in some series up to 20 % of the cases). This phenomenon is a nearly constant finding in primary follicular lymphomas of the skin.

Completely diffuse, growing follicular lymphomas are exceptional rare cases (e.g. Lieberman et al. 1986). At a workshop of the European Lymphoma Club, 80 % of cases that had been interpreted as diffuse centroblastic-centrocytic lymphoma proved to be immunocytomas/lymphocytic lymphomas or mantle cell lymphomas. Immunocytoma consists predominantly of lymphocytes, which can be misinterpreted as centrocytes on poorly prepared slides (!) and contains cIg-positive plasma cells or lymphoplasmacytoid cells. The larger blast cells do not correspond to centroblasts, but rather to immunoblasts or plasmablasts. Mantle cell lymphoma does not contain blast cells, with the exception of polyclonal plasma cell precursors or residual germinal center cells. The blastic variant of mantle cell lymphoma shows a monotonous-looking proliferation of cells with a morphological appearance between that of centrocytes and centroblasts. Typical centroblasts are found only in small numbers or not at all; immunoblasts do not occur. Mitotic activity is higher than in follicular lymphoma grades 1 and 2.

An individual case of a composite lymphoma, mantle cell lymphoma and follicular lymphoma has been described (Tsang et al. 1999).

Finally, as described below, a marginal zone differentiation can be observed in up to 10% of follicular lymphoma patients. This has to be kept in mind when studying the spleen, which can be secondary involved. In such cases the follicular lymphoma may involve the splenic marginal zone, mimicking a primary marginal zone lymphoma of the spleen (Alkan et al. 1996).

Some marginal zone lymphomas have a strong tendency to follicular colonization. This makes it difficult or even impossible in individual cases to distinguish between colonization of a marginal zone lymphoma and a primary follicular lymphoma with marginal zone differentiation (see Differential Diagnosis). Classical marginal zone lymphomas are CD10-negative; however, when they are colonizing the follicle they may become CD10-positive.

Finally nodular paragranuloma has to be kept in mind in the differential diagnosis as it may show a follicular growth pattern which can be identical to follicular lymphomas. The cytology is decisive in such cases as nodular paragranuloma consists mostly of IgD+ lymphocytes in the progressively transformed germinal centers.

Occurrence
Follicular lymphoma accounts for about one-fifth of all cases of NHL in Europe. In the United States, about 35% and in Italy (Milan) about 13% of all cases of NHL are of this type. The lowest frequency is found in Japan, with about 5%.

The most frequent subgroup is grade 1 (43%) followed by grades 2 and 3 (28% and 29%, respectively) (The Non-Hodgkin's Lymphoma Classification Project 1997).

Follicular lymphoma shows a peak around 60 years. The youngest patient was 13 years old and the oldest was 88. Hence follicular lymphoma does occur (<1%) in childhood (Frizzera and Murphy 1979; Winberg et al. 1979). A diagnosis of follicular lymphoma in a child must be substantiated, however, by the immunohistochemical or molecular demonstration of light-chain restriction or bcl-2 translocation. Interestingly, the median age of follicular lymphoma in Japan is significantly lower, 53 years. Follicular lymphoma is the only type of malignant lymphoma that shows a slight female preponderance (the male-to-female ratio is about 1:1.18).

Clinical Presentation and Prognosis
The disease begins insidiously and is therefore often in an advanced stage when the patient seeks medical care. About 65% of patients are in stage III or IV at the time of diagnosis, 54% in Japan. Bone marrow involvement is found in about 40%. B symptoms are noted by only 17% of patients. More than 80% are in the low risk group with respect to the IPI.

Cervical, axillary, and inguinal lymph nodes are involved most frequently, but lymph nodes in unusual sites (e.g. epitrochlear) may also be affected. Mediastinal lymph nodes are often bypassed and do not appear to be a site of primary involvement (Bartels 1980). Lymphoma in the retroperitoneal region frequently represents a follicular lymphoma.

There are no changes in blood protein levels for a long period of time; paraproteinemia (usually IgM) is seldom observed (about 1% of cases, Bartels 1980). About 33% of patients show a subleukemic blood picture, usually with only a slight increase in the number of centrocytes, at some time during the course of the disease. A very small number of patients may show a marked leukemic blood picture. The centrocytes can be recognized from their "notched" (Galton 1964) or "cleaved" nuclei.

In the Kiel collection, a significant primary extranodal localization was the *spleen* (Bartels 1980). In 70% of those patients, the spleen was the only infiltrated organ. Some of the patients recovered after splenectomy, while others later showed recurrence elsewhere. Diebold et al. (1987) also described a splenomegalic type of centroblastic-centrocytic lymphoma showing a relatively favorable prognosis.

Of all lymphomas of low-grade malignancy, the follicular lymphomas show the most favorable prognosis, although they are not curable by conventional therapeutic regimens. Long-term survival is relatively high when the disease is diagnosed in stages I or II (Brittinger et al. 1978, 1984; Kuse et al. 1983). The overall survival after 10 years is somewhat better than 50%. The major independent prognostic factors are age and serum lactate dehydrogenase (LDH) levels.

The growth pattern has hardly any influence on survival so long as more than 50% of the lymphoma exhibits a follicular pattern. However, more than 50% diffuse growth worsens the prognosis significantly (Hans et al. 2003). The purely diffuse variant apparently has a significantly poorer prognosis than do other types (Meugé et al. 1978; The Non-Hodgkin's Lymphoma Pathologic Classification Project 1982; Weisenburger et al. 2003). The available data on the prognostic significance of sclerosis are contradictory, but we presume that sclerosis does not have any significant influence on ultimate survival.

The size of the centrocytes and the number of centroblasts also have only a limited effect on survival: large centrocytes and numerous centroblasts seem to indicate a somewhat poorer prognosis (Rappaport et al. 1956; Jones et al. 1973; van Unnik et al. 1975; Molenaar et al. 1984). There was no statistically significant difference in survival between the small cleaved cell type and the mixed, small cleaved and large-cell type of follicular lymphoma as defined by the Working Formulation (WF) (Molenaar et al. 1984).

Looking at all three grades of follicular lymphoma from small cleaved to large cleaved, including stages III and IV, there is no difference in overall survival, which is 35–40% after 10 years. In addition, even the shapes of the survival curves are similar. There is no plateau for any of these three groups (Miller et al. 1997). Different results were obtained in earlier investigations and in a study by Lieberman et al. (1986). These differences may be a matter of definition: the large-cell type as defined in those studies may have corresponded to centroblastic lymphoma with a follicular growth pattern instead of follicular lymphoma (centroblastic-centrocytic lymphoma).

The survival rate is somewhat higher when the primary localization of the tumor is extranodal and when the patients are women. When the follicular lymphoma develops into a diffuse large-cell lymphoma-centroblastic-lymphoma, the survival rate drops considerably and lies between 10 and 20 months.

Also, in limited-stage disease the overall and event-free survival is not influenced by the grading system (Tezcan et al. 1999).

As grading of follicular lymphoma is not reproducible among different observers, it seems unlikely that such a subdivision has any predictive value with respect to the clinical prognosis. Most reports on prolonged survival shown so far, especially for follicular large-cell lymphoma, which in part is identical to follicular lymphoma grade 3, indicate that the differences in survival are due to other prognostic factors, especially to limited stage disease and the IPI (Kantarjian et al. 1984; Martin et al. 1995; Bartlett et al. 1994). Furthermore, the cellular proliferation index does not appear to add additional information regarding survival of patients (Martin et al. 1995).

Although Ott et al. (2002) could show a difference in chromosomal abnormalities between follicular lymphoma grade 3a and 2b it does not contribute to the estimation of the prognosis of patients. Hans et al. (2003) could not find a significant difference in overall survival for grade 3a and 3b. The more important difference lies obviously between grade 1 and 2 on the one hand and grade 3a on the other.

4.2.1.7 Mantle Cell Lymphoma (ICD-O: 9673/3)

Synonyms

- Kiel: Centrocytic lymphoma (mantle cell lymphoma)
- REAL: Mantle cell lymphoma
- WHO: Mantle cell lymphoma

Definition

Mantle cell lymphoma is characterized by monomorphic-appearing cells that are morphologically very much similar, although not identical to, germinal center centrocytes. This lymphoma type does not contain neoplastic centroblasts. The tumor cells are small to medium-sized with strongly irregular indented nuclei. In 5–10% of the cases, cytological variants of either blast-like (blastoid), lymphocytic, or large pleomorphic (anaplastic) cells are found. The growth pattern is either diffuse, nodular, or mantle zone.

Mantle cell lymphoma is derived from cells in the follicle, i.e. from follicular mantle cells. The cells correspond to naïve pre-germinal center B-cells. Mantle cell lymphoma is now generally accepted as a distinct clinical-pathological lymphoma entity.

Morphology

At low magnification, it is possible to make a tentative diagnosis of mantle cell lymphoma on Giemsa-stained slides: there is a monotonous-looking proliferation of small to, at most, medium-sized cells whose nuclei show weaker (grayer) staining than do those of lymphocytic lymphomas (Figs. 4.51–4.53). The nuclei are usually irregularly shaped and strongly indented or cleaved. The cytoplasm of the tumor cells is not visible. There are no monotypic blast cells (basophilic cells) of any type (centroblasts, immunoblasts). Polytypic blast cells (centroblasts, immunoblasts), however, may be

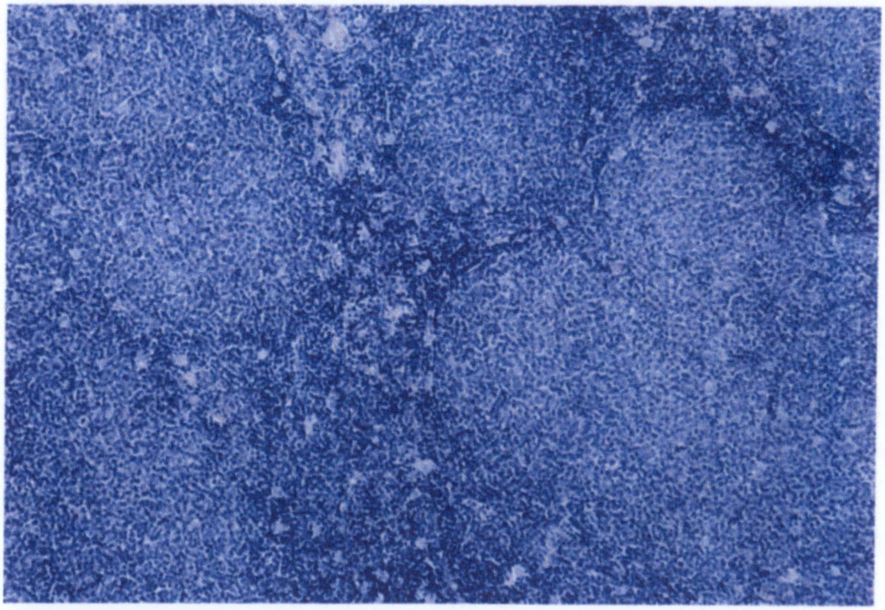

Fig. 4.51. Low-power view of a mantle cell lymphoma with a nodular growth pattern (Giemsa stain)

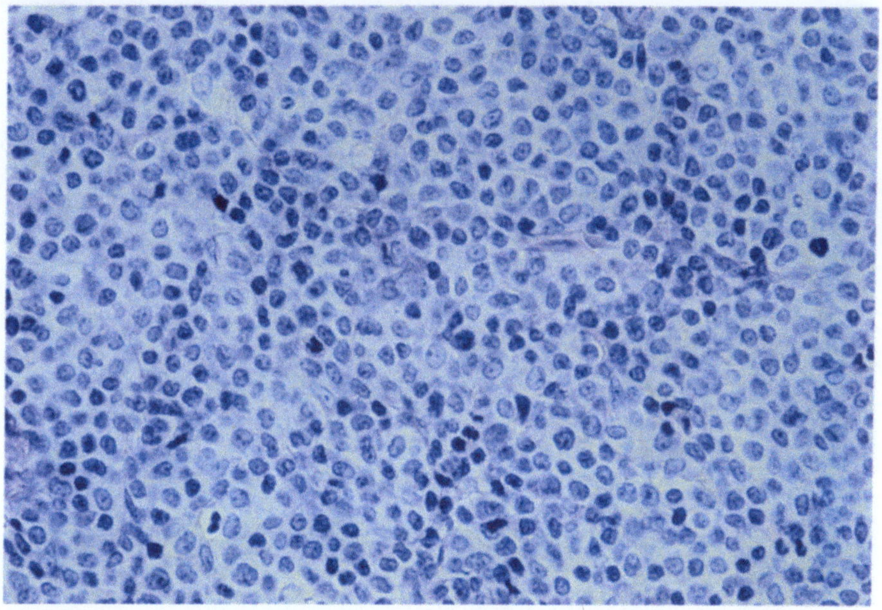

Fig. 4.52. Monomorphic infiltrate of a mantle cell lymphoma. Note the medium-sized cells with indented nuclei (Giemsa stain)

found as remnants of germinal centers. Plasmablasts, i.e. precursors of polytypic (reactive) plasma cells, are sometimes scattered among the tumor cells. The number of mitotic figures varies from case to case. The tumor cells are interspersed with macrophages and some small lymphocytes, e.g. T-lymphocytes. The number of T-cells is significantly lower than in follicular lymphomas. There is a loose, sometimes enlarged network of FDC, which usually show relatively large, round nuclei and solitary, medium-sized nucleoli (Fig. 4.54). These cells sometimes contain two or more nuclei and may finally turn into multinucleate giant cells, which Kjeldsberg and Kim (1981) reported to be similar to Warthin-Finkeldey giant cells. Such giant cells also occur in other types of neoplasms of the follicles (follicular lymphoma grade 1/centroblastic-cen-

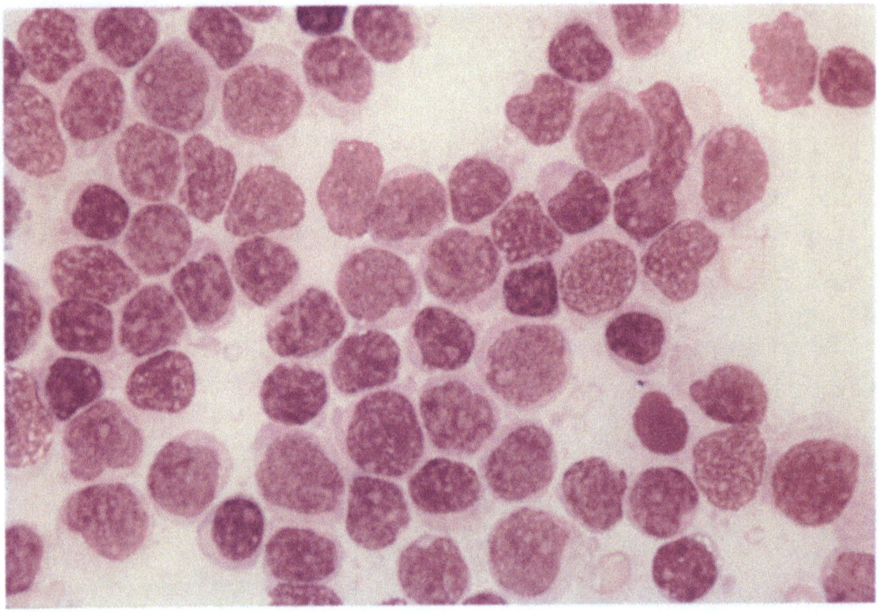

Fig. 4.53. Touch-imprint of a mantle cell lymphoma. The nuclei are irregularly shaped with inconspicuous nucleoli and a small cytoplasmic rim (Pappenheim stain)

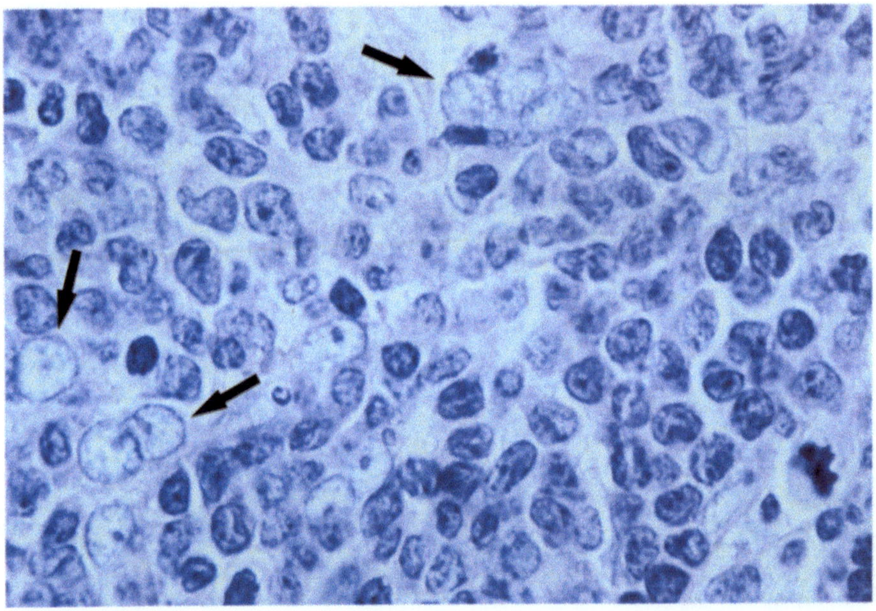

Fig. 4.54. High-power view of a mantle cell lymphoma. Note the centrocytes with irregularly shaped nuclei and accumulations of follicular dendritic cells (→) (Giemsa stain)

trocytic lymphoma, nodular paragranuloma) and in low-grade malignant B-cell lymphoma of MALT. They stain positive with antibodies for FDC.

Hyaline deposits are frequently found around small blood vessels (capillaries, not epithelioid venules); this finding is highly characteristic of mantle cell lymphoma. The reticulin fibers are usually thick and form a coarse alveolar network, which surrounds large, solid groups of tumor cells. Band-forming sclerosis or a diffuse increase in fibers is also occasionally found.

The growth pattern is either diffuse or nodular or both, as is readily appreciated with silver impregnation. In early stages, there may be a band-shaped infiltrate in the outer cortex of the node, which corresponds to a mantle zone pattern(surrounding remnants of

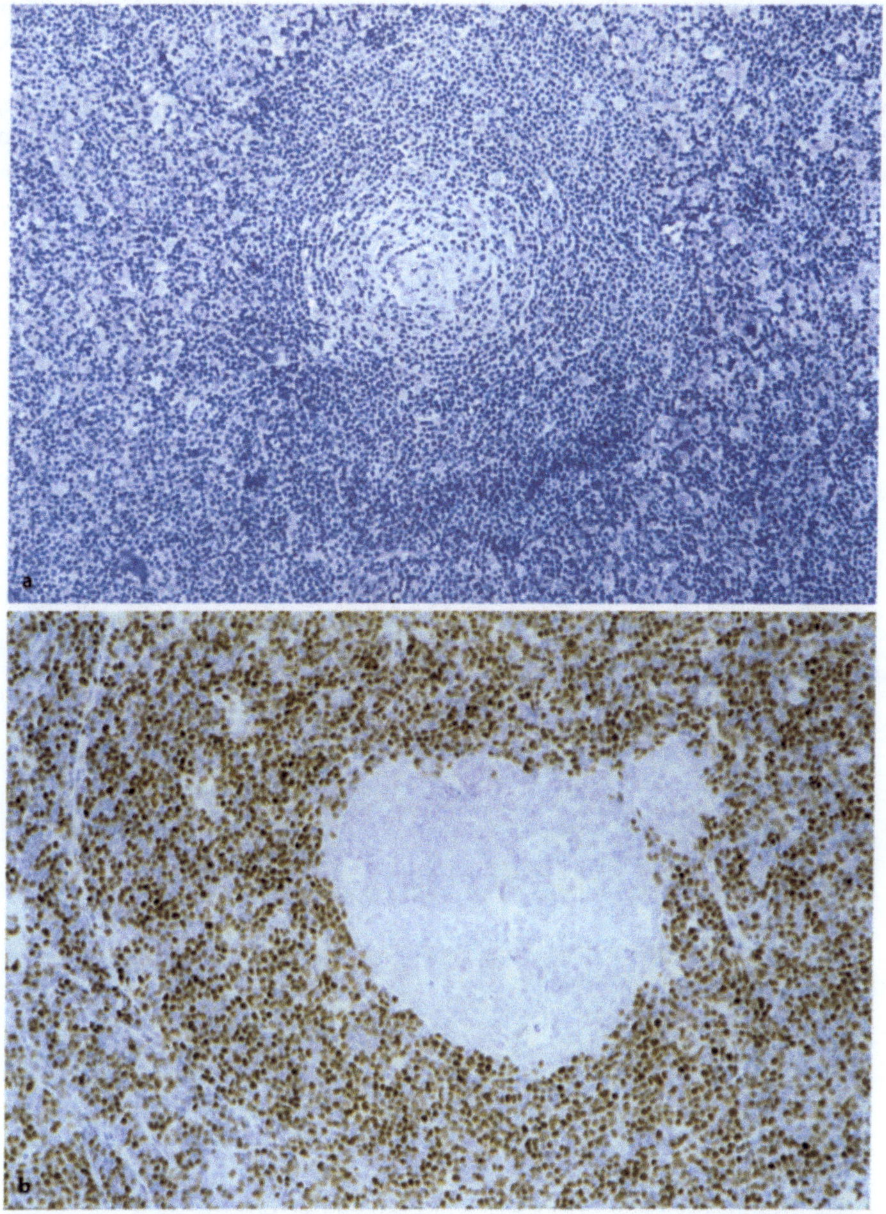

Fig. 4.55 a, b. Mantle cell lymphoma. The mantle zone growth pattern has a remnant of a germinal center. **a** Giemsa stain, **b** immunohistochemical staining for cyclin D1. Note the nuclear staining of the neoplastic centrocytes (immunoperoxidase)

germinal centers) (Fig. 4.55a, b). In a study from the Kiel Lymph Node Registry nodularity was found in slightly less than 50 % of patients as readily recognized by silver impregnation of the samples. In 17 % of the patients, the nodularity affected the whole lymph node section; in 28 % it was merely partial. In the same study, a mantle zone growth pattern, i.e. band-like growth of "centrocytes" around reactive (polyclonal) or residual germinal centers, was also investigated. In about 40 % of the patients, this growth pattern was detected at least in small areas of the node. A mantle zone growth pattern and nodularity were usually demonstrable in the same node. It is now well-accepted that proliferation of mantle cell lymphoma initially develops in the areas surrounding reactive germinal centers (mantle zone pattern; Fig. 4.56). Subsequently, the germinal centers may disappear, resulting in a nodular pattern. Finally, the tumor cells grow diffusely.

Variants. In the Kiel classification, small-cell and large-cell ("anaplastic") types were distinguished, although the borderline between the two types was not well-defined. The large-cell centrocytic lymphoma described by Stansfeld (1985) corresponded to the centrocytoid centroblastic lymphoma identified by the Kiel group (see Chap. 1.2) (A.G. Stansfeld 1988, personal communication). With the help of molecular genetics and immunohistochemistry, the morphological variants could be defined more precisely.

Centrocytoid/Blastoid/Lymphoblastoid Variant (Figs. 4.56–4.59). The term "centrocytoid centroblast" was originally chosen as it was thought that this variant belonged to the centroblastic lymphomas. Morphologically, the tumor cell lies between a centrocyte and a

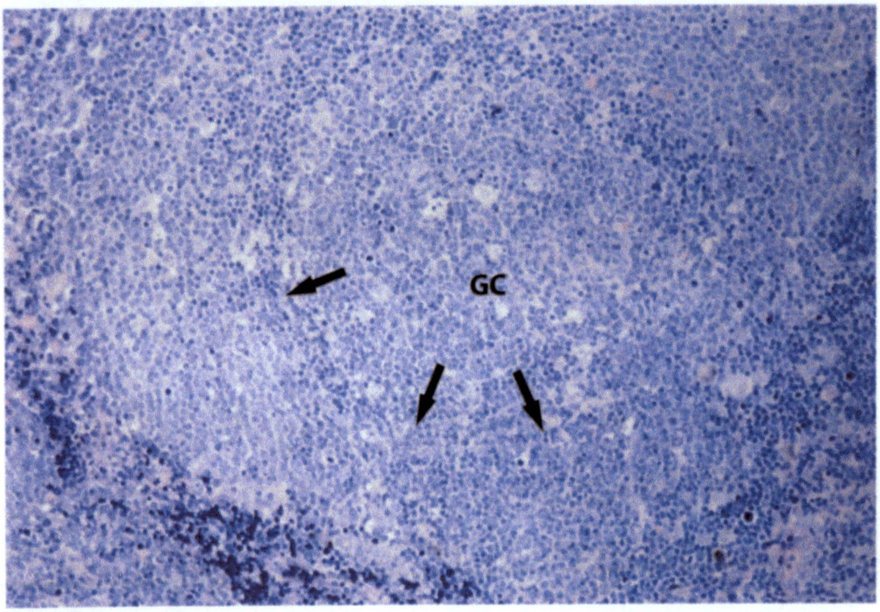

Fig. 4.56. Mantle zone growth pattern of a mantle cell lymphoma (→). Compare with Fig. 4.57 (blastic variant of mantle cell lymphoma) (Giemsa stain) (GC: germinal center)

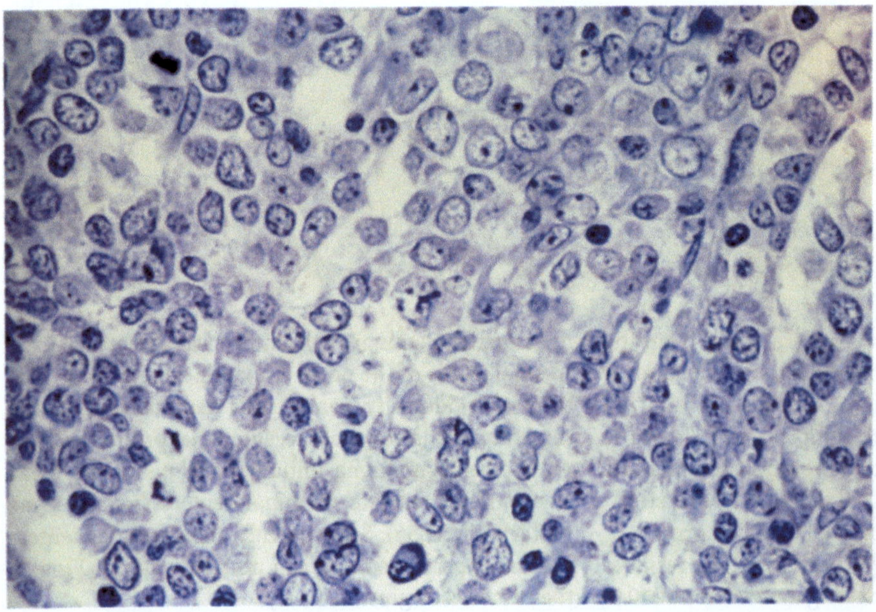

Fig. 4.57. Blastoid variant of mantle cell lymphoma. The cells have a light chromatin pattern, resembling that of centroblasts, with inconspicuous nucleoli, a small cytoplasmic rim and only slight nuclear indentations (Giemsa stain)

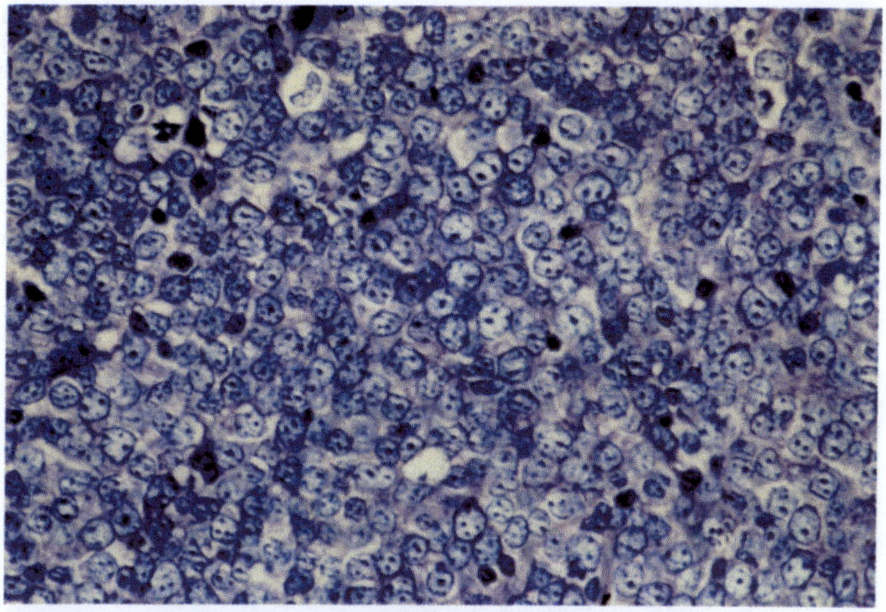

Fig. 4.58. Mantle cell lymphoma, blastoid variant. The chromatin pattern is similar to that of centroblasts; however, the nucleoli are multiple and small (Giemsa stain)

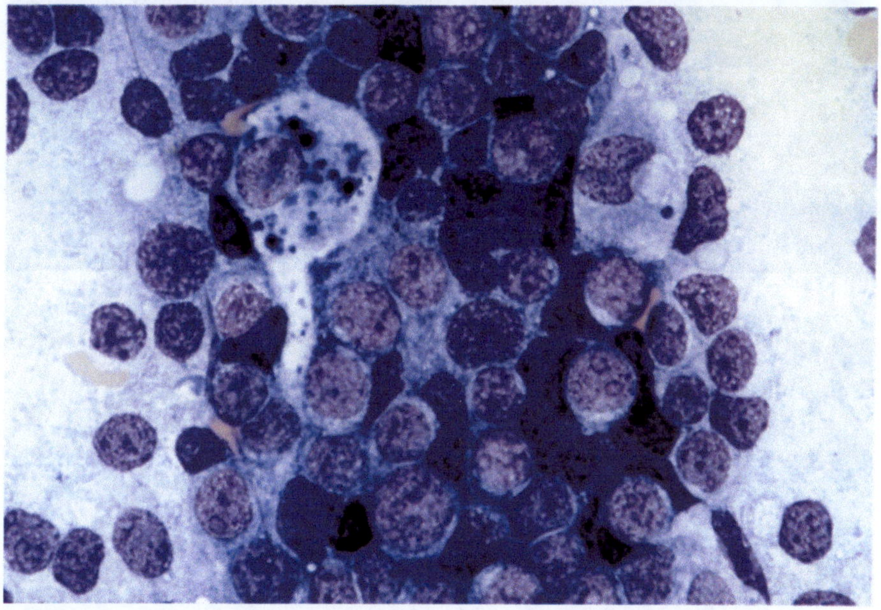

Fig. 4.59. Touch-imprint of a mantle cell lymphoma, blastoid variant. The nuclei are slightly smaller than those of typical centroblasts, with multiple small nucleoli and a small cytoplasmic rim (Pappenheim stain)

centroblast. The cell is *relatively* small (9–11 μm) and has mostly oval or round, rarely slightly irregular-shaped nuclei with two to five small, basophilic, slightly enlarged nucleoli. These are more prominent than in the classical type of mantle cell lymphoma. Nuclear indentations are hardly ever seen. The chromatin is more vesicular than in the classical type. The cytoplasm is scanty and only slightly basophilic in Giemsa stain. Sometimes the neoplastic cells resemble lymphoblasts with more prominent nucleoli. The mitotic rate is higher than in classical mantle cell lymphoma. It is easier to distinguish centrocytes from lymphoblasts in imprints than in sections, because the cytoplasm of lymphoblasts is more basophilic than that of centrocytes.

Pleomorphic Variant (Fig. 4.60). This type mostly corresponds to the anaplastic type of the Kiel classification. The nuclei are larger and show indentations. The nucleoli are not as prominent as in the blastoid variant. Sometimes a small, slightly basophilic cytoplasmic rim is visible. The cells usually have a high mitotic rate. There is a continuous spectrum ranging from cells of the classical type to the pleomorphic variant, making the distinction difficult and hardly reproducible. More frequently, this pleomorphic or anaplastic variant can be observed in patients who have relapsed (Norton et al. 1995).

Lymphocytic Variant (Fig. 4.61). Very few cases have been described which were morphologically diagnosed as a lymphocytic lymphoma. The tumors in these cases

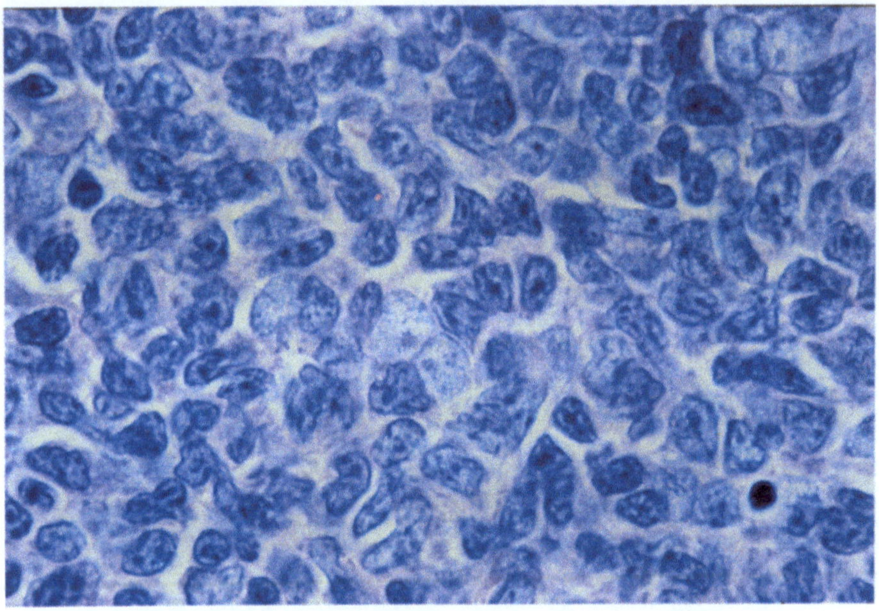

Fig. 4.60. Mantle cell lymphoma, pleomorphic variant. The nuclei are large and bizarre with a denser chromatin pattern than that of blasts; however, some of the nucleoli are prominent (Giemsa stain)

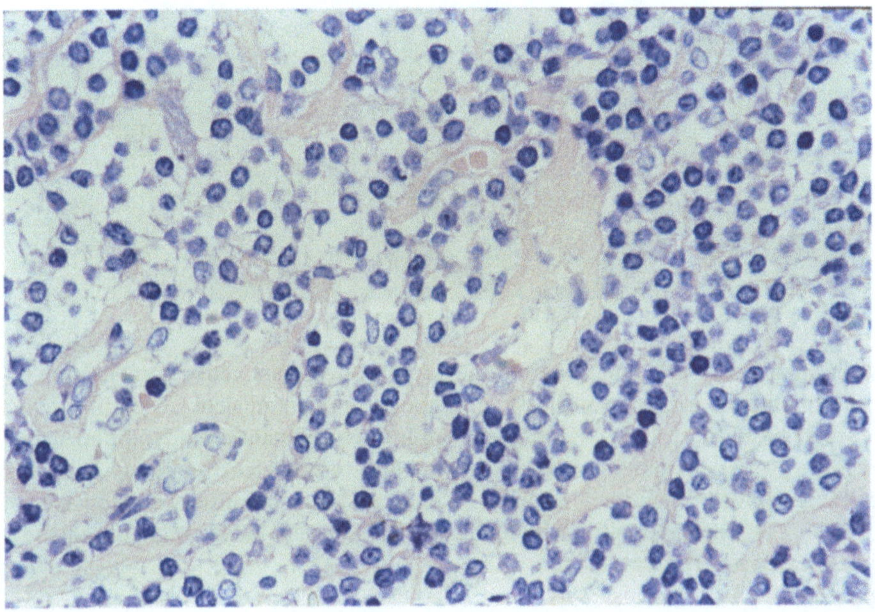

Fig. 4.61. Lymphocytic variant of mantle cell lymphoma with typical hyalinization of the vessel wall (Giemsa stain)

consisted of lymphocytes and prolymphocytes and were shown to carry the t(11;14) translocation and/or express cyclinD1 as demonstrated immunohistochemically. Although these tumors biologically belong to the group of mantle cell lymphomas, they may clinically behave as a lymphocytic lymphoma.

Some other cases appear at first glance as a lymphocytic lymphoma. However, at high magnification nuclear indentations are found and in other areas of the same section cells of the classical type of mantle cell lymphoma can be found.

In general, if a variant of a mantle cell lymphoma is included in the differential diagnosis, the whole section or all sections must be carefully evaluated, since usually at least small areas containing cells of the classical variant can be detected.

Today, it is not totally clear whether the detection of these variants has clinical importance. It has been stated that the blastoid variant shows a more aggressive growth pattern with a high proliferation index; however, a low proliferation index with this variant has also been described.

Finally, the fixation process may lead to artifacts if the central part is less well-fixed, and thus leads to a more blastic appearance of the neoplastic cells. Shrinking may result in smaller cells with a more lymphocytic picture. Thus, the detection of morphological variants should primarily be used to distinguish between the entire spectrum of mantle cell lymphomas.

Up to 70% of the patients may have a leukemic blood picture. This can be an important feature to include in the differential diagnosis of lymphocytic lymphomas as well as marginal zone lymphomas. Moreover, leukemic-type tumors are described to have a very aggressive clinical course. Most patients die within 18 months after onset of the disease. The cytological picture is highly variable, and all variants can be detected (Pittaluga et al. 1996; Wong et al. 1999). In other reports, the significance of a leukemic blood picture in relation to survival is unclear (Cohen et al. 1998).

Recently a new "nucleolated" leukemic variant of mantle cell lymphoma mimicking prolymphocytic leukemia has been described (Wong et al, 2002).

Evolution and Transformation. Occasionally, biopsies obtained some time after the primary diagnosis of mantle cell lymphoma disclose larger cells with more pronounced nuclear polymorphism and higher mitotic activity (anaplastic or pleomorphic variant). We consider these to be signs of advancing anaplasia and thus indications of an unfavorable progress.

The Kiel collection contained only one case in which a B-immunoblastic lymphoma with PAS-positive inclusions evolved out of a mantle cell lymphoma. We have never observed transformation of mantle cell lymphoma into centroblastic lymphoma (diffuse large-cell).

Immunohistochemistry

The hallmark antigen expression pattern is CD5-positive and CD23-negative; this constellation distinguishes mantle cell lymphoma from other low-grade malignant B-cell lymphomas. However up to 10% of mantle cell lymphomas with coexpression of cyclin D1 may express CD23 (Yatabe et al. 2000). The tumor cells show marked surface expression of Ig, chiefly IgM with light-chain restriction, predominately λ (60–70%). In 60% of the tumors, the cells simultaneously express IgD. In addition, the B-cell antigens CD22, CD19 and CD20 are found; 5% of the tumors may lack CD5 expression which is not confined to a distinct variant. This is important in the differential diagnosis of marginal zone lymphoma. CD10 is absent. A characteristic *nuclear* expression of cyclin D1 can be found in about 80–90% of mantle cell lymphomas (Yatabe et al. 2000) (Figs. 4.55, 4.62). The reliable detection of cyclin D1 strongly depends on good fixation of the tissue, as especially overfixation may lead to false-negative results. In 90% of tissue samples stained for complement receptors (CD35), CD23, or with Ki-M4p (FDC), mostly loose, slightly enlarged networks of FDC or, less frequently, small groups of FDC, i.e. remnants of germinal centers, can be identified. The T-cell content (a mixture of CD4-positive and CD8-positive cells) amounts to 5–10% and is thus usually much lower than that of follicular lymphoma grade I. The number of Ki-67-positive cells lies between 5% and 50%, with a mean of approximately 20%. Patients with ≥26% Ki67-positive cells have a worse prognosis (median survival 13 vs 45 months) (Raty et al. 2002). In a few cases, the centrocytes on paraffin sections show strongly stained monoclonal Ig in their scanty cytoplasm, without exhibiting a plasmacytoid morphology.

Genetic Features

The highly characteristic cytogenetic abnormality in mantle cell lymphoma is the translocation t(11;14)(q13;q32) (Williams et al. 1993). This translo-

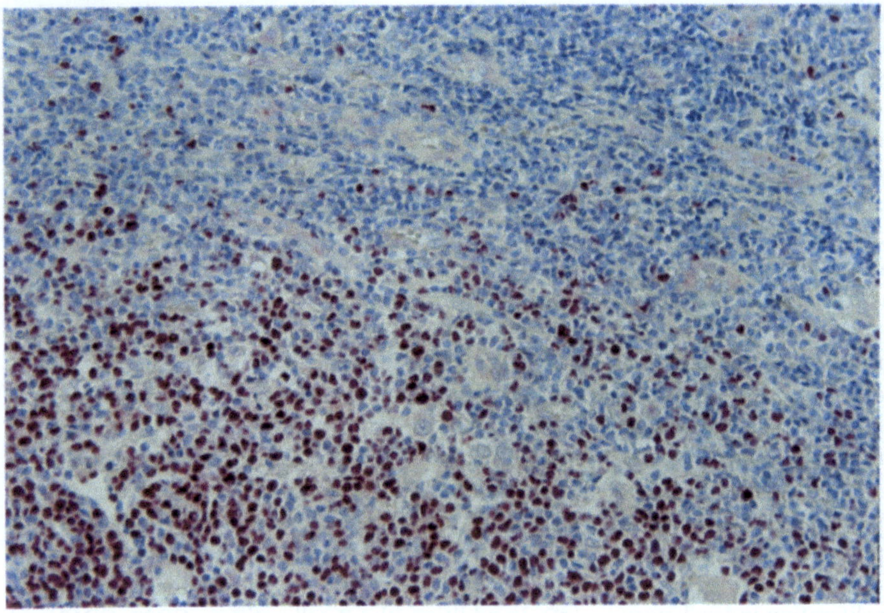

Fig. 4.62. Mantle cell lymphoma, immunohistochemical staining for cyclin D1 (alkaline phosphatase). Note the typical nuclear staining pattern

cation involves the IgH chain gene and the bcl-1 locus on chromosome 11, resulting in overexpression of cyclin D1 (see above). Depending on the method used, the translocation can be detected in the vast majority of cases.

p53 gene mutations are described to occur predominately in more aggressive (blastoid) variants of mantle cell lymphoma (Hernandez et al. 1996). Moreover the tumors more frequently have tetraploid chromosome clones (Ott et al. 1997) and a higher number of chromosomal imbalances, usually gains of chromosome 3q (50%). These chromosomal gains are described to be associated with a shorter survival of the patients (Bea et al. 1999). Additional chromosomal abnormalities, i.e. +12, 13q14, 17p–, were detected (Cuneo et al. 1999).

Diagnosis and Differential Diagnosis

The diagnosis is based on the monotony of the cell picture and the absence of markedly basophilic blast cells belonging to the same clone as the centrocytes. A similarly monotonous picture is found in *lymphoblastic lymphomas*, including ALL. In lymphoblastic lymphoma the nuclei are rounder than those of centrocytes, but they occasionally show protrusions. In mantle cell lymphoma the nuclei are generally more elongated or irregular, but they can sometimes be round. The cytoplasm of lymphoblastic lymphoma cells is clearly basophilic, but very scanty and thus hardly visible in sections. Lymphoblastic lymphoma shows, on the average, a larger number of mitotic figures than does centrocytic lymphoma. Imprints are helpful in the differential diagnosis. In lymphoblastic lymphoma the reticulin fiber pattern is finer and a vascular hyalinization is lacking.

Monocytic and myelomonocytic leukemias may also be confused with mantle cell lymphoma because of the polymorphic nuclei in the former neoplasms. Consideration of the following criteria should prevent misinterpretations. In monocytic leukemia the nuclei are occasionally reniform, deeply indented or folded and usually contain a larger nucleolus than do mantle cell nuclei. With Giemsa staining, the cytoplasm of monocytic leukemia cells is gray or grayish red and more abundant than that of centrocytes. Among these leukemic cells there are almost always a few, or even numerous, chloroacetate-esterase-positive myelocytes and promyelocytes. Reticulin fibers and capillaries are increased in number.

In a few cases, the borderline between mantle cell lymphoma and *follicular lymphoma grade 1* (centroblastic-centrocytic lymphoma) is not distinct. The presence of a few (markedly basophilic) centroblasts is required for a diagnosis of follicular lymphoma grade 1. One often has to search carefully for these cells. Nevertheless, it can be difficult to distinguish between neoplastic and reactive blasts. In that case immunohistochemistry is decisive. Follicular lymphoma is CD10-positive whereas mantle cell lymphoma stains positive for CD5.

Very rare cases of *small cell pleomorphic T-cell lymphoma* (peripheral T-cell lymphoma, unspecified) may be very similar to mantle cell lymphoma. The application of pan-B-cell or pan-T-cell antibodies is the only available aid in making a differential diagnostic decision. In almost all cases, however, small-cell T-cell lymphoma shows more pleomorphic nuclei and never a nodular or "mantle zone" growth pattern (see Chap. 5.2.2).

Nodal marginal zone lymphoma may sometimes also show a monotonous pattern; however, some blasts are always intermingled and the nuclear irregularities are less pronounced ("centrocyte-like cells"). Marginal zone lymphoma may exhibit a perifollicular pattern which may mimic a mantle zone pattern. Immunohistochemistry is decisive, with CD5 being negative in marginal zone lymphoma.

Occurrence

Mantle cell lymphoma accounts for 5–6% of the cases of NHL. The age curve shows a peak in the seventh decade. In the Kiel collection the youngest patient was 16 years old and the oldest was 86. There is a clear preponderance of males, with a male-to-female ratio of 2.7:1 (Argatoff et al. 1997).

Clinical Presentation and Prognosis

Most patients show generalized lymphoma (stage III or IV) at the time of diagnosis. Hepatosplenomegaly is observed in 30–60% of the patients (Pittaluga et al. 1996). Approximately 50% of patients present with B symptoms (Meusers et al. 1989). A small number of neoplastic cells are found in 40–60% of tumors, but an absolute count of neoplastic cells higher than 4.0/l is rare.

Extranodal involvement is a frequent finding. Bone marrow involvement is detected in 50–80% of the patients. It is more reliably found in bone marrow trephines than in aspirates. Moreover mantle cell lymphoma involves other extranodal sites including especially the GI tract and Waldeyer's ring. The GI tract is infiltrated in 10–20% of the cases either simultaneous with the primary diagnosis in the lymph node or during the course of the disease (see Chap. 6.2.1.3). In addition, in rare cases lymphomatoid polyposis may occur in the GI-tract, most often in the small and less frequently in the large bowel.

Mantle cell lymphoma shows a much poorer prognosis than either B-CLL, immunocytoma or follicular lymphoma. The median survival time was 32–43 months, depending in part on the treatment modality (Meusers et al. 1989; Bosch et al. 1998; Argatoff et al. 1997). Less than 10% of patients survived 5 years. The median overall survival is 28 months. However, patients with less than two residual lymphoma manifestations in remission experienced a relatively good prognosis, with an estimated 5-year survival of greater than 60% (Hiddemann et al. 1998). The prognosis is less favorable for patients whose tumors show high mitotic activity (or marked Ki-67 positivity) than for patients with tumors having a small number of mitotic figures. In the blastic variant, the increased number of chromosomal imbalances and the leukemic blood picture are unfavorable prognostic signs. The value of IPI in this entity is controversially discussed in the literature (Samaha et al. 1998; Zucca et al. 1995; Argatoff et al. 1997; Bosch et al. 1998). This may in part be due to the fact that most patients are within the high-risk categories. Yatabe et al. compared cyclin-D1-positive and -negative mantle cell lymphoma. They described the 5-year survival rate as being significantly different within the two groups (5-year survival: 30% vs 86%; Yatabe et al. 2000).

4.2.2 Large-B-Cell Lymphoma

4.2.2.1 Diffuse Large-B-Cell Lymphoma (ICD-O: 9680/3) – Common Features

Synonyms

- Kiel: Centroblastic, B-immunoblastic B-large-cell anaplastic
- Real: Diffuse large-B-cell
- WHO: Diffuse large-B-cell

Definition

These lymphomas occur in nodal and extranodal sites. They are defined as a diffuse infiltration of large-B-cells, in which the nucleus of an individual cell is the size of at least two lymphocyte nuclei or larger than the nucleus of a macrophage. The WHO classification (Jaffe et al. 2001) proposes that pathologists use the term "diffuse large-B-cell lymphoma", without other specification, only as a final diagnosis. The rationale of this proposal is the same as that proposed by the International Lymphoma Study Group and is contained within the REAL classification (Harris et al. 2000). According to this classification, the diagnosis of morphological subtypes of DLBCL is not reproducible between pathologists. On the other hand, the therapeutic strategy is more or less the same for all morphological subtypes and differences in the survival of patients with different subtypes are still controversial.

The WHO proposes that, for research purposes, pathologists distinguish between "morphological" and "clinical variants." The aim is to demonstrate differences in survival between these variants and, if possible, describe new entities particularly among the clinical variants. In this book, the morphological variants will be described together, but each clinical variant will be presented in the corresponding chapters based on organ pathology.

The *postulated normal counterpart* of the various subtypes of large-B-cell lymphomas is still not well-known but is probably represented by a peripheral B-cell showing a rearrangement of the variable heavy (V_H)-chain of the Ig gene (Küppers et al. 1999).

The study of gene expression profiles using DNA microarrays (Alizadeh et al. 2000) has revealed that DLBCL can be differentiated into two groups: a *germinal center B-cell-like* and an *activated B-cell-like*. Patients in the first group shows a better overall survival than those in the second. A precise correspondence between morphological groups and survival based on the up-dated Kiel classification has not yet been investigated.

Lossos et al. (2000a) distinguished two groups in DLBCL, one in which the tumor cells show ongoing somatic mutations of VH genes, in a pattern suggesting antigen selection pressure (Hsu and Levy 1995; Küppers et al. 1997; Ottensmeier et al. 1998; Hyland et al. 1998; Delecluze et al. 1999; Driessen et al. 1999; Thompsett et al. 1999), and another in which the tumor cells lack such mutations.

Correlations between the subtypes established by these two different methods have been evaluated (Lossos et al. 2000b). All DLBCLs classified as germinal center B-cell-like by gene expression showed ongoing mutations in the VH Ig genes while DLBCLs classified as activated B-cell-like had no such ongoing mutations. These findings validate the concept that lymphoid malignancies are derived from cells at variable stages of normal lymphocyte maturation and that the neoplastic cells retain the genetic program of their normal equivalents (Lossos et al. 2000b).

These results lead to the following conclusions:

1. The germinal center B cell-like type develops from cells belonging to *follicular B-cells.*
2. The activated B-cell-like type either derives from *post-germinal-center B-cells* in which somatic hypermutation no longer occurs or from *germinal center B-cells* by a "transformation event that changes germinal center gene expression pattern and stops the mutation process" (Lossos et al. 2000b). There is also a possibility of an additional type of DLBCL with gene expression features of *activated B-cell-like type*, but with also a low level of ongoing somatic mutation.
3. The results of further studies on DLBCL subtype should be compared with the morphology and the immunophenotype of the different subtypes of the WHO classification.

Morphology

The WHO classification proposed using the up-dated Kiel classification (Jaffe et al. 2001) to define the following variants: *centroblastic, immunoblastic* and *anaplastic large-cell B-cell lymphomas.* Since the publication of this classification, three other morphological variants have been described: *T-cell-rich/histiocyte-rich B-cell lymphoma, immunoblastic lymphoma expressing anaplastic large-cell-lymphoma kinase (ALK)-1, plasmablastic lymphoma* (mostly seen in HIV-positive patients).

All of these variants have in common the diffuse replacement and partial or total destruction of the normal architecture of the organ in which they develop, such that the tumors often become polycyclic masses compressing the adjacent normal tissue. Necrosis and hemorrhage may also be seen. In lymph nodes, interfollicular infiltrate and sinusal involvement can occur. Extension into the perinodal adipose tissue is often observed.

Immunohistochemistry

In DLBCL, CD45 and B-cell-associated antigens such as CD20 and CD79α are expressed, although one or more of these antigens may be lacking, particularly CD20 in the case of plasmacytic differentiation. Monotypic sIg is present in more than 75% of tumors. These markers are useful for the diagnosis (Stein et al. 1984; Melnyk et al. 1997). Other markers which can be expressed will be discussed during the presentation of each morphological variants (see Chap. 4.2.2.2). For example, expression of CD10 antigen correlates with the t(14;18)(q32;q21) major breakpoint region (Fang et al. 1999; Dogan et al. 2000). Other DLBCLs express CD5 and seem to represent a subtype seen in older patients, mostly women (Nakamura et al. 1999; Yamaguchi et al. 1999). Some DLBCLs are CD30-positive and have to be distinguished from anaplastic large-cell lymphomas (Piris et al. 1990). In the majority of the cases, DLBC comprises 40 to 60%, and sometimes even more up to 80%, of lymphoma cells positive for Mib-1 (Ki-67) (Miller et al. 1994). The expression of the following proteins has a certain prognostic value (see below): bcl-2 oncoprotein, demonstrated in about 40% of patients (Yunis et al. 1989; Hermine et al. 1996; Kramer et al. 1996; Monni et al. 1999; Gascoyne et al. 1997; Hill et al. 1996); bcl-6 protein, demonstrated in the majority of DLBCLs (71%), particularly those of the centroblastic subtype (82%) (Skinnider et al. 1999; Dogan et al. 2000); p53 protein, shown in about 17–40% of DLBCLs (Navaratnam et al. 1998; Piris et al. 1994; Sanchez et al. 1998; Kramer et al. 1996); CD44 isoforms, particularly CD44V6, expressed in about 30% of DLBCLs (Inagaki et al. 1999); caspase B, present in the cytoplasm of some DLBCLs (Donoghue et al. 1999); and survivin, an inhibitor of apoptosis, which is overexpressed in various human cancers, and detected in about 60% of the cases (Adida et al. 2000).

CD10 and bcl-6 are suitable for the diagnosis of the two types of DLBCLs described by microarrays techniques (see below; Chan and Huang 2001).

Summing up all immunohistochemical results and comparing them to DNA microarray profiles it becomes clear that the data may correlate with distinct clinicopathological features but do not predict clinical outcome (Colomo et al. 2003).

Genetics

In the majority of these tumors, a rearrangement of the heavy- and light-chain genes is demonstrated by PCR.

Chromosomal translocation leading to deregulation of specific oncogenes characterizes approximately 50% of cases of DLBCL (Rao et al. 1998). The three following translocations are most often detected: t(3;14)(q27;q32), t(8;14)(q24;q32), t(14;18)(q32;q21). Comparative genomic hybridization (CGH) analysis identified nine sites of chromosomal amplification. Six candidate amplified genes in a series of 96 DLBCLs were probed by quantitative Southern blotting (Rao et al. 1998). REL (2p12–16) amplification was associated with extranodal presentation. REL, MYC (8q24), BCL-2 (18q21), GLI, CDK4 and MDM 2 (12q13–14) amplifications were associated with advanced-stage disease (Rao et al. 1998).

The presence of a bcl-2 rearrangement was found more often in extensive (39%) and primary nodal (17%) lymphomas than in extranodal lymphomas (4%) (Kramer et al. 1998). This gene rearrangement did not significantly affect overall survival or disease-free survival. However, it correlates well with the germinal center B-cell gene expression signature and the expression of CD10 (Huang et al. 2002).

Rearrangement of bcl-6, which can occur with partners other than the Ig heavy-chain genes, is observed in about 20% (Muramatsu et al. 1996) to 30 or 35% of DLBCLs (Lo Cocco et al. 1994; Bastard et al. 1994; Otsuki et al. 1995b) and was found more often in patients with extranodal (36%) and advanced-stage (39%) presentation than in patients with primary nodal disease (28%), particularly in lymphomas expressing CD5 or CD30 (Capello et al. 2000) and in lymphoma with the morphology of centroblasts.

c-myc rearrangement is a relatively rare event (Levasseur et al. 1995) and have been shown in only 2% of primary nodal lymphomas and in 10% of primary extranodal lymphomas, particularly in gastrointestinal tract lymphomas (28%) which had a higher rate of complete remission (Kramer et al. 1998).

Using DNA-based techniques, mutations of p53 gene were disclosed in 22% of patients with DLBCL (Ichikawa et al. 1997).

Finally, translocations involving the IgH chain locus are more frequent in centroblastic (48.5%) than immunoblastic (25%) lymphoma according to Schlegelberger et al. (1999), who defined two distinct groups of DLBCL: one with translocations involving the IgH locus, corresponding mainly to the centroblastic group, and one showing chromosomal aberrations resembling those typically found in B-CLL and blastic mantle cell lymphoma, corresponding to B-cell lymphoma of pregerminal origin mainly presenting with an immunoblastic morphology.

Differential Diagnosis

The DLBCLs have to be distinguished from: *undifferentiated carcinoma*, *amelanotic malignant melanoma*, *acute myeloid leukemia*, *anaplastic large-cell lymphoma of T-cell type*, and *histiocytic sarcoma*.

More rarely, reactive inflammatory disorders with immunoblastic hyperplasia can mimic DLBCL. Particularly viral diseases (infectious mononucleosis) and hypersensitivity to drugs can be responsible for such hyperplasias. Some EBV-associated lymphoproliferative disorders occurring in patients with immunodeficiencies are very difficult to distinguish from DLBCL and even sometimes represent borderline lesions able to transform into true DLBCL.

In all these cases, the morphology of the cells on imprints or section as well as immunohistochemistry, and in some instances molecular biology, are mandatory for diagnosing DLBCL.

Occurrence

DLBCLs represent about 30–40% of non-Hodgkin's lymphomas. They often develop in extranodal sites (40%). All extranodal DLBCLs will be discussed in the chapters on the different organs.

The median age is in the sixth to seventh decade, but with a broad range. Many cases involve younger adults, adolescents and, less frequently, children, with a slight male predominance.

DLBCLs arise either primarily or secondarily from so-called small-B-cell malignant lymphoma (see Chaps. 4.2.1) or from lymphocyte-predominant Hodgkin's lymphoma, nodular type (Hansmann et al. 1989).

There is no known etiology, but the frequency of DLBCL seems to be increasing. The roles of pesticides, hair dyes, and various viruses are under discussion. For example, Epstein-Barr virus (EBV) in large-B-cell lymphomas has been demonstrated by in situ hybridization of EBER-1 in about 18% of centroblastic lymphomas, 32% of immunoblastic lymphomas, 37.5% of B-ALC and 31.6% of plasmablastic lymphomas (Hummel et al. 1995). The significance of these findings is not known.

Clinical Features and Prognosis

DLBCLs are responsible for large nodal masses that increase rapidly in size and which are often locally compressive. Patients can present B symptoms. A high level of LDH is often measured in the plasma.

All these lymphomas are aggressive, the secondary more than the primary ones. Primary DLBCLs are potentially curable (Armitage et al. 1998). They may have a good response to polychemotherapy, either alone or associated with radiotherapy. Patients with stage I or II, and patients without B symptoms have a significantly better overall survival and failure-free survival (Nakamine et al. 1991). Patients with a Karnofsky score of 70 or more have a significantly better overall survival (Nakamine et al. 1991). Many multicentric therapeutic trials are studying whether a difference exists in the prognosis of patients depending on morphological variant. The members of the ILSG ruled out any predictive value of the subtypes of large-B-cell lymphomas, as defined in the up-dated Kiel classification, based on the absence of good reproducibility between the members of their group. In fact, a precise classification in the Kiel group can only been made using a large-sized biopsy fixed in formalin solution, and with good histological technique, and good staining using Giemsa stain. Different studies have reported controversial results. Some of them have not demonstrated any difference in the survival between patients with the two main subtypes, centroblastic and immunoblastic, as defined in the up-dated Kiel classification or in the WF (Kwak et al. 1991; Stein et al. 1990; Salar et al. 1998; Neilly et al. 1995). In a study published by Engelhard et al. (1997) on cases reviewed by Karl Lennert, a difference in survival and prognosis between centroblastic, immunoblastic, and anaplastic large B-cell lymphoma was demonstrated, with patients with centroblastic lymphoma showing better survival. Immunoblastic morphology was shown to be of independent prognostic significance in a multivariate analysis. The NHL Classification Project carried out a retrospective study of 1,378 cases of NHL and identified 455 DLBCLs according to the REAL classification (Diebold et al. 2001). Centroblastic lymphomas represented the most frequent type (85.4%), consisting of polymorphic (58.6%), monomorphic (17.1%) and multilobated (9.7%). Immunoblastic lymphomas comprised 11.2% of the cases, 8.3% with and 2.9% without plasmablastic differentiation. Anaplastic large-cell lymphoma of B-cell type (ALC-B) consisted of only 3.4% of the cases. For the 401 patients with adequate data, the 5-year overall survival was 47% and the 5-year failure-free survival (FFS) 42%. There was no significant difference in the survival of patients with the three major histological types. The 5-year overall survival was 51% for patients with centroblastic, 45% for those with immunoblastic, and 33% for those with ALC-B. The 5-year FFS was 43% for patients with centroblastic, 38% for those with immunoblastic and 33% for those with ACL-B. The IPI score were found to predict survival for the entire group of

DLBCL patients. DLBCL with and without immunoblasts, that is, centroblastic polymorphic plus immunoblastic plus anaplastic large-B-cell lymphomas, on the one hand, and centroblastic monomorphic and multilobate on the other, were compared. The second group comprised 119 patients, and the first 325 patients. There were no significant differences between these two groups for all of the clinical features and for the IPI scores. Comparison of the 5-years overall survival and FFS of these groups demonstrated a better survival for patients in group 2 versus those group 1 with immunoblasts. The greatest differences in FFS between the two groups appeared to occur in patients with low-risk disease (Diebold et al. 2001).

In multivariate analysis, only patients older than 60 years, stage III/IV disease, a poor performance status, and an elevated serum LDH level were independent predictors of poor survival, whereas neither the histological group nor the other clinical features was predictive. In a separate multivariate analysis including just the IPI scores and the two histological groups, only the IPI scores were predictive of survival (Diebold et al. 2001).

The presence of immunoblasts seemed to predict for worse survival in this study. Very similar results have been presented by Baars et al. (1999). Ohshima et al. (1999) also stressed the fact that patients with immunoblastic lymphoma have a worse prognosis than those with centroblastic.

Also, the GELA group in France (Morel et al. 1997, 2002) showed that immunoblastic lymphoma was an independent predictor of a poor prognosis when compared to centroblastic lymphoma using the up-dated Kiel classification.

The most important question concerns the number (or percentage) of immunoblasts needed to subclassify the DLBCLs. In the up-dated Kiel classification (Stansfeld et al. 1988; Lennert 1981), an immunoblastic lymphoma comprises less than 10% centroblasts and about 60–90% immunoblasts, and a polymorphic centroblastic lymphoma more than 10% centroblasts and more than 10% immunoblasts. The estimation of the percentage of these two types of cells is very difficult in practice. It can be done reproducibly only with excellent histological technique, including Giemsa staining, and evaluation by a well-trained pathologist. Additional difficulties exist in reproducibly assigning DLBCL to subcategories. Further studies are needed to assess the possibility of stratifying DLBCL according to the number of immunoblasts.

The presence or absence of certain biological markers influence the prognosis (Montserrat 2001). CD5-positive DLBCLs have a very poor outcome, with frequent relapse and a FFS curve identical to that in mantle cell lymphoma (Yamaguchi et al. 1999). CD5-positive and CD5-negative but CD10-positive may constitute clinically relevant subtypes (Harada et al. 1999).

Expression of the proteins of CD44 isoforms (involved in tumor dissemination), particularly CD44V6, has emerged as a significant indicator of poorer overall survival (Drillenburg et al. 1999; Inagaki et al. 1999).

The expression of caspase B, an enzyme crucial to the apoptotic process, is correlated with a poor prognosis (Donoghue et al. 1999).

Survivin protein was demonstrated in about 134 (60%) of the 222 patients studied, 96% having centroblastic lymphoma and 4% immunoblastic lymphoma in virtually all tumor cells. The overall 5-year survival rate was significantly lower in patients with survivin expression than in those without (40% vs 54%, $p=0.02$). Multivariate analysis incorporating the IPI identified survivin expression as an independent predictive parameter of survival ($p=0.03$) in addition to LDH, stage and Eastern Cooperative Oncology Group (ECOG) scale. A second analysis incorporating IPI as a unique parameter demonstrated that survivin expression ($p=0.02$) remained a prognostic factor for survival independent of IPI ($p=0.001$). Thus, survivin expression may be considered as an unfavorable prognostic factor for patients with DLBCL (Adida et al. 2000).

The p53 status also seems to have prognostic significance (Nieder et al. 2001). In two studies, expression of p53 protein was associated with shorter survival (Navaratman et al. 1998; Piris et al. 1994). But this was not confirmed in two other studies f (Kramer et al. 1996; Sanchez et al. 1998). In a multivariate analysis, demonstration of p53 mutation was associated with a significantly shorter survival rate (Ichikawa et al. 1997).

Abnormal expression of p27 KIPI is associated with an adverse clinical outcome (Saez et al. 1999; Sanchez-Beato et al. 1999).

Expression of bcl-2 oncoprotein is associated with an aggressive course (Hermine et al. 1996; Hill et al. 1996; Kramer et al. 1996; Gascoyne et al. 1997; Monni et al. 1999).

bcl-6 rearrangement has no prognostic value,

whereas c-myc rearrangement is associated with a higher rate of complete remission (Kramer et al. 1996).

The 3q27 translocation seems to be associated with a better prognosis (Gascoyne et al. 1999).

New approaches would probably be useful, for example, studies of chromosomal and gene amplification (Rao et al. 1998; Capello et al. 2000) or DNA microarrays. Further studies combining morphology, immunophenotype and gene expression will also be of great interest.

Shipp et al. (2002) analyzed the DNA microarray expression of 6,817 genes in diagnostic tumor specimens from DLBCL patients treated by CHOP-based chemotherapy. They applied a supervised learning prediction method to identify patients who would be cured versus those with fatal or refractory disease. Two categories of patients showing very different 5-year overall survival rates (70% vs 12%) were distinguished. The authors recognized 13 genes implicated in DLBCL outcome including some that regulate responses to B-cell-receptor signaling, critical serine/threonine phosphorylation pathways, and apoptosis.

Of these 13 genes, nor1, pde4b and pkc-β2 isoform were correlated with outcome in the DLBCL patient series of Alizadeh et al. (2000).

The following genes were expressed at higher levels in DLBCL than in follicular lymphoma: lactate dehydrogenase, transferrin receptor, cyclin B1 and a CDC47 homolog (both associated with cellular proliferation) cathepsins B and D (associated with invasion and metastasis), high-mobility-group protein isoforms I and Y (HMGIY) (which are a myc protein target), hematopoietic cell kinase (HCK) (linked with CD44 signaling), and inhibitors of apoptosis such as galactine 3Ca (carbohydrate-binding protein), BFL1A1, also called BCL2A1 (a bcl2-related protein).

The authors then used immunohistochemistry to confirm these results. With a monoclonal antibody against PKC-β, they demonstrated the expression of this protein on paraffin-section. Expression was closely associated with a poor clinical outcome, while cured DLBCL patients were negative for pKC-β. These results validate the microarray measurement approach and confirm that microarray-based studies can be extended using methods that are more widely available in routine clinical practice.

4.2.2.2 Diffuse Large-B-Cell Lymphoma – Morphological Variants

The following variants are recognized:

1. Centroblastic lymphoma
2. Immunoblastic lymphoma
3. B-immunoblastic lymphoma expressing ALK-1
4. Anaplastic large-B-cell lymphoma
5. Plasmablastic lymphoma
6. T-cell-rich/histiocyte-rich large-B-cell lymphoma

4.2.2.2.1 Centroblastic Lymphoma

Synonyms

- Kiel: Centroblastic lymphoma
- REAL: Diffuse large-B-cell lymphoma

Definition

This category is applied in the updated Kiel classification to all high-grade/large-cell malignant lymphomas whose blast cells are exclusively or partially centroblasts. Centroblasts have round nuclei with a vesicular chromatin and two to four mostly marginal nucleoli. Within the category of centroblastic lymphoma, the number of admixed immunoblasts or multilobate cells and centroblast like cells is variable; the borderline between this type and B-immunoblastic lymphoma is not well-defined and has to be drawn arbitrarily (according to the number of immunoblasts; see Lukes and Collins 1975a, b). Only if immunoblasts clearly dominate the lymphoma is it described as immunoblastic B-cell lymphoma. Lymphomas with more than about 20% clearly recognizable centroblasts fall into the category of centroblastic lymphoma.

Morphology

The growth pattern is usually diffuse. In approximately 10% of tumors, however, a follicular growth pattern is recognizable. Such cases are borderline or equivalent to follicular lymphoma grade 3b (cohesive sheets of centroblasts) (see Chap. 4.2.1.6). Occasionally, there is show a follicular and diffuse proliferation of the tumor cells. The term follicular lymphoma is added to diffuse large-cell lymphoma if at least 25% of the infiltrated area shows a follicular growth pattern.

Scattered groups of epithelioid cells can sometimes be observed. A starry-sky cellular pattern and a certain degree of cohesiveness may also be present. FDC are rarely found.

There are a large number of mitotic figures (5–6/high-power field). Reticulin fibers are scanty. PAS staining rarely reveals positive globular inclusions in the tumor cells.

In the Kiel classification, four subtypes were cytologically characterized by Hui et al. (1987). The centrocytoid centroblastic lymphoma is omitted in this chapter as it has become clear that this subtype is a variant of mantle cell lymphoma. Today, it is also clear that there is a strong overlap between the three remaining categories of monomorphic, polymorphic, and multilobate centroblastic lymphoma of the Kiel classification, and a distinction is therefore arbitrary. Thus, we no longer use these subgroups in the diagnosis. The most important distinction also regarding the clinical aspects has to be made between centroblastic and immunoblastic B-cell lymphoma.

Centroblastic lymphoma covers a cytological spectrum which lies in between the previously described monomorphic subtype (Fig. 4.63) and the polymorphic subtype. In about 20% of centroblastic lymphomas, typical centroblasts dominate, which gives the tumor a monotonous-looking appearance (Fig. 4.64). The centroblasts may be medium-sized or large (10–14 µm). The nuclei are round and have fine chromatin, which makes them look relatively pale. In about one-third of the tumors, the cells have pleomorphic nuclei, whose appearance is otherwise identical to that of the round nuclei. The nuclei have two to four small or medium-sized nucleoli, which are frequently marginal. Cytoplasm is scanty and basophilic.

The centroblasts may be interspersed with a few centrocytes, centrocytoid cells, and immunoblasts. When more than 10% of the tumor cells are immunoblasts, the lymphoma is classified as belonging to the polymorphic subtype of centroblastic lymphoma (Fig. 4.65).

By examining a lymph node imprint it is very easy to recognize a typical centroblast because of its scanty, markedly basophilic cytoplasm and round nucleus with multiple nucleoli.

The majority of tumors clearly consist of a mixture of cells. All tumors show typical centroblasts and centrocytoid cells. There are often a few multilobate centroblasts as well. These cells are a strong indication of the germinal-center origin of the tumor. Immunoblasts are present in variable numbers. In most cases they stand out because of their size and morphology (large, central nucleoli; abundant, basophilic cytoplasm).

In about 10% of the tumors one may find a greater number of cells with lobate nuclei, i.e. nuclear lobations are evident at first glance (Fig. 4.66). As a rule, the

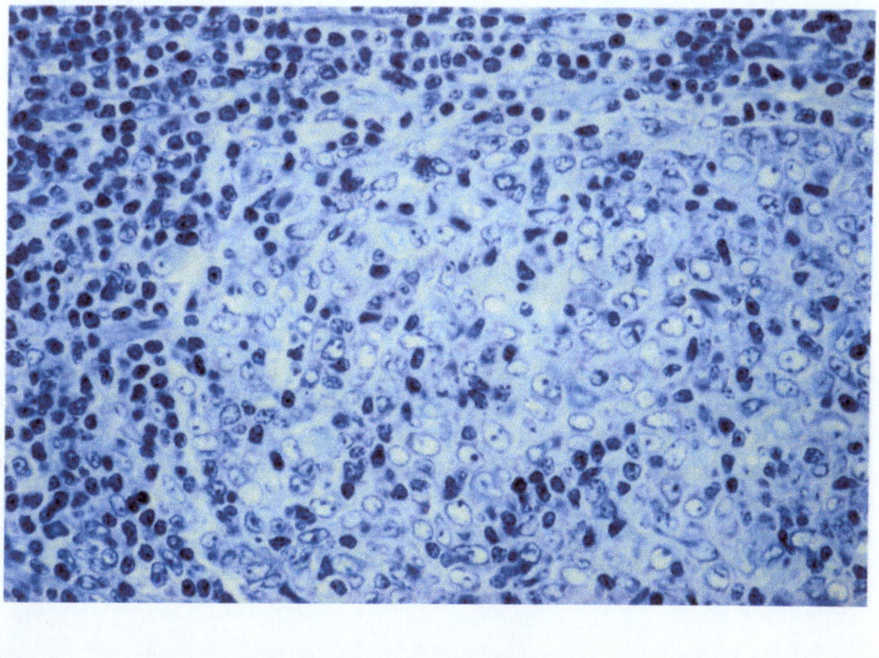

Fig. 4.63. Large-B-cell lymphoma, monomorphic centroblastic type, with a follicular growth pattern. The large cells in the follicles exhibit a typical centroblast morphology with pale chromatin, two to four medium-sized nucleoli symmetrically disposed, and a small basophilic cytoplasm (Giemsa stain)

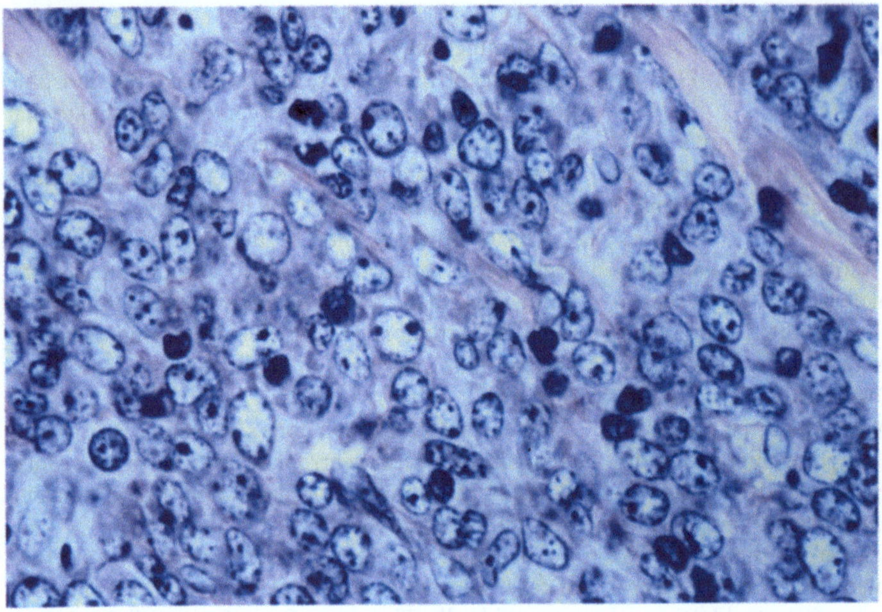

Fig. 4.64. Diffuse large-B-cell lymphoma, centroblastic type, monomorphic. The majority of the large or medium-sized lymphoma cells have a typical centroblast morphology (Giemsa stain)

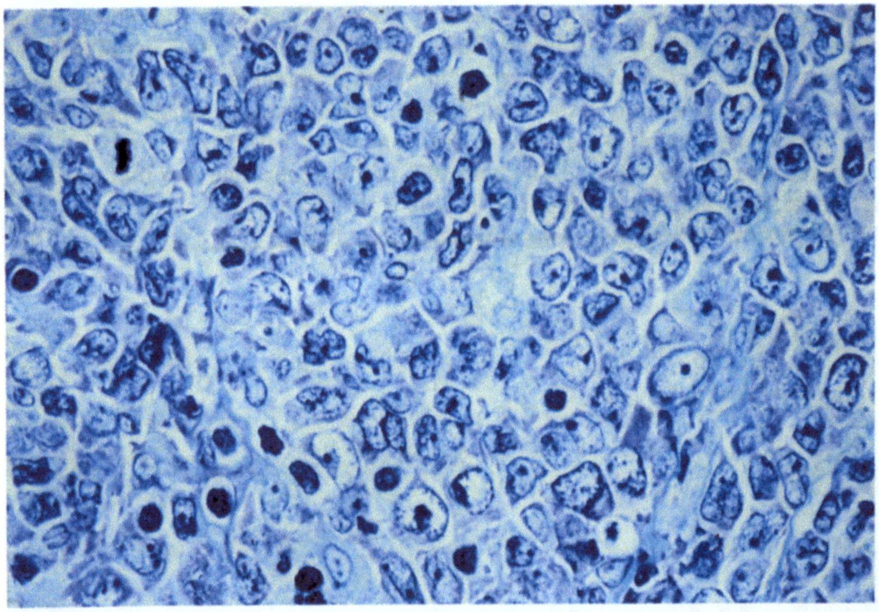

Fig. 4.65. Large-B-cell lymphoma, centroblastic type, polymorphic. Immunoblasts with a large, single, centrally situated nucleolus are associated with centroblasts (Giemsa stain)

nuclei have three or four lobations (Fig. 4.67). The cells are usually medium sized (11 – 13 μm). Occasionally, very large cells of otherwise identical appearance can be observed. The chromatin is fine. It is often difficult to recognize the nucleoli; when they are visible, they are usually medium-sized and marginal, like those of typical centroblasts. The cytoplasm is scanty to moderately abundant and moderately basophilic, but occasionally pale. Usually other types of germinal-center cells are also present in variable numbers and as mixtures, i.e. centroblasts, centrocytes, centrocytoid centroblasts and immunoblasts (Van Baarlen et al. 1988). Silver staining reveals that the tumor cells grow in narrow or large, compact complexes surrounded by thick fibers.

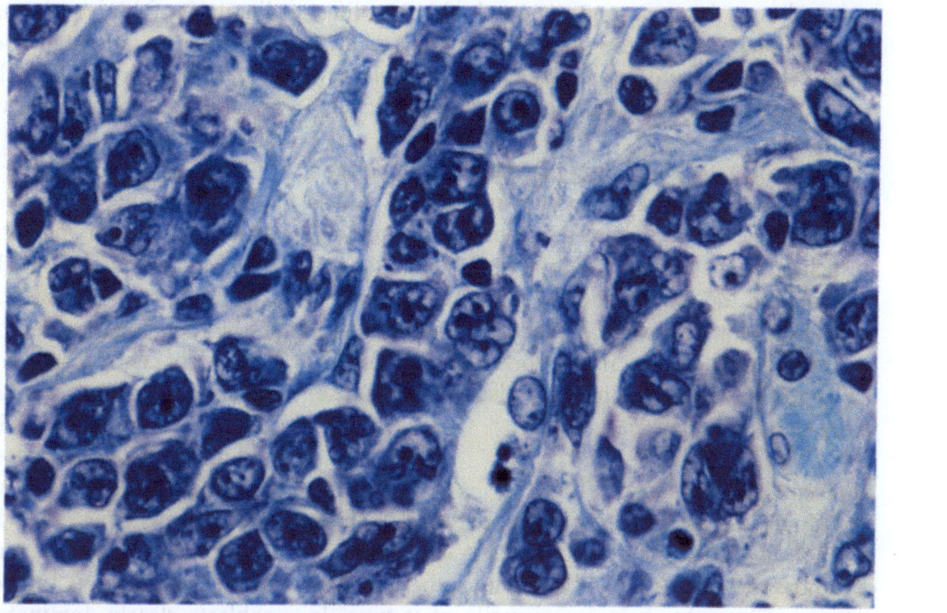

Fig. 4.66. Large-B-cell lymphoma, centroblastic type, multilobated. Some of the cells exhibit a multilobate nucleus (Giemsa stain)

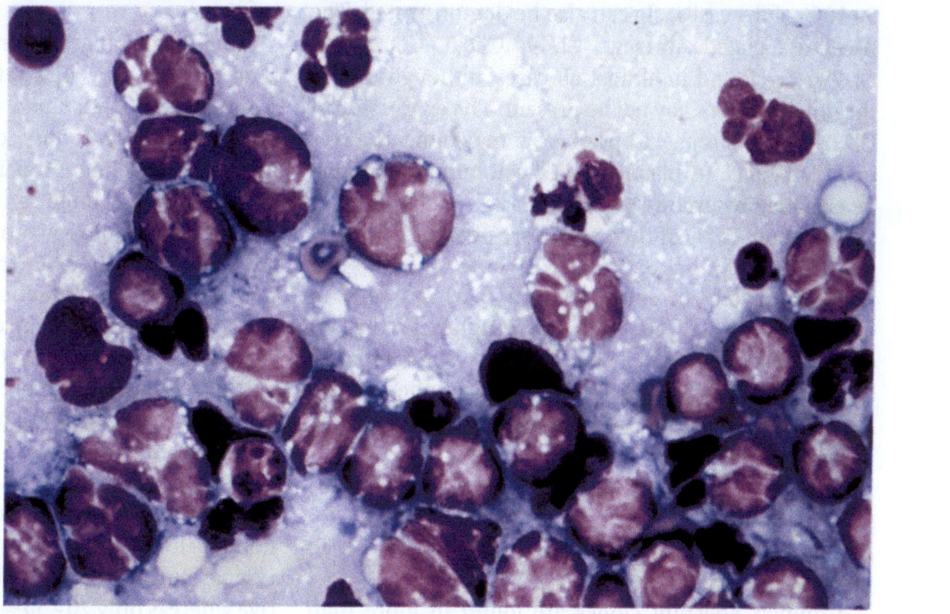

Fig. 4.67. Large-B-cell lymphoma, centroblastic type, multilobated. In this imprint, many cells have a nucleus divided in two to five lobes (May-Grünwald-Giemsa stain)

Transformation
The evolution of centroblastic cells is similar to that of most other diffuse large-cell lymphomas. Centroblastic lymphoma does not transform to other diffuse large-cell lymphomas during its clinical course or during relapse. However, this lymphoma type is the one which most frequently develops from low-grade follicular lymphoma grades 1 and 2 (Wendum et al. 1997).

As mentioned in Chap. 4.2.1.6, follicular lymphoma grades 1 and 2 may evolve into a centroblastic lymphoma in a considerable number of cases. The transformation may occur at the same time as the development of follicular lymphoma, that is, besides the typical follicular lymphoma, there are monotonous-looking proliferations of blast cells in the same lymph node or elsewhere. We designate such cases as *simultaneously* developed (in principle), secondary centroblastic lymphoma.

A centroblastic lymphoma may also develop after a number of months or a few or even many years; this is called *subsequent* secondary centroblastic lymphoma. In such cases, the follicular lymphoma is no longer recognizable in the lymph node. Occasionally, however, one can still find the original follicular lymphoma proliferation elsewhere, e.g. in the bone marrow. Secondary centroblastic lymphoma may also develop subsequent to immunocytoma.

Immunohistochemistry

sIg, chiefly of IgM type, can be demonstrated in 60–70% of centroblastic lymphomas. A small number of tumors show expression of IgG, while others are sIg-negative. The light-chains are usually of κ type. In 5–10% of the cases, cIg can also be demonstrated. The B-cell-associated antigens CD19, CD20, CD22 and CD79α are found in almost all cases, although one or the other antigen may not be present. The expression of CD23 and CD5 is an exception, as it may indicate a secondary DLBCL. A blastic mantle cell lymphoma must be excluded by cyclin D1 staining.

About 30–50% of the tumors are positive for bcl-2, and 70–90% for bcl-6.

FDC (usually in small residual foci) are seen in about one-third of centroblastic lymphomas that do not have a follicular growth pattern. Approximately 25% of the tumors express CD10. The number of cells expressing Ki-67 lies between 25 and 80% (mean: 50%).

Genetic Features

Heavy-chain Ig genes are rearranged in almost all cases.

Complex aberrant clones are found in more than 70% of centroblastic lymphomas; 30% of the cases carry the t(14;18) translocation. Deletions in 1q42, duplications in 1q23–32, trisomy 5 and changes in 15q were identified as independent prognostic markers (Schlegelberger et al. 1999).

Diagnosis and Differential Diagnosis

Typical centroblasts and multilobate centroblasts are unmistakable signs of centroblastic lymphoma. For a diagnosis of this lymphoma type among DLBCLs, these cells must be present in at least small numbers (>20%). A partial follicular growth pattern is also proof of a centroblastic lymphoma when the tumor cells are of blastic nature.

The indefinite borderline between centroblastic lymphoma and *immunoblastic B-cell lymphoma* is evident. Although the morphological distinction is arbitrary, so far some reports have shown that the distinction might be of clinical relevance. The definition used in the Kiel classification draws a line in relation to the number of centroblasts and immunoblasts. A centroblastic lymphomas is still diagnosed when at least 10–20% of the tumor cells are definitely centroblasts and multilobate centroblasts. One justification for this definition is the fact that such tumors may show a follicular growth pattern, which emphasizes the germinal-center nature of the tumor cells. An immunoblastic B-cell lymphoma is thus diagnosed when the immunoblasts clearly dominate over all other cells of the infiltrate.

Some centroblastic lymphomas with a monomorphic centroblastic infiltrate have to be distinguished from *Burkitt's lymphoma*. For this purpose it is absolutely necessary to use optimum histological techniques because inappropriate fixation and embedding of the tissue specimen can cause the central nucleoli of Burkitt's lymphoma to move to the nuclear membrane and hence to imitate centroblastic lymphoma cells. The nuclei of Burkitt's lymphoma cells are more intensely stained that those of centroblastic lymphoma cells and they have coarser chromatin. Cohesiveness and a starry-sky cellular pattern are typical features of Burkitt's lymphoma, but they are also found in a few cases of centroblastic lymphoma. There are certainly a few cases that cannot be clearly classified by morphological methods alone as being of one or the other type. Immunohistochemistry is very helpful for the diagnosis of typical Burkitt's lymphoma. The cells are CD10-positive whereas only 20–30% of centroblastic lymphomas express this antigen. They also do not express bcl-2, and 95% or more of the tumor cells are mib-1 (Ki67)-positive.

The *centrocytoid or blastoid/lymphoblastoid variant of mantle cell lymphoma* must be distinguished from diffuse centroblastic lymphoma. The cells in the variant of mantle cell lymphoma are smaller(9–11 μm). The nuclei are sometimes elongate or oval or even irregular, usually with two to five small, basophilic, central nuclei. The chromatin in the mantle cell variant is slightly coarser, and there is less cytoplasm. If the whole area of the infiltrate is carefully searched, one almost always finds smaller areas or foci of typical mantle cell lymphoma cells with strongly indented nuclei.

This differential diagnosis always has to be confirmed by immunohistochemistry. The mantle cell lymphoma variant is mostly CD5- and cyclin-D1-positive, in contrast to centroblastic lymphoma.

Follicular centroblastic lymphoma has to be distinguished from follicular lymphoma grade 3 and from other types of diffuse large-cell lymphoma, particularly from immunoblastic lymphoma.

When we draw the line in the Kiel classification between follicular lymphoma (centroblastic-centrocytic lymphoma) and centroblastic lymphoma, the actual number of centroblasts is not the only decisive factor. We diagnose centroblastic lymphoma only when solid sheets of centroblasts have replaced at least one circumscribed area of a lymph node. This is now more or less equivalent to follicular lymphoma grade 3b.

Occurrence

Centroblastic lymphoma is the most frequent type of high-grade malignant lymphoma. Among diffuse large-cell lymphomas, they make up about 75% of all cases (Engelhardt et al. 1997; The Non-Hodgkin's Lymphoma Classification Project 1997).

Primary centroblastic lymphoma occurs in all age groups, but there is a peak incidence in the seventh decade. Cases in childhood are exceptional but they do exist. In the Kiel collection the youngest patient was 1 year old, the oldest 97. The male-to-female ratio is about 1.2:1

Clinical Presentation and Prognosis

Schmalhorst et al. (1979; see also Stewart et al. 1986) published the first paper drawing attention to the clinical differences between centroblastic and immunoblastic lymphoma. In the present context it is interesting that 6% of patients with centroblastic lymphoma and 6% of those with immunoblastic lymphoma showed a leukemic blood picture or paraproteinemia. About 70% of patients with centroblastic lymphoma are in stage III and IV at the beginning of treatment. The relapse rate is around 30% compared to 70% in immunoblastic B-cell lymphomas (Engelhardt et al. 1997). Stewart et al. (1986) described the clinical findings in a relatively large series of American cases.

bcl-2 protein expression has been shown to be an independent prognostic risk factor but does not influence overall survival.

Patients with primary centroblastic lymphoma show a higher survival rate than do those with any other type of high-grade malignant lymphoma (Strauchen et al. 1978; Meusers et al. 1979). A comparison of the subtypes reveals that the monomorphic subtype has a significantly better prognosis than the others (Brittinger et al. 1984). *NB:* The "special cases" of centroblastic lymphoma described by Brittinger et al. largely correspond to what is now called the centrocytoid subtype.

The *prognosis* of simultaneous secondary centroblastic lymphoma corresponds to that of primary centroblastic lymphoma (all subtypes taken together), whereas subsequent secondary centroblastic lymphoma shows a much poorer prognosis (Brittinger et al. 1984; H. Bartels 1985, personal communication).

4.2.2.2.2 Immunoblastic Lymphoma

Synonyms

- Kiel: Immunoblastic lymphoma of B-cell type
- REAL: Diffuse large-B-cell lymphoma

Definition

This term is applied, in the up-dated Kiel classification, to a diffuse proliferation of large cells showing an abundant cytoplasm, often intensely basophilic (with Giemsa stain), surrounding an oval or round nucleus with open chromatin and a large, central, solitary nucleolus.

Definition of immunoblastic lymphoma is still not easy, most likely due to the poor reproducibility of the distinction between centroblastic and immunoblastic lymphomas. We think that this type of lymphoma should comprise less than 10% centroblasts and about 60–80% immunoblasts as well as a variable number of blast cells of variable sizes. Such blast cells may show a plasmacytic differentiation and are particularly numerous in immunoblastic lymphoma with "plasmacytoid" differentiation.

Morphology

B-immunoblastic lymphoma shows a diffuse growth pattern. A majority of the tumor cells are large, with basophilic cytoplasm in Giemsa stain and an oval or round pale nucleus containing a large, usually solitary, central nucleolus. In some cases the cytoplasm is clear and immunohistochemistry is needed to distinguish the cells from peripheral T-cells with an immunoblastic morphology (Nakamine et al. 1991). A few centroblasts (less than 10%) can be observed as well as cells presenting a plasmacytoid differentiation: plasmablasts, proplasma cells, even mature plasma cells. Mitoses are numerous (7–8/high-power field). Numerous reactive macrophages with abundant pale cytoplasm, containing debris of phagocytosed tumor cells (tingible bodies of macrophages) can be interspersed between the immunoblasts forming a starry-sky pattern. In some cases, groups of epithelioid cells with intensely acidophilic cytoplasm and no sign of phagocytosis of apoptotic debris can be observed.

Reticulum fibers in silver impregnation are sparse

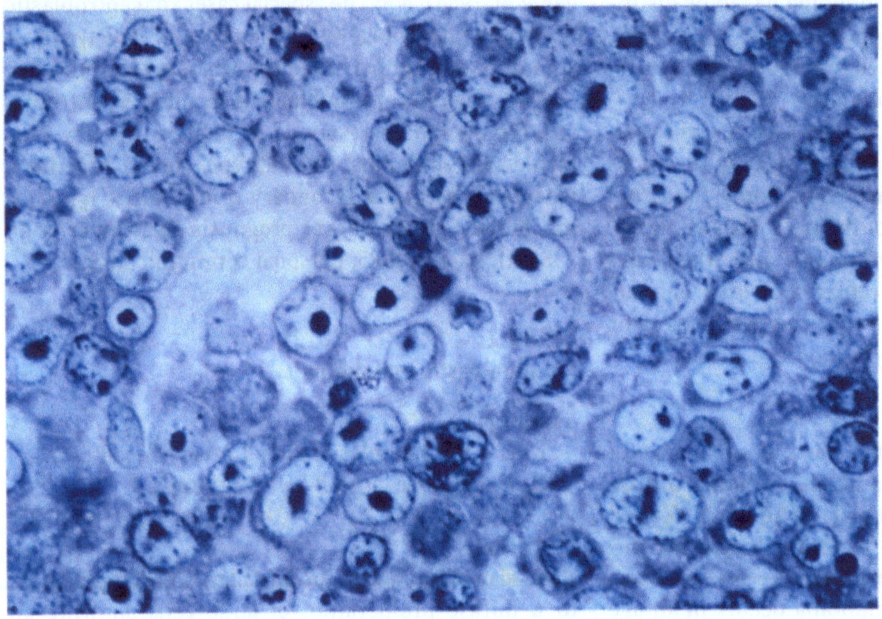

Fig. 4.68. Large-B-cell lymphoma, immunoblastic type without plasmablastic differentiation (Giemsa stain)

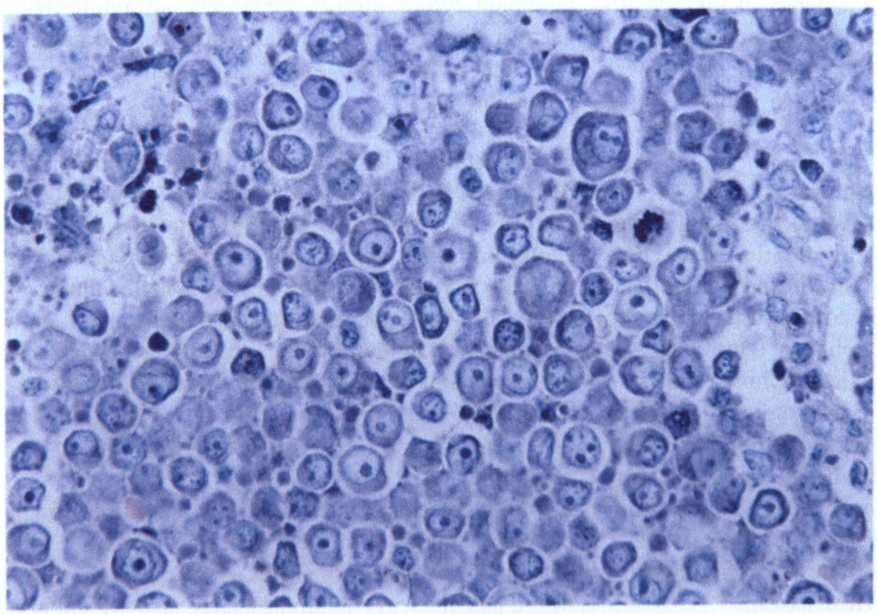

Fig. 4.69. Large-B-cell lymphoma, immunoblastic type with plasmablastic differentiation (Giemsa stain)

in half of the cases. In the other half, a slight to moderate increase in the number of fibers is observed. Necrosis can be present.

Finally, three subtypes can be recognized:

I. *B-immunoblastic lymphoma without plasmacytoid/plasmablastic differentiation* (Fig. 4.68)
The great majority of the cells present the morphology of typical B-immunoblasts. Centroblasts are absent or rare as are plasmablasts, proplasmocytes or plasma cells.

II. *B-immunoblastic lymphoma with plasmacytoid/plasmablastic differentiation* (Fig. 4.69)
In addition to typical immunoblasts, numerous cells with the same morphology are somewhat smaller. The cytoplasm is markedly basophilic and sometimes accumulates on one side of the nucleus, often with a perinuclear pale area corresponding to an enlarged Golgi apparatus. These cells often have multiple, central, medium sized nucleoli (plasmablasts). One always finds medium-sized cells (10–15 μm) with a plasma cell morphology, a perinuclear hof and a nucleus with small chromatin clumps, and a centrally situated, medium-sized, single nucleolus (proplasma cell) as well as typical plasma cells. Epithelioid cell groups and sometimes even Langhans' giant cells are more often present than in the other subtype.

III. *B-immunoblastic lymphoma lymphocyte-rich*
In this subtype, a variable number of small lymphocytes is associated with the immunoblasts. These tumors probably represent immunoblastic lymphoma secondary to a small-B-cell lymphoma (see Chap. 4.2.1).

Immunohistochemistry

About 80 % of the tumors present monotypic surface immunoglobulins. A large majority express B-cell-associated antigens: CD20, CD79α. Tumors with plasmacytoid/plasmablastic differentiation may lose CD20 expression, but they are mostly positive for CD79α, CD38, and CD138. EMA is also often positive, particularly when there is plasmacytoid/plasmablastic transformation. In numerous cases (60–70 %), and in almost all tumors with plasmacytoid/plasmablastic differentiation, it is possible to demonstrate the presence of intracytoplasmic immunoglobulins, with mostly μ heavy-chain and restricted light-chain. CD5 can be demonstrated, mainly secondary to B-CLL. bcl-2 and bcl-6 oncoproteins are less expressed than in centroblastic lymphoma (Skinnider et al. 1999). Finally, heterogeneous expression of CD30 can be observed such that the distinction from an anaplastic large-cell lymphoma can be very difficult (Piris et al. 1990).

Genetics

Heavy- and light-chain genes are rearranged. Heterogeneous and complex chromosomal changes have been reported (Nashelsky et al. 1994). The chromosomes most commonly gained were 3,11,6,18 and the most common structural abnormalities involved band 14q32, band 18q21 and bands 6q16–21. The loss of chromosomes 7,9, and Y and deletions of 6q were also observed (Nashelsky et al. 1994). No unique, common, primary cytogenetic abnormality has been disclosed but a translocation at 14q32 may be the primary cytogenetic lesion in some cases (Nashelsky et al. 1994), corresponding to a t(14;18)(q32;q21) or to a t(3;14)(q27;q32). These two translocations are responsible for overexpression of bcl-2 and bcl-6 oncogenes, respectively. Translocations involving the IgH chain locus are less frequent (25 %) than in centroblastic lymphoma (48.5 %) (Schlegelberger et al. 1999).

Differential Diagnosis

B-immunoblastic lymphomas must be distinguished from *hyperimmune reactions* and *virus infections*. In both conditions, numerous immunoblasts are present either dispersed or in small clusters, often associated with lymphoid cells at different phases of plasmacytic differentiation. Reed-Sternberg-like cells may be found. The architecture may be completely destroyed.

Drug hypersensitivity to various drugs (for example, hydantoin) represents one example of an hyperimmune reaction. In addition to immunoblastic hyperplasia, drug hypersensitivity results in fibrinoid necrosis and infiltration by numerous eosinophils.

Viral diseases are mostly represented by infectious mononucleosis (Fig. 4.70). Small foci of necrosis are often observed. Immunohistochemistry demonstrates that some immunoblasts express a B-cell phenotype and others a T-cell phenotype with marked increase of CD8-positive cells. In addition, lymphoid cells showing a plasmacytoid differentiation contain intracytoplasmic polytypic immunoglobulins.

Rare cases of bacterial diseases, for example pseudo-tuberculosis lymphadenitis due to *Yersinia enterocolitica* are responsible for B- and T-cell immunoblastic

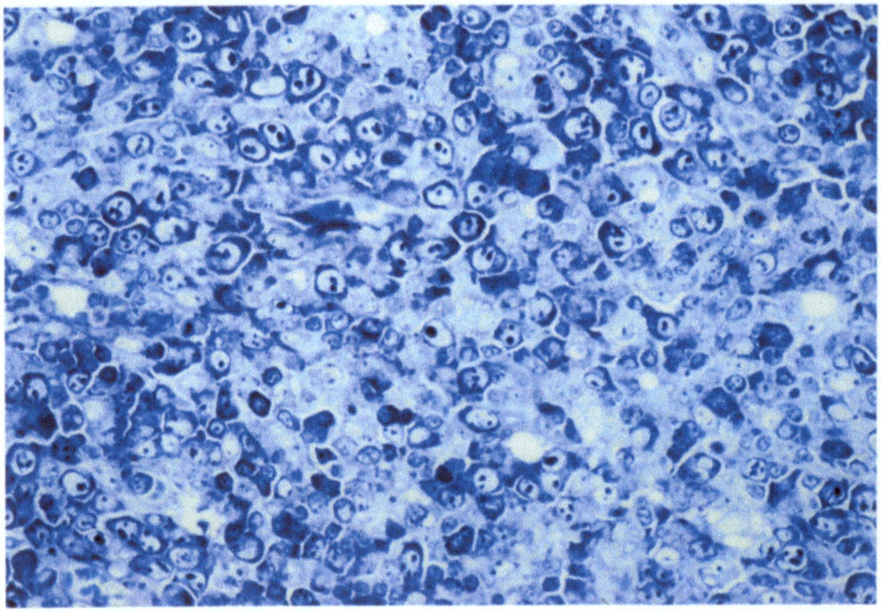

Fig. 4.70. Infectious mononucleosis. Diffuse infiltrate consisting of centroblasts immunoblasts, and many cells showing a plasmablastic and plasmacytic differentiation (Giemsa stain)

hyperplasia. The clinical presentation is very peculiar: fever with an abdominal syndrome simulating an acute appendicitis.

Finally, in some cases of necrotizing histiocytic lymphadenitis (Kikuchi-Fujimoto's lymphadenitis) which lack typical extensive apoptosis, immunoblastic hyperplasia can mimic a lymphoma; but apoptosis and a high content of histiocytes allow recognition of the disease.

Undifferentiated carcinomas, particularly lymphoepithelial carcinoma (Schmincke-Regaud's tumor of the nasopharynx), may be difficult to differentiate from immunoblastic lymphomas. The former are characterized by masses of large, moderately basophilic cells with strikingly pale nuclei (Lennert 1978). The nuclei contain large nucleoli, as do the nuclei of Hodgkin's cells. The tumor complexes in carcinoma contain numerous T-lymphocytes and interdigitating cells (S100-protein-positive). Between the tumor cell clusters there are often numerous inflammatory cells, especially eosinophils and plasma cells, and sometimes epithelioid cell granulomas as well. Even caseous-like necrosis is occasionally seen, mimicking tuberculosis (Rennke and Lennert 1973). With silver impregnation, the tumor-cell clusters, which are free of fibers, are often sharply demarcated from the fibrous regions of the residual lymphoid tissue. As a rule, the patient's blood serum shows elevated EBV-antibody titers, especially IgA viral capsid antigens (VCA). Immunohistochemistry demonstrates the absence of expression of CD45 and positivity for cytokeratins and EMA. Such cases of undifferentiated carcinoma are associated with an EBV infection and the neoplastic cells are LMP-1- and EBER-1-positive.

Other non-hematopoietic cell tumors, such as *malignant melanoma or malignant rhabdoid tumor*, can mimic immunoblastic lymphoma (Haas et al. 1981; Schmidt et al. 1989; Seo et al. 1988; Weeks et al. 1989). *Malignant rhabdoid tumor* is very similar to immunoblastic lymphoma, except that eosinophilic, round inclusions, either negative or weakly PAS-positive, are found in the cytoplasm of at least some tumor cells. Immunohistochemistry reveals vimentin as well as cytokeratin. This tumor originates in the kidney and usually affects children, but it can also occur in adults in soft tissues (Balaton et al. 1987).

Histiocytic neoplasms may look like immunoblastic lymphoma without plasmacytic differentiation, but often the cytoplasm is more abundant, gray and not basophilic. Again, immunohistochemistry is useful in showing the positivity of CD68, CD15, and lysozyme and the negativity of B-cell markers.

B-immunoblastic lymphoma can be distinguish from polymorphic centroblastic lymphoma by the presence of more than 10% typical centroblasts, from anaplastic plasmacytoma (myeloma) by the clinical presentation (multiple bone lesions, monoclonal serum component mainly IgA or IgG).

The distinction from anaplastic large-cell lymphoma may be difficult, particularly with the monomorphic type. In anaplastic large-cell lymphoma, the cells are large, and the cytoplasm has a more irregular outline and is more abundant. The basophilia is variable, from site to site, in the same cell and from cell to cell. Nuclei are larger, more irregular, often polylobulate. These cells are organized in small clusters, infiltrating the sinuses, or organized around arteries. The diagnosis is particularly difficult in the monomorphic subtype without or with a few horse-shoe like nuclei. Immunohistochemistry is only useful when tumor cells express some T-cell markers. The reason is that immunoblastic lymphomas express CD30 and even EMA, as does anaplastic large-cell lymphoma.

The diagnosis of anaplastic large-cell lymphoma of B-cell type is based only on the morphology of the tumor cells.

Some peripheral T-cell lymphomas, unspecified, with predominant large-cells may present with an immunoblastic morphology. In the up-dated Kiel classification these have been called T-immunoblastic lymphomas. Usually, the morphology of the cells of B and T-immunoblastic lymphomas is similar. Only immunohistochemistry allows them to be distinguished. Sometimes, a few differences can be observed between the two types (Nakamine et al. 1991). A clear cytoplasm is more frequently seen in T-cell immunoblastic lymphomas, which often show more pleomorphic nuclei with a higher mitotic rate. These tumors sometimes present as an interfollicular proliferation with an increase in capillary-sized blood vessels and infiltration by eosinophils. Necrosis and fibrosis are less frequent. T-cell immunoblastic lymphomas are more frequent in males, and occur at a younger age (fourth decade). Despite a lower stage disease in B-cell immunoblastic type, there is no difference in survival between the B-cell and T-cell types (Weisenburger 1991).

Occurrence

In the Kiel register of lymph nodes, about 4.3% of all cases of NHL were diagnosed as B-immunoblastic lymphoma. The disease shows a peak incidence in the seventh decade of life. The youngest patient was 43 months old, the oldest 91 years old. The male to female ratio is about 1.1:1.

Clinical Presentation and Prognosis

The clinical presentation and prognosis of B-immunoblastic lymphoma are very similar to that of other large-B-cell lymphomas (Schmalhorst et al. 1981). Superficial, often cervical lymph nodes are involved most frequently. In many cases, the lymph nodes are enlarged only on one side of the diaphragm. Bone marrow and liver are not infiltrated as often as they are in most other types of NHL (Schmalhorst et al. 1981).

A leukemic blood picture is very rare. Paraproteinemia, usually IgM, is evident in 10–15% of patients.

The evolution is aggressive and the prognosis in adult patients is poorer than that of most other types of large-B-cell lymphomas. The 5-year survival rate is approximately 50% or less.

Addendum: Secondary B-Immunoblastic Lymphoma

Synonyms

- Kiel: B-immunoblastic lymphoma with a high content of lymphocytes
- REAL: Not listed

Definition

This type of B-immunoblastic lymphoma is not well-known and has not been included in the new WHO classification. It represents a transformation of a small-B-cell lymphoma and is associated with an accelerated clinical disease course.

Morphology

Large immunoblastic cells associated with plasmablasts and a variable number of plasma cells are organized in dense groups or spread over a background comprising either numerous B-cells, sheets of lymphoplasmacytoid and plasma cells, or a more polymorphic cell population with medium to large T-lymphoid cells having a clear cytoplasm, plasma cells, histiocytes, and eosinophils.

This type of B-immunoblastic lymphoma can best be detected by immunohistochemistry. It occurs either in the setting of B-CLL, representing a transformation earlier described as Richter syndrome, or in transformation from lymphoplasmacytic lymphoma, MALT lymphoma or during an angioimmunoblastic T-cell lymphoma. It may also represent the most frequent type of lymphoma occurring in patients with auto-immune diseases: congenital immune deficiencies, immunosuppression in transplanted patients, Sjögren's syndrome, systemic lupus erythematosis, rheumatoid arthritis, and Hashimoto's disease (Lichtenstein).

Immunohistochemistry
Due to the frequent plasmacytoid differentiation, the lymphomatous cells may not express CD20, but are mostly positive for CD79α. Intracytoplasmic immunoglobulins with a light-chain restriction are often demonstrated, with a predominance of μ heavy-chain. Expression of CD5 is recognized in cases secondary to classic B-CLL or to its plasmacytoid variant. B-immunoblastic lymphoma secondary to angioimmunoblastic type T-cell lymphoma is often LMP-1 positive. bcl-2 or bcl-6 may be expressed. The number of Ki-67-positive cells is high (40–70%).

Genetics
Variable complex chromosomal abnormalities may be found. Immunoglobulin heavy- and light-chain genes are rearranged. The PCR-amplified IgH gene in DLBCL secondary to B-CLL and lymphoplasmacytic lymphoma may be either different or identical, indicating that in some cases the DLBCL arises from the same clone and that in other cases it represents a new malignant clone (Nakamura et al. 2000).

EBER-1 is positive in cases secondary to angioimmunoblastic T-cell lymphoma.

Differential Diagnosis
The diseases discussed for primary immunoblastic lymphoma are also discussed for secondary B-immunoblastic lymphoma.

The specific problem in this type of lymphoma is to recognize the transformation. The diagnosis of secondary immunoblastic lymphoma is easy when sheets of adjacent large cells (more than 20 or 50) are recognized, contrasting with the background constituted by the small-B-cell lymphoma. Transformation is less easy to recognize at an early phase and should only be diagnosed when more than 20% of large cells are discovered, and particularly when these large cells are organized in clusters.

The association of dispersed large cells and small lymphoid cells which occurs in small-B-cell lymphoma transforming into large-B-cell lymphoma has to be distinguished from large-B-cell lymphoma with a high content of T-cells.

Occurrence
Secondary immunoblastic lymphoma occurs in B-CLL, lymphoplasmacytic lymphoma, marginal zone lymphoma (either nodal, extranodal (MALT lymphoma) or primary splenic), and in angioimmunoblastic T-cell lymphoma type. It represents approximately 20% of all immunoblastic lymphomas.

Clinical Presentation and Prognosis
The disease can be diagnosed in a histopathological study of any biopsy at any moment of the evolution of small-B-cell lymphomas. In some cases, such transformation can be suspected when patients present B symptoms (fever, loss of weight, etc.) and/or develop a large bulky tumor mass. In patients with small-B-cell lymphoma, such a bulky mass should be biopsied or at least studied by needle aspiration and cytology.

Secondary immunoblastic lymphoma reflecting the transformation of the initial lymphoma has a poor prognosis and patients have a shorter survival rate than those with primary DLBCL.

4.2.2.2.3 B-Immunoblastic Lymphoma Expressing ALK-1

Synonyms
- Kiel: Not listed
- REAL: Not listed
- WHO: Diffuse large-B-cell lymphoma with full-length ALK

Definition
Lymphoma due to the proliferation of large cells with the morphology of immunoblasts, secreting immunoglobulins and expressing the ALK receptor kinase (Delsol et al. 1997). The normal cell counterpart is not known.

Morphology
The lymph node is diffusely infiltrated, either in part or completely destroyed, with invasion of the sinuses. The cell population is monomorphic, consisting of large cells resembling immunoblasts or anaplastic large cells (Fig. 4.71). The nucleus is round, pale with a large central nucleolus. The cytoplasm is abundant, amphophilic or basophilic with Giemsa stain (Fig. 4.71). Some cells exhibit a plasmablastic differentiation with a clear juxtanuclear area. A few giant cells with a Reed-Sternberg-like morphology may be recognized.

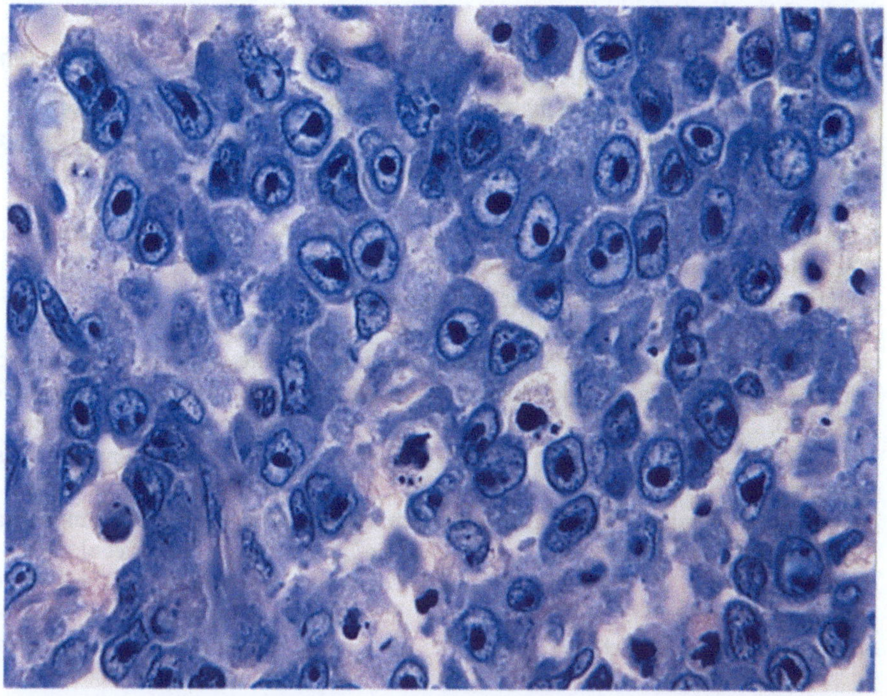

Fig. 4.71. B-immunoblastic-lymphoma, ALK-1-positive. The morphology of the cells is that of immunoblasts and sometimes that of large anaplastic cells, with an abundant, more or less basophilic cytoplasm (Giemsa stain)

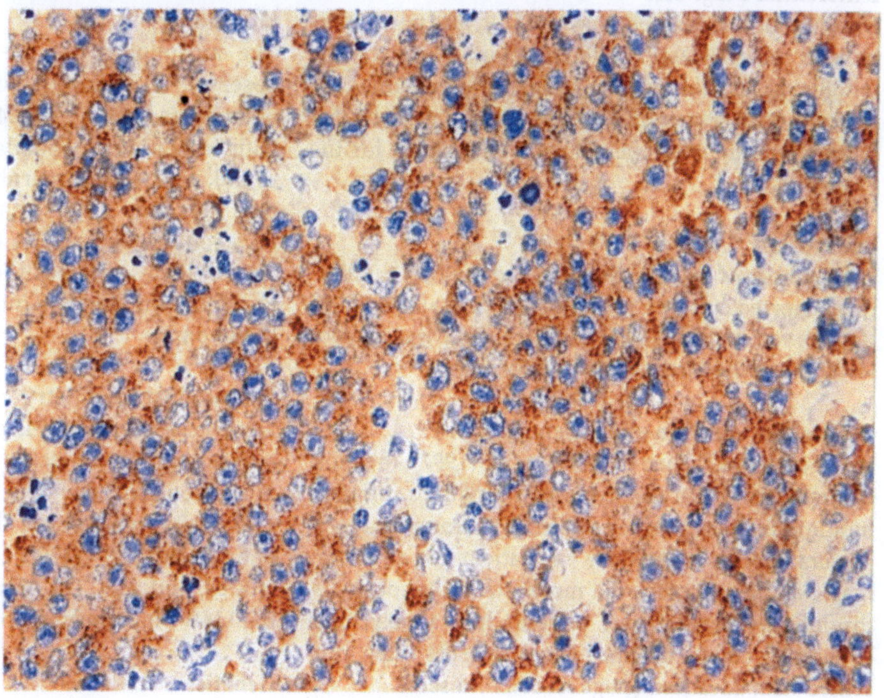

Fig. 4.72. Same patient as in Fig. 4.71. The tumor cells express ALK-1 (cytoplasmic positivity). They are also positive for EMA but not for CD30 or any B-cell markers. They contain intracytoplasmic IgA with a λ-light-chain restriction, demonstrating their B-cell origin (immunoperoxidase stain)

Immunohistochemistry

The large cells express CD45, often weakly, EMA strongly, but not CD30. They lack the B-markers CD20 and CD79α, but intracytoplasmic IgA with a light-chain restriction can be demonstrated. The tumor cells react also with the CD38 antibody detecting a plasma-cell-associated antigen. They also lack most of the T-cell markers, but are or may be positive for CD4 and CD57. They are typically labeled by antibodies (ALK-1) detecting both the intracytoplasmic and extracellular regions of the ALK receptor kinase. Positivity is observed in the cytoplasm by a granular pattern and near the nucleus by a dot-like pattern (Golgi area) (Fig. 4.72).

Genetics

Despite the expression of the ALK receptor kinase, the tumor cells do not have the t(2;5) translocation, and the resultant NPM-ALK fusion gene cannot be demonstrated. Only one patient with a trisomy 12 has been observed (Delsol et al. 1997).

Differential Diagnosis

B-immunoblastic lymphomas without, and particularly with plasmablastic differentiation, plasmablastic lymphoma and B-anaplastic large-cell lymphoma represent the three types of lymphomas that should be discussed. Immunohistochemistry is mandatory for the diagnosis.

Occurrence

The number of cases is very few, and the first publication reported on seven patients (Delsol et al. 1997). All but one was male. All were adult, only one was an adolescent, and the medium age was 51 years.

Clinical Presentation and Prognosis

In the series published by Delsol et al. (1997), the most common symptom was lymphadenopathies, often at multiple sites and even mediastinal. Splenomegaly was present in one patient. Only one patient had an abnormal hemogram: anemia, moderate lymphocytosis, thrombocytopenia. Three patients had a polyclonal hypergammaglobulinemia. Thus, patients often presented with advanced (stage III or IV) disease.

In most patients, the disease seems to follow an aggressive course despite polychemotherapy. One young patient with stage I disease remained in complete remission 13 years after treatment (Delsol et al. 1997).

4.2.2.2.4 Anaplastic Large-B-Cell Lymphoma

Synonyms

- Kiel: Large-cell anaplastic lymphoma of B-cell type
- REAL: Not listed
- WHO: Diffuse large-B-cell lymphoma, anaplastic variant

Definition

The existence of a B-cell diffuse large-cell lymphoma with anaplastic morphology and CD30 expression without the translocation t(2;5) or one of its variants has been recognized but is still controversial (Kuze et al. 1996; Engelhard et al. 1997; Tilly et al. 1997; The Non-Hodgkin's Lymphoma Classification Project 1997; Weisenburger et al. 2001). A recent publication finally recognized that some DLBCLs may present with a morphology mimicking anaplastic large-cell lymphoma associated with the expression of B-cell markers (Haralambieva et al. 2000).

Morphology

The morphology of the cells is identical to that observed in anaplastic large-cell lymphoma of T or null type (see Chap. 5.2.2.4). The tumor cells are large, with moderately abundant, gray cytoplasm, and round, oval or pleomorphic nuclei (Fig. 4.73). Some cells may have a horse-shoe-like nucleus. Giant cells occasionally occur. The carcinoma-like appearance predominates whereas the intrasinusoidal pattern is less common than in T/null type anaplastic large-cell lymphomas.

Immunohistochemistry

Large cells express CD45 and often CD30, but expression is sometimes weaker than in the T type and only intracytoplasmic, without membrane or dot-like Golgi area positivity. The cells also express B-cell-associated antigens (CD20, CD79α). EMA is not always demonstrated, and ALK-1 is negative. Some tumors expressing LMP-1 have been reported (Kuze et al. 1996).

Genetics

A Japanese report stresses the existence of a latent EBV infection of the tumor cells in 38% of the patients (Kuze et al. 1996).

The t(2;5) and related translocations have never

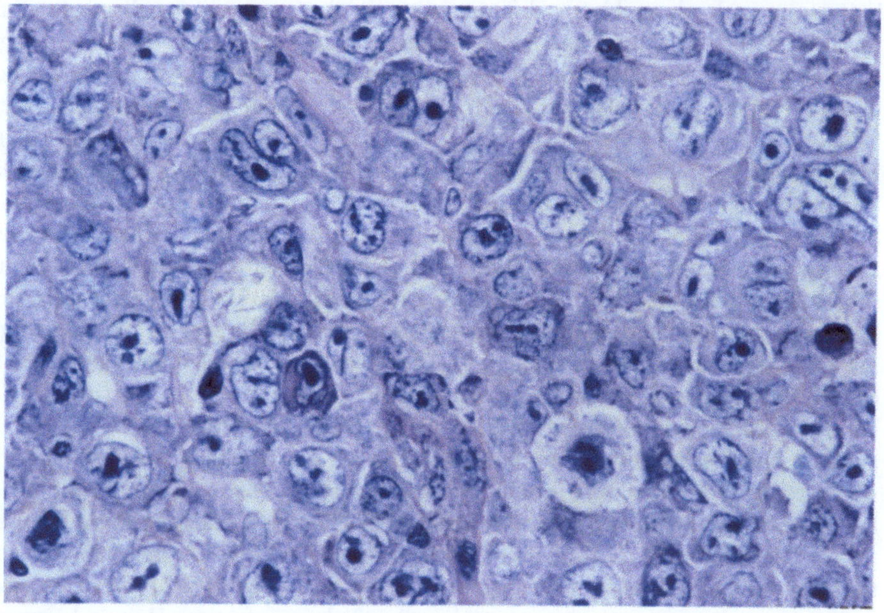

Fig. 4.73. Anaplastic large-B-cell lymphoma. The large tumor cells have an anaplastic morphology, but they express B-cell-associated antigens (Giemsa stain)

been demonstrated in these lymphomas (Haralambieva et al. 2000).

Differential Diagnosis

This type of anaplastic large-cell lymphoma should be clearly distinguished from the T- and/or null-type, which is defined by the immunophenotype and its molecular genetic profile.

The differential diagnosis includes other DLBCLs expressing CD30 and is based only on the morphology of the cells, i.e. centroblastic, immunoblastic or plasmablastic.

Occurrence

The number of cases is too small to have acquired sufficient data. The study of the Non-Hodgkin's Lymphoma Classification Project (1997) recognized 15 cases representing 3.4% of the patients (Weisenburger et al. 2001).

Clinical Presentation and Prognosis

The clinical presentation and prognosis of anaplastic large-B-cell lymphoma seem to be similar to that of other types of large-B-cell lymphomas.

The evolution is discussed controversially. The French GELA group reported on a series of anaplastic large-cell lymphomas, showing that the small number of patients with tumors of a B-cell immunophenotype have a poorer prognosis than those with the T or null type but a much better prognosis than those with other DLBCLs (Tilly et al. 1997). In other groups (Engelhard et al. 1997; The Non-Hodgkin's Classification Project 1997; Diebold et al. 2001; Weisenburger et al. 2001) the large-B-cell anaplastic lymphomas show the same poor evolution as other DLBCLs, particularly the immunoblastic type.

4.2.2.2.5 Plasmablastic Lymphoma

Synonyms

- Up-dated Kiel: Immunoblastic lymphoma with plasmablastic differentiation
- Real: Not listed
- WHO: Diffuse large-B-cell lymphoma, plasmablastic variant

Definition

Large-B-cell lymphoma with the morphology of immunoblastic lymphoma and plasmablastic differentiation presenting a peculiar immunophenotype (Delecluze et al. 1997; Brown et al. 1998; Dupin et al. 2000; Jaffe et al. 2001). This lymphoma is EBV-associated and occurs in HIV-positive patients, mainly in the oral cavity. The course is highly aggressive.

These types of lymphomas can also occur in HIV-negative patients, corresponding to immunoblastic lymphoma with plasmablastic differentiation in the up-dated Kiel classification, and have been included in a report on a series of HIV-positive patients with lymphoma (Raphaël et al. 1994; Diebold et al. 1997).

Morphology

The infiltration is diffuse, with destruction of the connective tissue and of the mucosa. The lymphoma cells are large, with an abundant amphophilic (with H and E) (Fig. 4.74) or basophilic (with Giemsa stain) cytoplasm. A clear paranuclear halo is often recognized as in plasmablasts (hypertrophic Golgi apparatus). The nucleus, eccentrically disposed, is round, oval or slightly irregular. The chromatin is dispersed giving a pale appearance. The nuclear membrane is often thick. There is a single, centrally situated, very prominent, large nucleolus in the majority of the cells. In other cells, often a little smaller, numerous medium-sized nucleoli occupy the center of the nucleus as in plasmablasts.

In many tumors, numerous apoptotic cells can be recognized, associated with many large macrophages containing tingible bodies. They are dispersed on a background of more or less cohesive tumor cells and form a starry-sky pattern. Mitoses are numerous.

Immunohistochemistry

The tumor cells are mostly CD45- (Delecluze et al. 1997; Jaffe et al. 2001) and CD20-negative or have a heterogeneous dispersion of only very faintly positive cells. By contrast, a stronger positivity is observed for CD79α and CD138, but not in all cells. Intracytoplasmic immunoglobulins are detected in the majority of the cells, with a light-chain restriction and expression of IgA or IgG. bcl-2 expression is heterogeneous with many negative cases; bcl-6 oncoprotein can be demonstrated in some cells in a very small number of patients. Ki-67-positive cells are numerous, often more than 90% of the tumor cells. In many patients, a few tumor cells express LMP-1. CD3-positive cells may be scarcely dispersed throughout the tumor cell sheets.

Genetics

Rearrangement of Ig heavy-chain, as demonstrated by PCR, confirms the monoclonality and the B-cell origin. No rearrangement of the bcl-2 gene can be found. EBER-1 is present in the nuclei of numerous cells in the majority of the cases, demonstrating a latent EBV infection. Human herpes virus 8 can also be demonstrated in HIV-positive patients (Dupin et al. 2000).

Differential Diagnosis

Plasmablastic lymphoma, as defined by Delecluze et al. (1997), represents a type of DLBCL occurring in HIV-positive patients. The same type of lymphoma can occur also in HIV patients, primarily in the serosa as a manifestation of the primary effusion lymphoma.

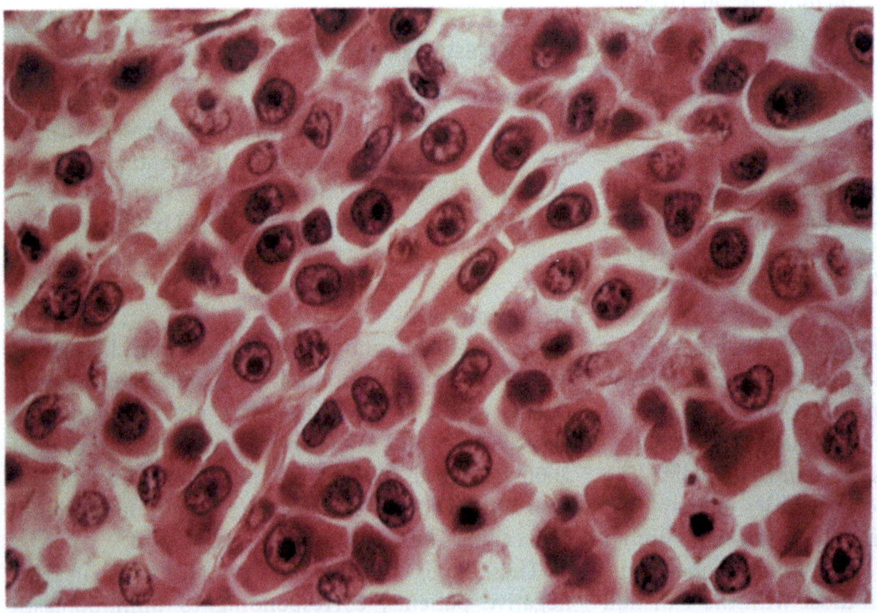

Fig. 4.74. Large-B-cell lymphoma, plasmablastic type. All of the tumor cells have a round nucleus with a single voluminous nucleolus and a very abundant cytoplasm containing monotypic IgA immunoglobulin (H and E stain)

The morphology and the immunophenotype are similar to those of immunoblastic lymphoma with plasmablastic differentiation, as described in the up-dated Kiel classification, particularly in HIV-positive patients (Raphaël et al. 1991, 1994; Diebold et al. 1997).

The most important differential diagnosis is represented by DLBCL secondary to transformation of multiple myeloma. Neither the morphology nor the immunophenotype allows differentiation between the two diseases. Only the presence of typical bone lesions and the presence of a monoclonal gammopathy demonstrate the origin as being from multiple myeloma. On the other hand, the presence of a latent EBV infection of the tumor cells, the absence of monoclonal gammopathy, and the demonstration of an HIV-positive serology strongly support a diagnosis of plasmablastic lymphoma.

Burkitt's lymphoma and even the variants should be easily excluded due to the large size of the tumor cells in plasmablastic lymphoma and the absence of typical medium-sized Burkitt's cells, even in the presence of a starry-sky cellular pattern, high mitotic rate, and a large number of Ki-67-positive cells.

Clinical Presentation and Prognosis

The majority of the patients (Delecluze et al. 1997) are HIV-positive homosexual males, drug addicts or both. Patients present with a tumor in the oral cavity, often localized on the gingiva, or sometimes involving the palatal mucosa. In some patients, early extension to the adjacent bone can be demonstrated on X-ray.

Staging of these patients sometimes discloses an extension to abdominal or retroperitoneal nodes which can develop during the course of the disease.

Bone involvement has also been shown by bone marrow biopsy at presentation or during evolution of the disease.

Despite the plasmablastic differentiation, no monoclonal Ig component can be detected in the serum.

A highly malignant behavior has been reported (Raphaël et al. 1991; Delecluze et al. 1997). As often observed in HIV-positive patients, the response to polychemotherapy with or without radiotherapy is poor. When the lymphoma is localized to the oral cavity, the response to radiotherapy alone may be good (Delecluze et al. 1997).

4.2.2.2.6 T-Cell-Rich/Histiocyte-Rich Large-B-Cell Lymphoma

Synonyms

- Kiel: Lymphocyte-rich B-cell lymphoma
- Real: B-cell lymphoma with a high content of T-cells

Definition

The *T-cell-rich large-B-cell lymphoma* was first designated as such by Ramsey et al. (1988) and is characterized by a diffuse infiltration of T-lymphocytes of small or medium size associated with a few dispersed large-B-cells (Scarpa et al. 1989; Chittal et al. 1991; Osborne et al. 1991a, b; Camilleri-Broët et al. 1996). The T-lymphocyte component should be quite numerous – at least 60–90% (Winberg et al. 1988; Ng et al. 1989; Baddoura and Chan 1991; Krishnan et al. 1991, 1994; Macon et al. 1992b; Rodriguez et al. 1993; De Wolf-Peeters and Pittaluga 1995). The large-B-cells show variable morphology (Camilleri-Broët et al. 1996), sometimes appearing as Reed-Sternberg-like cells (Chittal et al. 1990).

The *histiocyte-rich large-B-cell lymphoma* (Delabie et al. 1992; Sun et al. 1997) resembles T-cell-rich large-B-cell lymphoma, but in association with T-lymphocytes numerous histiocytes are seen (Delabie et al. 1992). The infiltration is mainly diffuse, although a faint nodularity may also be observed (Delabie et al. 1992).

Both lymphoma types are often misdiagnosed as Hodgkin's lymphoma or peripheral T-cell lymphoma.

The question whether such lymphomas represent a genuine specific entity or a peculiar presentation of DLBCL of follicular cell origin (Jaffe et al. 1991; Krishnan et al. 1991, 1994; Macon et al. 1992a, b; Camilleri-Broët et al. 1996; de Jong et al. 1996) is still controversial. An argument in favor of the second possibility is the association in some patients of both patterns, typical DLBCL in one site, T-cell rich or histiocyte-rich in another (Ng et al. 1989; Scarpa et al. 1989; Osborne et al. 1991a, b; Camilleri-Broët et al. 1996). The PCR finding in some patients of a rearrangement of bcl-2 due to a t(14;18) translocation is another argument (de Jong et al. 1996).

The relation to Hodgkin's disease lymphocyte-rich, nodular type (nodular paragranuloma), is also unclear, due to the fact that some tumors may transform into a diffuse pattern and others into a DLBCL, with an early stage that mimics a T-lymphocyte rich B-cell lymphoma. Borderline cases have been discussed (Chittal et al. 1990). The nosologic significance of T-cell-rich B-cell lymphoma (TcR-BCL) remains unclear and awaits clarification (Schmidt and Leder 1996). The postulated normal cellular counterpart is an activated peripheral B-lymphocyte of germinal-center origin (Bräuninger et al. 1999). The presence of a high number of T-lymphocytes can be explained either by the production of lymphokines by the tumor cells attracting T-lymphocytes, or by stimulation of cellular immunity by tumor antigens expressed by the neoplastic B-cells (Ohshima et al. 1994).

Morphology

These lymphomas are characterized by a diffuse infiltration of lymphocytes that obscures the normal architecture (Fig. 4.75) and extends into the perinodal fat. In a few cases, the predominance of an interfollicular involvement with persistence of normal follicles in various stages of activation has been reported. But, by definition, these lymphomas should not present a nodular pattern, which instead should lead to the discussion of a transformation of a Hodgkin's lymphoma, lymphocyte-predominant, nodular type, into a DLBCL still rich in lymphocytes.

The lymphocytes are small or medium-sized, sometimes with a clear chromatin corresponding to activated lymphocytes. In the histiocyte-rich variant (Delabie et al. 1992), sheets of histiocytes, sometimes with phagocytic activity, are associated with the lymphocytes. These histiocytes should not be confused with epithelioid cells. Plasma cell are not present in the majority of cases. A variable number of eosinophils may be observed, increasing the risk of misdiagnosing a classic Hodgkin's lymphoma. Post-capillary venules are often hypertrophic and more numerous than normally found. The large tumor cells present with the morphology of centroblast, immunoblast, anaplastic large cells, Hodgkin's cells, Reed-Sternberg-like giant cells, or even large cells with a multilobate or popcorn-like nucleus (Krishnan et al. 1991, 1994; Camilleri-Broët et al. 1996). It should be stressed that, as in classic Hodgkin's lymphoma, mixed cellularity, the tumor cells are rare, representing less than 10% of the total cell population, and dispersed in a sea of small lymphocytes or in sheets of histiocytes. Sometimes they are organized in small clusters.

Fibrosis, either intercellular or in large bands, can be seen, but without an annular pattern (Camilleri-Broët et al. 1996). Areas of necrosis are absent.

Immunohistochemistry

The large cells express B-cell markers (CD20, CD79α) (Fig. 4.76), surface or cytoplasmic immunoglobulins with a light-chain restriction (Ohshima et al. 1994),

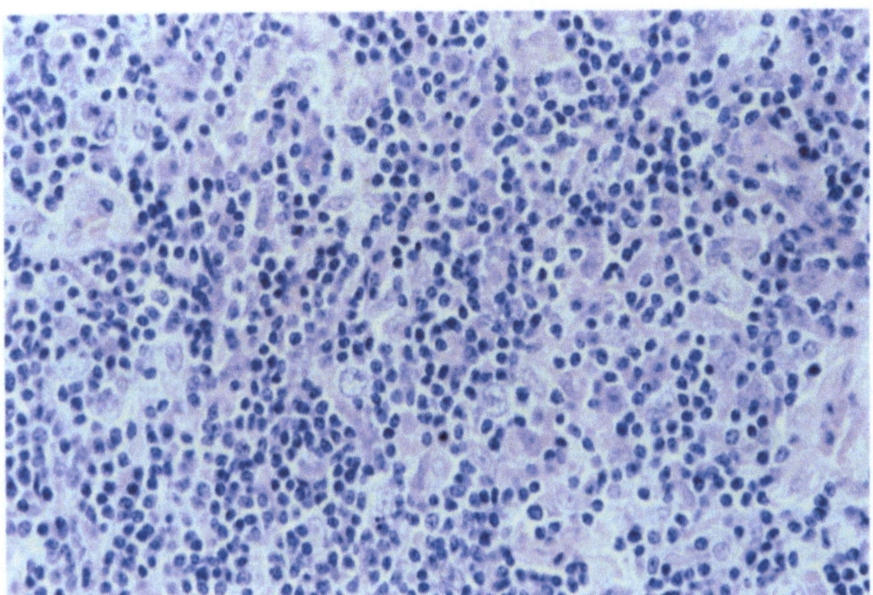

Fig. 4.75. T-cell-rich large-B-cell lymphoma. Diffuse infiltration by small and medium-sized lymphocytes (at least 60% with a T-cell phenotype), with rare, large tumor cells sometimes resembling Sternberg-Reed cells (Giemsa stain)

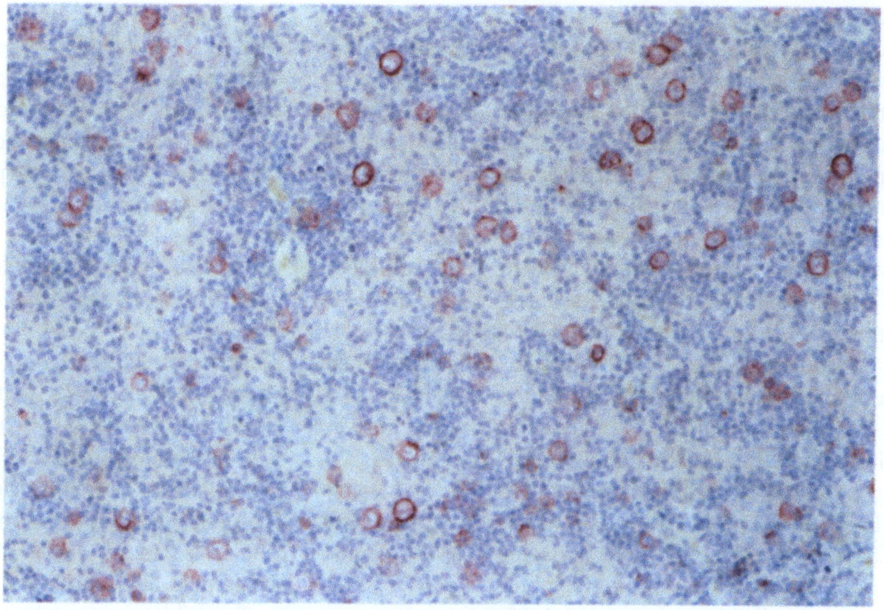

Fig. 4.76. T-cell-rich, histiocyte-rich, large-B-cell lymphoma. The rare tumor cells often resemble Sternberg-Reed cells, express CD20, and are surrounded by numerous lymphoid cells

Table 4.2. Comparison of the immunophenotype of T-cell-rich B-cell lymphoma (*TcR-BCL*), lymphocyte-predominant Hodgkin's lymphoma, nodular type (*LPHLN*), or diffuse (*LPHLD*) and classical Hodgkin's lymphoma, lymphocyte-rich (*CHLLR*)

		TcR-BCL	LPHLN	LPHLD	CHLLR
Pattern		Diffuse or interfollicular	Nodular with diffuse areas	Diffuse	Nodular
Lymphoid background	CD45	+	+	+	+
	CD20	−	+++	++ (?)	−/+
	IgD	−	+++	(?)	−
	CD3	+++	+ (patchy)	+ (?)	+++
	CD57	−/+	+++	(?)	−/+
Tumor cells	CD45	+	+	+	−
	CD20	+	+	+	+/−
	EMA	+	+	+	−
	J chain	?	+	(?)	−
	CD30	−/+	−	−	+
	CD15	−	−	−	+/−

EMA, sometimes CD30 (de Jong et al. 1996) but never CD15. The tumor cells are LMP-1-negative.

The reactive lymphocytes express a T-cell phenotype (CD3-, CD5-, CD7-, CD43-positive) with a variable number of CD4- and CD8-positive cells (ratio 2:1 to 1:1). In one study, the T-cell population mainly consisted of non-activated CD8-positive cytolytic αβT-cells expressing TiA-1 but not granzyme B (Felgar et al. 1998). There are only a few CD57-positive cells, in contrast to lymphocyte-predominant Hodgkin's lymphoma, nodular type (Kamel et al. 1993; Shahab et al. 1993). There is no rosetting pattern of small T-lymphocytes around large-B-cells as seen in classical Hodgkin's lymphoma. The number of small-B-cells is very low. Rare dispersed plasma cells are polytypic. There is no network of FDC or only small remnants of germinal centers (Fleming et al. 1998). The histiocytes express CD68 and all the common histiocyte markers but not S100 protein (Table 4.2).

Cytogenetics

In one case of TcR-BCL, a 14q+ chromosome marker involving 14q32 was observed (La Starza et al. 1996). One case of histiocyte-rich B-cell lymphoma showed complex clonal cytogenetic abnormalities including t(8;14)(q11;q32) (Sun et al. 1997).

In many cases, rearrangement of the Ig heavy-chain could be demonstrated (Osborne et al. 1991a, b; Macon et al. 1992a, b; La Starza et al. 1996; Sun et al. 1997; Ohshima et al. 1999). Sometimes, due to the very few number of tumor cells, PCR has failed to disclose this rearrangement. Krishnan et al. (1991, 1994) reported a rearrangement rate of 64 % in his series. By contrast, there is no rearrangement of the genes coding for the proteins of the antigen receptor of T-lymphocytes (de Jong et al. 1996).

Rearrangement of bcl-2 has been observed (Krishnan et al. 1991, 1994; Macon et al. 1992a, b).

Neoplastic large CD20-positive cells have been obtained by micromanipulation. In six TcR-BCLs, clonal Ig heavy- and light-chain gene rearrangements were identified; these harbored somatically mutated V gene rearrangements with an average mutation frequency of 15.5 % for heavy (VH)- and 5.9 % for light (VL)-chains, as well as intraclonal diversity. These results demonstrate that the precursors of the tumor cells are germinal center B-cells (Bräuninger et al. 1999).

Differential Diagnosis

In the majority of cases, *viral diseases, drug hypersensitivity,* and *autoimmune diseases* are easily eliminated based on morphology, immunohistochemistry, clinical data, and molecular biology (Ng et al. 1989).

This type of lymphoma should be distinguished from *T-cell lymphomas.* Early reports (Mirchandani et al. 1985; Jaffe 1985; Jaffe et al. 1984, 1991; Ramsay et al. 1988; Scarpa et al. 1989; Osborne et al. 1990) stressed the point that all of the respective cases primarily suggested a diagnosis of a T-cell neoplasia because of the morphology and the immunohistochemistry, which demonstrated that 60 – 90 % of the cells expressed a T-cell phenotype. However, genetic analysis did not show evidence of monoclonality of the T-cell population; rather, the few dispersed large cells were of the B-cell phenotype, and a rearrangement of immunoglobulin heavy- and/or light-chain was found.

Among the peripheral T-cell lymphomas, the *angioimmunoblastic type* is most the frequent lymphoma confused with T-cell-rich large-B-cell lymphomas. In both types of lymphoma, there is a background of T-cells associated with scattered large-B-cells. But, in the angioimmunoblastic type, the T-cell population comprises many large cells resembling immunoblasts with an abundant clear cytoplasm. In addition, B-blasts are dispersed and always associated with a variable number of plasma cells; these B-blasts often express LMP-1 and EBER-1, which is never observed in T-cell-rich large-B-cell lymphoma. On the other hand, burned-out follicles are frequently seen in the angioimmunoblastic type. Immunohistochemistry is not helpful in distinguishing between the two lymphomas. Only the presence of FDC hyperplasia (see Chap. 5.2.2.1) is a good argument in favor of the angioimmunoblastic type. Thus, in some cases, the differential diagnosis is dependent upon molecular genetics to show a TCR-γ gene rearrangement in the T-cell lymphoma, and in T-cell-rich large-B-cell lymphoma the absence of this rearrangement but an immunoglobulin heavy- or light-chain gene rearrangement. Nonetheless, we want to stress that, due to the low number of tumor cells, such B-cell rearrangements can be impossible to detect.

Peripheral T-cell unspecified, lymphoepithelioid type (Lennert's lymphoma), can also be discussed in relation to histiocyte-rich DLBC. The presence of a rearrangement of TCR-γ is the most important criteria.

T-cell/histiocyte-rich DLBCL also has to be distinguished from typical *large-B-cell lymphomas of centroblastic or immunoblastic* type with a higher content of reactive T-lymphocytes (Lennert 1978, 1981; Knowles et al. 1984). The precise definition given at the beginning of this section should be strictly used.

Histiocyte-rich large-B-cell lymphomas should also be distinguished from large-B-cell lymphomas associated with an epithelioid cell reaction (Lennert 1978, 1981; Kojima et al. 1996). Histiocytes and epithelioid cells should not be confused!

Classical Hodgkin's lymphoma, particularly lymphocyte-rich subtype, is included in the differential diagnosis of T-cell/histiocyte-rich DLBCL (Chittal et al. 1990, 1991; Macon et al. 1992a, b; Camilleri-Broët et al. 1996; de Jong et al. 1996; McBride et al. 1996). In the majority of cases, the presence of typical Reed-Sternberg cells, and/or of lacunar cells with a typical immunophenotype (CD30- and CD15-positive, often LMP-1-positive, CD20-positive in some cells only, EMA-negative) allows a clear-cut diagnosis.

Finally, the most difficult component of the differential diagnosis is *lymphocyte-rich Hodgkin's lymphoma, nodular type (nodular paragranuloma).* Sometimes, when the hypertrophic follicles are completely homogeneous and the tumor cells are numerous, the diagnosis of a T-cell-rich/histiocyte-rich large-B-cell lymphoma can be very difficult. Only demonstration of a nodular architecture, using silver impregnation, of a follicular dendritic cell network in the nodules where the large B-cells lie (Fleming et al. 1998), and the presence of both small B-lymphocytes expressing IgD and numerous CD57-positive lymphocytes can help. This differential diagnosis is particularly difficult when this type of Hodgkin's lymphoma is transforming into a large-B-cell lymphoma.

The most important point is related to the question whether a diffuse lymphocyte-predominant Hodgkin's lymphoma exists. This is still matter of controversial discussion. There may be borderline cases (Schmidt and Leder 1996).

Occurrence

These lymphomas develop mostly in adults (with a median age of 62.5 years), without or a slight male predominance. They make up 7% of all lymphomas and 3% of DLBCL (Lones et al. 2000). In a recent series of DLBCL in children, six cases out of 20 were TcR-BCLs.

Clinical Presentation and Prognosis

Patients present with superficial polyadenopathy, sometimes associated with mediastinal or abdominal involvement. Hepatosplenomegaly is seen in about half of the patients (Camilleri-Broët et al. 1996) due to lymphoma involvement of these organs (Khan et al. 1993; McBride et al. 1996). Other localizations have been published: Waldeyer's ring (Dargent et al. 1998), common bile duct (Brouland et al. 1993), and lung (Brousset et al. 1995). At necropsy, multiple localizations are often observed. Patients may have B symptoms. Peripheral blood cytopenia (anemia, thrombopenia) or pancytopenia may be present. Serum LDH is often elevated (Rodriguez et al. 1993). Bone marrow biopsy often discloses an involvement, even at presentation (Camilleri-Broët et al. 1996; McBride et al. 1996; Skinnider et al. 1997). The majority of the patients have, at presentation, stage III or stage IV disease (Ramsay et al. 1988; Baddoura and Chan 1991; Krishnan et al. 1991, 1994; Macon et al. 1992a, b; Camilleri-Broët et al. 1996).

T-cell-rich/histiocyte-rich large-B-cell lymphoma has an overall survival and a failure-free survival of 73 and 37%, respectively (Ripp et al. 2002). It should be clearly distinguished from Hodgkin's lymphoma (lymphocyte-predominant Hodgkin's disease) because the type of chemotherapy used to treat TcR-BCL has no curative effect on Hodgkin's lymphoma; thus, such patients must be treated like all other DLBCL patients (Chittal et al. 1990; Rodriguez et al. 1993; McBride et al. 1996; Ripp et al. 2002).

4.2.2.2.7 Unclassified Diffuse Large-B-Cell Lymphoma

Some diffuse large-cell lymphomas may be difficult to classify according to the morphological subtypes described above. For example, plasmablasts or other plasma cell precursors may be associated with centroblasts and immunoblasts, or numerous medium-sized cells can be associated with centroblasts (small centroblasts?), or numerous large centrocytes (anaplastic centrocytes) can be associated with centroblasts. Some other tumors show an individual cytological pattern which does not fit with the described cell types In the majority of these cases, however, at least the B-cell phenotype can be demonstrated.

Finally, some large-B-cell lymphomas cannot be properly classified due to insufficient biopsy material, crushed fragments or badly fixed specimens. As a result, the morphology cannot be well-recognized. In this situation, the term "DLBCL unclassified" can be proposed when the immunophenotype can be demonstrated. In cases in which immunohistochemistry fails to show the B-cell origin, the term "diffuse large-cell unclassified" should be used.

4.2.2.3 Diffuse Large-B-Cell Lymphoma – Clinical Variants

The following clinical variants of DLBCL proposed by the WHO classification (Jaffe et al. 2001) will be described in the organs or tissues in which they occur.

1. Primary mediastinal lymphoma (see Chap. 6.6.1)
2. Intravascular large-B-cell lymphoma (see Chap. 6.1.8)
3. PEL (see Chap. 6.8.1.1)
4. PAL (see Chap. 6.8.1.2)
5. Secondary to Liebow's lymphomatoid granulomatosis (see Chap. 6.7.1.4)

4.2.3 Burkitt's Lymphoma (ICD-O: 9687/3)

Synonyms

- Kiel: Burkitt's lymphoma, Burkitt's lymphoma with plasmacytoid differentiation
- Real: Burkitt's and Burkitt's-like lymphoma
- WHO: Burkitt's lymphoma, Burkitt's lymphoma with plasmacytoid differentiation and atypical/Burkitt's-like lymphoma

Definition

Burkitt's lymphoma is a B-cell neoplasia presenting as a voluminous solid tumor, often at extranodal sites, or less frequently as an acute leukemia. The tumor cells are monomorphic, cohesive, medium-sized with a basophilic cytoplasm, and round nuclei with multiple nucleoli. Burkitt's lymphoma is the fastest growing type of lymphoma, with a potential doubling time of 25.6 h (Iversen et al. 1974; Spina et al. 1997). A high number of mitoses can be recognized (Berard et al. 1969; Wright 1971), and the number of cells engaged in the cell cycle, as demonstrated by the expression of Ki67, is higher than 90% and may be up to 100%. The rate of apoptosis is very high also, responsible for a starry-sky cellular pattern. A constant genetic feature is represented by different translocations involving c-myc. Burkitt's lymphoma has a highly aggressive course but is curable by polychemotherapy, particularly when the disease is localized and treated early.

The postulated normal cell counterpart is a peripheral germinal center B-cells (Mann et al. 1976; Cario et al. 2000).

Morphology

Based on their morphology and immunohistochemistry, different types of Burkitt's lymphomas have been described. Today, these variants are summarized under the term "Burkitt's lymphoma."

Classical Burkitt's lymphoma. The tumor cells are "cohesive", i.e. they lie close together and thereby appear to form compact masses. Sometimes after fixation, they exhibit squared-off borders of retracted cytoplasm. The cells are very fragile and sensitive to necrosis and to fixation procedures. Inappropriate fixation (delayed fixation, insufficient quantity of fixative for the volume of tissue, prolonged fixation, etc.) are responsible for artifacts leading to difficulties in recognizing Burkitt's lymphoma.

The tumor cells have a monotonous appearance because of their uniform morphology and size (Fig. 4.77).They are medium-sized with nuclei approximately the same size as those of histiocytes, which are dispersed throughout the diffuse infiltration. The nuclei are round with coarsely reticulated, intensely stained chromatin (spotted) and two to four medium-sized basophilic central nucleoli (Fig. 4.77).

The cytoplasm is scanty or moderately abundant, markedly basophilic in Giemsa stain, often with a few small lipid vacuoles or droplets (Sudan-red-positive). The cells do not show any sign of maturation into plasmablasts or plasma cells.

As a rule, the tumor cells are interspersed with numerous starry-sky cells, i.e. large macrophages that

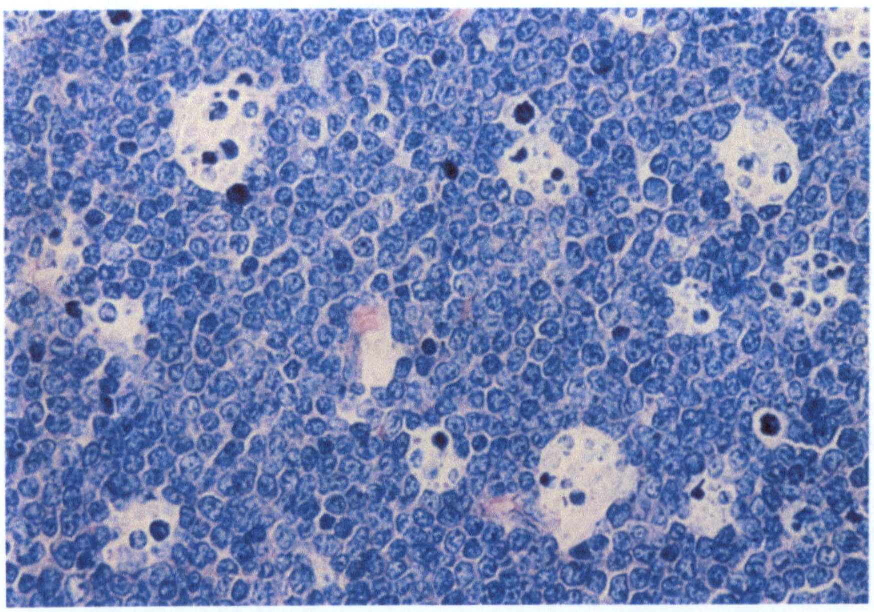

Fig. 4.77. Burkitt's lymphoma. Medium-sized lymphoid cells with multiple nucleoli, some mitoses, and numerous macrophages with apoptotic cells (Giemsa stain)

have phagocytosed many cells, including intact and apoptotic tumor cells (Fig. 4.77). Mitotic activity is high, with more than ten mitoses per high-power field. Argentaffin fibers are sparse. The lymphomatous infiltration is diffuse. Occasionally, Burkitt's lymphoma may proliferate in follicles that resemble active germinal centers (Mann et al. 1976). Two cases of mantle zone infiltration preceding infiltration of the germinal centers have been described (Pallesen 1983).

The PAS reaction is negative. Most of the cytoplasmic vacuoles can be identified as lipid droplets with Sudan red staining.

Variants. Variants of Burkitt's lymphoma can be divided into those involving plasmacytoid differentiation and atypical Burkitt/Burkitt-like conditions.

In *Burkitt's lymphoma with plasmacytoid differentiation*, the borderline between the variants with and without cIg is not distinct and must be drawn somewhat arbitrarily. Even in classic Burkitt's lymphoma there may be some Ig in nuclear pockets. However, under this term, we consider only the cases in which a large number or even all the tumor cells clearly show intracytoplasmic Ig deposits. This accumulation of Ig corresponds to a plasmacytoid differentiation (Fig. 4.78), with an eccentric, more abundant and more basophilic cytoplasm, and a large, pale juxtanuclear halo (Golgi apparatus).A certain degree of pleomorphism in the size and shape of the nucleus can be recognized (Hui et al. 1988; Lennert and Feller 1990). This morphological variant may be observed in sporadic and in immunodeficiency-associated Burkitt's lymphoma (Raphaël et al. 1991).

Atypical Burkitt's/Burkitt's-like disease comprises a majority of medium-sized Burkitt's cells. A high mitotic index and a high degree of apoptosis with a starry-sky pattern are also present as in classical Burkitt's lymphoma. But, there is a pleomorphism in both nuclear size and shape and the size and number of nucleoli (Harris et al. 1994, 1999). In addition, the cells have the morphology of small immunoblasts, or small centroblasts; there may also be a few large cells with the morphology of centroblasts or immunoblasts (less than 10%) (Fig. 4.79). The term " Atypical Burkitt/Burkitt-like" is reserved for lymphomas with a high number of cells expressing Ki67 (90–100%) and with a c-myc translocation. The distinction between this form of lymphoma and DLBCL is very difficult.

Cytology. The medium-sized cells have a monomorphous aspect with many mitoses. Starry-sky macrophages are numerous. The cell morphology is highly characteristic and often easier to identify as Burkitt's cells than in tissue sections. Thus, cytology plays an important role in the diagnosis of Burkitt's lymphoma.

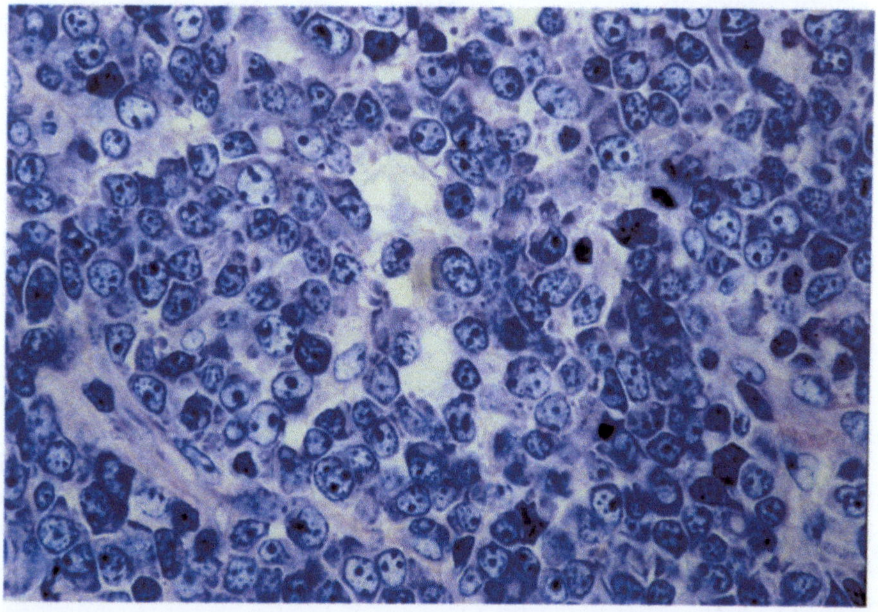

Fig. 4.78. Burkitt's lymphoma with plasmacytoid differentiation. Diffuse infiltration by medium-sized cells with a starry-sky pattern consisting of medium-sized cells with a typical morphology showing plasmacytoid differentiation (Giemsa stain)

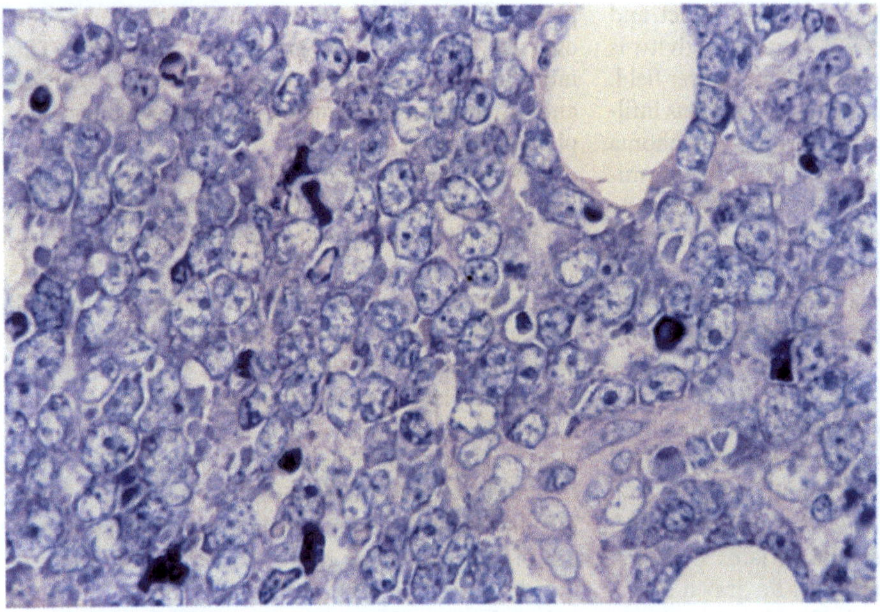

Fig. 4.79. Atypical Burkitt's/ Burkitt's-like lymphoma. In association with medium-sized cells typical for Burkitt's lymphoma, there are large cells, small immunoblasts, and cells with a plasmacytoid differentiation (Giemsa stain)

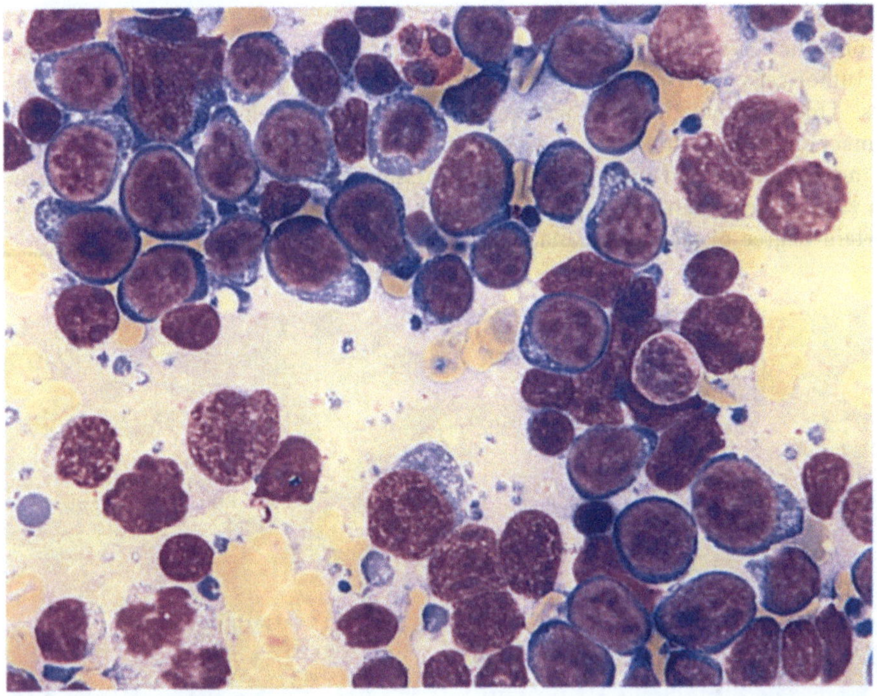

Fig. 4.80. Burkitt's lymphoma with plasmacytoid differentiation. Same patient as in Fig. 4.78. Some of the tumor cells have a more abundant, triangular cytoplasm with a pale juxtanuclear area, corresponding to the Golgi apparatus as in plasma cells (May-Grünwald-Giemsa stain)

The cells show a roundish nucleus with a thin membrane, clumped chromatin, and multiple medium-sized, centrally situated nucleoli. Around the nucleus, a small rim of intensely basophilic cytoplasm often contains lipid droplets.

In Burkitt's lymphoma with plasmacytoid differentiation the cytoplasm is more triangular, often with a pale juxtanuclear area corresponding to the Golgi apparatus (Fig. 4.80).

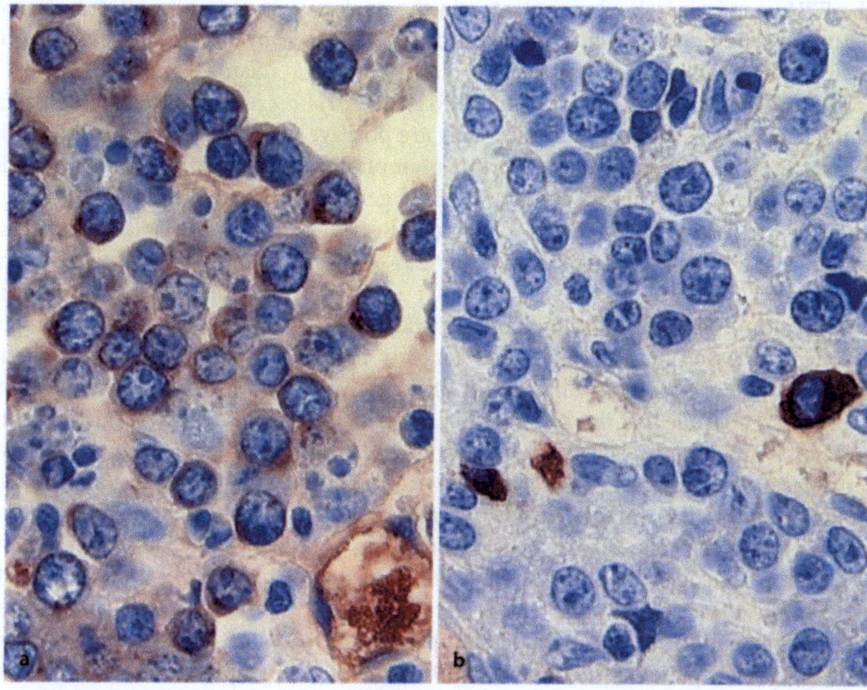

Fig. 4.81 a, b. Same patient as in Figs. 4.78 and 4.80. **a** The tumor cells contain λ monotypic intracytoplasmic immunoglobulin. **b** Only a few reactive plasma cells are positive for κ-light-chain, the tumor cells are negative (immunoperoxidase stain)

Immunohistochemistry

The tumor cells express the B-cell-associated antigens (CD20, CD79α) and surface immunoglobulins, mostly IgM, rarely IgA, with light-chain restriction. They are also positive for CD10, an argument supporting a follicular origin. They are negative for CD5, CD23 and TdT. The oncoprotein bcl-2 is not expressed but the cells are bcl-6-positive. CD10 is often, but not always, expressed often and the cells are sometimes CD23-positive (Payne et al. 1987). Only the plasmacytoid variant presents with monotypic intracytoplasmic immunoglobulins (Fig. 4.81).

One of the most important immunohistochemical findings is the demonstration of the expression of Ki67 (Mib1) by more than 90% (and up to 100%) of the tumor cells, reflecting the high number of cells engaged in the cell cycle.

Reactive cells are represented by a few CD3-positive T-cells and by CD68-positive starry-sky macrophages.

Cytogenetic Features

An early event in the development of Burkitt's lymphoma is a translocation leading to activation of the c-myc gene.

In the majority of patients there is a translocation of the c-myc gene at band q24 on chromosome 8 to the immunoglobulin heavy-chain gene on chromosome 14 at band q32, yielding a t(8;14). In other patients, the c-myc gene is translocated to the light-chains loci, either λ at 2p11 on chromosome 2 or κ at 22q11 on chromosome 22, resulting in two other types of translocations: t(2;8) and t(8;22).

The sites of the breakpoints are not the same in endemic and sporadic Burkitt's lymphoma. In endemic Burkitt's lymphoma, the breakpoint on chromosome 14 involves the heavy-chain joining region corresponding to an early B-cell. By contrast, the translocation in sporadic Burkitt's lymphoma involves the immunoglobulin switch region, corresponding to a later-stage B-cell (Pelicci et al. 1986; Neri et al. 1988; Shiramizu et al. 1991; Gutierrez et al. 1992; Cario et al. 2000).

The c-myc gene is stimulated as result of its proximity to genes on chromosomes 14, 2, or 22 responsible for the synthesis of immunoglobulin heavy- or light-chains λ or κ.

It is highly probable that this c-myc activation plays a primary role in lymphomagenesis, driving cells into the cell cycle (Gaidano et al. 1991). In addition, the activated c-myc gene stimulates specific target genes involved in apoptosis.

The EBV genome can be demonstrated in the nucleus of tumor cells by in situ hybridization on frozen or fixed paraffin-embedded tissue, particularly using a probe recognizing small EBV RNA (EBER-1). In African endemic cases, almost all tumor cells are positive (Prévot et al. 1992). In sporadic Burkitt's lymphoma, less than 30% of the tumors contain the EBV genome whereas in immunodeficiency-associated Burkitt's lymphoma, EBV is demonstrated in about 25–40% of patients.

The role of EBV in the development of Burkitt's lymphoma is not well-known (Facer and Playfair 1989). Since EBV is not present in all types of Burkitt's lymphoma, it is possible that this virus is not always necessary for lymphomagenesis and could be regarded in some cases as a passenger virus. Other environmental factors, such as other infections and immunosuppression may be involved in disease development.

Other genetic alterations have been demonstrated, for example, inactivation of p53; this is due to mutation of the gene in up to 30% of endemic and sporadic Burkitt's lymphoma patients (Gaidano et al. 1991; Bhatia et al. 1992; Preudhomme et al. 1995).

Differential Diagnosis

Endemic and sporadic Burkitt's lymphoma should first be distinguished from other lymphomas consisting of medium-sized lymphoid cells, such as *precursor B- or T-lymphoblastic lymphomas*. The morphology of the nucleus (often convoluted), of the nucleoli (often small), of the chromatin (with a washed-out aspect), of the cytoplasm (no deep basophilia) in lymphoblastic lymphoma is completely different than in Burkitt's lymphoma. In addition, the immunophenotype is different, often with expression of TdT and CD34, both of which are negative in Burkitt's lymphoma.

Granulocytic sarcoma may also represent a difficult differential diagnosis. This type of sarcoma can occur in children in the orbit and in the ovaries. The tissues are infiltrated by medium-sized cells with a more abundant, not deeply basophilic cytoplasm. On imprints or smears stained with May-Grünwald-Giemsa solutions, specific intracytoplasmic granules are easy to recognize, allowing the diagnosis. Such granules are not easily recognizable on tissue sections even with Giemsa stain. The presence of eosinophils may be of help. The diagnosis can be made with the Leder reaction, demonstrating in the cytoplasm a naphthol-ASD-chloracetate-esterase activity. Immunohistochemistry is also very useful, demonstrating the expression of myeloperoxidase, lysozyme, CD15 and other myeloid-related antigens.

All the histopathological variants of Burkitt's lymphoma should be differentiated from *diffuse large-B-cell lymphoma*. This is particularly true when the slides are not of optimal quality. Slight technical flaws may cause artificial displacement of the nucleoli toward the nuclear membrane, resulting in the erroneous diagnosis of monomorphic centroblastic lymphoma. It is also occasionally difficult to distinguish Burkitt's lymphoma from B-immunoblastic lymphoma comprising medium-sized cells with multiple central nucleoli, mimicking Burkitt's cells. The presence of numerous typical immunoblasts with extensive cytoplasm and a large central nucleolus allows recognition of a large-B-cell lymphoma.

The diagnosis is particularly difficult in cases of large-B-cell lymphoma, mainly centroblastic with a high level of apoptosis, a starry-sky pattern, numerous mitotic figures, and a large number of cells expressing Ki67. Such tumors may comprise a variable number of neoplastic medium-sized cells. These cases, or some of them, may correspond to "small non-cleaved non-Burkitt's lymphoma" in the Rappaport and WF classifications. The presence of a high number of large-B-cells is a good argument in favor of the diagnosis of large-B-cell lymphoma (Wright 1999). But sometimes the two conditions are difficult to distinguish (Harris et al. 1994, 1999). In these cases, immunohistochemistry and genetic studies are very useful.

Occurrence

In the areas of Africa where Burkitt's lymphoma (and malaria!) is endemic, there is an incidence of 1–12 cases per 100,000 children per year. R. Schmauz (1990, personal communication) observed that the percentage of Burkitt's lymphoma cases varies according to the incidence of malaria, from 23.2% to 44.6% of all malignant lymphomas in his series. In the United States, Levine et al. (1982) calculated a frequency of 1.4 cases per 1,000,000 white males and 0.4 cases per 1,000,000 white females. In the collection of the Lymph Node Register in Kiel, Burkitt's lymphoma of the lymph node, including cIg-positive cases, accounts for 2.6% of NHLs. If one includes the extranodal NHLs, which make up about 50% of the cases of Burkitt's lymphoma, one reaches a figure of about 3%. Among children in Germany, Burkitt's lymphoma of the lymph node accounts for at least 25% and at most 40% of NHLs.

The age peak is somewhat earlier in Africa (between the third and sixth year of life) than in the United States. In our collection, as in the American studies, there were several adults, whereas in African studies adult cases are a rarity. Nodal cases of Burkitt's lymphoma in our collection showed a first peak in the first two decades, a second peak in the fifth decade and a third peak in the seventh to eighth decade. Our youngest patient was 3 years old, our oldest 87. In the first two decades, males predominate highly, whereas in the eighth decade females are affected more frequently. All together, the male-to-female ratio is 1.5:1.

Clinical Presentation

Burkitt's lymphoma presents three clinical variants, showing differences in clinical presentation as well as in morphology and biology.

In all the three variants, patients present with a bulky mass that grows rapidly due to the short doubling time of the tumor cells. Variations in clinical presentation are explained by the epidemiology and the site of involvement. The majority of the patients present with high uric acid and high LDH levels. The staging procedure is somewhat different from the classic Ann Arbor system. Commonly, a modified system (Weitzman et al. 1991) initially described by Murphy (Murphy and Hustu 1980) is used (see Table 4.3). In 30% of the patients at presentation, localized stage I and stage II disease is found, whereas 70% of patients have extended-stage (III and IV) disease.

Ileocecal involvement represents one of the most frequent initial tumor sites of endemic and sporadic Burkitt's lymphoma.

The three variants have in common a high incidence of central nervous system involvement, a risk which should be considered during treatment.

Table 4.3. Staging system for Burkitt's lymphoma (Murphy and Hustu 1980, modified by Weitzman et al. 1991)

Stage I	A single tumor (extranodal) or single anatomic area (nodal) with the exclusion of mediastinum or abdomen.
Stage II	A single tumor (extranodal) with regional node involvement. Two or more nodal areas on the same side of the diaphragm. Two single (extranodal) tumors with or without regional node involvement on the same side of the diaphragm. Primary gastrointestinal tract tumor, usually in the ileocecal area, with or without involvement of associated mesenteric nodes only.
Stage II R	Completely resected abdominal disease.
Stage III	Two single tumors (extranodal) on opposite sites of the diaphragm. Two or more nodal areas above and below the diaphragm. All primary intrathoracic tumors (mediastinal, pleural, thymic). All paraspinal or epidural tumors, regardless of other tumor site(s). All extensive primary intra-abdominal disease.
Stage III A	Localized but non-resectable abdominal disease.
Stage III B	Widespread multiorgan abdominal disease.
Stage IV	Any of the above with initial CNS and/or bone marrow involvement (>25%).

Endemic Burkitt's lymphoma. This variant, described by the surgeon Dennis Burkitt (1958, 1970), represents the most common malignancy of childhood in equatorial Africa. The incidence peak is between 4 and 7 years with a male to female ratio of 2:1. In other equatorial ("intertropical") areas of the world, endemic Burkitt's lymphoma has been observed, for example, in Papua, New Guinea, and in the Amazon region. There is a strong correlation in all these places with climatic factors, such as rainfall and altitude, which also correspond with the occurrence of endemic malaria (Facer and Playfair 1989).

In earlier reports on African endemic Burkitt's lymphoma, the most frequent site of primary manifestation was the jaw (Burkitt 1958, 1970; Wright 1971, 1997; Wright et al. 1997), but in the meantime the incidence of primary manifestation in the abdomen has increased markedly. Approximately 50% of the patients present with facial bone involvement: jaw and orbit. Intra-abdominal presentations are due to ileocecal, omentum, ovary, or kidney involvement. The breast may also be involved during puberty or pregnancy. In almost all patients, EBV can be demonstrated (Prévot et al. 1992; Tao et al. 1998).

Sporadic Burkitt's lymphoma. This variant is observed mainly in children and in young adults in any other part of the world (Magrath and Sariban 1985; Wright et al. 1997). Sporadic Burkitt's lymphoma in Western Europe and North America has a low incidence, representing about 1–2% of all lymphomas in patients with a median age of 30 years, but accounting approximately for 30–50% of all lymphomas occurring in children. The association with EBV is low, less than 30% of the cases.

In North Africa and South America, the incidence of Burkitt's lymphoma is intermediate between that of sporadic and endemic Burkitt's lymphoma. In these regions, as in endemic Burkitt's lymphoma, a low socio-economic status and early EBV infection are associated with a higher number of Burkitt's lymphoma tumors with latent infection of the tumor cells by EBV.

In this clinical variant, jaw localizations are less frequent, representing, for example, only 33% of Burkitt's lymphoma patients in the United States (Wright 1971). Instead, the lymphoma usually develops as an abdominal tumor (Arseneau et al. 1975; Banks et al. 1975; Levine et al. 1982).

Ileocecal involvement is the most frequent site in patients in western Europe (Levine et al. 1982). Other sites are the abdominal lymph nodes or the retroperitoneum. Such retroperitoneal tumors can be responsible for spinal cord compression and paraplegia. Ovaries and kidneys are also frequently involved. Breast localization, sometimes bilateral, has been observed, often during puberty, pregnancy or lactation. Waldeyer's ring and mediastinal involvement remain rare. Primary lymph node presentation is not frequent and is seen more often in adult than in children.

Immunodeficiency-Associated Burkitt's lymphoma. This variant is the most frequent type of lymphoma observed in patients with immunodeficiencies (Raphaël et al. 1991). In acquired immunodeficiency, due to HIV infection, Burkitt's lymphoma is often observed and may present as the initial manifestation of AIDS (Raphaël et al. 1991; Hamilton-Dutoit et al. 1993). A latent EBV infection is found in 25–40% of patients. Primary nodal and bone marrow involvement are frequent in this variant (Ziegler et al. 1984; Raphaël et al. 1991; Hamilton-Dutoit et al. 1993).

Evolution

Spontaneous, endemic, and sporadic types of Burkitt's lymphoma have a rapid, aggressive course. A polychemotherapy regimen associated with treatment protecting the central nervous system (Magrath et al. 1984; Soussain et al. 1995) can result in complete remission after 1 year, particularly when treatment is given rapidly to patients with localized stages I and II, according to the system proposed by Murphy and Hustu (1980). Complete remission cannot be obtained in about 70% of the patients with stage III or IV disease. Relapse occurs often during the first or second year after treatment.

During the early treatment period, rapid tumor cell death in tumors with a high rate proliferation is responsible for a *tumor lysis syndrome*. The extensive cell death results in release into the blood of phosphates, potassium, purine, xanthine, hypoxanthine, and uric acid. Patients suffer severe hyperkalemia with possible cardiac arrest, hyperphosphatemia with secondary hypocalcemia, and severe renal failure due to precipitation of uric acid, xanthine, and/or phosphate in renal tubules (Cohen et al. 1980; Weitzman et al. 1991).

Tumor lysis syndrome can be prevented by careful monitoring during the initial period of chemotherapy (Weitzman et al. 1991).

Prognosis

The most important factors regarding prognosis are related to disease stage according to the system of Murphy and Hustu (1980) (Table 4.3), as modified by Weitzman et al. (1991).

Bone marrow involvement (Wright and Pike 1968; Brunning et al. 1977) or the development of central nervous system symptoms are indicative of a poor prognosis.

Addendum: Acute Burkitt's Leukemia (ICD-O: 9826/3)

Synonyms

- FAB classification: L3

Definition

Acute leukemia with proliferation of medium-sized B-blasts resembling Burkitt's cells has been included in the FAB classification as an acute lymphoblastic leukemia, L3 type (Bennett et al. 1976). This type of leukemic blood picture develops in about 5–10% of patients with non-endemic Burkitt's lymphoma, accounting for approximately 2–3% of patients with L3 acute lymphoblastic leukemia (Clift et al. 1963; Stevens et al. 1972; Flandrin et al. 1975; Prokocimer et al. 1980; Abe et al. 1982; Gluck et al. 1986).

Morphology

The medium-sized blasts are often larger than neutrophils. The nucleus is round or ovoid, with spotted chromatin, and two to four medium-sized nucleoli, often centrally situated. The cytoplasm, moderately and rarely abundant, is deeply basophilic, or sometimes basophilic to gray. Prominent well-defined vacuoles are often present. Some variability in the size of the cells and in the degree of chromatin condensation can be observed.

On biopsy, the diffuse infiltration shows the same morphology as the tumor.

Immunophenotype

The blasts express membrane Ig with light-chain restriction and several B-cell markers (CD19, 20, 22 and 79a). The expression of CD45 is much stronger than in blasts of acute lymphoblastic leukemias. These cells do not express TdT or CD34. Rarely, acute Burkitt's leukemia cells have a typical precursor B-ALL phenotype (Flandrin et al. 1975).

Genetics

Acute Burkitt's leukemia have the same cytogenetic abnormalities as seen in Burkitt's lymphoma (Abe et al. 1982; Gluck et al. 1986).

Clinical Presentation and Evolution

In the majority of the cases, acute Burkitt's leukemia is observed in patients presenting with Burkitt's lymphoma and with voluminous tumors. There is a male predominance. High levels of uric acid and LDH are measured in the serum.

Evolution

Intensive chemotherapy, different from the regimen used to treat acute lymphoblastic leukemia, results in a complete remission in 80–90% of the patients. At the beginning of the treatment, a tumor lysis syndrome may be observed (Cohen et al. 1980). The rate of relapse is low in patients surviving 1 year.

References

Abe R, Tebbi CK, Yasuda H, Sandberg AA (1982) North American Burkitt-type ALL with a variant translocation t(8;22). Cancer Genet Cytogenet 7:185–195

Adida C, Haioun C, Gaulard P, Lepage E, Morel P, Brière J, Dombret H, Reyes F, Diebold J, Gisselbrecht C, Salles G, Altieri DC, Molina T (2000) Prognostic significance of survivin expression in diffuse large B-cell lymphomas. Blood 96:1921–1925

Alberti VN, Neiman RS (1984) Lymphoplasmacytic lymphoma. A clinicopathologic study of a previously unrecognised composite variant. Cancer 53:1103–1108

Alizadeh AA, Eisen MB, Davis RE, Ma C, Lossus IS, Rosenwald A, Boldrick JC, Sabet H, Tran T, Yu X et al (2000) Distinct types of diffuse large B-cell lymphoma indentified by gene expression profiling. Nature 403:503–511

Aljurf M, Cornbleet J, Michel F (1994) CD5+ chronic B-cell leukemia with features intermediate to chronic lymphocytic leukemia and hairy cell leukemia. Hematol Pathol 8:99–109

Alkan S, Ross CW, Hanson CA, Schnitzer B (1996) Follicular lymphoma with involvement of the splenic marginal zone: a pitfall in the differential diagnosis of splenic marginal zone cell lymphoma. Hum Pathol 27:503–506

Almasri NM, Iturraspe JA, Braylan RC (1998) CD10 expression in follicular lymphoma and large cell lymphoma is different from that of reactive lymph node follicles. Arch Pathol Lab Med 122:539–544

Alsabeh R, Medeiros LJ, Glackin C, Weiss LM (1997) Transformation of follicular lymphoma into CD30-large cell lymphoma with anaplastic cytologic features. Am J Surg Pathol 21:528–536

Amor DJ, Algar EM, Slater HR, Smith PJ (1998) High frequency of t(12;21) in childhood acute lymphoblastic leukemia detected by RT-PCR. Pathology 30:381–385

Andriko JAW, Swerdlow SH, Aguilera NI, Abbondanzo SL (2001) Is lymphoplasmacytic lymphoma/immunocytoma a distinct entity? A clinicopathologic study of 20 cases. Am J Surg Pathol 25:742–751

Argatoff LH, Connors JM, Klasa RJ, Horsman DE, Gascoyne RD (1997) Mantle cell lymphoma: a clinicopathologic study of 80 cases. Blood 89:2067–2078

Armitage JA, Weisenburger DD for the Non-Hodgkin's lymphoma classification Project (1998) New approach to classifying non-Hodgkin's lymphomas: clinical features of the major histologic subtypes. J Clin Oncol 16:2780–2795

Arseneau JC, Canellos GP, Banks PM, Berard CW, Gralnick HR, Devita VT Jr (1975) American Burkitt's lymphoma: a clinicopathologic study of 30 cases. I Clinical factors relating to prolonged survival. Am J Med 58:314–321

Baars JW, de Jong D, Willemse EM, Gras L, Dalesio O, van Heerde P, Huygens PC, van den Lelie H, van den Borne AEGKR (1999) Diffuse large B-cell non-Hodgkin lymphomas: the clinical relevance of histological subclassification. Br J Cancer 79:1770–1774

Baddoura FK, Chan WC (1991) T-cell rich B-cell lymphoma: a clinicopathologic study. Mod Pathol 4:68A

Bahler DW, Aguilera NS, Chen CC, Abbondanzo SL, Swerdlow SH (2000) Histological and immunoglobulin VH gene analysis of interfollicular small lymphocytic lymphoma provides evidence for two types. Am J Pathol 157:1063–1070

Balaton AJ, Vaury P, Videgrain M (1987) Paravertebral malignant rhabdoid tumor in an adult. A case report with immunocytochemical study. Pathol Res Pract 182:713–716

Banks PM, Arseneau JC, Gralnick HR, Canellos GP, Devita Jr VT, Berard CW (1975) American Burkitt's lymphoma: a clinicopathologic study of 30 cases. II. Pathologic correlations. Am J Med 58:322–329

Barekman CL, Aguilera NSI, Abbondanzo SL (2001) Low-grade B-cell lymphoma with coexpression of both CD5 and CD10. A report of 33 cases. Arch Pathol Lab Med 125:951–953
Bartels H (1980) Prognose der malignen Lymphome der Keimzentren. Habilitationsschrift, Lübeck
Bartlett NL, Rizeq M, Dorfman RF, Halpern J, Horning SJ (1994) Follicular large-cell lymphoma: intermediate or low grade? J Clin Oncol 12: 1349–1357
Bastard C, Deweindt C, Kerckaert JP, Lenormand B, Bossi A, Pezella F, Fruchart C, Duval C, Monconduit M, Tilly H (1994) LA23 rearrangements in non-Hodgkin's lymphoma: correlation with histology, immunophenotype, karyotype and clinical outcome in 217 patients. Blood 83:2423–2427
Bea S, Ribas M, Hernandez JM, Bosch F, Pinyol M, Hernandez L, Garcia JL, Flores T, Gonzalez M, Lopez-Guillermo A, Piris MA, Cardesa A, Montserrat E, Miro R, Campo E (1999) Increased number of chromosomal imbalances and high-level DNA amplifications in mantle cell lymphoma are associated with blastoid variants. Blood 93:4365–4374
Ben-Ezra J, Burke JS, Swartz WG, Brownell MD, Brynes RK, Hill R, Nathwani BN, Oken MM, Wolf BC, Woodruff R, Rappaport H (1989) Small lymphocytic lymphoma: a clinicopathologic analysis of 268 cases. Blood 73:579–587
Bennet MH, Millett YL (1969) Nodular sclerotic lymphosarcoma. A possible new clinicopathological entity. Clin Radiol 20:339–343
Bennett JM, Catovsky D, Daniel MT, Flandrin G, Galton DA, Gralnick HR, Sultan C (1976) Proposals for the classification of the acute leukaemias. French-American British (FAB) cooperative group. Br J Haematol 33:451–458
Berard C, O'Conor GT, Thomas LB, Torloni H (1969) Memoranda: Histopathological definition of Burkitt's tumor. Bull WHO 40:601–607
Bernard A, Boumsell L, Reinherz EL, Nadler LM, Ritz J, Coppin H, Richard Y, Valensi F, Dausset J, Flandrin G, Lemerle J, Schlossmman SF (1981) Cell surface characterization of malignant T cells from lymphoblastic lymphoma using monoclonal antibodies: evidence for phenotypic differences between malignant T cells from patients with acute lymphoblastic leukemia and lymphoblastic lymphoma. Blood 57:1105–1110
Bernell P, Jacobsson B, Lilienmark J, Hjalmar V, Arvidsson I, Hast R (1998) Gain of chromosome 7 marks the progression from indolent to aggressive follicle centre lymphoma and is a common finding in patients with diffuse large B-cell lymphoma: a study by FISH. Br J Haematol 101:487–491
Bhatia KG, Gutierrez MI, Huppi K, Siwarski D, Magrath IT (1992) The pattern of p53 mutations in Burkitt's lymphoma differs from that of solid tumors. Cancer Res 52:4273–4276
Bollum FJ (1979) Terminal deoxynucleotide transferase as a hematopoietic cell marker. Blood 54:1203–1215
Bosch F, Lopez-Guillermo A, Campo E, Ribera JM, Conde E, Piris MA, Vallespi T, Woessner S, Montserrat E (1998) Mantle cell lymphoma: presenting features, response to therapy, and prognostic factors. Cancer 82:567–575
Bräuninger A, Küppers R, Spiekers T, Siebert R, Strickler JG, Schlegelberger B, Rajewski K, Hansmann ML (1999) Molecular analysis of single B cells from T-cell-rich B-cell lymphoma shows the derivation of the tumor cells from mutating germinal center B cells and exemplifies means by which immunoglobulin genes are modified in germinal center B cells. Blood 93:2679–2687
Brittinger G, Bartels H, Bremer K, Burger A, Dühmke E, Gunzer U, König E, Schmalhorst U, Stacher A, Stein H, Theml H, Waldner R (Kieler Lymphomgruppe) (1978) Klinische Bedeutung der Kiel-Klassifikation der malignen Non-Hodgkin-Lymphome. Ergebnisse einer retrospektiven Studie. In: Hartwich G (ed) Diagnose und Therapie von Leukämien und malignen Lymphomen. Straube, Erlangen, pp 57–66
Brittinger G, Bartels H, Common H, Dühmke E, Fülle HH, Gunzer U, Gyenes T, Heinz R, König E, Meusers P, Paukstat M, Pralle H, Theml H, Köpcke W, Thieme C, Zwingers T, Musshoff K, Stacher A, Brücher H, Herrmann F, Ludwig WD, Pribilla W, Burger-Schüler A, Löhr GW, Gremmel H, Oertel J, Gerhartz H, Koeppen K-M, Boll I, Huhn D, Binder T, Schoengen A, Nowicki L, Pees HW, Scheurlen PG, Leopold H, Wannenmacher M, Schmidt M, Löffler H, Michlmayr G, Thiel E, Zettel R, Rühl U, Wilke HJ, Schwarze E-W, Stein H, Feller AC, Lennert K (Kiel Lymphoma Study Group) (1984) Clinical and prognostic relevance of the Kiel classification of non-Hodgkin lymphomas: results of a prospective multicenter study by the Kiel Lymphoma Study Group. Hematol Oncol 2:269–306
Brouland JP, Molimard J, Nemeth J, Valleur P, Galian A (1993) Primary T-cell rich B-cell lymphoma of the common bile duct. Virchows Arch A Pathol Anat 423:513–517
Brousset P, Chittal SM, Schlaifer D, Delsol G (1995) T-cell rich B-cell lymphoma in the lung. Histopathology 26:371–373
Brown RS, Campbell C, Lishman SC, Spittle MF, Miller RF (1998) Plasmablastic lymphoma: a new subcategory of human immunodeficiency virus-related non-Hodgkin's lymphoma. Clin Oncol (R Coll Radiol) 10:327–329
Brunning RD, McKenna RW, Bloomfield CD, Coccia P, Gajl-Peczalska J (1977) Bone marrow involvement in Burkitt's lymphoma. Cancer 40:1771–1779
Brynes RK, Almaguer PD, Leathery KE, McCourty A, Arber DA, Medeiros LJ, Nathwani BN (1996) Numerical cytogenetic abnormalities of chromosomes 3, 7, and 12 in marginal zone B-cell lymphomas. Mod Pathol 9:995–1000
Burkitt D (1958) A sarcoma involving the jaws in African children. Br J Surg 46:218
Burkitt DP (1970) General features and facial tumours. In: Burkitt DP, Wright DH (eds) Burkitt's lymphoma. Livingstone, Edinburgh
Callet-Bauchu E, Salles G, Gazzo S, Poncet C, Morel D, Pages J, Coiffier B, Coeur P, Felman P (1999) Translocations involving the short arm of chromosome 17 in chronic B-lymphoid disorders: frequent occurrence of dicentric rearrangements and possible association with adverse outcome. Leukemia 13:460–468
Camilleri-Broët S, Molina T, Audouin J, Le Tourneau A, Diebold J (1996) Morphological variability of tumour cells in T-cell-rich B-cell lymphoma. A histopathological study of 14 cases. Virchows Arch 429:243–248
Campo E, Miquel R, Krenacs L, Sorbara L, Raffeld M, Jaffe ES (1999a) Primary nodal marginal zone lymphomas of splenic and MALT. Am J Surg Pathol 23:59–68
Campo E, Raffeld M, Jaffe ES (1999b) Mantle-cell lymphoma. Semin Hematol 36:115–127
Capello D, Vitolo U, Pasqualucci L, Quattrone S, Migliaretti G,

Fassone L, Arriatti C, Vivenza D, Gloghini A, Pastore C, Lanza C, Nomdedeu J, Butto B, Freilone R, Buonaivto D, Zagonel V, Gallo E, Palestro G, Saglio G, Dalla-Favera R (2000) Distribution and pattern of bcl-6 mutations throughout the spectrum of B-cell neoplasia. Blood 95:651–659

Carbone A, Gloghini A, Pinto A, Attadia V, Zagonel V, Volpe R (1989) Monocytoid B-cell lymphoma with bone marrow and peripheral blood involvement at presentation. Am J Clin Pathol 92:228–236

Cario G, Stadt VZ, Reiter A, Welte K, Sykora KW (2000) Variant translocation in sporadic Burkitt's lymphoma detected in fresh tumour material: analysis of three cases. Br J Haematol 110:537–546

Chan WC, Huang JZ (2001) Gene expression analysis in aggressive NHL. Ann Hematol 80:B38–B41

Chen Z, Le Paslier D, Dausset J, Degos L, Flandrin G, Cohen D, Sigaux F (1987) Human T-cell γ-genes are frequently rearranged in B-lineage acute lymphoblastic leukemias but not in chronic B-cell proliferations. J Exp Med 165: 1000–1015

Chittal SM, Caverivière P, Voigt J-J, Dumont J, Nenévent B, Fauré P, Bordessoule GD, Delsol G (1987) Follicular lymphoma with abundant PAS-positive extracellular material. Immunohistochemical and ultrastructural observations. Am J Surg Pathol 11:618–624

Chittal SM, Alard C, Rossi JF, Saati TA, Le Tourneau A, Diebold J, Delsol G (1990) Further phenotypic evidence that nodular lymphocyte predominant Hodgkin's disease is a large B-cell lymphoma in evolution. Am J Surg Pathol 14:1024–1035

Chittal SM, Brousset P, Voigt JJ, Delsol G (1991) Large B-cell lymphoma rich in T-Cells and simulating Hodgkin's disease. Histopathology 19:211–220

Clift RA, Wright DH, Clifford P (1963) Leukemia in Burkitt's lymphoma. Blood 22:243–251

Cogliatti SB, Lennert K, Hansmann M-L, Zwingers TL (1990) Monocytoid B cell lymphoma. Clinical and prognostic features of 21 patients. J Clin Pathol 43:619–625

Cohen LF, Balow JE, Magrath IT, Poplack DG, Ziegler JL (1980) Acute tumor lysis syndrome. A review of 37 patients with Burkitt's lymphoma. Am J Med 68:486–490

Cohen PL, Kurtin PJ, Donovan KA, Hanson CA (1998) Bone marrow and peripheral blood involvement in mantle cell lymphoma. Br J Haematol 101:302–310

Coiffier B, Thieblemont C, Felman P, Salles G, Berger F (1999) Indolent nonfollicular lymphomas: characteristics, treatment, and outcome. Semin Oncol 36:198–208

Cooper K, Haffajee Z (1997) bcl2 and p53 protein expression in follicular lymphoma. J Pathol 182:307–310

Cousar JB, McGinn DL, Glick AD, List AF, Collins RD (1987) Report of an unusual lymphoma arising from parafollicular B-lymphocytes (PBLs) or so-called "monocytoid" lymphocytes. Am J Clin Pathol 87:121–128

Crist WM, Carroll AJ, Shuster JJ, Behm FG, Whitehead M, Vietti TJ, Look AT, Mahoney D, Ragab A, Pullen DJ, Land VJ (1990) Poor prognosis of children with pre-B acute lymphoblastic leukemia is associated with the t(1;19)(q23;p13): a Pediatric Oncology Group study. Blood 76:117–122

Cuneo A, Bigoni R, Rigolin GM, Roberti MG, Bardi A, Piva N, Milani R, Bullrich F, Veronese ML, Croce C, Birg F, Döhner H, Hagemeijer A, Castoldi G (1999) Cytogenetic profile of lymphoma of follicle mantle lineage: correlation with clinicobiologic features. Blood 93:1372–1380

Damle RN, Wasil T, Fais F, Ghiotto F, Valetto A, Allen SL, Buchbinder A, Budman D, Dittmar K, Kolitz J, Lichtman SM, Schulman P, Vinciguerra VP, Rai KR, Ferrarini M, Chiorazi N (1999) Ig V gene mutation status and CD38 expression as novel prognostic indicators in chronic lymphocytic leukemia. Blood 94:1840–1847

Dargent JL, Roufosse C, Remmelink M, Neve P (1998) Primary T-cell-rich B-cell lymphoma of the Waldeyer's ring. A pathologic condition more frequent than presupposed? Am J Surg Pathol 22:638–640

Davis GG, York JC, Glick AD, McCurley TL, Collins RD, Cousar JB (1992) Plasmacytic differentiation in parafollicular (monocytoid) B-cell lymphoma: a study of 12 cases. Am J Surg Pathol 16:1066–1074

De Jong ED, van Gorp J, Sie-Go D, van Heerde P (1996) T-cell rich B-cell non-Hodgkin's lymphoma: a progressed form of follicle centre cell lymphoma and lymphocyte predominance Hodgkin's disease. Histopathology 28:15–24

De Man JCH, Meiners WBH (1962) Crystals of protein nature in the cytoplasm of lymphatic cells in a case of lymphoreticular malignancy. Blood 20(4)

Delabie J, Vandenberghe E, Kennes C, Verhoef G, Foschini MP, Stul M, Cassiman JJ, de Wolf-Peeters C (1992) Histiocyte-rich B-cell lymphoma. A distinct clinicopathologic entity possibly related to lymphocyte predominant Hodgkin's disease, paragranuloma subtype. Am J Surg Pathol 16:37–48

Delecluze HJ, Anagnostopoulos I, Dallenbach F, Hummel M, Marafioti T, Schneider U, Kuhn D, Schmidt-Westhausen A, Reichart PA, Gross U, Stein H (1997) Plasmablastic lymphomas of the oral cavity: a new entity associated with the Human Immunodeficiency Virus Infection. Blood 89:1413–1420

Delecluze HJ, Hummel M, Marafioti T, Anagnostopoulos I, Stein H (1999) Comon and HIV-related diffuse large B-cell lymphomas differ in their immunoglobulin gene mutation pattern. J Pathol 188:133–138

De Leon ED, Alkan S, Huang JC, His ED (1998) Usefulness of an immunohistochemical panel in paraffin-embedded tissues for the differentiation of B-cell Non-Hodgkin's lymphomas of small lymphocytes. Mod Pathol 11:1046–1051

Delsol G, Lamant L, Mariame B, Pulford K, Dastugue N, Brousset P, Rigal-Huguet F, Al Saati T, Cerreti DP, Morris SW, Mason DY (1997) A new subtype of large B-cell lymphoma expressing the ALK kinase and lacking the 2;5 translocation. Blood 89:1483–1490

De Wolf-Peeters C, Pittaluga S (1995) T-cell rich B-cell lymphoma: a morphological variant of a variety of non-Hodgkin's lymphomas or a clinico-pathological entity? Histopathology 26:383–385

Diebold J, Tulliez M, Bernadou A, Audouin J, Tricot G, Reynes M, Bilski-Pasquier G (1980) Angiofollicular and plasmacytic polyadenopathy: a pseudotumourous syndrome with dysimmunity. J Clin Pathol 33:1068–1076

Diebold J, Kanavaros P, Audouin J, Bernadou A, Zittoun R (1987) Les lymphomes malins centroblastiques centrocytiques et centroblastiques à prédominance splénique (ou primitifs de la rate). Etude anatomo-clinique de 17 cas. Bull Cancer (Paris) 74:437–453

Diebold J, Raphaël M, Prévot S, Audouin J (1997) Lymphomas associated with HIV infection. In: Wotherspoon AC (ed) Lymphoma cancer surveys series, vol 30. Cold Spring Harbor Laboratory Press, Cold Spring Harbor, pp 263–294
Diebold J, Anderson JR, Armitage JO, Connors J, Maclennan KA, Müller-Hermelink HK, Nathwanni BN, Ullrich F, Weisenburger DD, for the non-Hodgkin's lymphoma classification project (2002) Diffuse large B-cell lymphoma: a clinicopathologic analysis of 444 cases classified according to the up-dated Kiel classification. Leukemia Lymphoma 43: 97–104
Dierlamm J, Pittaluga S, Wlodarska I, Stul M, Thomas J, Boogaerts M, Michaux L, Driessen A, Mecucci C, Cassiman J-J, de Wolf-Peeters C, van den Berghe H (1996) Marginal zone B-cell lymphomas of different sites share similar cytogenetic and morphologic features. Blood 87:299–307
Dogan A, Du MQ, Aiello A, Diss TC, Ye HAT, Pan LX, Isaacson PG (1998) Follicular lymphomas contain a clonally linked but phenotypically distinct neoplastic B-cell population in the interfollicular zone. Blood 91:4708–4714
Dogan A, Bagdi E, Munson P, Isaacson PG (2000) CD10 and BCL-6 expression in paraffin sections of normal lymphoid tissue and B-cell lymphomas. Am J Surg Pathol 24:846–852
Döhner H, Stilgenbauer S, James MR, Benner A, Weilguni T, Bentz M, Fischer K, Hunstein W, Lichter P (1997) 11q deletions identify a new subset of B-cell chronic lymphocytic leukemia characterized by extensive nodal involvement and inferior prognosis. Blood 89:2516–2522
Döhner H, Stilgenbauer S, Döhner K, Bentz M, Lichter P (1999) Chromosome aberrations in B-cell chronic lymphocytic leukemia: reassessment based on molecular cytogenetic analysis. J Mol Med 77:266–281
Donoghue S, Baden HS, Lauder I, Sobolewski S, Pringle JH (1999) Immunohistochemical localization of caspase-3 correlates with clinical outcome in B-cell diffuse large-cell lymphoma. Cancer Res 59:5386–5391
Driessen A, Tierens A, Ectors N, Stul M, Pittaluga S, Geboes K, Delabie J, De Wolf-Peeters C (1999) Primary diffuse large B-cell lymphoma of the stomach: analysis of somatic mutations in the rearranged immunoglobulin heavy chain variable genes indicates antigen selection. Leukemia 13:1085–1092
Drillenburg P, Wielenga VJM, Kramer MHH, van Krieken JHJM, Kluin-Nellemans HC, Hermans J, Heisterkamp S, Noordijk EM, Kluin PM, Pals ST (1999) CD44 expression predicts disease outcome in localized large B-cell lymphoma. Leukemia 13:1448–1455
Dunphy CH, Oza YV, Skelly ME (1999) An otherwise typical case of non-Japanese hairy cell leukemia with CD10 and CDw75 expression: response to cladaribine phosphate therapy. J Clin Lab Anal 13:141–144
Dupin N, Diss TL, Kellam P, Tulliez M, Du MQ, Sicard D, Weiss RA, Isaacson PG, Boshoff C (2000) HHV-8 is associated with a plasmablastic variant of Castleman disease that is linked to HHV-8 positive plasmablastic lymphoma. Blood 95:1406–1412
Ellison KJ, Nathwani BN, Cho SY, Martin SE (1989) Interfollicular small lymphocytic lymphoma: the diagnostic significance of pseudofollicles. Hum Pathol 20:1108–1118
Engelhard M, Brittinger G, Huhn D, Gerhartz HH, Meusers P, Siegert W, Thiel E, Wilmanns W, Aydemir U, Bierwolf S, Griesser H, Tiemann M, Lennert K (1997) Subclassification of diffuse large B-cell lymphomas according to the Kiel classification: distinction of centroblastic and immunoblastic lymphomas is a significant prognostic risk factor. Blood 89:2291–2297
Facer CA, Playfair JHL (1989) Malaria, Epstein-Barr virus and the genesis of lymphomas. Adv Cancer Res 53:33–71
Fang JM, Finn WG, Hussong JW, Goolsby CL, Cubbon AR, Variakojis D (1999) CD10 antigen expression correlates with the t(14;18)(q32;q21) major breakpoint region in diffuse large B-cell lymphoma. Mod Pathol 12:295–300
Felgar RE, Steward KR, Cousar JB, Macon WR (1998) T-cell-rich large B-cell lymphomas contain non-activated CD8+ cytolytic T-cells, show increased tumor cell apoptosis and have lower Bcl-2 expression than diffuse large-B-cell lymphomas. Am J Pathol 153:1707–1715
Felix CA, Wright JJ, Poplack DG, Reaman GH, Cole D, Goldman P, Korsmeyer SJ (1987) T cell receptor α-, β-, and γ-genes in T cell and pre-B cell acute lymphoblastic leukemia. J Clin Invest 80:545–556
Finn WG, Singleton TP, Schnitzer B, Ross CW, Stoolman LM (2001) Adhesion molecule expression in CD5-negative/CD10-negative chronic B-cell leukemias: comparison with Non-Hodgkin's lymphomas and CD5-positive B-cell chronic lymphocytic leukemia. Hum Pathol 32:66–73
Flandrin G, Brouet JC, Daniel MT, Preud'Homme JL (1975) Acute leukemia with Burkitt's tumor cells: a study of six cases with special reference to lymphocyte surface markers. Blood 45:183–188
Fleming MD, Shahsafaei A, Dorfman DM (1998) Absence of dendritic reticulum cell staining is helpful for distinguishing T-cell-rich B-cell lymphoma from lymphocyte predominance Hodgkin's disease. Appl Immunohistochem 6:16–22
French Cooperative Group on Chronic Lymphocytic Leukaemia (1986) Effectiveness of "CHOP" regimen in advanced untreated chronic lymphocytic leukaemia. Lance I:1346–1349
Frizzera G, Murphy SB (1979) Follicular (nodular) lymphoma in childhood: a rare clinical-pathological entity. Report of eight cases from four cancer centers. Cancer 44:2218–2235
Frizzera G, Massarelli G, Banks PM, Rosai J (1983) A systemic lymphoproliferative disorder with morphologic features of Castleman's disease. Pathologic findings in 15 patients. Am J Surg Pathol 7:211–231
Frizzera G, Anaya JS, Banks PM (1986) Neoplastic plasma cells in follicular lymphomas. Clinical and pathologic findings in six cases. Virchows Arch [A]:409:149–162
Gaba AR, Stein RS, Sweet DL, Variakojis D (1978) Multicentric giant lymph node hyperplasia. Am J Clin Pathol 69:86–90
Gaidano G, Ballerini P, Gong JZ, Inghirami G, Neri A, Newcomb EW, Magrath IT, Knowles DM, Dalla-Favera R (1991) p53 mutations in human lymphoid malignancies association with Burkitt lymphoma and chronic lymphocytic leukemia. Proc Natl Acad Sci USA 88:5413–5417
Galton DAG (1964) Chronic lymphocytic leukaemia: its pathogenesis and relationship to lymphosarcoma. In: Roulet FC (ed) Symposium on lymphoreticular tumours in Africa. Karger, Basel, pp 163–172
Galton DAG, Goldman JM, Wiltshaw E, Catovsky D, Henry K,

Goldenberg GJ (1974) Prolymphocytic leukaemia. Br J Haematol 27:7–23

Gascoyne RD, Adomat SA, Krajewsa S, Krajewski M, Horsman DE, Tolcher AW, O'Reilly SE, Hoskins P, Coldman AJ, Reed JC, Connors JM (1997) Prognostic significance of Bcl-2 protein expression and Bcl-2 gene rearrangement in diffuse aggressive non-Hodgkin's lymphoma. Blood 90:244

Gascoyne RD, Aoun P, Wu D, Chhanabhai M, Skinnider BF, Greiner TC, Morris SW, Connors JM, Vose JM, Viswanatha DS, Coldman A, Weisenburger DD (1999) Prognostic significance of anaplastic lymphoma kinase (ALK) protein expression in adults with anaplastic large cell lymphoma. Blood 93:3913–3921

Gluck WL, Bigner SH, Borowitz MJ, Brenckman WD (1986) Acute lymphoblastic leukemia of Burkitt's type (L3 ALL) with 8;22 and 14;18 translocations and absent surface immunoglobulins. Am J Clin Pathol 85:636–640

Goates JJ, Kamel OW, LeBrun DP, Benharroch D, Dorfman RF (1994) Floral variant of follicular lymphoma: immunological and molecular studies support a neoplastic process. Am J Surg Pathol 18:37–47

Greaves MF, Chan LC, Furley AJW, Watt SM, Molgaard HV (1986) Lineage promiscuity in hemopoietic differentiation and leukemia. Blood 67:1–11

Greenberg JM, Quertermous T, Seidman JG, Kersey JH (1986) Human T cell γ-chain gene rearrangements in acute lymphoid and nonlymphoid leukemia: comparison with the T cell receptor β-chain gene. J Immunol 137:2043–2049

Groves FD, Travis LB, Devesa SS, Ries LA, Fraumeni JF (1998) Waldenström's macroglobulinemia: incidence patterns in the United States, 1988–1994. Cancer 82:1078–1081

Gupta D, Lim MS, Medeiros LJ, Elenitoba-Johnson KSJ (2000) Small lymphocytic lymphoma with perifollicular, marginal zone, or interfollicular distribution. Mod Pathol 13:1161–1166

Gutierrez M, Bahitta K, Barraga R, Diez B, Sackmann NF, de Andreas M (1992) Molecular epidemiology of Burkitt's lymphoma from South America: differences in breakpoint locations and EB association from tumours in other world regions. Blood 79:3261–3266

Haas JE, Palmer NF, Weinberg AG, Beckwith JB (1981) Ultrastructure and malignant rhabdoid tumor of the kidney: a distinctive renal tumor of children. Hum Pathol 12:646–657

Hall PA, D'Ardenne AJ, Richards M A, Stansfeld AG (1987) Lymphoplasmacytoid lymphoma: an immunohistological study. J Pathol 153:213–223

Hamblin TJ, Davis Z, Gardiner A, Oscier DG, Stevenson FK (1999) Unmutated Ig V(H) genes are associated with a more aggressive form of chronic lymphocytic leukemia. Blood 94:1848–1854

Hamilton-Dutoit SJ, Raphaël M, Audouin J, Diebold J, Lisse I, Pedersen C, Oksenhendler E, Marelle L, Pallesen G (1993) *In situ* demonstration of Epstein-Barr virus small RNAs (EBER1) in acquired immunodeficiency syndrome-related lymphomas: correlation with tumor morphology and primary site. Blood 82:619–624

Hans CP, Weisenburger DD, Vose JM, Hock LM, Lynch JC, Aoun P, Greiner TC, Chan WC, Bociek RG, Bierman PJ, Armitage JO (2003) A significant diffuse component predicts for inferior survival grade 3 follicular lymphoma, but cytologic subtypes do not predict survival. Blood 101:2363–2367

Hansmann ML, Stein H, Fellbaum C, Hui PK, Parwaresch MR, Lennert K (1989) Nodular paragranuloma can transform into high-grade malignant lymphoma of B-type. Hum Pathol 20:1169–1175

Harada S, Suzuki R, Uehira K, Yatabe Y, Kagami Y, Ogura M, Suzuki H, Oyama A, Kodera Y, Ueda R, Morishima Y, Nakamura S, Seto M (1999) Molecular and immunological dissection of diffuse large cell lymphoma: CD5+ and CD5- with CD10+ groups may constitute clinically relevant subtypes. Leukemia 13:1441–1447

Haralambieva E, Pulford KA, Lamant L, Pileri S, Roncador G, Gatter RC, Delsol G, Mason DY (2000) Anaplastic large-cell lymphoma of B-cell phenotype are anaplastic lymphoma kinase (ALK) negative and belong to the spectrum of diffuse large-B-cell lymphomas. Brit J Haematol 109:584–591

Harris M, Eyden B, Read G (1981) Signet ring cell lymphoma. A rare variant of follicular lymphoma. J Clin Pathol 34:884–895

Harris NL, Bhan AK (1985) B-cell neoplasms of the lymphocytic, lymphoplasmacytoid, and plasma cell types: immunologic analysis and clinical correlation. Hum Pathol 16:829–837

Harris NL, Jaffe ES, Stein H, Banks PM, Chan JKC, Cleary ML, Delsol G, De Wolf-Peeters C, Falini B, Gatter KC, Grogan TM, Isaacson PG, Knowles DM, Mason DY, Muller-Hermelink HK, Pileri S, Piris MA, Ralfkiaer E, Warnke RA (1994) A revised European-American classification of lymphoid neoplasms: a proposal from the International Lymphoma Study Group. Blood 84:1361–1392

Harris NL, Jaffe ES, Diebold J, Flandrin G, Müller-Hermelink HK, Vardiman J, Lister TA, Bloomfield CD (1999) World Health Organization classification of neoplastic diseases of the hematopoietic and lymphoid tissue: report of the clinical advisory committee meeting. Airlie House, Virginia, Nov 1997. J Clin Oncol 17:3835–3849

Harris NL, Jaffe ES, Diebold J, Flandrin G, Müller-Hermelink HK, Vardiman J (2000) Lymphoma classification – from controversy to consensus: The R.E.A.L. and WHO Classification of lymphoid neoplasms. Ann Oncol 11 [Suppl 1]:3–10

Heinz R, Stacher A, Theml H, Pralle H, Bremer K, Brunswicker F, Burkert M, Common H, Fülle HH, Grüneisen A, Hermann F, Leopold H, Liffers R, Nowicki L, Nürnberger R, Rengshausen H, Rühl U, Schoengen A, Schmidt M, Wirthmüller R, Schwarze E-W (Kiel Lymphoma Study Group) (1979) Immunocytic lymphoma, a clinical entity distinct from chronic lymphocytic leukaemia. 5th meeting of the International Society of Haematology, European and African Division, Hamburg, 26–31 Aug 1979

Hermine O, Haioun C, Lepage E, d'Agay MF, Brière J, Lavignac C, Fillet G, Salles G, Marolleau JJP, Diebold J, Reyes F, Gaulard P (1996) Prognostic significance of bcl-2 protein expression in aggressive non-Hodgkin's lymphoma. Blood 87:265–272

Hernandez L, Fest T, Cazorla M, Teruya-Feldstein J, Bosch F, Peinado MA, Piris MA, Montserrat E, Cardesa A, Jaffe ES, Campo E, Raffeld M (1996) p53 gene mutations and protein overexpression are associated with aggressive variants of mantle cell lymphomas. Blood 87:3351–3359

Hiddemann W, Unterhalt M, Herrmann R, Wöltjen HH, Kreuser ED, Trümper L, Reuss-Borst M, Terhardt-Kasten E, Busch M, Neubauer A, Kaiser U, Hanrath RD, Moddeke H, Helm G, Freund M, Stein H, Tiemann M, Parwaresch R (1998) Mantle-cell lymphomas have more widespread disease and a slower response to chemotherapy compared with follicle-center lymphomas: results of a prospective comparative analysis of the German Low-Grade Lymphoma Study Group. J Clin Oncol 16:1922–1930

Hill ME, Maclennan KA, Cunningham DC et al (1996) Prognostic significance of BCL-2 expression and bcl-2 major breakpoint region rearrangement in diffuse large cell non-Hodgkin's lymphoma: a British National Lymphoma Investigation Study. Blood 88:1046–1051

Hoelzer D, Thiel E, Löffler H, Bodenstein H, Plaumann L, Büchner T, Urbanitz D, Koch P, Heimpel H, Engelhardt R, Müller U, Wendt F-C, Sodomann H, Rühl H, Herrmann F, Kaboth W, Dietzfelbinger H, Pralle H, Lunschen C, Hellriegel K-P, Spors S, Nowrousian RM, Fischer J, Fülle H, Mitrous PS, Pfreundschuh M, Görg C, Emmerich B, Queisser W, Meyer P, Labedzki L, Essers U, König H, Mainzer K, Herrmann R, Messerer D, Zwingers T (1984) Intensified therapy in acute lymphoblastic and acute undifferentiated leukemia in adults. Blood 64:38–47

Hoelzer D, Ludwig WD, Thiel E, Gaßmann W, Löffler H, Fonatsch C, Rieder H, Heil G, Heinze B, Arnold R, Hossfeld D, Büchner T, Koch P, Freund M, Hiddemann W, Maschmeyer G, Heyll A, Aul C, Faak T, Kuse R, Ittel TH, Gramatzki M, Diedrich H, Kolbe K, Fuhr HG, Fischer K, Schadeck-Gressel C, Weiss A, Strohscheer I, Metzner B, Fabry U, Gökbuget N, Völkers B, Messerer D, Überla K (1996) Improved outcome in adult B-cell acute lymphoblastic leukemia. Blood 87:495–508

Hsu FJ, Levy R (1995) Preferential use of the VH4 Ig gene family by diffuse large-cell lymphoma. Blood 86:3072–3082

Huang JC, Finn WG, Goolsby CL, Variakojis D, Peterson LC (1999) CD5$^-$ small B-cell leukemias are rarely classifiable as chronic lymphocytic leukaemia. Am J Clin Pathol 111:123–130

Hui PK, Feller AC, Pileri S, Gobbi M, Lennert K (1987) New aggressive variant of suppressor/cytotoxic T-CLL. Am J Clin Pathol 87:55–59

Hui PK, Feller AC, Lennert K (1988) High grade non-Hodgkin's lymphoma of B-cell type. I. Histopathology. Histopathology 12:127–143

Hummel M, Anagnostopoulos I, Korbjuhn P, Stein H (1995) Epstein-Barr virus in B-cell non-Hodgkin's lymphomas: unexpected infection patterns and different infection incidence in low- and high-grade types. J Pathol 175:263–271

Hyland J, Lasota J, Jasinski M, Petersen RO, Nordling S, Miettinen M (1998) Molecular pathological analysis of testicular diffuse large cell lymphomas. Hum Pathol 29:1231–1239

Ichikawa A, Kinoshita T, Watanabe T, Kato H, Nagai H, Tsushita K, Saito H, Hotta T (1997) Mutations of the p53 gene as a prognostic factor in aggressive B-cell lymphoma. N Engl J Med 337:529–534

Iida S, Rao PH, Nallasivam P, Hibshoosh H, Butler M, Louie DC, Dyomin V, Ohno H, Chaganti RS, Dalla-Favera R (1996) The t(9;14)(p13;q32) chromosomal translocation associated with lymphoplasmacytoid lymphoma involves the PAX-5 gene. Blood 88:4110–4117

Inagaki H, Banno S, Wakita A, Veda R, Eimotu T (1999) Prognostic significance of CD44V6 in diffuse large B-cell lymphoma. Mod Pathol 12:546–552

Isobe T, Ikeda Y, Ohta H (1979) Comparison of sizes and shapes of tumor cells in plasma cell leukemia and plasma cell myeloma. Blood 53:1028–1030

Iversen OH, Iversen U, Ziegler JL, Bluming AZ (1974) Cell kinetics in Burkitt lymphoma. Eur J Cancer 10:155–163

Jacobs RH, Vokes EE, Golomb HM (1985) Second malignancies in hairy cell leukemia. Cancer 56:1462–1467

Jaffe ES (1985) Pseudoperipheral T cell lymphomas. In: Jaffe ES (ed) Surgical pathology of the lymph nodes and related organs. Saunders, Philadelphia, pp 230–231

Jaffe ES, Longo DL, Cossman J, Hsu SM, Arnold A, Kors-meyer SJ (1984) Diffuse B cell lymphomas with T cell predominance in patients with follicular lymphoma or "pseudo T cell lymphoma". Lab Invest 50:27A–28A

Jaffe ES, Gonzalez CL, Medeiros LJ, Raffeld M (1991) T-cell-rich B-cell lymphomas (letter). Am J Clin Pathol 15:491–492

Jaffe ES, Harris NL, Stein H, Vardiman JW (eds) (2001) World Health Organization classification of tumours pathology and genetics of tumours of hematopoietic and lymphoid tissues. IARC Press, Lyon

Jones SE, Fuks Z, Bull M, Kadin ME, Dorfman RF, Kaplan HS, Rosenberg SA, Kim H (1973) Non-Hodgkin's lymphomas. IV. Clinicopathologic correlation in 405 cases. Cancer 31:806–823

Kamel OW, Gelb AB, Shibuya RB, Warnke RA (1993) Leu 7 (CD57) reactivity distinguishes nodular lymphocyte predominance Hodgkin's disease from nodular sclerosing Hodgkin's disease, T-cell rich B-cell lymphoma and follicular lymphoma. Am J Pathol 142:541–546

Kampmeier P, Spielberger R, Dickstein J, Mick R, Golomb H, Vardiman JW (1994) Increases incidence of second neoplasms in patients treated with interferon α 2b for hairy cell leukemia: a clinicopathologic assessment. Blood 83:2931–2938

Kantarjian HM, McLaughlin P, Fuller LM, Dixon DO, Osborne BM, Cabanillas FF (1984) Follicular large cell lymphoma: analysis and prognostic factors in 62 patients. J Clin Oncol 2:811–819

Keating MJ (1999) Chronic lymphocytic leukemia. Semin Oncol 26 [Suppl 14]:107–114

Kersey J, Abramson C, Perry G, Goldman A, Nesbit M, Gajl-Peczalska K, LeBien T (1982) Clinical usefulness of monoclonal-antibody phenotyping in childhood acute lymphoblastic leukaemia. Lancet ii:1419–1423

Khalidi HS, Chang KL, Medeiros LJ, Brynes RK, Slovak ML, Murata-Collins JL, Arber DA (1999) Acute lymphoblastic leukemia. Survey of immunophenotype, French-American-British classification, frequency of myeloid antigen expression, and karyotypic abnormalities in 210 pediatric and adult cases. Am J Clin Pathol 111:467–476

Khan SM, Cottrell BJ, Millward-Sadler GH, Wright DH (1993) T-cell-rich B-cell lymphoma presenting as liver disease. Histopathology 23:217–224

Kim H, Dorfman RF (1974) Morphological studies of 84 untreated patients subjected to laparotomy for the staging of non-Hodgkin's lymphomas. Cancer 33:657–674

Kim H, Dorfman RF, Rappaport H (1978) Signet ring cell lymphoma. A rare morphologic and functional expression of nodular (follicular) lymphoma. Am J Surg Pathol 2:119–132

Kimby E, Mellstedt H for the Lymphoma Group of Central Sweden (1991) Chlorambucil/Prednisone versus CHOP in symptomatic chronic lymphocytic leukemia of B-cell type. A randomised trial. Leuk Lymph 5 [Suppl]:93–96

Kjeldsberg CR, Kim H (1981) Polykaryocytes resembling Warthin-Finkeldey giant cells in reactive and neoplastic lymphoid disorders. Hum Pathol 12:267–272

Kjeldsberg CR, Wilson JF, Berard CW (1983) Non-Hodgkin's lymphoma in children. Hum Pathol 14:612–627

Knowles DM II, Halper JP, Jakobiec FA (1984) T-lymphocyte subpopulations in B-cell-derived non-Hodgkin's lymphomas and Hodgkin's disease. Cancer 54:644–651

Kojima M, Sakuma H, Mori N (1983) Histopathological features of plasma cell dyscrasia with polyneuropathy and endocrine disturbances, with special reference to germinal center lesions. Jpn J Clin Oncol 13:557–576

Kojima M, Nakamura S, Motoori T, Kurabayashi Y, Hosomura Y, Itoh H, Yoshida K, Suzuki R, Seto M, Koshikawa T, Suchi T, Joshita T (1996) Centroblastic and centroblastic-centrocytic lymphomas associated with prominent epithelioid granulomatous response without plasma cell differentiation: a clinicopathologic study of 12 cases. Hum Pathol 27:660–667

Korsmeyer SJ, Arnold A, Bakhshi A, Ravetch JV, Siebenlist U, Hieter PA, Sharrow SO, LeBien TW, Kersey JH, Poplack DG, Leder P, Waldmann TA (1983) Immunoglobulin gene rearrangement and cell surface antigen expression in acute lymphocytic leukemias of T cell and B cell precursor origins. J Clin Invest 71:301–313

Kramer MH, Hermans J, Parker J, Krol AD, Kluin-Nelemans JC, Haak HL, van Krieken JH, de Jong D, Kluin PM (1996) Clinical significance of bcl-2 and p53 protein expression in diffuse large B-cell lymphoma: a population based study. J Clin Oncol 14:2131–2138

Kramer MHH, Hermans J, Wijburg E, Philippo K, Geelen E, Van Krieken JHJM, de Jong D, Maartense E, Schuuring E, Kluin PM (1998) Clinical relevance of Bcl-2, Bcl-6 and MYC rearrangements in diffuse large B-cell lymphoma. Blood 92:3152–3162

Krishnan J, Ventre K, Reid A, O'Leary T, Frizzera G (1991) T cell rich large B cell lymphoma: a study of clinical morphologic and immunohistochemical features, and PCR analysis of bcl-2 rearrangements. Mod Pathol 4:76A

Krishnan J, Walberg K, Frizzera G (1994) T-cell-rich large B-cell lymphoma. A study of 30 cases supporting its histologic heterogeneity and lack of clinical distinctiveness. Am J Surg Pathol 18:455–465

Kumar S, Green GA, Teruya-Feldstein J, Raffeld M, Jaffe ES (1996) Use of CD23 (BU38) on paraffin sections in the diagnosis of small lymphocytic lymphoma and mantle cell lymphoma. Mod Pathol 9:925–929

Kung PC, Long JC, McCaffrey RP, Ratliff RL, Harrison TA, Baltimore D (1978) Terminal deoxynucleotidyl transferase in the diagnosis of leukemia and malignant lymphoma. Am J Med 64:788–794

Küppers R, Rajewski K, Hansmann ML (1997) Diffuse large cell lymphomas are derived from mature B-cells carrying V region genes with a high load of somatic mutation and evidence of selection for antibody expression. Eur J Immunol 27:1398–1405

Küppers R, Klein U, Hansmann MI, Rajewsky K (1999) Cellular origin of human B-cell lymphomas. N Engl J Med 341:1520–1529

Kuse R, Heilmann HP, Calavrezos A, Hausmann K (1983) Prognostic differences in low-malignancy germinal center cell lymphomas and immunocytomas. Relationship to histological subtypes, stages and therapy. Dtsch Med Wochenschr 108:1948–1954

Kuze T, Nakamura N, Hashimoto Y, Abe M, Wakasa H (1996) Clinicopathological, immunological and genetic studies of CD30+ anaplastic large cell lymphoma of B-cell type: association with Epstein-Barr virus in a Japanese population. J Pathol 180:236–242

Kwak LW, Wilson M, Weiss LM, Horning SJ, Warnke RA, Dorfman RF (1991) Clinical significance of morphologic subdivision in diffuse large cell lymphoma. Cancer 68:1988–1993

La Starza R, Aventin A, Falzetti D, Stul M, Martelli MF, Falini B, Mecucci C (1996) 14q+ chromosome marker in a T-cell-rich B-cell lymphoma. J Pathol 178:227–231

Lai R, Arber DA, Chang KL, Wilson CS, Weiss LM (1998) Frequency of bcl-2 expression in non-Hodgkin's lymphoma: a study of 778 cases with comparison of marginal zone lymphoma and monocytoid B-cell hyperplasia. Mod Pathol 11:864–869

Leibetseder F, Thurner J (1973) Angiofollikuläre Lymphknotenhyperplasie (Zwiebelschalen-Lymphom). Med Klin 68: 817–820

Lennert K (1958) Die Frühveränderungen der Lymphogranulomatose. Frankf Z Pathol 69:103–122

Lennert K (1961) Lymphknoten. Diagnostik in Schnitt und Ausstrich. Cytologie und Lymphadenitis. Handbuch der speziellen pathologischen Anatomie und Histologie, vol 1. Springer, Berlin Göttingen Heidleberg

Lennert K in collaboration with Mohri N, Stein H, Kaiserling E, Müller-Hermelink HK (1978) Malignant lymphomas other than Hodgkin's disease. Springer, Berlin Heidelberg New York (Handbuch der speziellen pathologischen Anatomie und Histologie, vol 1/3B)

Lennert K (1981) Histopathologie der non-Hodgkin Lymphome (nach der Kiel-Klassification). In Zusammenarbeit mit H. Stein. Springer, Berlin Heidelberg New York

Lennert K, Feller AC (1990) Histopathologie der Non-Hodgkin Lymphome, 2nd edn. Springer, Berlin Heidelberg New York

Lens D, Matutes E, Catovsky D, Coignet LJA (2000) Frequent deletions at 11q23 and 13q14 in B cell prolymphocytic leukemia (B-PLL). Leukemia 14:427–430

Levasseur M, Middleton PG, Angus B, Proctor SJ, Norden J, Howard MR (1995) C-MYC Gene abnormalities in high grade and centroblastic-centrocytic non-Hodgkin's lymphoma. Leuk Lymph 18:131–136

Levine PH, Kamaraju LS, Connelly RR, Berard CW, Dorfman RF, Magrath I, Easton JM (1982) The American Burkitt's lymphoma registry: eight years experience. Cancer 49:1016–1022

Lichtenstein A, Levine AM, Lukes RJ (1979) Immunoblastic sarcoma. A clinical description. Cancer 43:343–352

Liebermann PH, Filippa DA, Straus DJ, Thaler HT, Cirrincione C, Clarkson BD (1986) Evaluation of malignant lymphomas using three classifications and the Working Formulation. 482 cases with median follow-up of 11.9 years. Am J Med 81:365–380

Lo Cocco F, Ye BH, Lista F, Corradini P, Offit K, Knowles DM, Chaganti RSK, Dalla Favera R (1994) Rearrangement of the bcl-6 gene in diffuse large cell non-Hodgkin's lymphoma. Blood 83:1757

Lones MA, Cairo MS, Perkins SL (2000) T-cell-rich large B-cell lymphoma in children and adolescents: a clinicopathologic report of six cases from the Children's Cancer Group Study CCG-5961. Cancer 88:2378–2386

Look AT, Roberson PK, Williams DL, Rivera G, Bowman WP, Pui CH, Ochs J, Abromowitch M, Kalwinsky D, Dahl GV, George S, Murphy SB (1985) Prognostic importance of blast cell DNA content in childhood acute lymphoblastic leukemia. Blood 65:1079–1086

Lossos IS, Okada CY, Tibshirani R, Warnke R, Vose J, Grreiner T, Levy R (2000a) Molecular analysis of immunoglobulin genes in diffuse large B-cell lymphomas. Blood 95:1797–1803

Lossos IS, Alizadeh AA, Eisen MB, Chan WC, Brown PO, Botstein D, Staudt LM, Levy R (2000b) Ongoing immunoglobulin somatic mutation in germinal center B cell-like but not in activated B cell-like diffuse large cell lymphomas. Proc Natl Acad Sci USA 97:10.209–10.213

Lukes RJ, Collins RD (1975a) New approaches to the classification of the lymphomata. Br J Cancer 31 [Suppl 1]:1–28

Lukes RJ, Collins RD (1975b) A functional classification of malignant lymphomas. In: Rebuck JW, Berard CW, Abell MR (eds) The reticuloendothelial system. Monographs in pathology, no 16. Williams and Wilkins, Baltimore, pp 213–242

Mabuchi H, Fujii H, Calin G, Alder H, Negrini M, Rassenti L, Kipps TJ, Bullrich F, Croce CM (2001) Cloning and characterization of CLLD6, CLLD7, and CLLD8, novel candidate genes for leukemogenesis at chromosome 13q14, a region commonly deleted in B-cell chronic lymphocytic leukemia. Cancer Res 61:2870–2877

Macon WR, Cousar JB, Waldron JA, Hsu SM (1992a) Interleukin-4 may contribute to the abundant T-cell reaction and paucity of neoplastic B cells in T-cell-rich B-cell lymphomas. Am J Pathol 141:1031–1036

Macon WR, Williams ME, Greer JP, Stein RS, Collins RD, Cousar JB (1992b) T-cell-rich B-cell lymphomas: a clinicopathologic study of 19 cases. Am J Surg Pathol 16:351–363

Magrath IT, Sariban E (1985) Clinical features of Burkitt's lymphoma in the USA. IARC Sci Publ 60:119–127

Magrath IT, Janus C, Edwards BK, Spiegel R, Jaffe ES, Berard CW, Miliauskas J, Morris K, Barnwell R (1984) An effective therapy for both undifferentiated (including Burkitt's lymphomas) and lymphoblastic lymphomas in children and young adults. Blood 63:1102–1111

Malik STA, Amess J, D'Ardenne AJ, Lister TA (1989) Hairy cell leukemia – mediastinal involvement. A report of two cases and review of the literature. Hematol Oncol 7:303–306

Mann RB, Berard CW (1983) Criteria for the cytological subclassification of follicular lymphomas: a proposed alternative method. Hematol Oncol 1:187–192

Mann RB, Jaffe ES, Braylan RC, Nanba K, Frank MM, Ziegler JL, Berard CW (1976) Non-endemic Burkitt's lymphoma: a B-cell tumor related to germinal centers. N Engl J Med 295:685–691

Mann RB, Jaffe ES, Berard CW (1979) Malignant lymphomas – a conceptual understanding of morphologic diversity. Am J Pathol 94:104–192

Mann RB (1985) Follicular lymphoma and lymphocytic lymphoma of intermediate differentiation. In: Jaffe ES (ed) Surgical pathology of the lymph nodes and related organs. Major problems in pathology, vol 16. Saunders, Philadelphia, pp 165-202

Martin AR, Weisenburger DD, Chan WC, Ruby EI, Anderson JR, Vose JM, Bierman PJ, Bast MA, Daley DT, Armitage JO (1995) Prognostic value of cellular proliferation and histologic grade in follicular lymphoma. Blood 85:3671–3678

McBride JA, Rodriguez J, Luthra R, Ordonez G, Cabanillas F, Pugh WC (1996) T-cell-rich B large-cell lymphoma simulating lymphocyte-rich Hodgkin's disease. Am J Surg Pathol 20:193–201

Melnyk A, Rodriguez A, Pugh WC, Cabannillas F (1997) Evaluation of the Revised European-American Lymphoma classification confirms the clinical relevance of immunophenotype in 560 cases of aggressive non-Hodgkin's lymphoma. Blood 89:4514–4520

Mercieca J, Puga M, Matutes E, Moskovic E, Salim S, Catovsky D (1994) Incidence and significance of abdominal lymphadenopathy in hairy cell leukaemia. Leuk Lymph 14 [Suppl 1]:79–83

Meugé C, Hoerni B, de Mascarel A, Durand M, Richaud P, Hoerni-Simon G, Chauvergne J, Lagarde C (1978) Non-Hodgkin malignant lymphomas. Clinico-pathologic correlations with the Kiel classification. Retrospective analysis of a series of 274 cases. Eur J Cancer 14:587–592

Meusers P, Bartels H, Brittinger G, Common H, Dühmke E, Fülle HH, Gunzer U, Heinz R, König E, Musshoff K, Pralle H, Schmalhorst U, Theml H, Krüger GR, Lennert K (1979) Heterogeneity of diffuse "histiocytic" lymphoma according to the Kiel classification. N Engl J Med 301:384

Meusers P, Engelhard M, Bartels H, Binder T, Füller HH, Görg K, Gunzer U, Havemann K, Kayser W, König E, König HJ, Kuse R, Löffler H, Ludwig W-D, Mainzer K, Martin H, Pralle H, Schoppe WD, Staiger HJ, Theml H, Zurborn KH, Zwingers T, Lennert K, Brittinger G (1989) Multicentre randomized therapeutic trial for advanced centrocytic lymphoma: anthracycline does not improve the prognosis. Hematol Oncol 7:365–380

Lagios MD, Friedlander LM, Wallerstein RO, Bohannon RA (1974) Atypical azurophilic crystals in chronic lymphocytic leukemia. A case report and comparison with other crystalline inclusions. Am J Clin Pathol 62:342–349

Migliazza A, Bosch F, Komatsu H, Cayanis E, Martinotti S, Toniato E, Guccione E, Qu X, Chien M, Murty VVV, Gaidano G, Inghirami G, Zhang P, Fischer S, Kalachikov SM, Russo J, Edelman I, Efstratiadis A, Dalla-Favera R (2001) Nucleotide sequence, transcription map, and mutation analysis of the 13q14 chromosomal region deleted in B-cell chronic lymphocytic leukemia. Blood 97:2098–2103

Miller TP, Grogan TM, Dahlbert S, Spier CM, Braziel RM, Banks PM, Foucar K, Kjeldsberg CR, Levy N, Nathwani BN (1994) Prognostic significance of the Ki-67-associated proliferative antigen in aggressive non-Hodgkin's lymphomas:

a prospective Southwest Oncology Group trial. Blood 83:1460–1466

Miller TP, LeBlanc M, Grogan TM, Fisher RI (1997) Follicular lymphomas: do histologic subtypes predict outcome? Hematol Oncol 11:893–900

Miranda RN, Cousar JB, Hammer RD, Collins RD, Vnencak-Jones CL (1999) Somatic mutation analysis of IgH variable regions reveals that tumor cells of most parafollicular (monocytoid) B-cell lymphoma, splenic marginal zone B-cell lymphoma, and some hairy cell leukemia are composed of memory B lymphocytes. Hum Pathol 30:306–312

Miranda RN, Briggs RC, Kinney MC, Veno PA, Hammer RD, Cousar JB (2000) Immunohistochemical detection of Cyclin D1 using optimised conditions is highly specific for mantle cell lymphoma and hairy cell leukemia. Mod Pathol 13:1308–1314

Mirchandani I, Palutke M, Tabaczka P, Foldfarb S, Eisenberg L, Pak MSY (1985) B-cell lymphomas morphologically resembling T-cell lymphomas. Cancer 56:1578–1583

Molenaar WM, Bartels H, Koudstaal J (1984) Histological, epidemiological and clinical aspects of centroblastic-centrocytic lymphomas subdivided according to the "working formulation". Br J Cancer 49:263–268

Mollejo M, Menarguez J, Cristobal E, Algara P, Sanchez-Diaz E, Fraga M, Piris MA (1994) Monocytoid B cells. A comparative clinical pathological study of their distribution in different types of low-grade lymphomas. Am J Surg Pathol 1131–1139

Monni O, Franssila K, Joensuu H, Knuutila S (1999) BCL2 overexpression in diffuse large B-cell lymphoma. Leuk Lymph 34:45–52

Montserrat E (2001) Prognostic factors in aggressive lymphoma: the contribution of novel biological markers. Ann Hematol 80:B42–B44

Montserrat E, Sanchez-Bisono J, Vinolas N, Rozman C (1986) Lymphocyte doubling time in chronic lymphocytic leukaemia: analysis of its prognostic significance. Br J Haematol 62:567–575

Morel P, Xerri L, Cojean I et al (1997) Prognostic value of subclassification of diffuse large B-cell lymphomas according to the Kiel classification: a GELA studdy on 1487 patients. Blood 90:336a

Morel P, Besuschio S, Cojean I, Gaulard P, Casanovas O, Diebold J (2002) Prognosis value of subclassification of diffuse large B-cell lymphomas according to the Kiel classification : a GELA study of 1492 patients (in press)

Muramatsu M, Akasaka T, Kadowaki N, Ohno H, Yamabe H, Edamura S, Doi S, Mori T, Okuma M, Fukuhara S (1996) Rearrangement of the Bcl-6 gene in B-cell lymphoid neoplasms : comparison with lymphomas associated with Bcl-2 rearrangement. Br J Haematol 93:911–920

Murphy SB, Hustu HO (1980) A randomized trial of combined modality therapy of childhood non-Hodgkin's lymphoma. Cancer 45:630–637

Nakamine H, Masih AS, Scott-Strobach R, Duggan MJ, Bast MA, Armitage JO, Weisenburger DD (1991) Immunoblastic lymphoma with abundant clear-cytoplasm. A comparative study of B- and T-cell types. Am J Clin Pathol 96:177–183

Nakamura N, Hashimoto Y, Kuze T, Tasaki K, Sasaki Y, Sato M, Abe M (1999) Analysis of the immunoglobulin heavy chain gene variable region of CD5-positive diffuse large B-cell lymphoma. Lab Invest 79:925–933

Nakamura N, Kuze T, Hashimoto Y, Hoshis S, Tominaga K, Sasaki Y, Shirakawa A, Sato M, Maeda K, Abe M (2000) Analysis of the immunoglobulins heavy chains gene of secondary diffuse large B-cell lymphoma that subsequently developped in four cases with B-cell chronic lymphocytic leukemia or lymphoplasmacytoid lymphoma (Richter's syndrome). Pathol Int 50:636–643

Nashelsky MB, Hess MM, Weisenburger DD, Pierson JL, Bast MA, Armitage JO, Sanger WG (1994) Cytogenetic abnormalities in B-immunoblastic lymphoma. Leuk Lymph 14:415–420

Nathwani BN, Winberg CD, Diamond LW, Bearman RM, Kim H (1981a) Morphologic criteria for the differentiation of follicular lymphoma from florid reactive follicular hyperplasia: a study of 80 cases. Cancer 48:1794–1806

Nathwani BN, Diamond LW, Winberg CD, Kim H, Bearman RM, Glick JH, Jones SE, Gams RA, Nissen NI, Rappaport H (1981b) Lymphoblastic lymphoma: a clinicopathologic study of 95 patients. Cancer 48:2347–2357

Nathwani BN, Mohrmann RL, Brynes RK, Taylor CR, Hansmann ML, Sheibani K (1992) Monocytoid B-cell lymphomas: an assessment of diagnostic criteria and a perspective on histogenesis. Hum Pathol 23:1061–1071

Nathwani BN, Anderson JR, Armitage JO, Cavalli F, Diebold J, Drachenberg MR, Harris NL, MacLennan KA, Müller-Hermelink HK, Ullrich FA, Weisenburger DD (1999a) Clinical significance of follicular lymphoma with monocytoid B cells. Non-Hodgkin's Lymphoma Classification Projekt. Hum Pathol 30:263–268

Nathwani BN, Drachenberg MR, Hernandez AM, Levine AM, Sheibani K (1999b) Nodal monocytoid B-cell lymphoma (nodal marginal-zone B-cell lymphoma). Semin Hematol 36:128–138

Navaratnam S, Williams GJ, Rubinger M, Pettigrew NM, Mowat MR, Begleiter A, Johnston JB (1998) Expression of p53 predicts treatment failure in aggressive non-Hodgkin's lymphomas. Leuk Lymph 29:139–144

Nazeer T, Burkart P, Dunn H, Jennings TA, Wolf B (1997) Blastic transformation of hairy cell leukemia. Arch Pathol Lab Med 121:707–713

Neilly IJ, Ogston M, Bennett B, Dawson AA (1995) High grade non-Hodgkin's lymphoma in the elderly-12 years experience in the Grampian region of Scotland. Hematol Oncol 13:99–106

Neri A, Barega F, Knowles D, Magrath I, Dalla-Favera R (1988) Different regions of the immunoglobulin heavy-chain locus are involved in chromosomal translocation in distinct pathogenetic forms of Burkitt lymphoma. Proc Nat Acad Sci USA 85:2748–2754

Neth O, Seidemán K, Jansen P, Mann G, Tiemann M, Ludwig WD, Riehm H, Reiter A (2000) Precursor B-cell lymphoblastic lymphoma in childhood and adolescence: clinical features, treatment, and results in trials NHL-BFM 86 and 90. Med Pediatr Oncol 35:20–27

Newland JR, Linke RP, Lennert K (1986) Amyloid deposits in lymph nodes: a morphologic and immunohistochemical study. Hum Pathol 17:1245–1249

Ng CS, Chan JKC (1987) Monocytoid B-cell lymphoma. Hum Pathol 18:1069–1071

Ng CS, Chan JKC, Hui PK, Lau WH (1989) Large B-cell lymphomas with a high content of reactive T cells. Hum Pathol 20:1145–1154

Nguyen DT, Diamond LW, Schwonzen M, Bohlen H, Diehl V (1995) Chronic lymphocytic leukemia with an interfollicular architecture: avoiding diagnostic confusion with monocytoid B-cell lymphoma. Leuk Lymph 18:179–184

Nieder C, Petersen S, Petersen C, Thames HD (2001) The challenge of p53 as prognostic and predictive factor in Hodgkin's or non-Hodgkin's lymphoma. Ann Hematol 80:2–8

Nizze H, Cogliatti SB, von Schillin C, Feller AC, Lennert K (1991) Monocytoid B-cell lymphoma: morphological variants and relationship to low-grade B-cell lymphoma of the mucosa-associated lymphoid tissue. Histopathology 18:403–424

Norton AJ, Matthews J, Pappa V, Shamash J, Love S, Rohatiner AZ, Lister TA (1995) Mantle cell lymphoma: natural history defined in a serially biopsied population over a 20-year period. Ann Oncol 6:249–256

Offit K, Jhanwar SC, Ladanyi M, Filippa DA, Chaganti RSK (1991) Cytogenetic analysis of 434 consecutively ascertained specimens of Non-Hodgkin's lymphoma: correlations between recurrent aberrations, histology, and exposure to cytotoxic treatment. Genes Chromosomes Cancer 3:189–201

Offit K, Parsa NZ, Filippa D, Jhanwar SC, Chaganti RSK (1992) t(9;14)(p13;q32) denotes a subset of low-grade Non-Hodgkin's lymphoma with plasmacytoid differentiation. Blood 80:2594–2599

Offit K, Louie DC, Parsa NZ, Noy A, Chaganti RSK (1995) Del(7)(q32) is associated with a subset of small lymphocytic lymphoma with plasmacytoid features. Blood 86:2365–2370

Ohno H, Ueda C, Akasaka T (2000) The t(9;14)(p13;q32) translocation in B-cell non-Hodgkin's lymphoma. Leuk Lymphoma 36:435–445.

Ohshima K, Masuda Y, Kikuchi M, Sumiyoshi Y, Kobari S, Yoneda S, Takeshita M, Kimura N (1994) Monoclonal B cells and restricted oligoclonal T cells in T-cell-rich B-cell lymphoma. Pathol Res Pract 190:15–24

Ohshima K, Suzumiya J, Sato K, Kanta M, Haraoka S, Kikuchi M (1999) B-cell lymphoma of 708 cases in Japan: incidence rates and clinical prognosis according to the REAL classification. Cancer Lett 135:73–81

Okuda T, Fisher R, Downing JR (1996) Molecular diagnostics in pediatric acute lymphoblastic leukemia. Mol Diagn 1:139–151

Osborne BM, Butler JJ (1987) Follicular lymphoma mimicking progressive transformation of germinal centers. Am J Clin Pathol 88: 264–269

Osborne BM, Butler JJ, Pugh WC (1990) The value of immunophenotyping on paraffin sections in the identification of T-cell rich B-cell large-cell lymphomas: lineage confirmed by JH rearrangement. Am J Surg Pathol 14: 933–938

Osborne BM, Butler JJ, Pugh WC (1991a) The value of immunophenotyping on paraffin sections in the identification of T-cell rich B-cell large-cell lymphomas: lineage confirmed by J_h rearrangment. Am J Surg Pathol 14:933–938

Osborne BM, Buttler JJ, Pugh WC (1991b) The authors's response (letter to the editor). Am J Surg Pathol 15:492

Oscier DG, Thompsett A, Zhu D, Stevenson FK (1997) Differential rates of somatic hypermutation in V_H genes among subsets of chronic lymphocytic leukemia defined by chromosomal abnormalities. Blood 89:4153–4160

Otsuki T, Yano T, Clark HM, Bastard C, Kerckaert JP, Jaffe ES, Raffeld M (1995b) Analysis of LAZ3 (BCL-6) status in B-cell non-Hodgkin's lymphomas: results of rearrangement and gene expression studies and a mutational analysis of coding region sequences. Blood 85:2877–2884

Ott G, Kalla J, Ott M, Schryen B, Katzenberger T, Müller JG, Müller-Hermelink HK (1997) Blastoid variants of mantle cell lymphoma: frequent bcl-1 rearrangements at the major translocation cluster region and tetraploid chromosome clones. Blood 89:1421–1429

Ott G, Katzenberger T, Lohr A, Kindelberger S, Rudiger T, Wilhelm M, Kalla J, Rosenwald A, Muller JG, Ott MM, Muller-Hermelink HK (2002) Cytomorphologic, immunohistochemical, and cytogenetic profiles of follicular lymphoma: 2 types of follicular lymphoma grade 3. Blood 99:3806–12

Ottensmeier CH, Thompsett AR, Zhu D, Wilkins BS, Sweetenham JW, Stevenson FR (1998) Analysis of VH genes in follicular and diffuse lymphoma shows ongoing somatic mutation and multiple isotype transcripts in early disease with changes during disease progression. Blood 91:4292–4299

Oviat DL, Cousar JB, Collins RD, Flexner JM, Stein RS (1984) Malignant lymphomas of follicular center cell origin in humans. Cancer 53:1109–1114

Ozdemirli M, Fanburg-Smith JC, Hartmann DP, Shad AT, Lage JM, Magrath IT, Azumi N, Harris NL, Cossman J, Jaffe ES (1998) Precursor B-lymphoblastic lymphoma presenting as a solitary bone tumor and mimicking Ewing's sarcoma. Am J Surg Pathol 22:795–804

Pallesen G (1983) Burkitt's lymphoma: diagnostic and taxonomic aspects. In: Molander DW (ed) Diseases of the lymphatic system. Diagnosis and therapy. Springer, Berlin Heidelberg New York, pp 89–102

Pangalis GA, Angelopoulou MK, Vassilakopoulos TP, Siakantaris MP, Kittas C (1999) B-chronic lymphocytic leukaemia, small lymphocytic lymphoma, and lymphoplasmacytic lymphoma, including Waldenström's macroglobulinemia: a clinical, morphologic, and biologic spectrum of similar disorders. Semin Hematol 36:104–114

Papamichael D, Norton AJ, Foran JM, Mulatero C, Mathews J, Amess JAL, Bradburn M, Lister TA, Rohatiner AZS (1999) Immunocytoma: a retrospective analysis from St. Bartholomew's Hospital – 1972 to 1996. J Clin Oncol 17:2847–2853

Payne CM, Grogan TM, Cromey DW, Bjore CG Jr, Kerrigan DP (1987) An ultrastructural, morphometric and immunophenotypic evaluation of Burkitt's and Burkitt's-like lymphomas. Lab Invest 57:200–218

Pelicci PG, Knowles DM, Favera RD (1985) Lymphoid tumors displaying rearrangements of both immunoglobulin and T cell receptor genes. J Exp Med 162:1015–1024

Pelicci PG, Knowles D, Magrath I, Dalla-Favera R (1986) Chromosomal breakpoint and structural alterations of the c-myc locus differ in endemic and sporadic forms of Burkitt lymphoma. Proc Nat Acad Sci USA 83:2984–2990

Pezella F, Gatter KC, Mason DY, Bastard C, Duval C, Krajewski A, Turner GE, Ross FM, Clark H, Jones DB, Leroux D, Le Marc'Hadour F (1990) Bcl-2 protein expression in follicular lymphomas in absence of 14;18 translocation. Lancet 336:1510–1511

Piris MA, Rivas C, Morente M, Cruz MA, Rubio C, Oliva H (1988) Monocytoid B-cell lymphoma, a tumour related to the marginal zone. Histopathology 12:383–392

Piris M, Brown DC, Gatter KC, Mason DY (1990) CD30 expression in non-Hodgkin's lymphoma. Histopathology 17:211–218

Piris MA, Pezella F, Martinez-Montero JC, Orradre JL, Vilvendas R, Cuena R, Cruz MA, Martinez B, Pezella F (1994) p53 and bcl-2 expression in high grade B-cell lymphomas. Correlation with survival time. Br J Cancer 69:337–341

Piris MA, Mollejo M, Campo E, Menarguez J, Flores T, Issacson PG (1998) A marginal zone pattern may be found in different varieties of Non-Hodgkin's lymphoma: the morphology and immunohistology of splenic involvement by B-cell lymphomas simulating splenic marginal zone lymphoma. Histopathology 33:230–239

Pittaluga S, Verhoef G, Criel A, Maes A, Nuyts J, Boogaerts M, de Wolf Peeters C (1996) Prognostic significance of bone marrow trephine and peripheral blood smears in 55 patients with mantle cell lymphoma. Leuk Lymph 21:115–125

Pittaluga S, Verhoef G, Criel A, Wlodarska I, Dierlamm J, Mecucci C, van den Berghe H, de Wolf Peeters C (1996) "Small" B-cell non-Hodgkin's lymphomas with splenomegaly at presentation are either mantle cell lymphoma or marginal zone cell lymphoma. A study based on histology, cytology, immunohistochemistry, and cytogenetic analysis. Am J Surg Pathol 20:211–223

Preudhomme C, Dervite I, Wattel E, Vanrumbeke M, Flactif M, Lai JL, Hecquet B, Coppin MC, Nelken B, Gosselin B, Fenaux P (1995) Clinical signification of p53 mutations in newly diagnosed Burkitt's lymphoma and acute lymphoblastic leukemia. A report of 48 cases. J Clin Oncol 13:812–820

Prévot S, Hamilton-Dutoit S, Audouin J, Walter P, Pallesen G, Diebold J (1992) Analysis of African Burkitt's and high-grade B-cell non Burkitt's lymphoma for Epstein-Barr virus genomes using in situ hybridization. Br J Haematol 80:27–32

Prokocimer M, Matzner Y, Ben-Bassat H, Polliack A (1980) Burkitt's lymphoma presenting as acute leukemia (Burkitt's lymphoma cell leukemia). Report of two cases in Israel. Cancer 45:2884–2889

Pugh WC, Manning JT, Butler JJ (1988) Paraimmunoblastic variant of small lymphocytic lymphoma/leukemia. Am J Surg Pathol 12:907–917

Pui CH (1995) Childhood leukemias. N Engl J Med 332:1618–1630

Radzun HJ, Hansmann M-L, Heidebrecht HJ, Bödewadt-Radzun S, Wacker HH, Kreipe H, Lumbeck H, Hernandez C, Kuhn C, Parwaresch MR (1991) Detection of a monocyte/macrophage differentiation antigen in routinely processed paraffin-embedded tissues by monoclonal antibody Ki-M1P. Lab Invest 65:306–315

Raghoebier S, Kibbelaar RE, Kleiverda JK, Kluin-Nelemans JC, van Krieken JH, Kok F, Kluin PM (1992) Mosaicism of trisomy 12 in chronic lymphocytic leukemia detected by non-radioactive in situ hybridization. Leukemia 6:1220–1226

Rai KR, Sawitsky A, Cronkite EP, Chanana AD, Levy RN, Pasternack BS (1975) Clinical staging of chronic lymphocytic leukemia. Blood 46:219–234

Raimondi SC (1993) Current status of cytogenetic research in childhood acute lymphoblastic leukemia. Blood 81:2237–2251

Ramsay AD, Smith WJ, Isaacson PG (1988) T-cell-rich B-cell lymphoma. Am J Surg Pathol 12:433–443

Rao PH, Houldsworth J, Dyomina K, Parsa NZ, Cigudosa JC, Louie DC, Popplewell L, Offit K, Jhanwar SC, Chaganti RSK (1998) Chromosomal and gene amplification in diffuse large B-cell lymphoma. Blood 92:234–240

Raphaël M, Gentilhomme O, Tulliez M, Bryon PA, Diebold J (1991) Histopathologic features of high-grade non-Hodgkin's lymphomas in acquired immunodeficiency syndrome. The French Study Group of Pathology for Human Immunodeficiency Virus-Associated Tumors. Arch Pathol Lab Med 115:15–20

Raphaël M, Audouin J, Lamine M, Delecluze HJ, Vuillaume M, Lenoir GM, Gisselbrecht C, Lennert K, Diebold J (1994) Immunophenotype and genotypic analysis of acquired immunodeficiency syndrome-related non-Hodgkin's lymphomas. Am J Clin Pathol 101:773–782

Rappaport H, Winter WJ, Hicks EB (1956) Follicular lymphoma. A re-evaluation of its position in the scheme of malignant lymphoma, based on a survey of 253 cases. Cancer 9:792–821

Raty R, Franssila K, Joensuu H, Teerenhovi L, Elonen E (2002) Ki-67 expression level, histological subtype, and the International Prognostic Index as outcome predictors in mantle cell lymphoma. Eur J Haematol 69:11–20

Reiter A, Schrappe M, Tiemann M, Ludwig WD, Yakisan E, Zimmermann M, Mann G, Chott A, Ebell W, Klingebiel T, Graf N, Kremens B, Müller-Weihrich S, Plüss HJ, Zintl F, Henze G, Riehm H (1999) Improved treatment results in childhood B-cell neoplasms with tailored intensification of therapy: a report of the Berlin-Frankfurt-Münster Group trial NHL-BFM 90. Blood 94:3294–3306

Rennke H, Lennert K (1973) Käsig-tuberkuloide Reaktion bei Lymphknotenmetastasen lymphoepitheliler Carcinome (Schmincke-Tumoren). Virchows Arch (A) 358:241–247

Rice L, Shenkenberg T, Lynch EC, Wheeler TM (1982) Granulomatous infections complicating hairy cell leukaemia. Cancer 49:1924–1928

Ripp JA, Loiue DC, Chan W, Nawaz H, Portlock CS (2002) T-cell rich B-cell lymphoma: clinical distinctiveness and response to treatment in 45 patients. Leuk Lymphoma 43:1573-1580

Robbins BA, Ellison DJ, Spinosa JC, Carey CA, Lukes RJ, Poppema S, Saven A, Piro LD (1993) Diagnostic application of two-color flow cytometry in 161 cases of hairy cell leukemia. Blood 82:1277–1287

Rodriguez J, Pugh WC, Cabanillas F (1993) T-cell-rich B-cell lymphoma. Blood 82:1586–1589

Rodriguez J, McLaughlin P, Fayad L, Santiago M, Hess M, Rodriguez MA, Romaguera J, Hagemeister F, Kantarjian H, Cabanillas F (2000) Follicular large cell lymphoma: long-term follow-up of 62 patients treated between 1973–1981. Ann Oncol 11:1551–1556

Saez AI, Sanchez E, Sanchez-Beato M, Cruz MA, Chacon I, Munoz E, Camacho FI, Martinez-Montero JC, Mollejo M, Garcia JF, Piris MA (1999) $p27^{KIP1}$ is abnormally expressed in diffuse large B-cell lymphomas and is associated with an adverse clinical outcome. Br J Cancer 89:1427–1434

Salar A, Fernandez de Sevilla A, Romagosa V, Domingo-Claros A, Gonzalez-Barca E, Pera J, Climent J, Granema A (1998)

Diffuse large B-cell lymphoma: is morphologic subdivision useful in clinical management? Eur J Haematol 60: 202–208

Samaha H, Dumontet C, Ketterer N, Moullet I, Thieblemont C, Bouafia F, Callet-Bauchu E, Felman P, Berger F, Salles G, Coiffier B (1998) Mantle cell lymphoma: a retrospective study of 121 cases. Leukemia 12:1281–1287

Sanchez E, Chacon I, Plaza MM, Munoz E, Cruz MA, Martinez B, Martinez-Montero JC, Saez AL, Garcia JF, Piris MA (1998) Clinical outcome in diffuse large B-cell lymphoma is dependent on the relationship between different cell-cycle regulator proteins. J Clin Oncol 16:1931–1939

Sanchez-Beato M, Camacho FI, Martinez-Montero JCM, Saez AI, Villuendas R, Sanchez-Verde L, Garcia JF, Piris MA (1999) Anomalous high $p27^{KIP1}$ expression in a subset of aggressive B-cell lymphomas is associated with cyclin D3 overexpression. $P27^{KIP1}$-cyclin D3 colocalization in tumor cells. Blood 94:765–772

Scarpa A, Bonetti F, Zamboni G, Menestrina F, Chilosi M (1989) T-cell-rich B-cell lymphoma (letter to the editor). Am J Surg Pathol 13:335–337

Schlegelberger B, Zwingers T, Harder L, Nowotny H, Siebert R, Vesely M, Bartels H, Sonnen R, Hopfinger G, Nader A, Ott G, Muller-Hermelink K, Feller A, Heinz R (1999) Clinicopathogenetic significance of chromosomal abnormalities in patients with blastic peripheral B-cell lymphoma. Kiel-Wien-Lymphoma Study Group. Blood 94:3114–3120

Schlette E, Bueso-Ramos C, Giles F, Glassman A, Hayes K, Medeiros LJ (2001) Mature B-cell leukemias with more than 55% prolymphocytes. A heterogeneous group that includes an unusual variant of mantle cell lymphoma. Am J Clin Pathol 115:571–581

Schmalhorst U, Bartels H, Boll I, Burger-Schüler A, Common H, Fülle HH, Graubner M, Heinz R, Huhn D, Leopold H, Meusers P, Nowicki L, Nürnberger R, Oertel J, Rühl U, Sieber G, Schmidt M, Schoengen A, Strassner A, Schwarze EW (Kiel Lymphoma Study Group) (1979) Clinical and prognostic heterogeneity of high-grade malignant lymphomas. 5th meeting of the International Society of Haematology, European and African Division, Hamburg, 26–31 Aug 1979

Schmalhorst U, Bartels H, Boll I, Burger-Schüler A, Common H, Fülle HH, Graubner M, Heinz R, Huhn D, Leopold H, Meusers P, Nowicki L, Nürnberger R, Oertel J, Rühl U, Sieber G, Schmidt M, Schoengen A, Strassner A, Schwarze EW, Brittinger G (1981) Clinical and prognostic heterogeneity of non-Hodgkin's lymphomas of high-grade malignancy. Blut 43:201–211

Schmid U, Helbron D, Lennert K (1982) Development of malignant lymphoma in myeopithelial sialadenitis (Sjögren's syndrome). Virchows Arch [A] 395:11–43

Schmid U, Karow J, Lennert K (1985) Follicular malignant non-Hodgkin's lymphoma with pronounced plasmacytic differentiation: a plasmacytoma-like lymphoma. Virchows Arch [A] 405:473–481

Schmidt D, Leuschner I, Harms D, Sprenger E, Schäfer H-J (1989) Malignant rhabdoid tumor. A morphological and flow cytometric study. Pathol Res Pract 184:202–210

Schmidt V, Leder LD (1996) T-cell-rich B-cell lymphoma. A distinct clinicopathologic entity, Leuk Lymphoma 23:17–24

Seo IS, Min KW, Brodhecker C, Mirkin LD (1988) Malignant renal rhabdoid tumour. Immunohistochemical and ultrastructural studies. Histopathology 13:657–666

Shahab I, Manning JT, Pugh WC (1993) Utility of CD57 immunostaining in the differential diagnosis of T-cell rich B-cell lymphoma and nodular lymphocyte predominant Hodgkin's disease. Mod Pathol 6:100A

Sham RL, Phatak P, Carignan J, Janas J, Olson JP (1989) Progression of follicular large cell lymphoma to Burkitt's lymphoma. Cancer 63:700–702

Sheibani K, Burke JS, Swartz WG, Nademanee A, Winberg CD (1988) Monocytoid B-cell lymphoma: clinicopathologic study of 21 cases of a unique type of low-grade lymphoma. Cancer 62:1531–1538

Shipp MA, Ross KN, Tamayo P, Weng AP, Kutok JL, Aguiar RCT, Gaasenbeek M, Angelo M, Reich M, Pinkus g, Ray TS, Koval MA, Last KW, Norton A, Lister TA, Mesirov J, Neuberg DS, Lander ES, Aster JC, Golub TR (2002) Diffuse large B-cell lymphoma outcome prediction by gene-expression profiling and supervised machine learning. Nature Med 8:68–74

Shiramizu B, Barriga F, Neequaye J, Jafri A, Dalla-Favera R, Neri A, Gutierrez M, Levine P, Magrath I (1991) Pattern of chromosomal breakpoint locations in Burkitt's lymphoma: relevance to geography and Epstein-Barr virus association. Blood 77:1516–1526

Shvidel L, Shtalrid M, Bassous L, Klepfish A, Vorst E, Berrebi A (1999) B-cell prolymphocytic leukemia: a survey of 35 patients emphasizing heterogeneity, prognostic factors and evidence for a group with an indolent course. Leuk Lymphoma 33:169–179

Singh N, Wright DH (1997) The value of immunohistochemistry on paraffin wax embedded tissue sections in the differentiation of small lymphocytic and mantle cell lymphomas. J Clin Pathol 50:16–21

Skinnider BF, Connors JM, Gascoyne RD (1997) Bone marrow involvement in T-cell-rich B-cell lymphoma. Am J Clin Pathol 108:570–578

Skinnider BF, Horsman DE, Dupuis B, Gascoyne RD (1999) Bcl-6 and Bcl-2 protein expression in diffuse large B-cell lymphoma and follicular lymphoma: correlation with 3q27 and 18q21 chromosomal abnormalities. Hum Pathol 30:803–808

Sobol RE, Mick R, Royston I, Davey FR, Ellison RR, Newman R, Cuttner J, Griffin JD, Collins H, Nelson DA, Bloomfield CD (1987) Clinical importance of myeloid antigen expression in adult acute lymphoblastic leukemia. N Engl J Med 316:1111–1117

Soussain C, Patte C, Ostronoff M, Delmer A, Rigal-Huguet F, Cambier N, Leprise PY, François S, Cony-Makhoul P, Harousseau JL, Janvier M, Chauvenet L, Witz F, Pico J (1995) Small noncleaved cell lymphoma and leukemia in adults. A retrospective study of 65 adults treated with the LMB pediatric protocols. Blood 85:664–674

Spina D, Leoncini L, Megha T, Gallorini M, Disanto A, Tosin P, Abinya O, Nyong'o A, Pileri S, Kraft R, Laissue JA, Cottier H (1997) Cellular kinetic and phenotypic heterogeneity in and among Burkitt's and Burkitt-like lymphomas. J Pathol 182:145–150

Stansfeld AG (ed) (1985) Lymph node biopsy interpretation. Churchill Livingstone, Edinburgh

Stansfeld AG, Diebold J, Kapanci Y, Kelényi G, Lennert K, Mioduszewska O, Noel H, Rilke F, Sundstrom C, Van Unnik JAM, Wright DH (1988) Updated Kiel classifcation for lymphomas (letter to the editor). Lancet i:292–293 and 603

Stark AN, Limbert HJ, Roberts BE, Jones RA, Scott CS (1986) Prolymphocytoid transformation of CLL: a clinical and immunological study of 22 cases. Leuk Res 10:1225–1232

Stein H, Lennert K, Feller AC, Mason DY (1984) Immunohistological analysis of human lymphoma: correlation of histological and immunological categories. Adv Cancer Res 42:67–147

Stein RS, Greer JP, Flexner JM, Hainsworth JD, Collins RD, Macon WR, Cousar JD (1990) Large-cell lymphomas: clinical and prognostic features. J Clin Oncol 8:1370–1379

Stevens DA, O'Conor GT, Levine PH, Rosen RB (1972) Acute leukemia with "Burkitt's lymphoma cells" and Burkitt lymphoma. Ann Intern Med 76:967–973

Stewart ML, Felman IE, Nichols PW, Panignin-Hill A, Lukes RJ, Levine AM (1986) Large noncleaved follicular center cell lymphoma. Clinical features in 53 patients. Cancer 57:288–297

Stilgenbauer S, Döhner H, Bulgay-Morschel M, Weitz S, Bentz M, Lichter P (1993) High frequency of monoallelic retinoblastoma gene deletion in B-cell chronic lymphoid leukemia shown by interphase cytogenetics. Blood 81:2118–2124

Strauchen JA, Young RC, DeVita Jr VT, Anderson T, fantone JC, Berard CW (1978) Clinical relevance of the histopathological subclassification of diffuse "histiocytic" lymphoma. N Engl J Med 299:1382–1387

Sun T, Susin M, Tomao FA, Brody J, Koduru P, Hajdu SI (1997) Histiocyte-rich B-cell lymphoma. Hum Pathol 28:1321–1324

Suryanarayan K, Hunger SP, Kohler S, Carroll AJ, Crist W, Link MP, Cleary ML (1991) Consistent involvement of the BCR gene by 9;22 breakpoints in pediatric acute leukemias. Blood 77:324–330

Takatsuki K, Sanada I (1983) Plasma cell dyscrasia with polyneuropathy and endocrine disorder: clinical and laboratory features of 109 reported cases. Jpn J Clin Oncol 13:543–556

Takatsuki K, Uchiyama T, Sagawa K, Yodoi J (1976) Plasma cell dyscrasia with polyneuropathy and endocrine disorder: review of 32 patients. Excerpta Medica Int Congr Ser 415:454–457

Tao Q, Robertson KD, Manns A, Hildesheim A, Ambinder RF (1998) Epstein-Barr virus (EBV) in endemic Burkitt's lymphoma: molecular analysis of primary tumor tissue. Blood 91:1373–1381

Tawa A, Benedict SH, Hara J, Hoizumi N. Gelfand EW (1987) Rearrangement of the T-cell receptor γ-chain gene in childhood acute lymphoblastic leukemia. Blood 70:1933–1999

Tezcan H, Vose JM, Bast M, Bierman PJ, Kessinger A, Armitage JO (1999) Limited stage I and II follicular non-Hodgkin's lymphoma: the Nebraska Lymphoma Study Group experience. Leuk Lymph 34:273–285

The Non-Hodgkin's Lymphoma Pathologic Classifcation Project (1982) National Cancer Institute sponsored study of classifications of non-Hodgkin's lymphomas: summary and description of a working formulation for clinical usage. Cancer 49:2112–2135

The Non-Hodgkin's Lymphoma Classification Project (1997) A clinical evaluation of the International Lymphoma Study Group classification of non-Hodgkin's lymphoma. The Non-Hodgkin's Lymphoma Classification Project. Blood 89: 3909–3918

Thomas X, Archimbaud E, Charrin C, Magaud JP, Fiere D (1995) CD34 expression is associated with major adverse prognostic factors in adult acute lymphoblastic leukemia. Leukemia 9:249–253

Thompsett AR, Ellison DW, Stevenson FK, Zhu D (1999) V_H gene sequences from primary central nervous system lymphomas indicate derivation from highly mutated germinal center B cells with ongoing mutational activity. Blood 94:1738–1746

Tierens A, Delabie J, Pittaluga S, Driessen A, De Wolf-Peeters C (1998) Mutation analysis of the rearranged immunoglobulin heavy chain genes of marginal zone cell lymphomas indicates an origin from different marginal zone B lymphocyte subsets. Blood 91:2381–2386

Tiesinga JJ, Wu CD, Inghirami G (2000) CD5+ follicle center lymphoma. Immunophenotyping detects a unique subset of "floral" follicular lymphoma. Am J Clin Pathol 114:912–921

Tilly H, Gaulard P, Lepage E et al (1997) Primary anaplastic large-cell lymphoma in adults: clinical presentation, immunophenotype and outcome. Blood 90:3727–3734

Traweek T, Sheibani K, Winberg CD, Mena RR, Wu AM, Rappaport H (1989) Monocytoid B-cell lymphoma: its evolution and relationship to other low-grade B-cell neoplasms. Blood 73:573–578

Tsang P, Pan L, Cesarman E, Tepler J, Knowles DM (1999) A distinctive composite lymphoma consisting of clonally related mantle cell lymphoma and follicle center cell lymphoma. Hum Pathol 30:988–992

Tworek JA, Singleton TP, Schnitzer B, His ED, Ross CW (1998) Flow cytometric and immunohistochemical analysis of small lymphocytic lymphoma, mantle cell lymphoma, and plasmacytoid small lymphocytic lymphoma. Am J Clin Pathol 110:582–589

Uckun FM, Sather H, Gaynon P, Arthur D, Nachman J, Sensel M, Steinherz P, Hutchinson R, Trigg M, Reaman G (1997) Prognostic significance of the $CD10^+CD19^+CD34^+$ B-progenitor immunophenotype in children with acute lymphoblastic leukemia: a report from the Children's Cancer Group. Leuk Lymph 27:445–457

Usha L, Bradlow B, Stock W, Platanias LC (2000) CD5+ immunophenotype in the bone marrow but not in the peripheral blood in a patient with hairy cell leukemia. Acta Haematol 103:210–213

Van Baarlen J, Schuurman HJ, van Unnik JA (1988) Multilobated non-Hodgkin's lymphoma. A clinicopathologic entity. Cancer 61:1371–1376

Van der Putte SCJ, Schuurman HJ, Rademakers LHPM, Kluin P, van Unnik JAM (1984) Malignant lymphoma of follicle centre cells with marked nuclear lobation. Virchows Arch [B]46:93–107

Van Unnik JAM, Breur K, Burgers JMV, Cleton F, Hart AAM, Stenfert Kroese WF, Somers R, van Turnhout JMM (1975) Non-Hodgkin's lymphomata: clinical features in relation to histology. Br J Cancer 31 [Suppl II]:201–207

Vannier JP, Bene MC, Faure GC, Bastard C, Garand R, Bernard A (1989) Investigation of the CD10 (cALLA) negative acute lymphoblastic leukaemia: further description of a group with a poor prognosis. Br J Haematol 72:156–160

Vardiman JW, Golomb HM (1984) Autopsy findings in hairy cell leukaemia. Semin Oncol 11:370–379
Waldenström JG (1958) Die Makroglobulinämie. Ergebn Inn Med Kinderheil 9:586–621
Watson P, Wood KM, Lodge A, McIntosh GG, Milton I, Piggott NH, Proctor SJ, Taylor PR, Smith S, Jack F, Bell H, Steward M, Anderson JJ, Horne CHW, Angus B (2000) Monoclonal antibodies recognizing CD5, CD10 and CD23 in formalin-fixed, paraffin-embedded tissue: production and assessment of their value in the diagnosis of small B-cell lymphoma. Histology 36:145–150
Weeks DA, Beckwith JB, Mierau GW, Luckey DW (1989) Rhabdoid tumor of kidney. A report of 111 cases from the National Wilms' Tumor Study Pathology Center. Am J Surg Pathol 13:439–458
Weisenberg E, Anastasi J, Adeyanju M, Variakojis D, Vardiman JW (1995) Hodgkin's disease associated with chronic lymphocytic leukaemia. Eight additional cases, including two of the nodular lymphocyte predominant type. Am J Clin Pathol 103:479–484
Weisenburger DD, Anderson JR, Diebold J, Gascoyne RD, MacLennan KA, Müller-Hermelink HK, Nathwani BN, Ullrich F, Armitage JO for the Non-Hodgkin's Lymphoma Classification Project (2001) Systemic anaplastic large-cell lymphoma: results from the Non-Hodgkin's Lymphoma Classification Project. Am J Hematol 67:172–178
Weisenburger DD, Nathwani BN, Winberg CD, Rappaport H (1985) Multicentric angiofollicular lymph node hyperplasia: a clinicopathologic study of 16 cases. Hum Pathol 16:162–172
Weisenburger DD, Sanger WG, Armitage JO, Purtilo DT (1987) Intermediate lymphocytic lymphoma: immunophenotypic and cytogenetic findings. Blood 69:1617–1621
Weiss LM, Wood GS, Dorfman RF (1985) T-cell signet-ring cell lymphoma. A histologic, ultrastructural, and immunohistochemical study of two cases. Am J Surg Pathol 9:273–280
Weiss LM, Bindl JM, Picozzi VJ, Link MP, Warnke RA (1986) Lymphoblastic lymphoma: an immunophenotype study of 26 cases with comparison to T cell acute lymphoblastic leukemia. Blood 67:474–478
Weitzmann S, Greenberg ML, Thorner P (1991) Treatment of non-Hodgkin's lymphoma in childhood. In: Wiernik PH, Canellos GP, Kyle RA, Schiffer CA (eds) Neoplastic diseases of blood, vol 1, 2nd edn. Churchill Livingstone, New York
Wendum D, Sebban C, Gaulard P, Coiffier B, Tilly H, Cazals D, Boehn A, Casasnovas RO, Bouabdallah R, Jaubert J, Ferrant A, Diebold J, de Mascarel A, Gisselbrecht C (1997) Follicular large-cell lymphoma treated with intensive chemotherapy: an analysis of 89 cases included in the LNH87 trial and comparison with the outcome of diffuse large B-cell lymphoma. Groupe d'Etude des Lymphomes de l'Adulte. J Clin Oncol 15:1654–1663
Williams DL, Tsiatis A, Brodeur GM, Look AT, Melvin SL, Bowman WP, Kalwinsky DK, Rivera G, Dahl GV (1982) Prognostic importance of chromosome number in 136 untreated children with acute lymphoblastic leukemia. Blood 60:864–871
Williams ME, Swerdlow SH, Rosenberg CL, Arnold A (1993) Chromosome 11 translocation breakpoints at the PRAD1/Cyclin D1 gene locus in centrocytic lymphoma. Leukemia 7:241–245
Wiltshaw E (1971) Extramedullary plasmacytoma. Br Med J 11:319–328
Winberg CD, Nathwani BN, Rappaport H (1979) Nodular (follicular) lymphomas in children and young adults: a clinicopathologic study of 64 patients (abstract). Lab Invest 40:292
Winberg CD, Sheibani K, Burke JS, Wu A, Rappaport H (1988) T-cell rich lymphoproliferative disorders. Morphologic and immunologic differential diagnoses. Cancer 62:1539–1555
Wong KF, Chan JKC, So JCC, Yu PH (1999) Mantle cell lymphoma in leukemic phase: characterization of its broad cytologic spectrum with emphasis on the importance of distinction from other chronic lymphoproliferative disorders. Cancer 86:850–857
Wong KF, So CC Chan JK (2002) Nucleolated variant of mantle cell lymphoma with leukemic manifestations mimicking prolymphocytic leukemia. Am J Clin Pathol 117:246–51
Wright DH (1971) Burkitt's lymphoma; a review of the pathology, immunology and possible aetiological factors. In: Sommers SC (ed) Pathology annual. Appletton-Century-Crofts, New York, pp 337–363
Wright DH (1997) What is Burkitt's lymphoma. J Pathol 182:125–127
Wright DH (1999) What is Burkitt's lymphoma and when is it endemic? Blood 93:758
Wright DH, Pike PA (1968) Bone marrow involvement in Burkitt's tumour. Br J Haematol 15:409–416
Wright DH, MacKeever P, Carter R (1997) Childhood non-Hodgkin's lymphoma in the United Kingdom: Findings from UK children's cancer study group. J Clin Pathol 50:128–134
Yamaguchi M, Ohno T, Oka K, Taniguchi M, Ito M, Kita K, Shiku H (1999) De novo CD5-positive diffuse large B-cell lymphoma: clinical characteristics and therapeutic outcome. Br J Haematol 105:1133–1139
Yatabe Y, Suzuki R, Tobinai K, Matsuno Y, Ichinohasama R, Okamoto M, Yamaguchi M, Tamaru JI, Uike N, Hashimoto Y, Morishima Y, Suchi T, Seto M, Nakamura S (2000) Significance of cyclin D1 overexpression for the diagnosis of mantle cell lymphoma: a clinicopathologic comparison of cyclin D1-positive MCL and cyclin D1-negative MCL-like B-cell lymphoma. Blood 95:2253–2261
York JC, Glick AD, Cousar JB, Collins RD (1984) Changes in the appearance of hematopoietic and lymphoid neoplasms: clinical, pathologic, and biologic implications. Hum Pathol 15:11–38
Yunis JJ, Mayer MG, Arnesen MA, Aeppli DP, Oken MM, Frrizzera G (1989) bcl-2 and other genomic alterations in the prognosis of large-cell lymphoma. N Engl J Med 20:1047–1054
Ziegler JL, Beckstead JA, Volberding PA, Abrams DI, Levine AM, Lukes RJ, Gill PS, Burkes RL, Meyer PR, Metroka CE et al (1984) Non-Hodgkin's lymphoma in 90 homosexual men. Relation to generalised lymphadenopathy and the acquired immunodeficiency syndrome. N Engl J Med 311:565–570
Zinzani PL, Bendandi M, Visani G, Gherlinzoni F, Frezza G, Merla E, Manfroi S, Gozzetti A, Tura S (1996) Adult lymphoblastic lymphoma: clinical features and prognostic factors in 53 patients. Leuk Lymph 23:577–582
Zucca E, Roggero E, Pinotti G, Pedrinis E, Capella C, Venco A, Cavalli F (1995) Patterns of survival in mantle cell lymphoma. Ann Oncol 6:257–262

Chapter 5

Nodal and Leukemic NK/T-Cell Lymphoma

The same subdivision is used for NK/T-cell lymphomas as for B-cell lymphomas. Precursor types (lymphoblastic) are differentiated from peripheral types, nodal from extranodal ones.

In the sections covering nodal NK/T-cell lymphomas the entities are roughly distinguished between either a *predominately leukemic* or a *predominately nodal* manifestation. All entities with a *predominately extranodal* manifestation are described in the chapters on the different organs.

Concerning peripheral NK/T-cell lymphomas, about two-thirds of the cases are primary nodal lymphomas and one-third primary extranodal ones. The frequency of the different subtypes of nodal lymphomas is given in Table 3.3 according to the Kiel classification. The International Lymphoma Study Group (ILSG) found that the different subtypes within the Kiel classification can not be reproducibly diagnosed and thus placed the pleomorphic type of nodal lymphoma together with T-zone and lymphoepithelioid lymphomas, describing it as peripheral T-cell lymphoma, unspecified. This led to the phenomenon that today 55% of peripheral T-cell lymphomas are within this category.

Among nodal lymphomas, the angioimmunoblastic type is the second most frequent. In extranodal sites, the natural killer (NK)/T-cell lymphoma, nasal type is the most frequent one (Rüdiger et al. 2002). The overall survival rate is poor, about 30% after 5 years. There is no significant difference between the different subtypes (Gisselbrecht et al. 1998; Rüdiger et al. 2002). The only exception is anaplastic large-cell lymphomas (ALCL),which has a more favorable prognosis especially in children and young adults (see Chap. 5.2.2.4)

5.1 Precursor T-Lymphoblastic Leukemia[1]/ Lymphoma[2] (ICD-O: 9837/3[1]; 9729/3[2])

Synonyms

- Kiel: Lymphoblastic lymphoma of T-cell type
- REAL: Precursor T-lymphoblastic leukemia/ lymphoma
- WHO: Precursor T-lymphoblastic leukemia/ lymphoma

Definition

T-lymphoblastic leukemia/lymphoma is derived from precursor cells of peripheral T-lymphocytes (for general remarks see B-lymphoblastic leukemia/lymphoma, Chap. 4.1). According to their antigen profile, these cells originate in the bone marrow ("prethymic type") or the thymus ("early" and "late thymus cortex type"). T-lymphoblasts mostly have round nuclei with fine chromatin and a scanty cytoplasm. In most cases, some of the cells have nuclei with a gyrate (convoluted) outline. This nuclear configuration is not specific, however, since it sometimes occurs in B-lymphoblastic lymphomas as well.

Histologically, it is impossible to distinguish a T-lymphoblastic lymphoma, i.e. the genuine tumor variant, from T-lymphoblastic leukemia [acute lymphoblastic leukemia of T-cell type(T-ALL)].

Morphology

The cells are relatively small or medium sized. They are spread apart (not cohesive; Figs. 5.1, 5.2). The cytoplasm of T-lymphoblasts is scanty and only moderately basophilic. In most cases, some of the nuclei have a gyrate (convoluted) outline and show only very small, inconspicuous nucleoli and very fine chromatin. Convolution means that there are deep clefts in the nuclei (Fig. 5.3). These convoluted nuclei can be found in about 90% of T-lymphoblastic lymphomas. There is usually high mitotic activity. The tumor cells are occasionally interspersed with eosinophils. The reticulin fibers are very fine and usually sparse. The lymph node architecture is diffusely destroyed by the monotonous infiltrate of the tumor cells. There is usually an infiltration of the capsule, sometimes with extension into the adipose tissue. Alternatively, there may primarily be an interfollicular infiltrate, leaving some remnants of follicles intact. The sinuses may be preserved. A starry-sky like pattern is usually not prominent.

Cytologically leukemic lymphoblasts have a typical L2 morphology with round or convoluted nuclei and prominent nucleoli. The cytoplasm is more prominent than seen in tissue sections. Cytoplasmic vacuoles are rare.

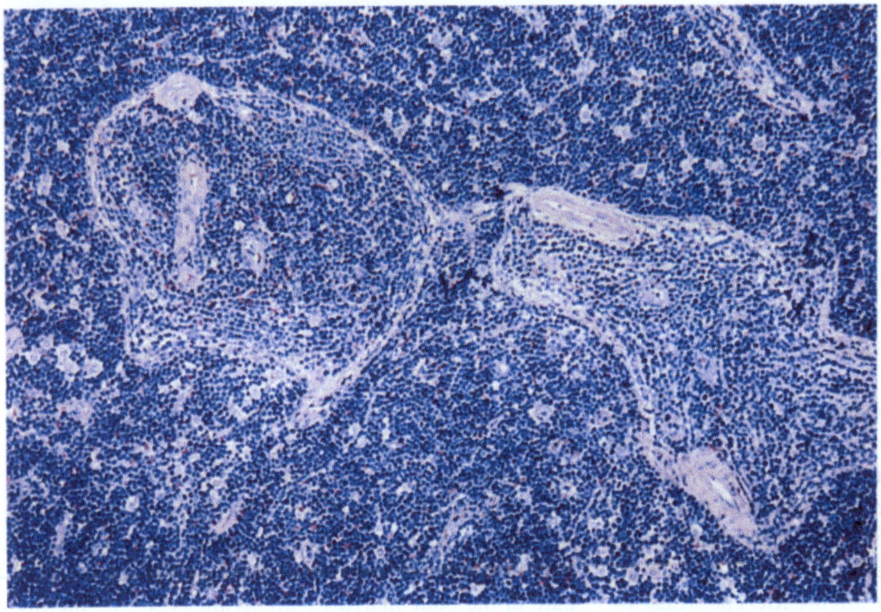

Fig. 5.1. Low-power view of a T-lymphoblastic lymphoma. The infiltrate is monotonous, a slightly developed starry sky pattern is visible. The sinuses are filled with neoplastic lymphoblasts (Giemsa stain)

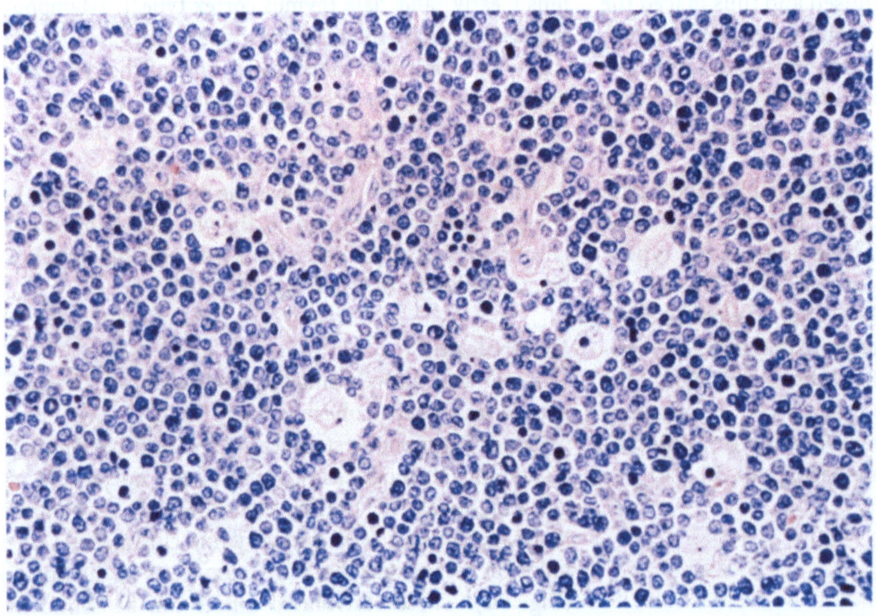

Fig. 5.2. Monotonous infiltrate of a lymphoblastic lymphoma with mostly round nuclei and some intermingled macrophages (Giemsa stain)

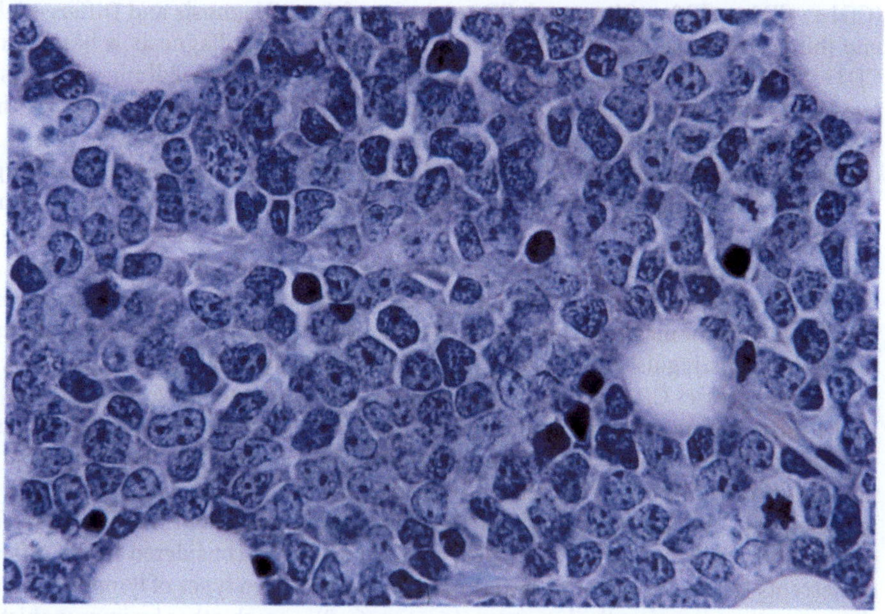

Fig. 5.3. High-power view of a T-lymphoblastic lymphoma. Nuclear convolutions are hardly recognizable (Giemsa stain)

Immunohistochemistry is necessary to distinguish the T-cell type from the B-cell type with certainty.

Immunohistochemistry

A feature that all T-lymphoblastic leukemias/lymphomas have in common is the expression of CD7 antigen. However, if this is the only antigen expressed, then one must remember that it can also be demonstrated in about 20 % of immature myelomonocytic neoplasms. More than 90 % of the tumors express terminal deoxynucleotide transferase (TdT), and cytoplasmic CD3. CD10, on paraffin sections, can be detected in about 60 % of the tumors (Conde-Sterling et al. 2000). Other antigens found in immature T-lymphoblastic lymphomas are CD2 and CD5. The mature thymus cortex type is characterized by CD1a expression and by simultaneous expression of CD4 and CD8. With increasing maturation into peripheral T-cells, CD4 *or* CD8 expression is lost.

Some 40 % of tumors are positive for CD34, and more than 70 % express CD99. There may be coexpression of CD79α together with T-cell antigens, which does not indicate lineage infidelity but a non-lineage-specific cross reactivity.

The number of proliferating cells (Ki-67+) is similar to that for B-lymphoblastic lymphoma, with a median of about 45 %.

Roughly one-third of T-ALL/T-lymphoblastic (LB) coexpress at least one myelomonocytic antigen, such as CD13,CD15, CD33, and CD65. The most frequently expressed myeloid antigen is CD13 followed by CD33 and CD15 (Pui et al. 1998; Khalidi et al. 1999).

Immunohistochemistry has made it possible to assign all lymphoblastic lymphomas to the B-cell or T-cell series. Blast-cell infiltrates that express neither the B-cell-associated antigens CD19 and/or CD22 nor the T-cell-associated antigen CD7 or CD3 are of myelomonocytic or of true NK-cell origin. Even when the T-cell or B-cell nature of the lymphoma is certain, however, one should still search for the expression of myelomonocytic antigens, because it is possible to find antigen coexpression on the same cell or a mixed blast-cell infiltration. This would have other therapeutic and prognostic consequences.

In exceptional cases, tumors have been described which additionally express NK-cell antigens. These are mostly CD2+, CD5–, CD56+. The tumor cells have a lymphoblastic morphology (Nakamura et al. 1998; Koita et al. 1997; Ichinohasama et al. 1996). Such cases have been designated as either lymphoblastic or immature blastic NK/T-cell lymphomas (ICD-O:9727/3). Characteristically, there is coexpression of TdT without detection of cytotoxic granules (granzyme B).

According to Knowles (1988), the prothymic phenotype (CD2+, CD7+) is expressed in about two-thirds of all T-ALLs, whereas the thymus cortex phenotype

(CD1+, CD2+, CD3+, CD4+ and CD8+) is found in one-third; rarely, the medullary thymus type (CD1+, CD3+, CD4+ or CD8+) is expressed. In contrast, about two-third of the (non-leukemic) T-lymphoblastic lymphomas must be classified as belonging to the thymus cortex phenotype and one-third to the medullary thymus type. Prethymic phenotypes are almost entirely limited to T-ALL.

Very detailed immunohistochemical investigations allow eight stages of differentiation among the T-lymphoblastic lymphomas and leukemias (Feller et al. 1986b) to be distinguished. The least mature (prethymic) type expresses CD7 and HLA-DR simultaneously. In the most mature type of T-lymphoblastic lymphoma/leukemia, the partial loss of CD4 or CD8 and CD1 indicates transformation of the cells into peripheral T-lymphocytes. A comparison of these phenotypic groups with clinical data revealed that children and adolescents (up to the age of 15 years) predominantly show a more mature cell phenotype (groups 6–8), while in older patients there is a preponderance of the immature differentiation types. It was possible to demonstrate a mediastinal tumor only in differentiation groups 5–7, and not in groups 1–4. Leukemic blood pictures, however, were chiefly associated with an immature degree of differentiation (Feller et al. 1988).

Genetic Features

About 80% of T-lymphoblastic leukemia/lymphomas have a T-cell receptor (TCR)-γ rearrangement; of these, an additional 10–15% show a rearrangement of the Ig heavy-chain gene (Hara et al. 1988; Greenberg et al. 1986; Tawa et al. 1987; Pelicci et al. 1985; Pilozzi et al. 1999). The number of observed rearrangements is higher in frozen section than in formalin-fixed tissue. Some especially immature prothymocyte phenotypes (CD7+, TdT+) may lack a TCR rearrangement.

About three quarters of T-ALLs/T-LBs are characterized by an abnormal karyotype. Most of these tumors are hyperdiploid (Mittelman 1981); 25% have abnormalities involving regions of the TCR genes. The most frequent abnormality involves chromosome bands 14q11.2, 1p32, 7q35,10q24, 11p13, and 11p14, involving areas coding for transcription factors TAL1 and RBTN1 and 2 (Petkovic et al. 1996; Kaneko et al. 1989; Khalidi et al. 1999; Chen et al. 1990). The Philadelphia chromosome translocation is rare in T-LB.

Diagnosis and Differential Diagnosis

The diagnosis is based on a monotonous infiltrate of mostly medium-sized blastic cells with round or convoluted nuclei. Each case has to be analyzed immunohistochemically to clarify the nature of the lymphoblasts and to exclude lineage infidelity, e.g. coexpression especially of myelomonocytic antigens.

The most important distinction in the differential diagnosis is that between T-lymphoblastic lymphoma and *lymphoblastic lymphoma of B-cell type*. Although the nuclear convolutions are usually less pronounced in B-lymphoblastic lymphoma, the nuclear configuration cannot serve as a basis for the decision as to whether a lymphoblastic lymphoma is of B-cell or T-cell nature.

Mantle cell lymphoma (see Chap. 4.2.1.7), *acute myeloid and myelomonocytic leukemias*, and *blastic NK-cell or NK/T-cell lymphomas* (see above) must also be considered in the differential diagnosis. The latter two types of lymphomas have to be differentiated from each other by immunohistochemistry as the morphology can be identical. The lymphoblastic NK/T-cell type is positive for TdT, otherwise this lymphoma has to be designated as peripheral NK/T-cell lymphoma.

Occurrence

T-lymphoblastic lymphoma accounts for about 3–4% of all cases of NHL among adults. In childhood it is the most frequent NHL. Cases are about equally divided between the first two decades of life, with a median age of 9 years; in later life, up to and including the eighth decade, T-lymphoblastic lymphoma occurs infrequently. The male-to-female ratio is about 6–4:1 (Reiter et al. 1995, 2000).

Non-leukemic lymphoblastic lymphoma of T-cell type is much more common than that of B-cell type.

Clinical Presentation and Prognosis

In about 90% of the cases, T-lymphoblastic lymphoma begins with a ventral mediastinal tumor (generally originating from the thymus) that is often associated with pleural effusions. In addition, lymph nodes in the supraclavicular region or elsewhere may be enlarged. Lymph nodes are sometimes also the first site of visible manifestation of T-lymphoblastic lymphoma. Most childhood patients present in stage III. About 20% have a primary bone marrow infiltration, but in 80% of the patients the bone marrow is eventually included in the tumor process, and, as a result, a leukemic blood picture appears. At this stage, various extranodal organs, including the central nervous system, may be involved as well.

In a minority of cases, the lymphoblastic proliferation begins in the bone marrow and results in the development of leukemia.

During the last 15 years a complete remission rate of up to 75% of children with lymphoblastic lymphoma or ALL of the T-cell type has been achieved (Anderson et al. 1983; Eden et al. 1992; Tubergen et al. 1995). Recently, intensified ALL-type therapy has led to 90% event-free survival at 5 years (Reiter et al. 2000); in adults, the prognosis is probably somewhat less favorable.

Addendum: Unclassified Lymphoblastic Lymphoma

In the Kiel classification, the unclassified type of lymphoblastic lymphoma was listed as a category of its own. Even today, this term is still used for a T- or B-lymphoblastic lymphoma when there is no material available to investigate the surface antigens and thus determine the origin of the tumor cells. However, using current immunohistochemical techniques, all lymphoblastic lymphomas can be assigned to either a B-or T-cell origin.

5.2 Peripheral NK/T-Cell Lymphoma

5.2.1 Peripheral NK/T-Cell Lymphoma – Predominately Leukemic

The subtypes of the different T-cell lymphomas/predominately leukemic including their immunophenotypic characteristics are detailed in Table 5.1. With the exception of T-cell chronic lymphocytic/prolymphocytic leukemia (T-CLL/T-PLL), these types of lymphoma do not significantly infiltrate the lymph node. Thus, in this section only T-PLL/T-CLL is described in detail.

5.2.1.1 T-Cell Chronic Lymphocytic/Prolymphocytic Leukemia (ICD-O: 9834/3)

Synonyms

- Kiel: Chronic lymphocytic leukemia of T-cell type
- REAL: T-cell chronic lymphocytic leukemia/prolymphocytic leukemia
- WHO: T-cell prolymphocytic leukemia

Table 5.1. Characteristics of T-cell leukemias/leukemic T-cell lymphomas. *T-PLL* T-cell prolymphocytic leukemia, *T-LGL* T-cell large granular lymphocytic leukemia, *ATL* Adult T-cell leukemia

	T-PLL[a]	T-LGL[b]	NK-cell[c]	ATL[d]
Nuclei	Humped/ round	Round	Round, slightly irregular	Pleomorphic
Azurophil granules	–	+	+	–
Cytoplasm	Basophilic	Pale	Pale-slightly basophilic	Slightly basophilic
CD 2	+	+	–	+
CD 3	+	+	–	+
CD 4	+	–/+	–	+
CD 8	–	+/–	–	–
CD4/CD8	–/+	–	–	–
CD 7	+/–	–	–	–
CD 56	–	–/+	+	–
CD 57	–	+	–	–
TIA 1	–	+	+	–

[a] See Figs. 5.8, 5.9, [b] see Fig. 5.10, [c] see Figs. 5.11a, 5.11b, [d] see Fig. 5.12

Definition

So far, only T-CLL/T-PLL is known to significantly infiltrate the lymph node. The infiltrate consists of small, only slightly pleomorphic cells and is characterized by a marked increase of epithelioid venules.

Morphology

There is always a marked increase in the number of epithelioid venules in T-CLL (Figs. 5.4, 5.5), whereas in B-cell chronic lymphocytic leukemia (B-CLL) it is less pronounced or not seen at all. The nuclei of the lymphocytes are more variable in shape than those of B-CLL. The few blast cells often have multiple, large, central nucleoli (Fig. 5.6). In contrast to B-CLL, T-CLL does not show a pseudofollicular pattern (proliferation centers). The T lymphocytes migrate through the walls of the venules and partially destroy them (Fig. 5.7). When this happens, the venules can be more readily recognized from their fibers and basement membranes. Occasionally, a marked increase in the number of so-called plasmacytoid monocytes cells has been seen.

T-CLL may transform into a T-immunoblastic lymphoma.

In lymph node sections it is almost impossible to distinguish between a lymphocytic- and a prolymphocytic-dominated lymphoma; only the nuclei look somewhat larger in T-PLL.

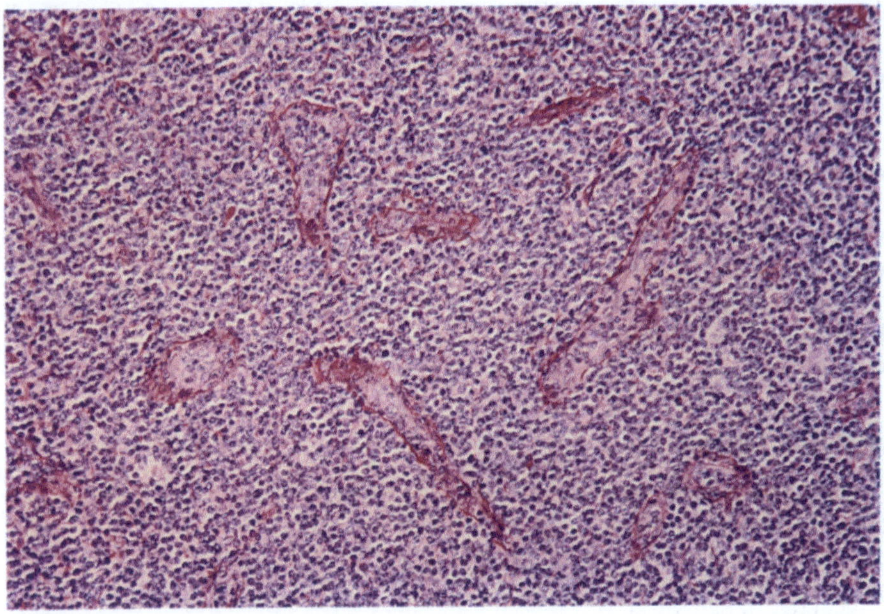

Fig. 5.4. T-cell chronic lymphocytic/prolymphocytic leukemia (T-CLL/PLL). Note the increased number of epithelioid venules. The PAS-positive basement membrane is partly filled with neoplastic T-cells

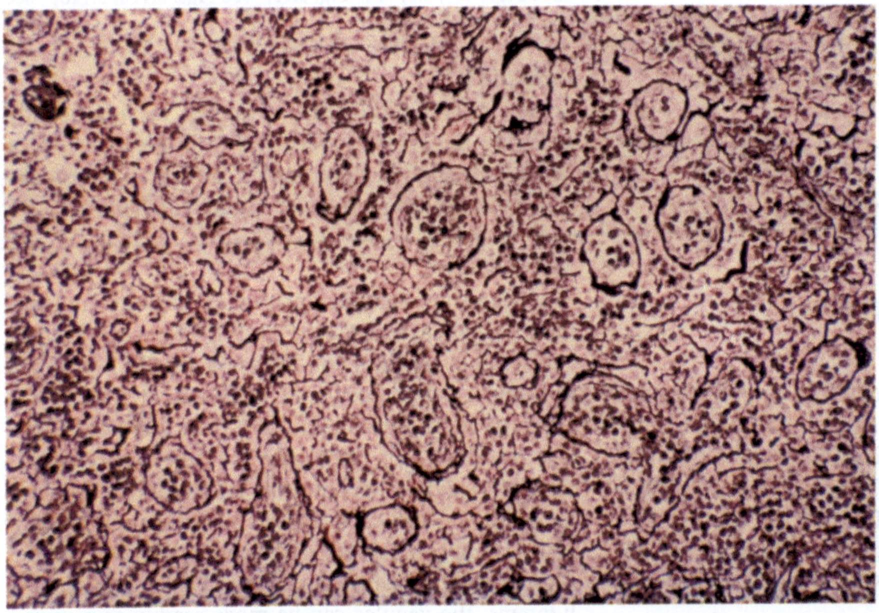

Fig. 5.5. Silver impregnation of a T-CLL/PLL biopsy. The number of small epithelioid venules is markedly increased

T-CLL and T-PLL can easily be distinguished in blood smears (Figs. 5.8, 5.9). However mostly a mixture of both cell types is found in these neoplasms.

Immunohistochemistry
See Table 5.1.

Occurrence
The relative frequency of T-CLL among all cases of CLL is about 3%. T-CLL generally occurs in middle and old age, but it has been observed in a 19-year-old patient.

Clinical Picture and Prognosis
Infiltration of the bone marrow is not always present, and when it occurs it is not as heavy as in B-CLL. Infil-

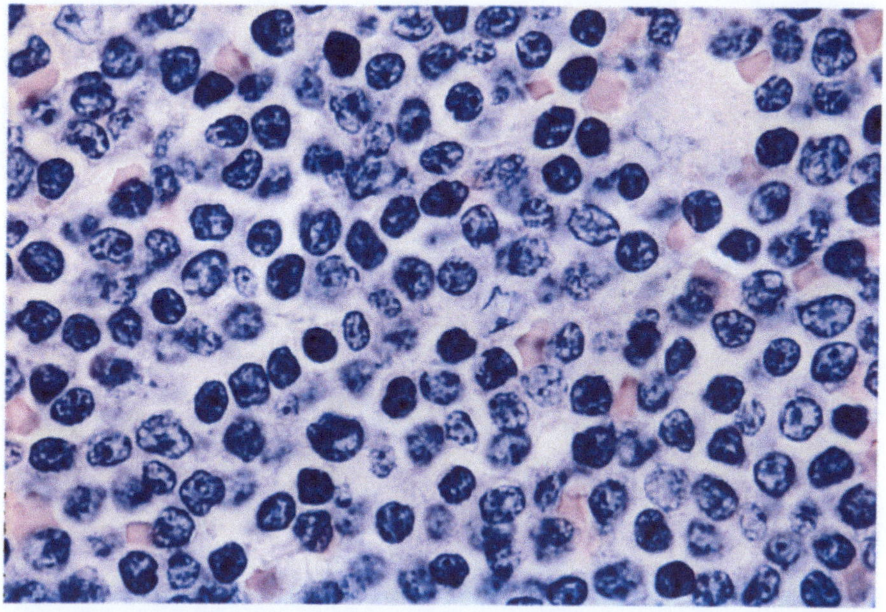

Fig. 5.6. High-power view of a T-CLL/PLL with a quite homogenous infiltrate of cells with slightly pleomorphic nuclei, a dense chromatin pattern, and small nucleoli (Giemsa stain)

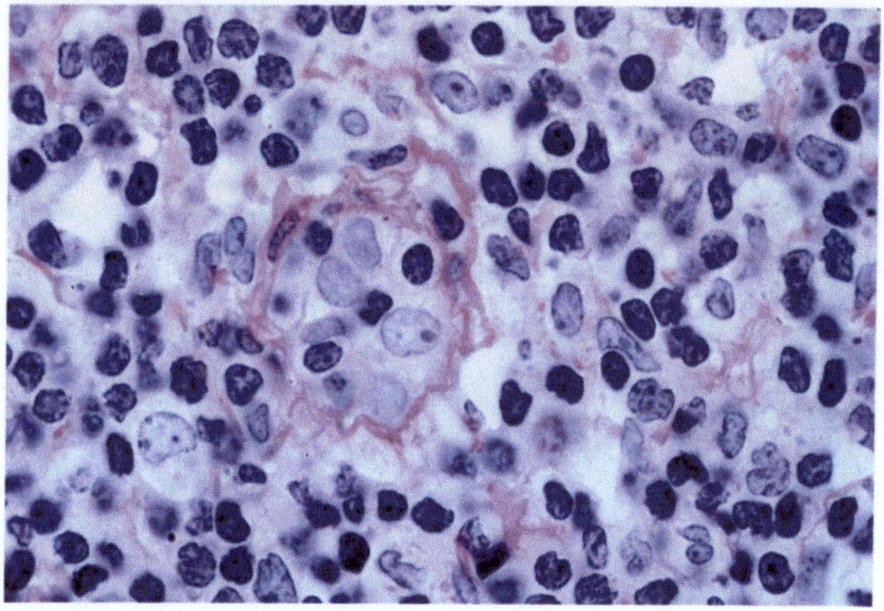

Fig. 5.7. PAS-staining of an epithelioid venule in a T-CLL/PLL biopsy. The wall of the venule is partly destroyed. The nuclei of the tumor cells show a more pronounced pleomorphism.

tration of the skin is, however, frequently observed ("dermatotropism" of T-lymphocytes). Involvement of lymph nodes is often slight. In contrast, marked splenomegaly is seen in almost all patients.

Addendum: Prolymphocytic Variant of T-CLL

In the prolymphocytic variant (T-PLL), the leukemic cells are somewhat larger and have round or pleomorphic nuclei. These contain medium-sized, very prominent, solitary nucleoli. Cytoplasm is abundant and markedly basophilic (in contrast to the grayish blue cytoplasm in all types of T-CLL!; see Fig. 5.9).

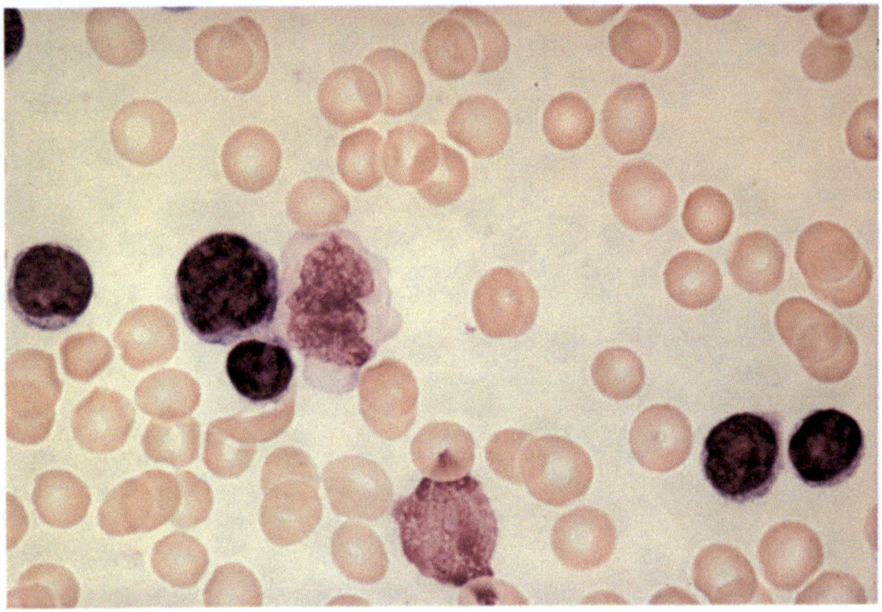

Fig. 5.8. Blood smear of a T-CLL/PLL. Most of the cells are quite small with a small cytoplasmic rim. The cells shows marked nuclear indentations (Pappenheim stain)

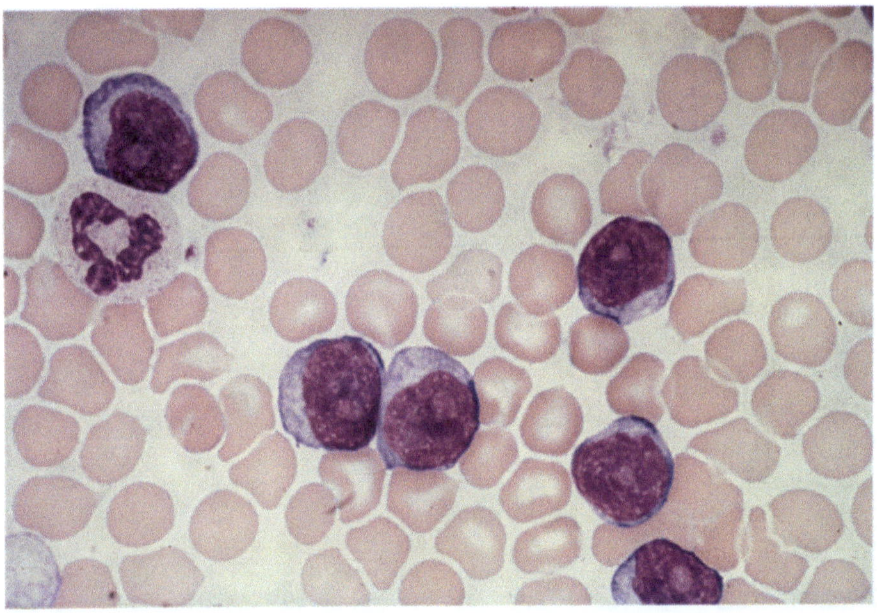

Fig. 5.9. Blood smear of a T-PLL. The cells have typical round nuclei, prominent nucleoli and a broad cytoplasmic rim (Pappenheim stain)

In the WHO Classification T-CLL and T-PLL are summarized to T-PLL. As the content of T lymphocytes and prolymphocytes is variable in this disease both terms may be used or given as T-CLL/T-PLL.

The cytology of T-cell large granular lymphocytic leukemia (LGL) (see Chap. 6.10.1.8) and aggressive NK/T-cell leukemia is shown in Figs. 5.10 and 5.11.

5.2.1.2 Adult T-Cell Leukemia/Lymphoma

This particular type of T-cell lymphoma was discovered by Takatsuki et al. (1976) and found to be endemic in certain parts of southwestern Japan, particularly Kyushu. Shortly thereafter, endemic cases were recognized in the Caribbean basin and in immigrants from

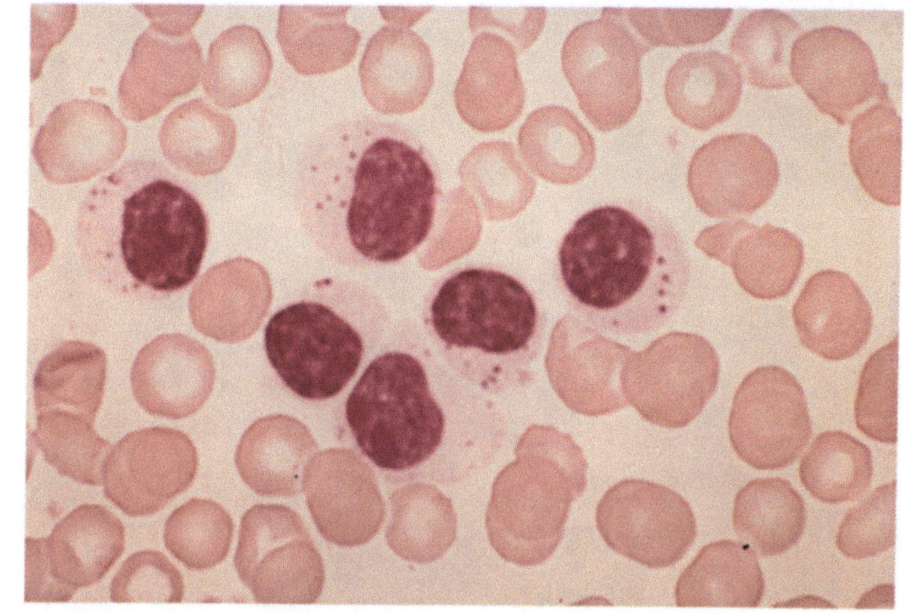

Fig. 5.10. Blood smear of a T-cell large granular lymphocytic leukemia (LGL). Note the monomorphic neoplastic cells containing azurophilic granules (Pappenheim stain)

this region in England and Holland (Catovsky et al. 1982; Vyth-Dreese and de Vries 1982). Sporadic cases have also been reported in the United States (Grossman et al. 1981; Kadin and Kamoun 1982). The lymphoma is caused by the retrovirus human T-cell leukemiavirus type 1 (HTLV-1) (Poiesz et al. 1980; Blattner et al. 1982).

A variable proportion (up to 40%) of the inhabitants of the endemic areas are healthy carriers of HTLV-1. These persons are seropositive for the adult T-cell leukemia/lymphoma (ATLL) antigen and have polyclonally integrated viral genomes in their T-cells. The virus is transmitted mainly from mother to child and from husband to wife. It has been estimated that one of every 900 male carriers of the virus and one of every 2,000 female carriers older than 40 years develop ATLL each year (Tajima et al. 1986; Tajima and Kuoishi 1985; Manns et al. 1999; Tsukasaki et al. 2000; Siegel et al. 2001).

Synonyms

- Kiel: Pleomorphic small-cell, medium-sized and large-cell lymphoma
- REAL: Adult T-cell leukemia/lymphoma
- WHO: Adult T-cell leukemia/lymphoma

Definition

Adult T-cell lymphoma/leukemia is a lymphatic malignancy of mostly medium and large pleomorphic T-cells associated with HTLV-1.

Morphology

The nuclei are extremely pleomorphic, even more so than those seen in virus-negative cases (Figs. 5.12, 5.13a, b). Particularly striking is the marked variation in the size of the nuclei. The nuclei of medium-sized cells are approximately 6–9 μm in diameter, the large ones about 10–12 μm. The medium-sized cells have dense chromatin. The large cells show round or oval nuclei with a distinct nuclear membrane and from two to five large, basophilic nucleoli. In all cases, large cells with nuclei that have multiple indentations on one side ("jellyfish" appearance) are found. The cytoplasm is moderately abundant and gray or blue (basophilic) with Giemsa staining. Many mitotic figures are present. Some tumors have a more monotonous blastic appearance (Fig. 5.14).

Giant cells are often found in ATLL (Fig. 5.13a, 5.15), and two kinds are recognizable: giant cells of the Reed-Sternberg type and those of the cerebriform type. Cells of the first type show large, often lobulated nuclei with a pale nuclear membrane, very fine, weakly stained chromatin and very large, violet, occasionally vacuolated nucleoli. The cytoplasm is abundant and grayish blue with Giemsa staining. Such cells may occur in early infiltrates of the lymph node together with T-cells with absent or only minimal pleomorphism mimicking Hodgkin's disease. In such cases the Hodgkin- and Sternberg-like cells are B-cells, have episomal or inte-

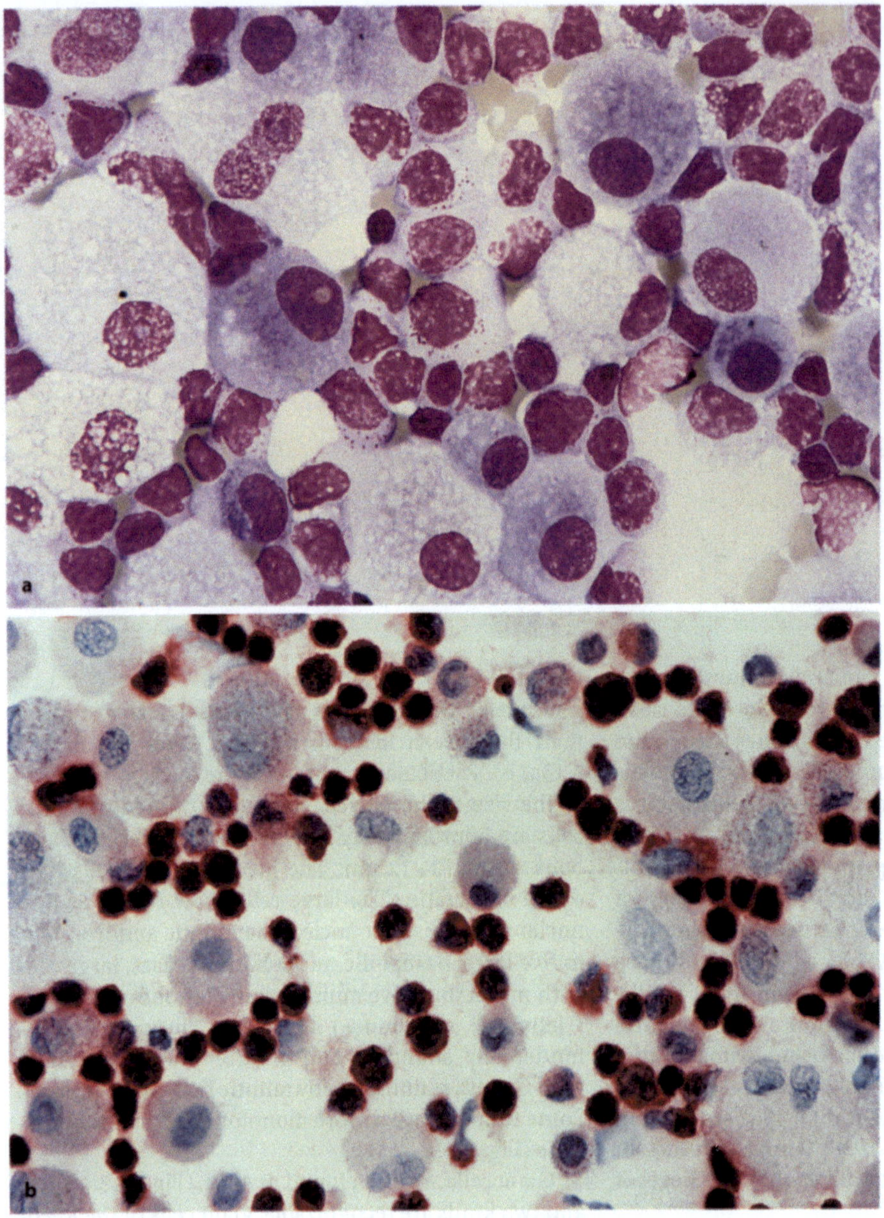

Fig. 5.11 a, b. Bronchoalveolar lavage from an aggressive natural killer (NK)-T-cell leukemia. **a** The cells have round slightly irregular nuclei and the cytoplasmic contains many coarse azurophilic granules (Pappenheim stain). **b** Immunohistochemical staining for cytotoxic granules (T-cell-restricted intracellular antigen-1, TIA1) (immunohistochemistry, alkaline phosphatase)

grated EBV and are CD30-positive (Ohshima et al. 1997).

Giant cells of the cerebriform type (Kikuchi et al. 1986) show deep indentations in the nuclear membrane, coarse, basophilic chromatin and two or three large, basophilic nucleoli. This second type appears to be very characteristic of, if not specific to, HTLV-1-positive T-cell lymphomas (Kikuchi et al. 1986).

The tumors are generally interspersed with a fair number of macrophages. Plasma cells are rare. Eosinophils, however, are occasionally plentiful. Epithelioid venules may be conspicuous, but generally they are not arborizing.

Some tumors may show necrosis (Fig. 5.16).

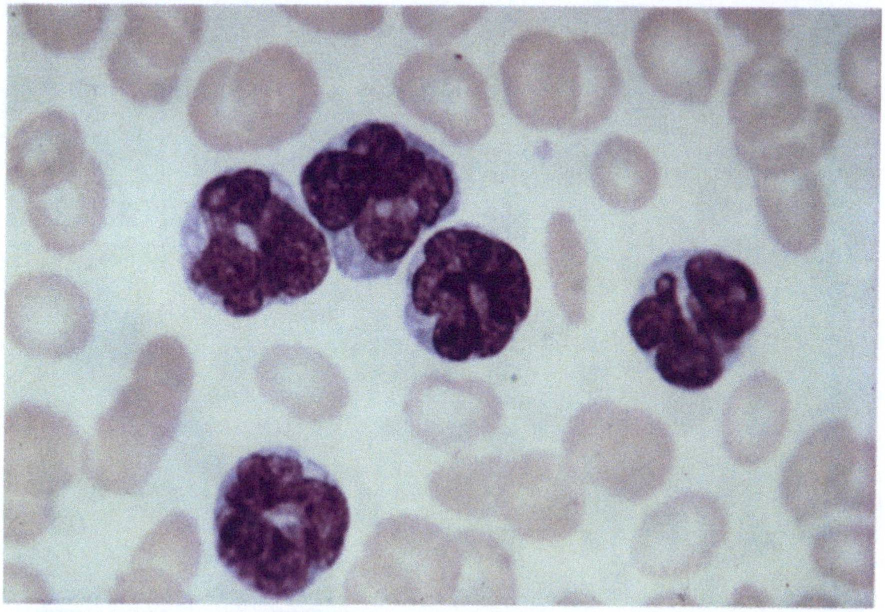

Fig. 5.12. ATLL with leukemic cells. Note the marked nuclear indentations (flower cells) (Pappenheim stain)

Immunohistochemistry

As a rule, the phenotype is that of peripheral helper/inducer T-cells (CD2+, CD3+, CD4+) with simultaneous expression of antigens associated with cell activation, HLA-DR, CD30 (especially large cells) and CD25. Only a few cells are of suppressor/cytotoxic subtype (CD8+). A few tumors have shown coexpression of CD4 and CD8, but were CD1a-negative. All tumors are CD7-negative. Thus, CD2+, CD25+, CD4+, CD7– is a quite characteristic immunophenotype.

Genetic Features

All tumors show clonal rearrangement of TCR genes and have HTLV-1 clonally integrated.

Occurrence

ATLL affects adults; the mean age is 57 years. There is only a slight male preponderance (male-to-female ratio is approx. 1.4:1). This contrasts with most other types of lymphoma in Japan, which affect men much more frequently. In endemic areas, ATLL makes up about 50% of all T-cell neoplasms (Ohshima et al. 2002).

Clinical Features and Prognosis

ATLL is usually leukemic or subleukemic. The neoplastic cells in the peripheral blood have highly lobulated nuclei (Hanaoka 1984).

Since the bone marrow is usually involved only slightly, anemia is not a significant symptom. Lymphadenopathy is common and it is often generalized. Hepatomegaly and splenomegaly are also found in many patients. The skin is often affected, with lesions in the form of erythematous patches and papules (histologically, the skin lesions resemble those of mycosis fungoides, since they often show epidermal infiltration and Pautrier's microabscesses!). Hypercalcemia is associated with ATLL in up to 50% of patients and may result in renal failure. Most patients have hypogammaglobulinemia, but a few show a polyclonal or even a monoclonal increase in Ig. Cellular immunity is markedly reduced. Due to the considerable reduction in both humoral and cellular immunity, patients are very susceptible to bacterial and viral infections, including opportunistic ones. Hence infections are a common cause of death.

The prognosis is less favorable than that of virus-negative pleomorphic, medium-sized, and large-cell T-cell lymphomas (peripheral T-cell lymphoma, unspecified). The median survival time is 4.7 months (Suchi et al. 1987). This may be due in part to hypercalcemia. Another reason for the early deaths is the patients' increased susceptibility to bacterial and viral infections. In addition to the rapidly progressive types of ATLL, there is a chronic or even smoldering type characterized by fewer leukemic cells in the

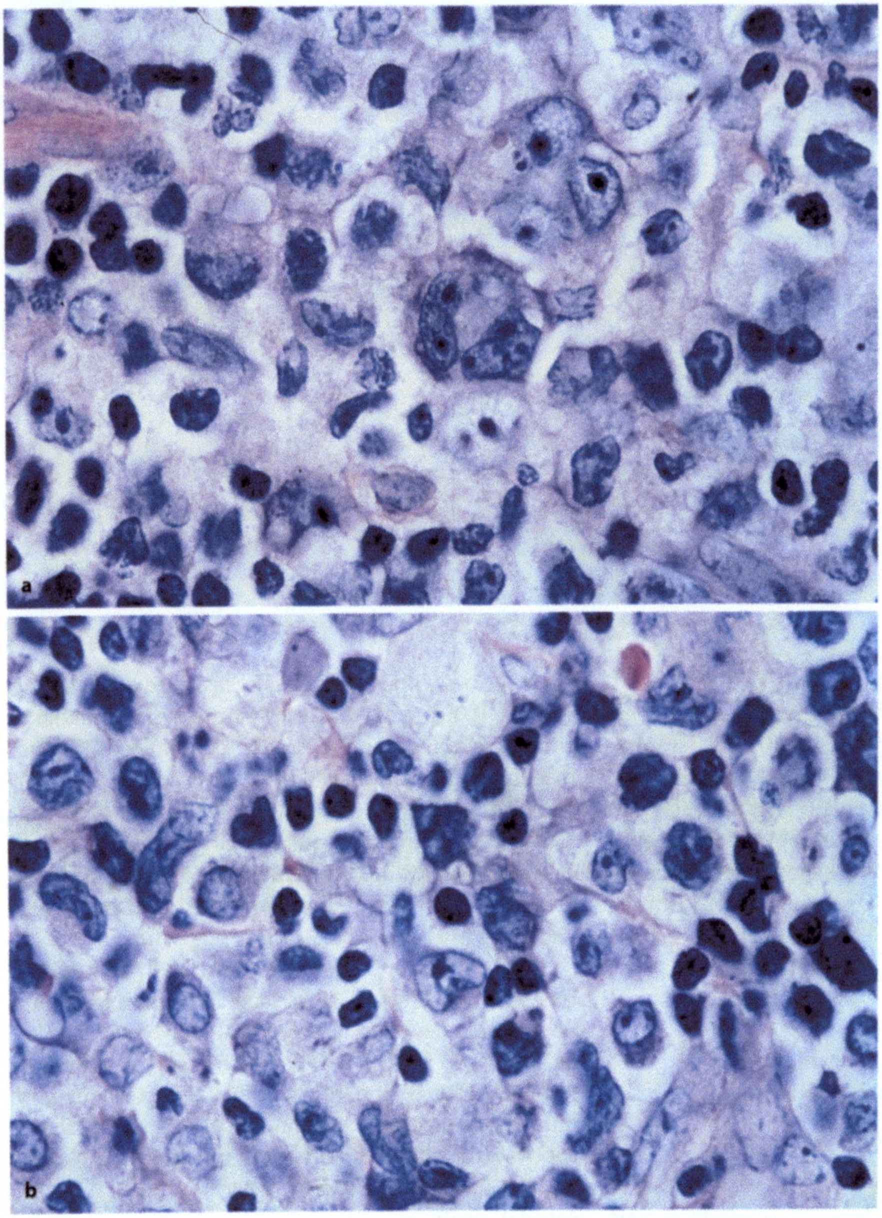

Fig. 5.13. a ATLL with a blastic infiltrate. Some cells show marked nuclear pleomorphism, some cells resemble Reed-Sternberg. **b** ATLL with a clear-cell appearance and blasts

peripheral blood and a prolonged clinical course. Histologically, this type corresponds to the pleomorphic, small-cell type of the Kiel classification (see Chap. 5.2.2.2).

5.2.2 Peripheral NK/T-Cell Lymphoma Predominately Nodal

5.2.2.1 Angioimmunoblastic T-Cell Lymphoma (ICD-O: 9705/3)

Although angioimmunoblastic T-cell lymphoma (AIBTCL) is one of the best defined entities among

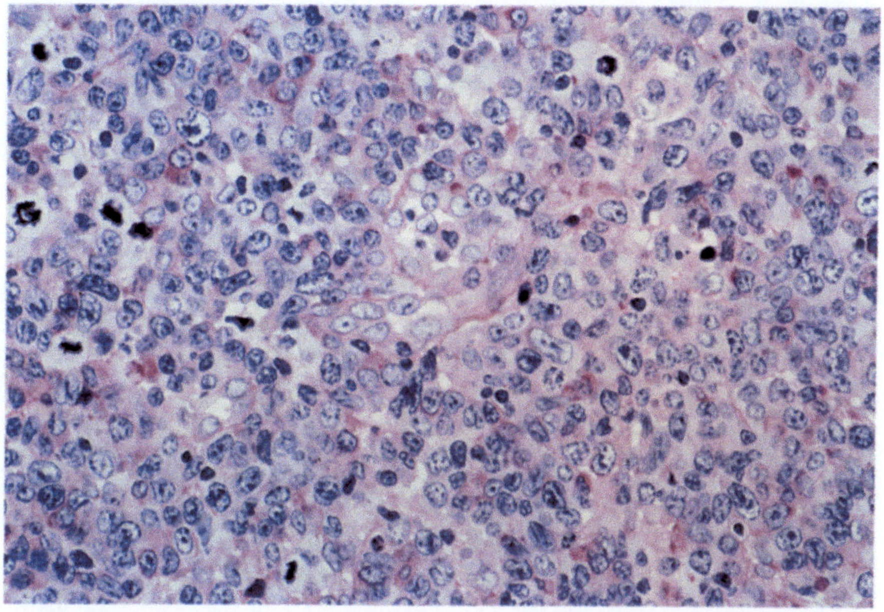

Fig. 5.14. ATLL with a quite monotonous blastic infiltrate (Giemsa stain)

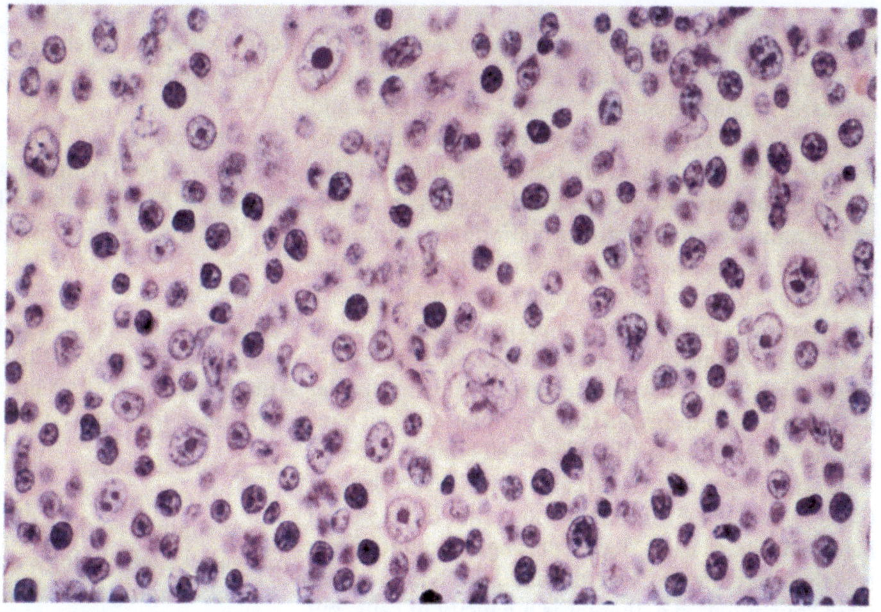

Fig. 5.15. ATLL with small and medium-sized cells, and some Hodgkin- and Reed-Sternberg-like cells (H and E stain)

peripheral T-cell lymphomas, it has an interesting history. Initially described as a hyperimmune reaction and premalignant disease, it is now recognized as a well-defined malignant lymphoma.

In 1971, at a workshop of US and Japanese lymphoma study groups in Nagoya (Lennert 1992, personal communication), Dorfman described a distinct histological lesion that he had observed in four patients (Dorfman and Warnke 1974). This observation was published 1 year later by Liao et al. (1972), who called the lesion "malignant histiocytosis with cutaneous involvement and eosinophilia". At the same workshop, two of the participating pathologists reported similar lesions, but under different names. Lennert called the lesion "lymphogranulomatosis X" (LgX) because its morphology resembled that of Hodgkin's

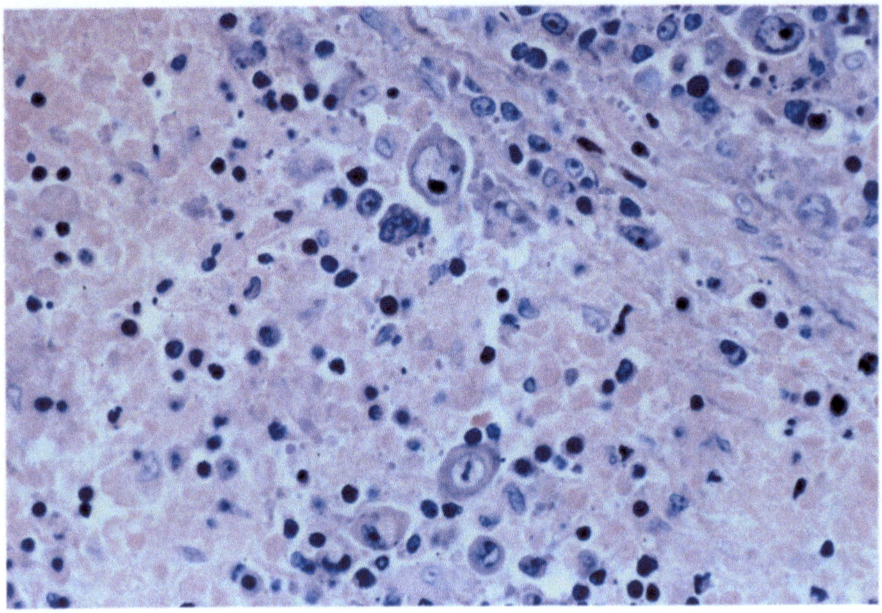

Fig. 5.16. ATLL with some blasts and necrosis (Giemsa stain)

lymphoma (also called "lymphogranulomatosis" in German). Lukes and Tindle (1973) named it "immunoblastic lymphadenopathy" (IBL). Later, Frizzera and Rappaport (1974) proposed the term "angioimmunoblastic lymphadenopathy with dysproteinemia" (AILD). All of the authors interpreted the disease as an abnormal immune reaction. Transformation into immunoblastic sarcoma has been described in a number of publications, although with varying frequency. Hence LgX was eventually interpreted as a prelymphoma.

In 1979, Shimoyama et al., in Tokyo, described a lymph node lesion that they regarded as being similar to IBL but they interpreted it as a peripheral T-cell lymphoma. They called it "IBL-like T-cell lymphoma".

From autopsy reports on cases in the Kiel collection (Knecht et al. 1985), it was obvious that there should be a non-neoplastic "LgX" or angioimmunoblastic lymphadenopathy. In several cases, the lymph nodes were "burnt out", i.e. there was a paucity of cells, but there was an abundance of fibers and vessels. The lymphoid cell proliferation had disappeared without a trace, even without chemotherapy. This picture is somewhat similar to the phase of cellular depletion in late-stage HIV infection.

A favorable course over a period of years or spontaneous remission does not necessarily mean, however, that there is no underlying T-cell lymphoma.

Today more than 90% of the tumors have been shown to be monoclonal T-cell proliferations and were thus called T-cell lymphoma of AILD type.

Synonyms

- Kiel: T-cell lymphoma of AILD (LgX) type
- REAL: Angioimmunoblastic T-cell lymphoma
- WHO: Angioimmunoblastic T-cell lymphoma

Definition

Angioimmunoblastic T-cell lymphoma is a morphologically and clinically distinct entity. It primarily occurs in the lymph node. The major morphological diagnostic criteria in fully developed cases are defined as follows:

1. Total effacement of the architecture and frequent infiltration and overgrowth of the lymph node capsule mostly with absence of germinal centers.
2. Variegated cytology, dominated by pleomorphic T-cells ranging from small to medium-sized and some large cells with clear cytoplasm (clear cells).
3. Admixture of small lymphocytes, plasma cells, eosinophilic granulocytes, histiocytes, and sometimes epithelioid cells.
4. Marked increase in the number of arborizing vessels, mostly epithelioid venules, with thickened PAS-positive basement membranes.
5. Large, irregular-shaped accumulations of follicular dendritic cells (immunohistochemistry).

Morphology

In fully developed AIBTCL, the lymph node architecture is effaced and replaced by a highly vascularized infiltration that frequently bypasses the capsule and spreads into the surrounding adipose tissue (Figs. 5.17, 5.18). The follicles and germinal centers are missing. However, as the infiltrate starts in the T-zone or in the interfollicular areas, early infiltrates may still exhibit follicles, sometimes with even florid germinal centers (Fig. 5.19) (Kojima et al. 2001a). The subcapsular sinus is often recognizable and contrasts with the diffuse infiltration of the nodal and perinodal tissue.

Usually, there are a few poorly defined foci of B lymphocytes as remnants of follicles. In most cases the number of follicular dendritic cells is markedly increased. They sometimes form concentrically arranged,

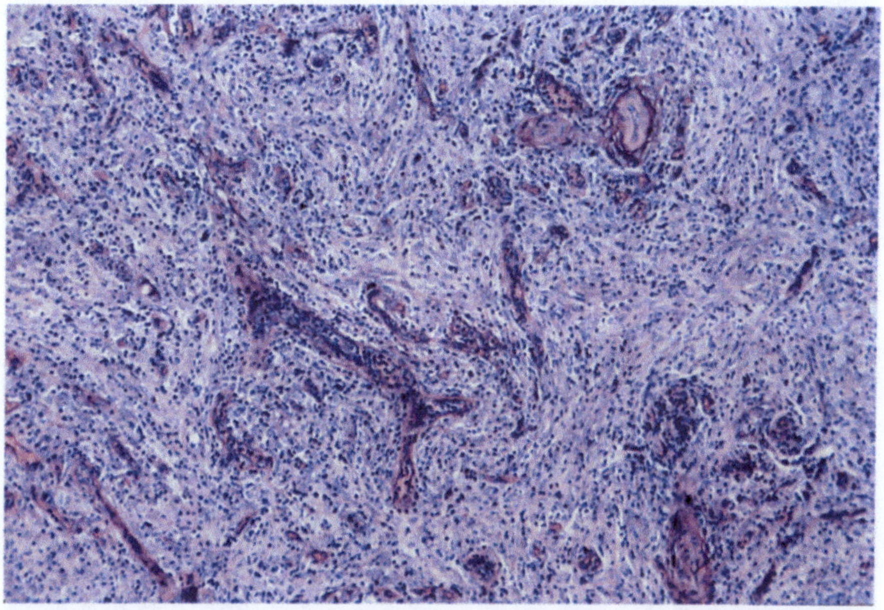

Fig. 5.17. Angioimmunoblastic T-cell lymphoma. Note the marked increase of epithelioid venules which show typical branching (Giemsa-stain)

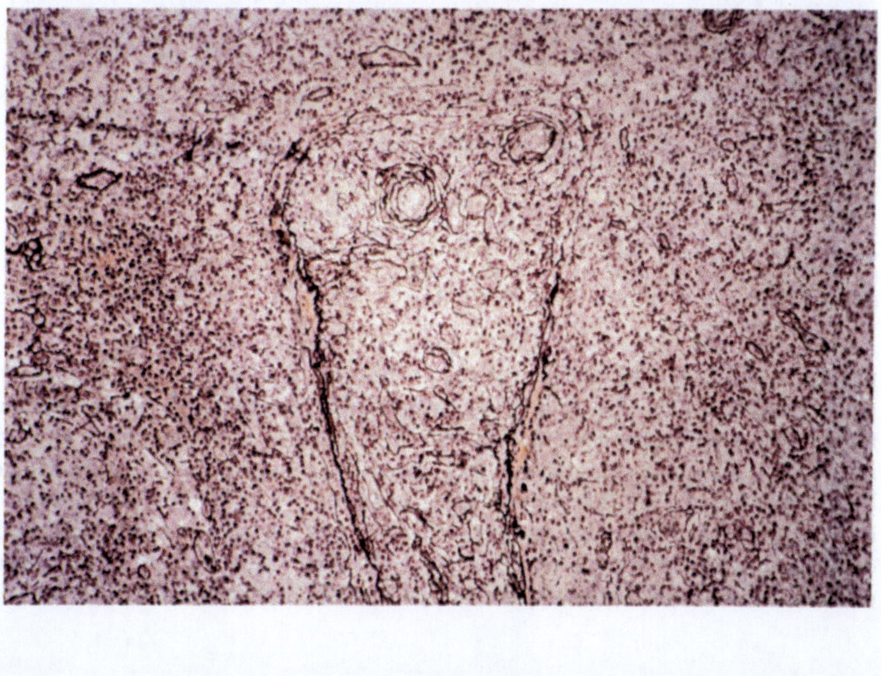

Fig. 5.18. Silver impregnation of the capsular area in an angioimmunoblastic T-cell lymphoma. The trabecular and capsular network is partly destroyed

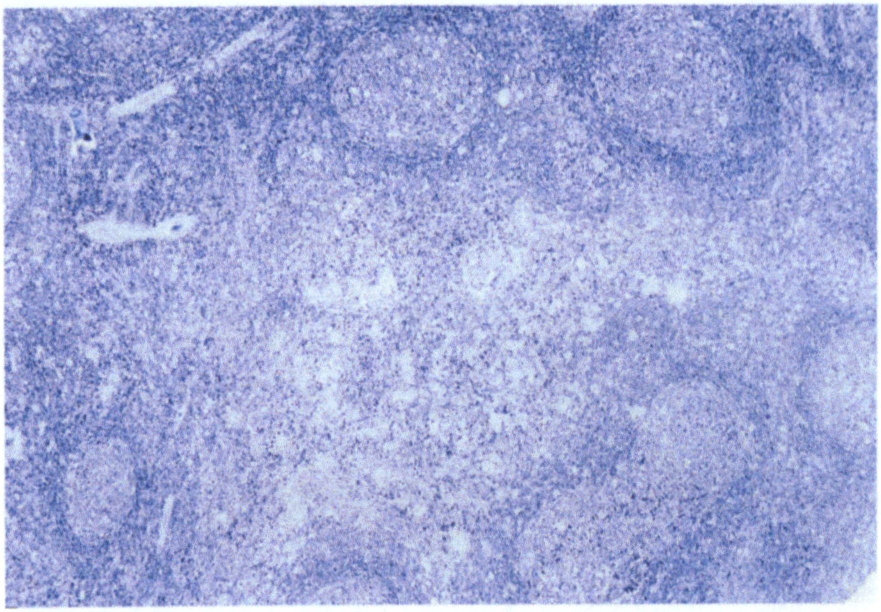

Fig. 5.19. Early infiltrate of angioimmunoblastic T-cell lymphoma. There is follicular hyperplasia and an infiltrate in the interfollicular area (Giemsa stain)

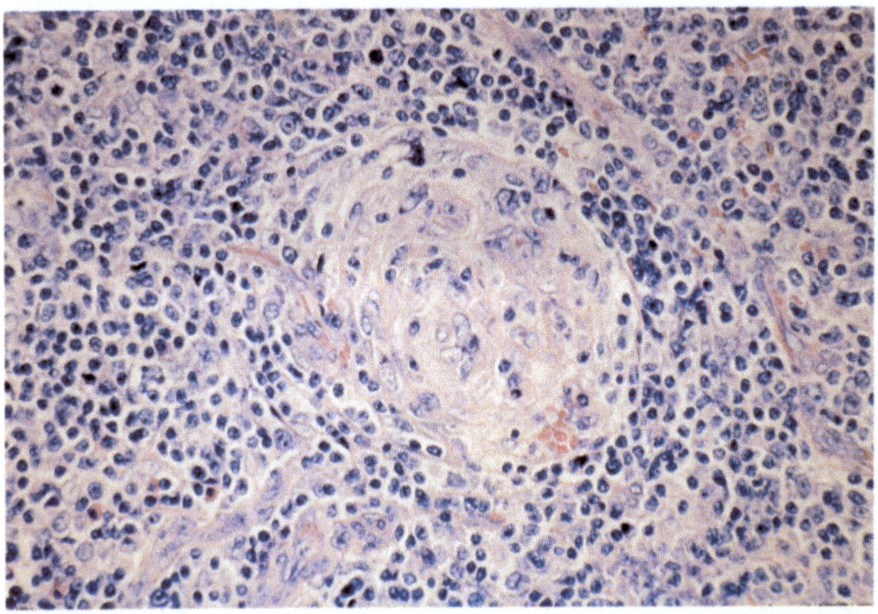

Fig. 5.20. Angioimmunoblastic T-cell lymphoma with a burned-out germinal center (Giemsa stain)

pale foci, which were initially interpreted as "burned-out" germinal centers (Fig. 5.20). We now know that, more often, the follicular dendritic cells collect in large, irregularly shaped accumulations that extend far beyond the original B-cell areas, spreading out in the tumor tissue which has a high content of venules. It is difficult to recognize the follicular dendritic cells with conventional stains, whereas they are easily identified with appropriate immunohistochemical staining (Fig. 5.21). These follicular dendritic cells may even actively proliferate and evidently lose their functional contact with B-lymphocytes.

The tumor infiltration is usually not as dense and homogeneous as that of other T- or B-cell lymphomas. In many cases, areas with lots of cells alternate with other areas that are more depleted. The spaces between

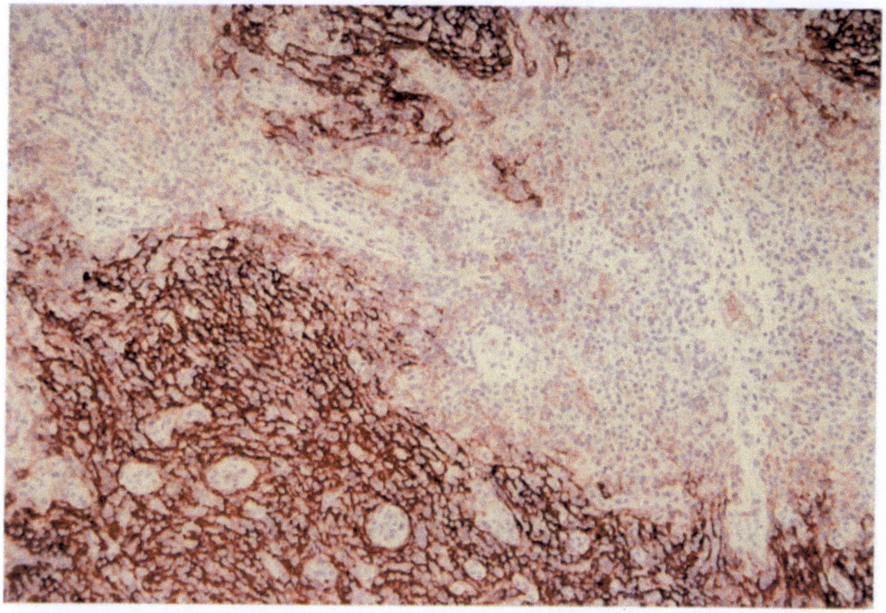

Fig. 5.21. Angioimmunoblastic T-cell lymphoma. Note the large, irregular shaped network of follicular dendritic cells spreading within the T-zones, and the many epithelioid venules (immunohistochemical stain, alkaline phosphatase)

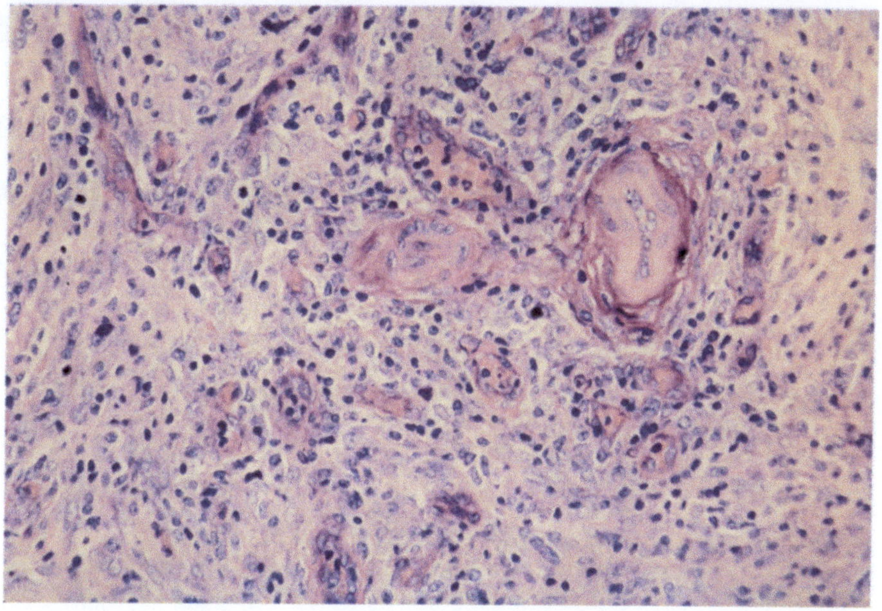

Fig. 5.22. Angioimmunoblastic T-cell lymphoma. Note the many epithelioid venules with marked thickening of the basement membrane in a hypocellular area (Giemsa stain)

the tumor cells often contain small, amorphous, weakly PAS-positive deposits, which prove to be mostly reticulin fibers and collagenous fibers (Knecht and Lennert 1981c).

As a hallmark, the infiltrated areas show a very large number of vessels, mostly so-called epithelioid or high endothelial venules, which are frequently branched. A distinctive feature of the epithelioid venules is their PAS-positive walls, which vary in thickness and represent (Fig. 5.22, 5.23) thickened multilayered basement membranes and collagenous fibers. Arterioles and arteries are also often surrounded by a broad, hyalinized layer of PAS-positive material or by concentrically arranged, thick bundles of collagenous fibers.

The tumor cells vary to some extent in their cytology (Figs. 5.24–5.26). The majority of the tumor cells

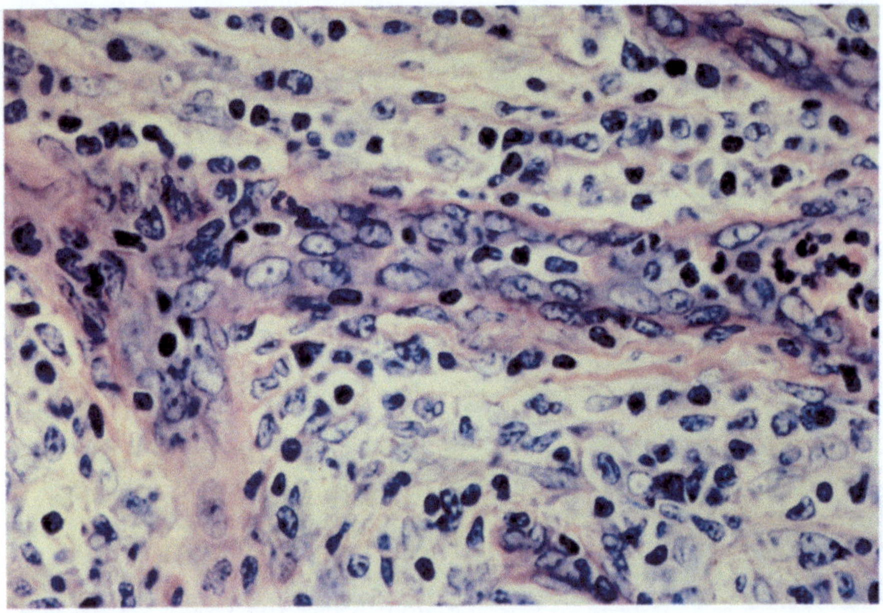

Fig. 5.23. A branching epithelioid venule in an angioimmunoblastic T-cell lymphoma. The vessel wall is infiltrated by neoplastic T-cells (Giemsa stain)

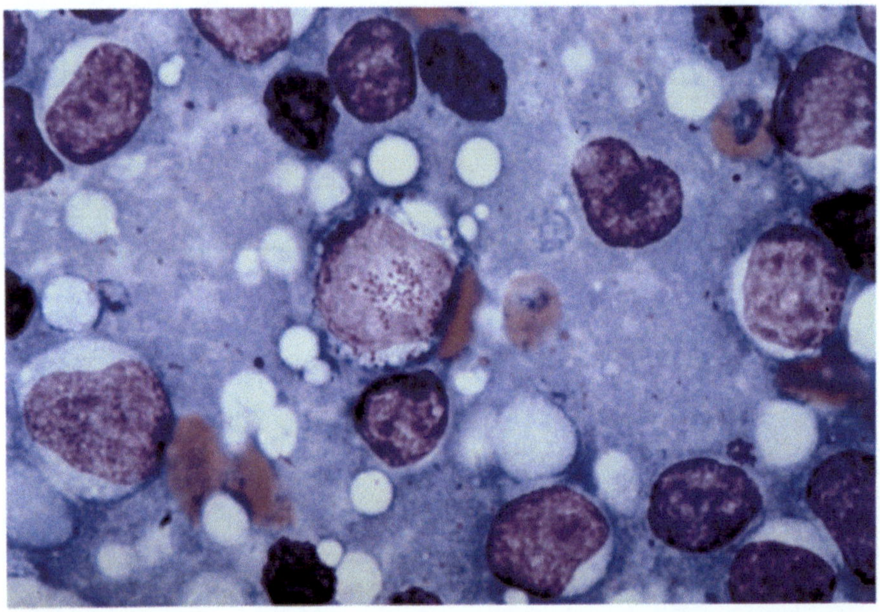

Fig. 5.24. Imprint of an angioimmunoblastic T-cell lymphoma. Note the medium sized and large pleomorphic cells, some of which have azurophilic granules in their cytoplasm (Pappenheim stain)

are small or medium-sized. They have more or less polymorphic nuclei with small or medium-sized nucleoli and scanty, pale gray to grayish blue cytoplasm. Cells with abundant, "transparent" cytoplasm (clear cells) are frequently found, mostly in small clusters (Fig. 5.27). These cells are PAS-negative. Their nuclei are less pleomorphic. In addition, there are usually some diffusely distributed, large basophilic blast cells that vary in their appearance, some of which are typical immunoblasts. On immunohistochemistry they can be identified as B-blasts, mostly EBV-positive (Fig. 5.28). One may also find sporadic multinucleate cells, occasionally resembling Reed-Sternberg cells. Mitotic figures are found in moderate or large numbers.

The tumor cells are often interspersed with many plasma cells (mostly polyclonal), plasmablasts, and

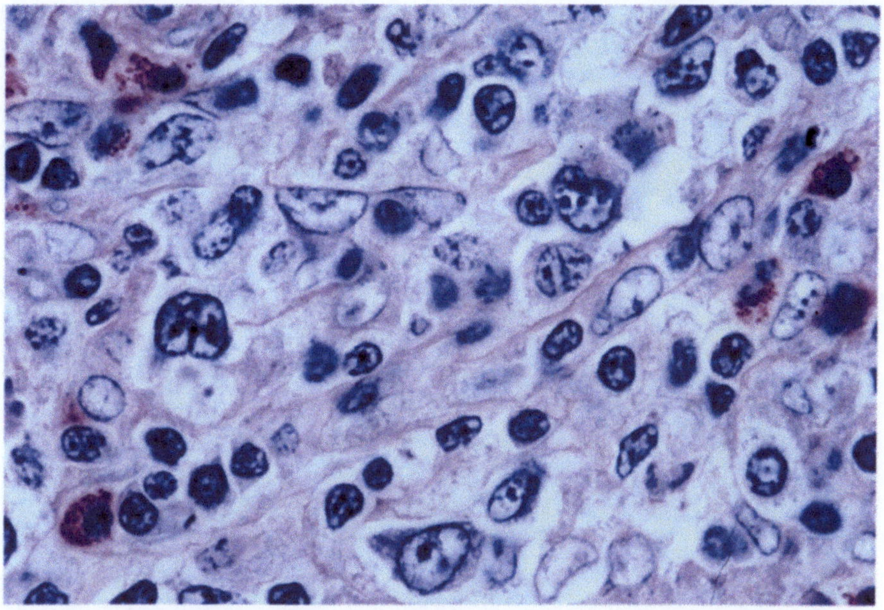

Fig. 5.25. Angioimmunoblastic T-cell lymphoma with neoplastic cells of various size. The nuclei are mostly pleomorphic, with a binucleate cell (Giemsa stain)

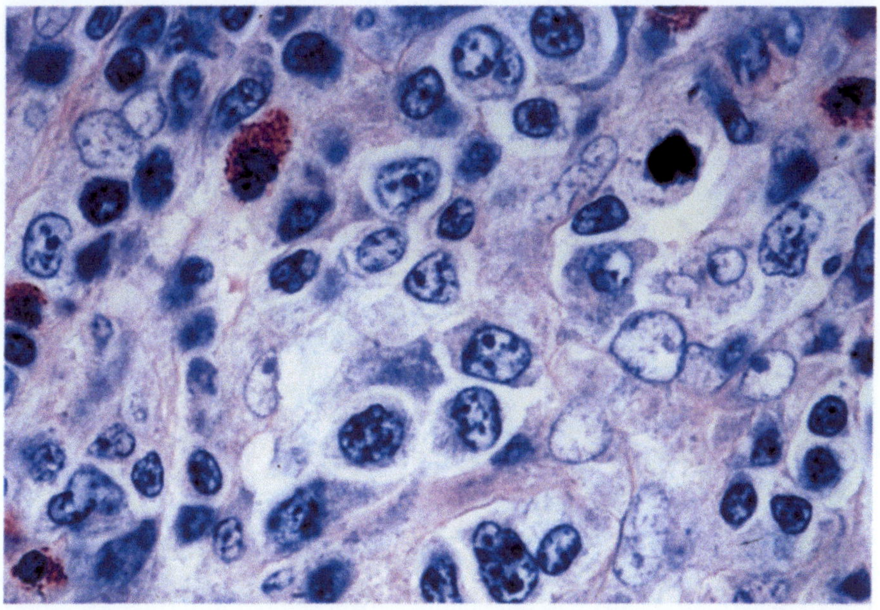

Fig. 5.26. Angioimmunoblastic T-cell lymphoma with neoplastic cells of various size. The nuclei are mostly pleomorphic, sometimes round; there is marked eosinophilia, some cells have a clear cytoplasm (Giemsa stain)

with numerous eosinophils as well as a varying number of histiocytes. A special morphological variant of AIBTCL shows epithelioid cells arranged in small foci (see Chap. 5.2.2.2) similar or identical to the epithelioid cell clusters seen in lymphoepithelioid lymphoma (see Differential Diagnosis) (Fig. 5.29).

Beside this typical histological picture, AIBTCL may exhibit a morphological spectrum, which on the one hand has to be differentiated from reactive "hyperimmune reactions" and on the other from peripheral T-cell lymphomas, unspecified.

The former is usually accompanied by the presence of follicles, mostly with florid germinal centers. The interfollicular infiltrate with the typical features mentioned above mostly consists of predominately smaller but already pleomorphic lymphoid cells, which leads to

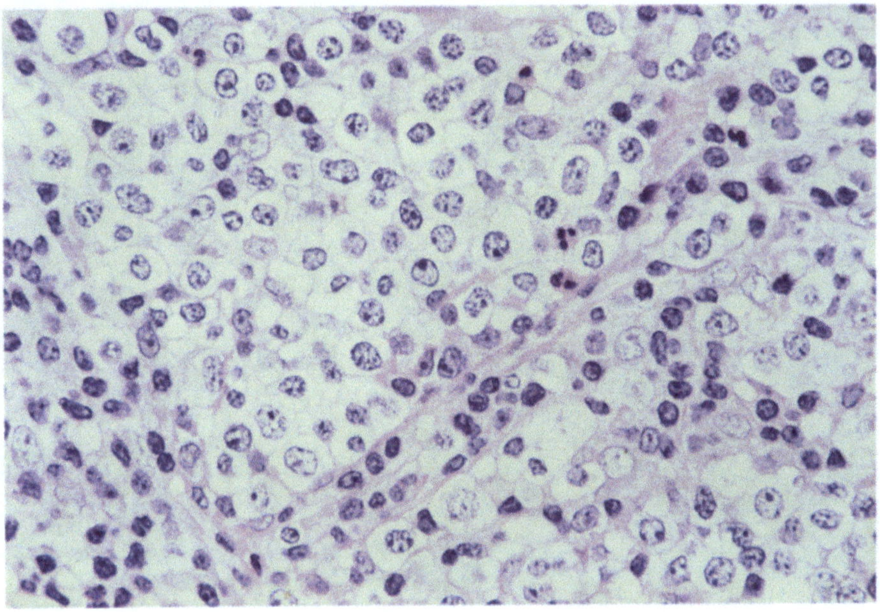

Fig. 5.27. Angioimmunoblastic T-cell lymphoma with a sheet of clear cells (Giemsa stain)

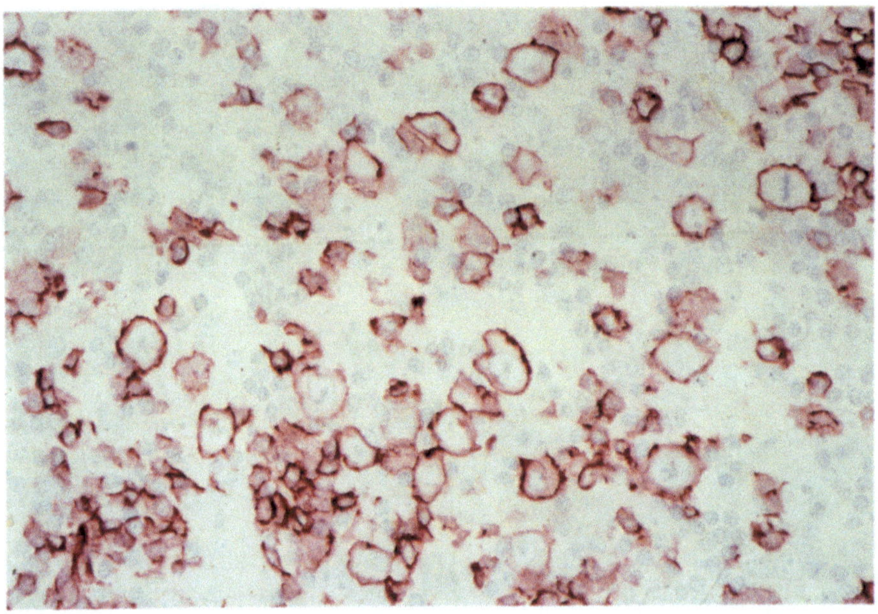

Fig. 5.28. Immunohistochemical staining for CD20 in angioimmunoblastic T-cell lymphoma (alkaline phosphatase). Note the CD20-positive blasts which are also EBV-positive (not shown)

a slightly monotonous appearing infiltrate among arborizing vessels (Figs. 5.29–5.31). In most of these cases the sinuses are at least partially preserved, indicating an early infiltrate of AIBTCL.

At the other end of the spectrum are more cellular types, with a decreasing number of typical vessels and more large pleomorphic cells. In these cases, the diagnosis of AIBTCL requires the detection of an enlarged network of follicular dendritic cells by immunohistochemistry (see Differential Diagnosis).

Evolution and Transformation. In some patients, already at the onset of the disease or as seen on a second biopsy subsequent to recurrence, the tumor cells are medium-sized or large and densely packed (at least in places); they also show high mitotic activity. This is

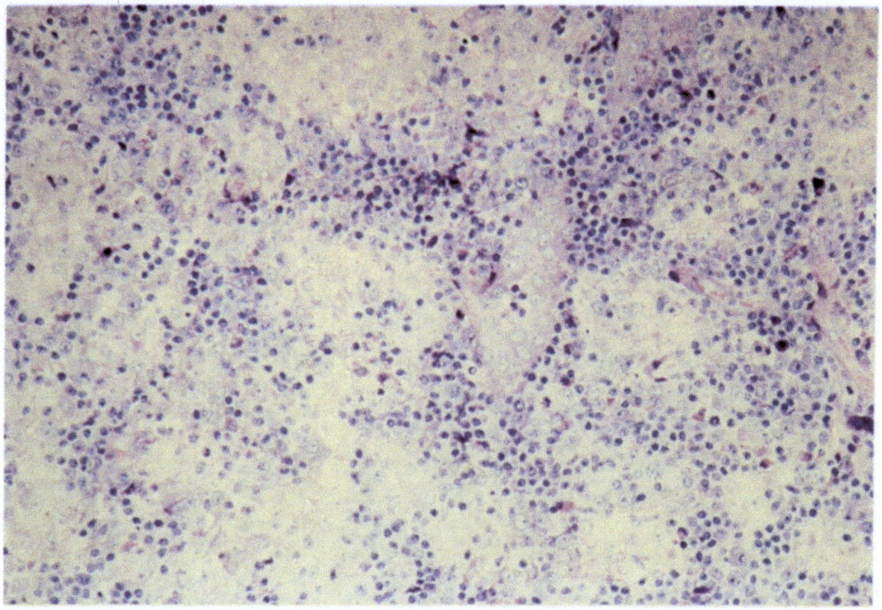

Fig. 5.29. Angioimmunoblastic T-cell lymphoma. Note the marked increase of epithelioid cells which mimic lymphoepithelioid lymphoma (Lennert's lymphoma). A prominent epithelioid venule is visible (Giemsa stain)

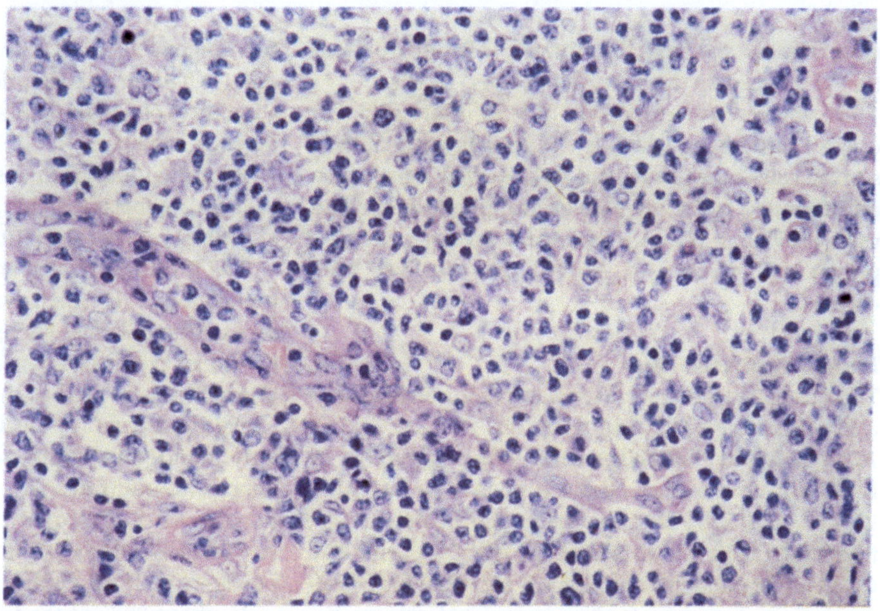

Fig. 5.30. High-power view of the early infiltrate of angioimmunoblastic T-cell lymphoma shown in Fig. 5.19. The lymphoid infiltrate is quite pleomorphic, some prominent high endothelial venules are visible

accompanied by a decrease of arborizing vessels and the lack of a typical follicular dendritic cell network. These features indicate transformation into a peripheral T-cell lymphoma, unspecified (Kiel: high-grade pleomorphic T-cell lymphoma). This occurs in approximately 10% of patients.

In about the same percentage of patients there is an increase in monotypic plasma cells and a in the number of B-immunoblasts. Some of these patients may develop a diffuse large-B-cell lymphoma – B-immunoblastic (Abruzzo et al. 1993). In a majority of patients, however, the monotypic immunoblasts (and plasma cells) are still intermingled with a large number of neoplastic T-cells, without forming cohesive tumor cell clusters. In such cases it is not clear whether a genuine secondary neoplasm has developed, or whether it

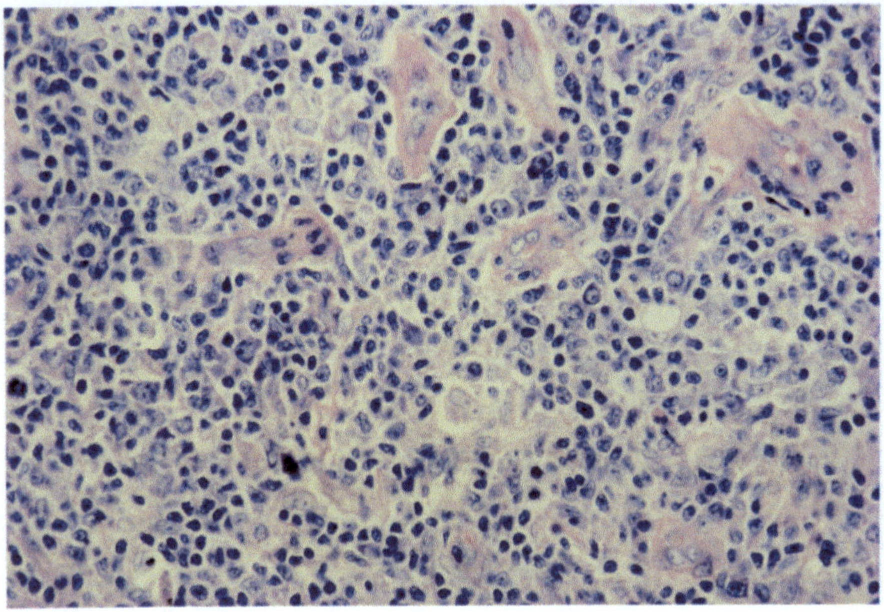

Fig. 5.31. High-power view of the early infiltrate of angioimmunoblastic T-cell lymphoma shown in Fig. 5.29. The lymphoid infiltrate is quite pleomorphic, some prominent high endothelial venules are visible

should be assumed that the monotypic B-cell proliferation is induced by the neoplastic helper-T-cells.

During its course AIBTCL may infiltrate different organ sites, among which is the skin. In such cases, a similar cellular infiltrate can be observed mostly also accompanied by an increase of prominent epithelioid venules. This is always a secondary involvement, as a primary occurrence of AIBTCL has not yet been observed.

Immunohistochemistry

The variegated infiltration shows a predominance of T-cells with a mature phenotype(CD3+, CD2+, CD5+). Antigen loss is rare. Whereas all other mature T- or NK/T-cell lymphomas exhibit a phenotype of either CD4 *or* CD8, AIBTCL, although predominately CD4+, frequently has a higher admixture of CD8+ cells. The CD4 to CD8 quotient was 3.9 ± 2.7. Simultaneous demonstration of the proliferation-associated antigen Ki-67 shows that CD4-positive cells proliferate almost exclusively in about two-thirds of the tumors, whereas in the other third there is an increased number of proliferating CD8-positive cells in addition to CD4-positive cells. Whether CD8-positive cells also belong to the neoplastic T-cell clone remains controversial. By cytogenetics it could be shown that a trisomy 3 is found in CD4- and CD8-positive cells (Schlegelberger et al. 1996). Willenbrock et al. (2001) reported that a clonal rearrangement for TCR is found only in CD4-positive cells. Whatever the significance of these findings, the admixture of a high number of CD8-positive cells is of diagnostic help.

Recently it has been described that, in the majority of cases, neoplastic T-cells, to some extent, (between 5 and 30%) coexpress CD10 (Attygalle et al. 2002).

The B-cell-associated antigen CD20 is found on two populations: (1) small lymphocytes as remnants of preexisting follicles. These cells frequently form small band-like aggregates beneath the lymph node capsule. These B cells as well as the plasma cells show a polyclonal Ig pattern. (2) CD20-positive B-blasts are regularly found, mostly diffusely intermingled within the neoplastic infiltrate. These B-cells are almost always positive for EBV. Moreover, EBV can also be demonstrated in T-cells or in both B- and T-cells (Anagnostopoulos et al. 1992; Zettl et al. 2002).

In about 80% of the tumors, there is an extensive, irregularly defined network of follicular dendritic cells (CD35+, Ki-M4p+, CD23+, CD21+), with the expression of CD35 being most prominent. This follicular dendritic cell network can be regarded as a diagnostic feature.

Genetic Features

DNA analysis of the TCR genes shows that clonal T-cell proliferations are present in more than 90% of patients. By PCR analysis, about 15% additionally show a clonal Ig heavy-chain gene rearrangement (Feller et al. 1988).

Cytogenetic studies showed that in about 40% of patients there is a trisomy 3 and less frequently trisomy 5 and +X. Compared to peripheral T-cell lymphomas, unspecified (pleomorphic, small-, medium- and large-cell), a higher rate of normal metaphases and the occurrence of unrelated clones can be detected in AIBTCL (Schlegelberger et al. 1994).

Complex aberrant clones could be shown to be of independent prognostic significance (Schlegelberger et al. 1996).

Differential Diagnosis

Of great importance is the distinction between an early infiltrate of AIBTCL with preserved germinal centers and an abnormal immune ("hyperimmune") reaction (Knecht and Lennert 1981a,b) that shows active germinal centers and a hyperplastic pulp containing numerous venules. Such conditions may appear in autoimmune diseases (Kojima et al. 2001b). Hence the cytology of the pulp and the interfollicular areas must be studied carefully. In a hyperimmune reaction, the pulp and interfollicular areas do not contain any accumulations of atypical T-lymphocytes with pronounced nuclear pleomorphism (Fig. 5.30). In early phases of AIBTCL, small clusters of more monotonous-appearing pleomorphic lymphocytes can be detected associated with a focal proliferation of epithelioid venules (Fig. 5.19). In all ambiguous cases, clonality studies and very careful clinical observation is necessary; in addition, if possible, a new biopsy should be obtained after a few weeks.

Occasionally, it is impossible to draw a clear borderline between angioimmunoblastic T-cell lymphoma on the one hand and *T-zone lymphoma* and *lymphoepithelioid lymphoma* on the other, especially when follicles are no longer present. A hallmark for the differentiation is staining for follicular dendritic cells, which only show remnants or well-preserved networks in the latter two lymphoma types. The cellular infiltrate is more monotonous, consisting of mostly smaller lymphoid cells with less nuclear pleomorphism. In lymphoepithelioid lymphoma, the proliferation of epithelioid venules can be masked by a high number of epithelioid cells.

Peripheral T-cell lymphoma, unspecified, which, among others, comprises the Kiel category of pleomorphic T-cell lymphoma, has a more monotonous cellular infiltrate with a higher cell density and hardly any plasma cells or eosinophils. Also, arborizing vessels are either an exception or they are absent.

In exceptional cases, in which an *immunocytoma* shows a marked increase in the number of venules, this lymphoma can bear a certain resemblance to AIBTCL with many epithelioid cells. A false diagnosis is prevented by the observation of a greater cell density of the infiltration, which is composed of small lymphocytes that have round nuclei and are interspersed with *monotypic* plasma cells or lymphoplasmacytoid cells. Moreover, such tumors should have a higher number of diffusely distributed small-B-lymphocytes.

Occurrence

Angioimmunoblastic T-cell lymphoma accounts among nodal lymphomas for 20.9% of the peripheral NK/T-cell lymphomas in the Kiel collection and is thus the most frequent nodal type of peripheral NK/T-cell lymphoma. Among all NK/T-cell lymphomas, it makes up about 8% and 3%. In a prospective study of unselected cases by the Kiel Lymphoma Study Group (Brittinger et al. 1984), there were 1,127 patients with NHL and 32 patients with "AILD-type T-cell lymphoma", which is equivalent to 2.7%.

The GELA group found 24% of peripheral NK/T-cell lymphomas to be AIBTCL (Gisselbrecht et al. 1998).

Following the WHO or REAL classification, the Non-Hodgkin's Lymphoma Classification Project arrived at a nearly identical percentage of cases among peripheral NK/T-cell lymphomas (18% out of 129 cases) (Rüdiger et al. 2002).

Angioimmunoblastic T-cell lymphoma tends to be a disease of older people, with a steep peak in the seventh decade of life. The youngest patient was 16 years old, the oldest 84. One should be extremely careful with a diagnosis of this disease in children or young adults; as a rule, viral infections or hyperimmune reactions are more likely in this age group. There is a slight male preponderance (the male-to-female ratio is approx. 1.18:1).

Clinical Presentation

In general, patients present with a generalized lymphadenopathy and thus stage III or IV disease. Usually cervical, axillary, mediastinal, and abdominal lymph nodes are involved. Patients frequently report rapid growth of the affected area and a history of recurrent lymph node enlargement (Knecht and Lennert 1981a).

B symptoms were recorded in two-thirds of the patients. Half the patients had skin rashes and pruritus. Hepatomegaly and splenomegaly were also seen in two-thirds of the patients. A third of the patients showed a remarkable tendency to develop edema, particularly in the upper extremities and the face. Pleural effusions, ascites, and lung infiltrates were seldom observed (Siegert et al. 1995).

The laboratory findings were generally those of a hyperimmune process. Two-thirds of the patients were anemic; 30 % had a positive Coombs' test, in which case the patients could be said to have either hemolytic anemia or, if the marrow was depleted and reticulocytosis was missing, aplastic anemia. An analysis of blood smears showed that the numbers of large granular lymphocytes (CD8+), hyperbasophilic cells (plasma cells, proplasmacytes, plasmablasts) and basophilic granulocytes were increased. The ESR varied within a wide range; in 11 % of patients it was normal, in 23 % highly elevated. There was almost always a polyclonal increase immunoglobulins in the blood. Rheumatoid factors, cryoglobulin, and antibodies against smooth muscle cells (vimentin) were reported in 5–20 % of the patients (Pautier et al. 1999).

Dellagi et al. (1984) found antivimentin autoantibodies in 75 % of their patients with AILD. Circulating immune complexes appear to be a frequent phenomenon. An important feature is drug hypersensitivity (chiefly, antibiotics, antiphlogistics and cytostatic drugs), which is not uncommon and can appear prior to, simultaneously with, or during the course of the disease and which then leads to the skin lesions described above. In 11 of 172 patients, another malignant tumor (usually carcinoma) was found in addition to the lymphoma (Knecht et al. 1985). HTLV-1 antibodies are not detectable.

It is of importance to keep in mind that most patients primarily respond to immunosuppressive therapy. Some patients show spontaneous remissions even over months or without any recurrence.

The older data (Knecht and Lennert 1981b) on prognosis probably give the wrong impression. They were collected at a time when AIBTCL was still considered to be an abnormal immune reaction. Patients were often treated only with corticosteroids and received cytostatic drugs much too late, if at all. The results were accordingly poor. Patients treated with corticosteroids alone showed a median survival period of 5.3 months, while with polychemotherapy it was 13.3 months.

Angioimmunoblastic T-cell lymphoma runs an aggressive course in more than 70 % of patients. As in other large-cell or aggressive lymphomas, a younger age and a limited stage of disease may indicate a slightly better outcome. The same is true for a low LDH. Individual patients respond without any predictive signs to an immunosuppressive therapy with corticoids, sometimes even with stable remission. Another few patients show spontaneous remission without any therapy. Overall, about 80 % of patients die within 5 years, 60 % already within the first 2 years.

Chromosomal analysis indicated that the presence of complex aberrant clones was an independent prognostic factor, with a lower incidence of therapy-induced remission. Thus, the International Prognostic Index (IPI)is currently the best predictor of prognosis (Gisselbrecht et al. 1998).

A prospective study of 53 patients showed complete remission in 29 % of those treated with prednisone alone (Siegert et al. 1989). With subsequent chemotherapy (COPLAM/IMVP16), complete remission was achieved in 57 %. Chemotherapy alone led to full remission in only 37 %. The remission periods were short, 4.5, 3.5 and 8.5 months, respectively. The mean survival period was almost 24 months. In a new prospective study, the median survival was 15 months. The survival curve showed a plateau (at 40 %) after 2 years. Treatment with low doses of interferon-α has been recommended (Trinkler et al. 1989; Siegert et al. 1991). This agent has been reported to be useful as salvage treatment for patients who are refractory to combination therapy or when the latter is contra-indicated. Also, successful treatment with purine analogues (Hast et al. 1999) and with cyclosporin (Yamamura et al. 1996) has been reported.

5.2.2.2 Peripheral T-Cell Lymphoma, Unspecified (ICD-O: 9702/3)

This category groups together different subtypes, variants, and entities that were separated, somewhat arbitrarily, in the Kiel classification. It is commonly understood that this group does not cover a clinically or pathologically homogeneous group of lymphomas. Although it includes more than 50 % of the nodal peripheral NK/T-cell lymphomas, a unifying approach was chosen, since, as stated previously, the entities of the Kiel classification cannot be reproducibly diagnosed and their separation has no clinical relevance with respect to outcome. Thus, these lymphomas should be considered together, at least until new studies provide a basis upon which to separate them. In other words, if the lymphomas within this group cannot be otherwise subtyped, then "peripheral T-cell lymphoma, unspecified" serves as a diagnosis that excludes everything else.

When the REAL and the WHO classifications were formulated, it was obvious that a specific treatment for one or the other lymphomas in this category was not available and the number of cases investigated was small. Thus it was acceptable to group these lymphomas into one which category, since all of them have a poor prognosis. However, as new therapeutic strategies emerge the need will arise for a more stratified classification.

According to the Kiel classification, this category comprises the following lymphomas:

- Pleomorphic small-cell, medium-sized and large-cell as well as immunoblastic
- Lymphoepithelioid lymphoma/Lennert's lymphoma
- T-zone lymphoma
- Nodal NK/T-cell lymphoma, nasal type (not listed in the Kiel classification)

These groups are discussed in the individual sections that follow below.

5.2.2.2.1 Pleomorphic, Small-Cell, Medium-Sized and Large-Cell T-Cell Lymphoma

This category mostly consist of a mixture of medium and large cells with a marked pleomorphism of their nuclei. The cells have an unsharp border compared with that of the small-cell pleomorphic type on the one hand, and the immunoblastic type on the other. The pure small-cell pleomorphic type is a category of its own. In a lymph node, it is rare and may be associated with HTLV-1 positivity. The transition to the immunoblastic type is also indistinct, and tumors with a predominance of true immunoblasts such as B-immunoblasts exist but are extremely rare.

Finally, this category comprises a high percentage of tumors with a cytotoxic or sometimes even NK-cell phenotype. This is documented by the frequent detection of azurophilic granules. These tumors have to be differentiated from the extremely rare, primary nodal manifestation of a NK/T-cell lymphoma, nasal type, with angiocentricity.

Thus, the pleomorphic medium-sized and large-cell type of lymphoma will be the focus of the next section.

Synonyms

- Kiel: Pleomorphic small-cell, medium-sized and large-cell
- REAL: Peripheral T-cell lymphoma, unspecified – medium sized cell, mixed medium and large (provisional cytological category)
- WHO: Peripheral T-cell lymphoma, unspecified

Definition

The tumor is composed of medium-sized, large, or medium-sized and large cells showing a considerable degree of nuclear pleomorphism. The patients may be HTLV-1 positive (in endemic areas). In the tumors of these patients, the nuclear pleomorphism often tends to be more pronounced and appears as "polymorphism", i.e. variations in shape among cells of the same type. During a 1984 workshop, Japanese experts on ATLL were often (about 60% of the cases), but not always, able to make a histological distinction between virus-positive and virus-negative tumors (Lennert et al. 1985). Thus, these cases are described together. Further information on ATLL are given in Chap. 5.2.1.2.

Pleomorphic, small-T-cell lymphoma is composed of a relatively monotonous-looking proliferation of small T-cells with pleomorphic nuclei and without a significant admixture of large, basophilic blast cells.

Table 5.2. Histological characteristics of peripheral T-cell lymphomas

1.	Primary infiltration of T regions
2.	Epithelioid venules are often increased in number and sometimes atypical
3.	Tumor cells Mostly pleomorphic (to a variable degree) Rarely basophilic Occasionally "clear" cells Occasionally giant cells, including Sternberg-Reed type
4.	Sometimes admixture of: Interdigitating cells Epithelioid cells Eosinophils Plasma cells (polytypic)
5.	Low-grade malignant lymphoma frequently transforms into high-grade malignant lymphoma

This tumor may be HTLV-1 positive, especially in Japanese and Caribbean patients, in which case it often presents with the clinical picture of *chronic* ATLL (see Chap. 5.2.1.2) or is within the differential diagnosis of T-PLL or mycosis fungoides/Sézary's syndrome.

Some general histological characteristics of peripheral T-cell lymphoma, unspecified, are given in Table 5.2.

Morphology

The tumor cells are sometimes predominately medium-sized, or large; more often, however, there is a mixture of medium-sized and large cells intermingled with small cells and blasts. Typically, there is an extraordinary variety of nuclear configurations. Often the nucleus is convex and smooth on one side, while the opposite side is concave and has many irregular indenta-

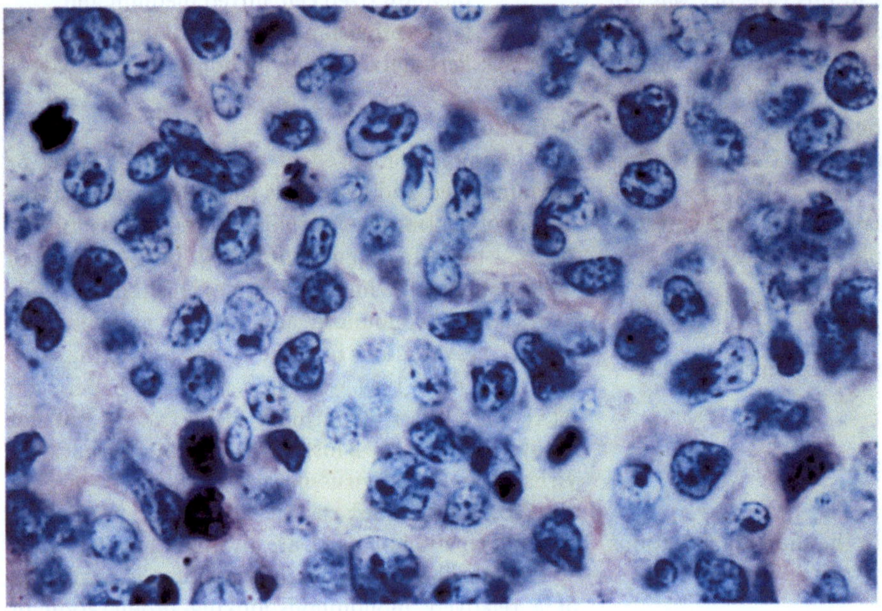

Fig. 5.32. Peripheral T-cell lymphoma, unspecified. Note the medium and large cells with pleomorphic nuclei (Giemsa stain)

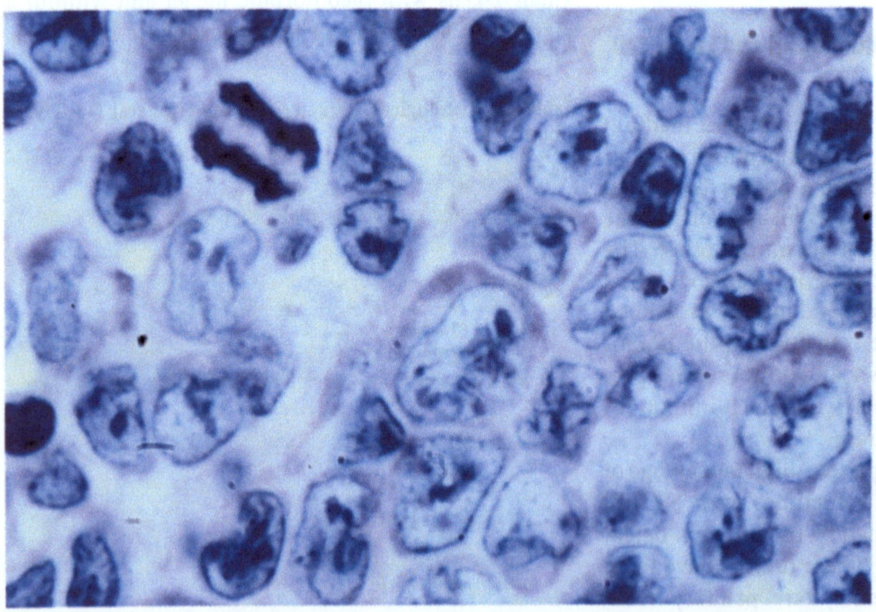

Fig. 5.33. Peripheral T-cell lymphoma, unspecified. Note the blastic pleomorphic cells with jellyfish appearance (Giemsa stain)

tions (Figs. 5.32–5.35). The resulting images are often very bizarre, occasionally reminding one of jellyfish or embryos. There are also nuclei that could be described as cerebriform (Weisenburger et al. 1982). The chromatin is moderately fine or coarse. The nucleoli are large, of varying shape and number, and basophilic. In imprints the cells frequently exhibit azurophilic granules (Fig. 5.36). The cytoplasm is moderately abundant and moderately basophilic. The tumor cells are mostly densely packed. The vascularity is not prominent. Epithelioid venules are, for the most part, missing. Occasionally, a small to moderate number of eosinophils and sporadic mast cells are interspersed among the tumor cells. Now and again, one sees interdigitating cells, which also have bizarre-looking nuclei. These cells show very fine chromatin, however, and the nucle-

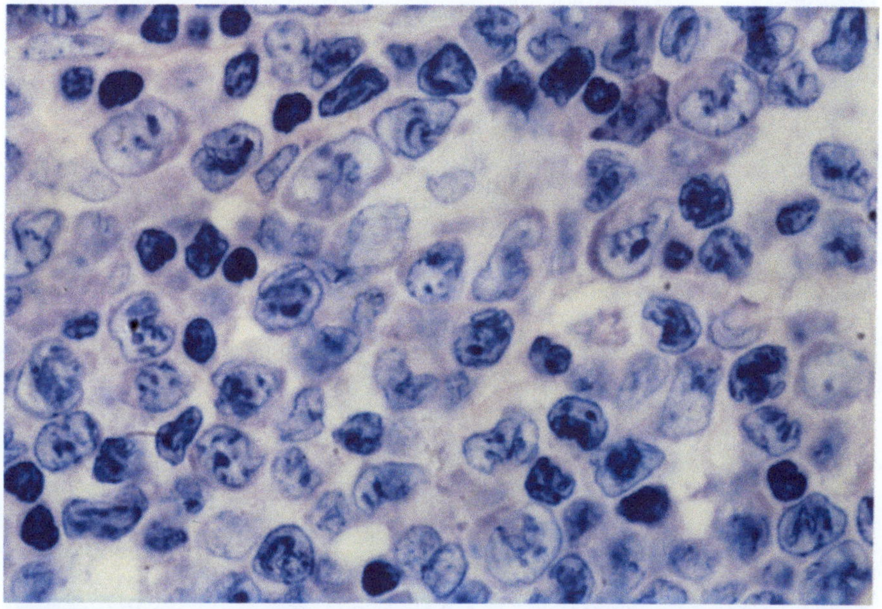

Fig. 5.34. Peripheral T-cell lymphoma, unspecified. Note the highly pleomorphic nuclei with many bizarre configurations (Giemsa stain)

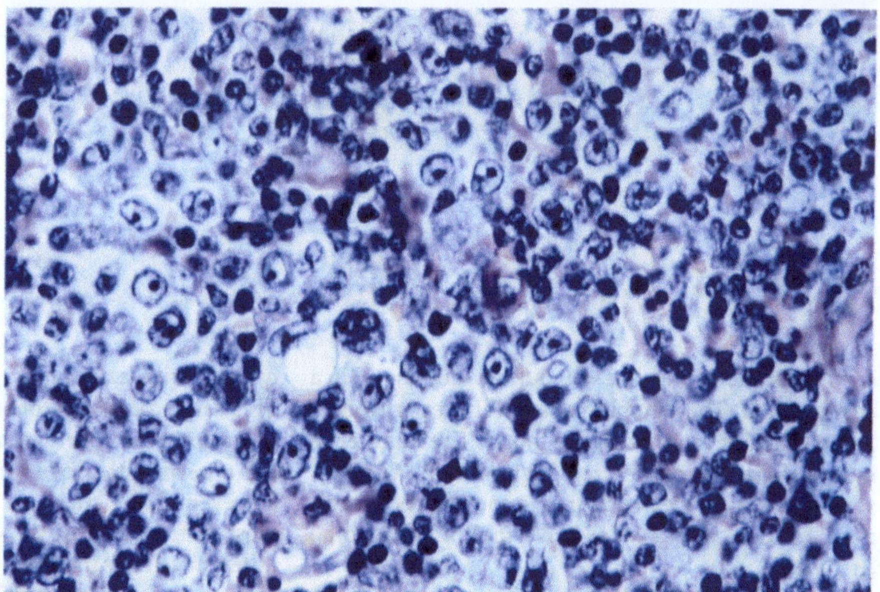

Fig. 5.35. Peripheral T-cell lymphoma, unspecified. Note the pleomorphic cells and the large number of T-immunoblasts

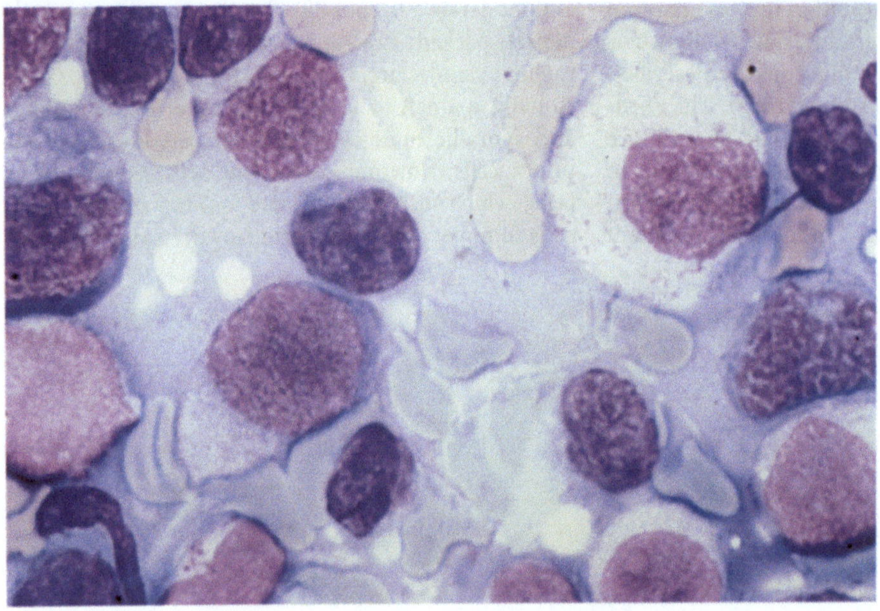

Fig. 5.36. Imprint of a peripheral T-cell lymphoma, unspecified. Note the medium-sized and large cells, some of which have azurophilic granules (Pappenheim stain)

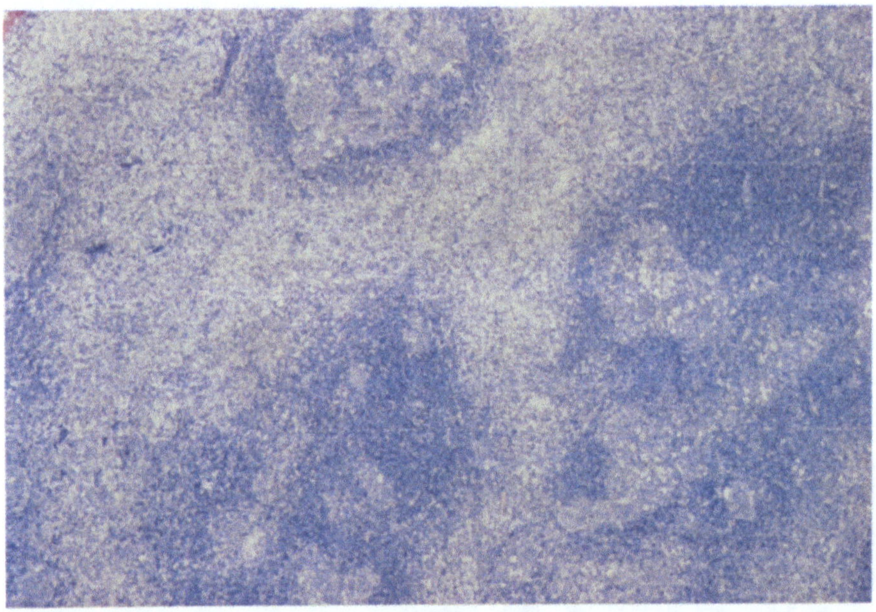

Fig. 5.37. Peripheral T-cell lymphoma, unspecified, with a T-zone growth pattern (Giemsa stain)

ar membrane looks like an outline drawn with a sharp pencil. The cytoplasm is hardly recognizable. At times, giant tumor cells are found. The number of mitotic figures is moderately high to high. Angioinvasion and angiodestruction are sometimes prominent. In such cases a NK/T-cell lymphoma has to be excluded.

In imprints, the cells have large irregular nuclei, frequently with azurophilic granules in the cytoplasm. This can indicate a cytotoxic phenotype.

As for other peripheral nodal T-cell lymphomas, this type may start to infiltrate in the T-zone (Fig. 5.37); however, this pattern of growth should be distinguished from that of T-zone lymphoma, which has a different cellular infiltrate.

Despite the pleomorphism of the tumor cell nuclei,

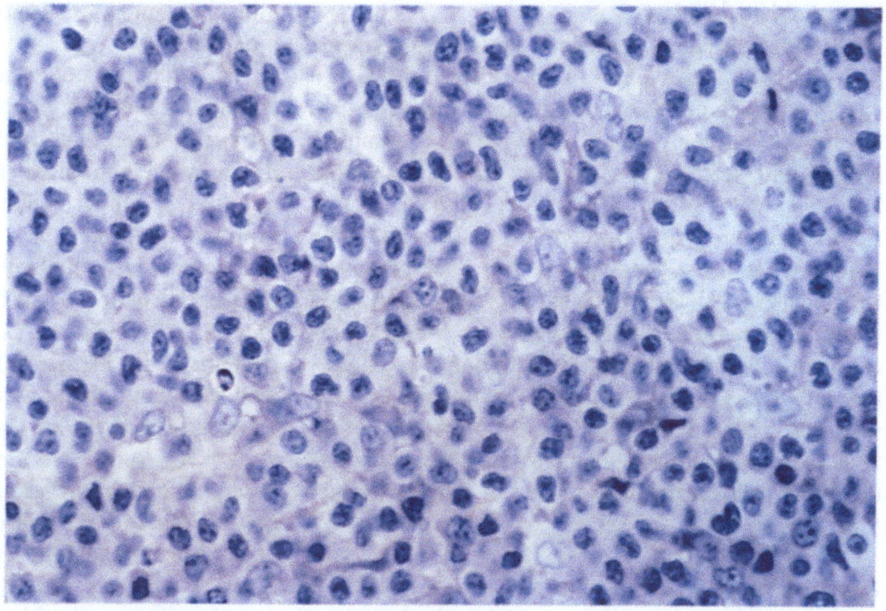

Fig. 5.38. Peripheral T-cell lymphoma, unspecified. This is a pleomorphic small-cell lymphoma consisting of a more homogenous appearing cell population than seen in the medium sized and large cell types (Giemsa stain)

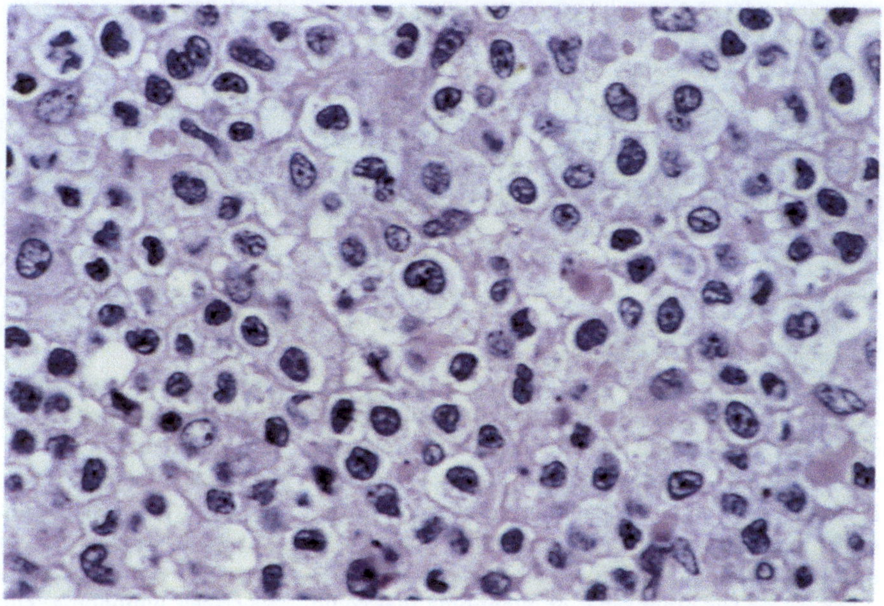

Fig. 5.39. Peripheral T-cell lymphoma featuring clear cells (Giemsa stain)

the small-cell type has a relatively monotonous appearance. The tumor cells are generally small and vary only slightly in size (Fig. 5.38); they all have scanty, pale gray cytoplasm. In some cases, the cytoplasm is abundant and as clear as water (clear cells; Fig. 5.39). The nuclei are irregularly shaped, and assume a wide range of forms. They often appear serrated on the concave side, while the convex side looks smooth. The chromatin is moderately dense. The nucleoli are usually solitary and small. There are practically no other cells interspersed among these cells. The number of mitotic figures is low. Venules are not very conspicuous. Sometimes there is a noticeable infiltration of small to medium-sized vessels, often with angiodestruction. This must lead to careful exclusion of a primary extranodal NK/T-cell lymphoma.

Immunohistochemistry

The tumor cells characteristically show the phenotype of peripheral T-cells (CD2+, CD3+, CD5+, and CD4+ or CD8+). In about 20% of the tumors, there is a partial loss of antigens, which results in an incomplete immunophenotype. Approximately 30% of the tumors have cells with features of activated cells, i.e. expression of interleukin (IL)-2 receptors (CD25) and CD30. Tumors that are CD25-positive are simultaneously CD7-positive. The lack of the latter antigen, combined with the expression of IL-2 receptors, may be an indication of HTLV-1 positivity. The number of proliferating cells (Ki-67+) also increases as the tumor cells increase in size. Proliferation rates between 15 and 80% are found, with a median of about 60%. Follicular dendritic cells occasionally occur in small, residual foci.

Genetic Features

The TCR genes are usually rearranged, the Ig heavy-chain genes are in a germline configuration.

Although specific chromosomal abnormalities do not exist more frequently than in other peripheral T-cell lymphomas, a polyploid chromosome number is found. In contrast to AILD, Lennert's lymphoma and T-zone lymphoma, peripheral T-cell lymphomas (unspecified) have complex aberrant clones with abnormalities in chromosomes 6p, 7/7q, 8, and 13. They do not carry a trisomy 3, unlike the three above-mentioned entities (Schlegelberger et al. 1994).

Diagnosis and Differential Diagnosis

Despite the pleomorphism of the nuclei, the appearance of the tumor cells is relatively monotonous (in contrast to those of the HTLV-1-induced tumor in the same category!). This type of pleomorphism is so characteristic, providing the quality of the slides is impeccable, that this type of T-cell lymphoma can even be diagnosed without immunological staining.

There are few other types of lymphoma that could be confused with pleomorphic, medium-sized and large-cell T-cell lymphoma. The *tumor phase of mycosis fungoides* resembles pleomorphic, medium-sized and large-cell T-cell lymphoma. In such cases, the history is of importance. As AILD may transform into *peripheral T-cell lymphoma, unspecified,* an indistinct border may be found in such cases. The cells in pleomorphic lymphomas are more densely packed, and the inflammatory infiltrate is much less pronounced. Finally, enlarged follicular dendritic cell networks are absent in the pleomorphic type.

It is often, but not always possible for an expert to distinguish between virus-positive and virus-negative tumors (Lennert et al. 1985). In virus-positive tumors, the variation in the size of the nuclei is much more pronounced than the irregularity of the nuclear configuration. (see Chap. 5.2.1.2)

Pleomorphic, small-cell T-cell lymphoma must be differentiated first of all from *T-zone lymphoma* and *mantle cell lymphoma.* Mantle cell lymphoma never contains clear cells. The reticulin fibers are thicker and less abundant. Small vessels often contain hyaline deposits. The nuclei are not as pleomorphic as those in T-cell lymphoma, since they tend to be round or indented and are never serrated. Nevertheless, there are mantle cell lymphomas that cannot be distinguished morphologically from pleomorphic, small-cell T-cell lymphoma. Finally, *lymphoblastic lymphoma* occasionally poses problems in a differential diagnosis (see Chap. 5.1).

Occurrence

Pleomorphic, medium-sized and large-cell T-cell lymphoma accounts for only about 2.6% of the nodal lymphomas in our collection. It makes up 15.5% of the NK/T-cell lymphomas. The youngest patient in our collection was 13 years old, while the oldest was 87. The age curve reveals a peak incidence in the eighth decade of life. There is a slight predominance of males, with a male-to-female ratio of approximately 1.35:1.

Clinical Presentation and Prognosis

The tumor is often first diagnosed on a biopsy of an enlarged lymph node. It is not uncommon, however, for the first biopsy to come from the skin, tonsils, soft-tissues, or stomach. In such cases, however, a primary extranodal NK/T-cell lymphoma is highly probable. Particular attention should be paid to the nasal type of NK/T-cell lymphoma, clinically called *lethal midline granuloma* (see Chap. 6.2.2.2).

The survival rates of our patients with pleomorphic, medium-sized cell T-cell lymphoma were clearly lower than those of with pleomorphic, small-cell-type and T-zone lymphoma, but somewhat better than those with the pleomorphic, large-cell type. Pleomorphic, medium-sized and large-cell T-cell lymphomas hence show the clinical behavior of high-grade aggressive lymphoma.

Addendum: Nodal Peripheral Cytotoxic NK/T-Cell Lymphoma, Nasal Type

Synonyms

- Kiel: Not listed
- REAL: Not listed
- WHO: Not listed

Definition

This type of lymphoma consists mostly of medium sized or large pleomorphic T-cells with an admixture of inflammatory cells and focal necrosis. Angiocentrism and angiodestruction may be found. Immunohistochemical detection of the cytotoxic granules T-cell-restricted intracellular antigen-1 (TIA1) and/or granzyme B is essential for the diagnosis (Jaffe 1996).

Morphology

Almost all of these rare tumors are characterized by tumor cells which exhibit a marked nuclear pleomorphism of medium-sized and large cells. The lymph node is diffusely infiltrated by tumor cells and shows a complete effacement of its architecture. Intermingled with the tumor cells are reactive histiocytes, which sometimes show hemophagocytosis. Small lymphocytes can also be intermingled. Eosinophilic granulocytes are rare, as are plasma cells. A focal necrosis and many apoptotic cells are frequently found. Angiocentrism and angiodestruction can be detected in some cases (Figs. 5.40, 5.41). Touch imprints exhibit numerous tumor cells with azurophilic granules (Jaffe et al. 1996).

In general, the cellular composition points to a T-cell lymphoma. The focal necrosis may further indicate a NK/T-cell origin. This morphological picture makes it always necessary to exclude a primary extranodal NK/T-cell lymphoma with secondary lymph node involvement.

Immunohistochemistry

The phenotype is similar to that of the extranodal NK/T-cell lymphomas(see Chap. 6.2.2.2). Mostly the tumor cells express CD2. They are TIA1-positive and less frequently granzyme-B-positive. CD3 is variable, CD8 is more frequently found than CD4. Some tumors have a NK-cell phenotype (CD56+).

The majority of tumors stain positive for late membrane protein (LMP).

Genetic Features

In these rare lymphomas, no specific chromosomal abnormalities are described.

True NK-cell lymphomas have their TCR gene in a germline configuration; thus, they are CD3-negative. All other tumors are TCR-γ-chain rearrangement.

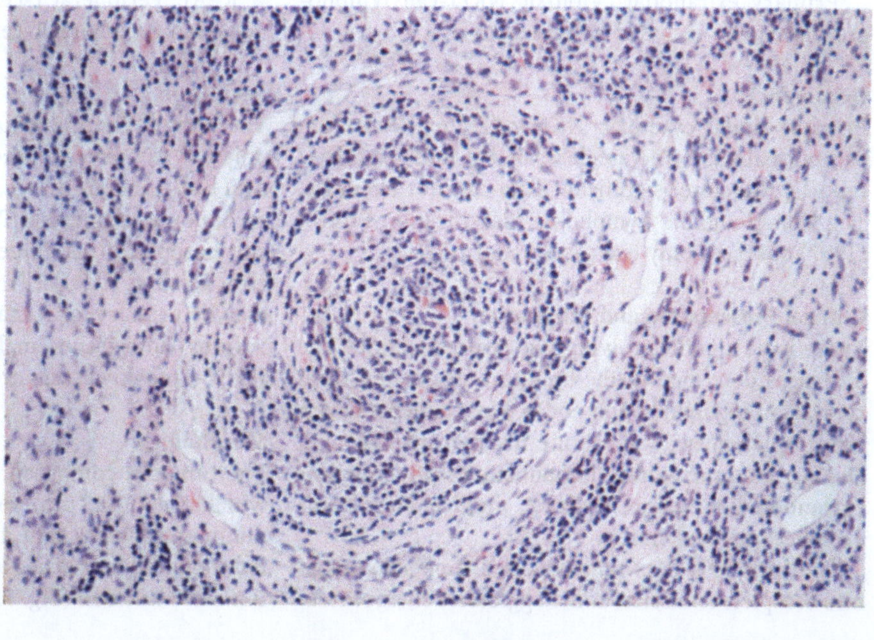

Fig. 5.40. Nodal peripheral NK-/T-cell lymphoma, nasal type. There is marked angiocentricity and angiodestruction (H and E stain)

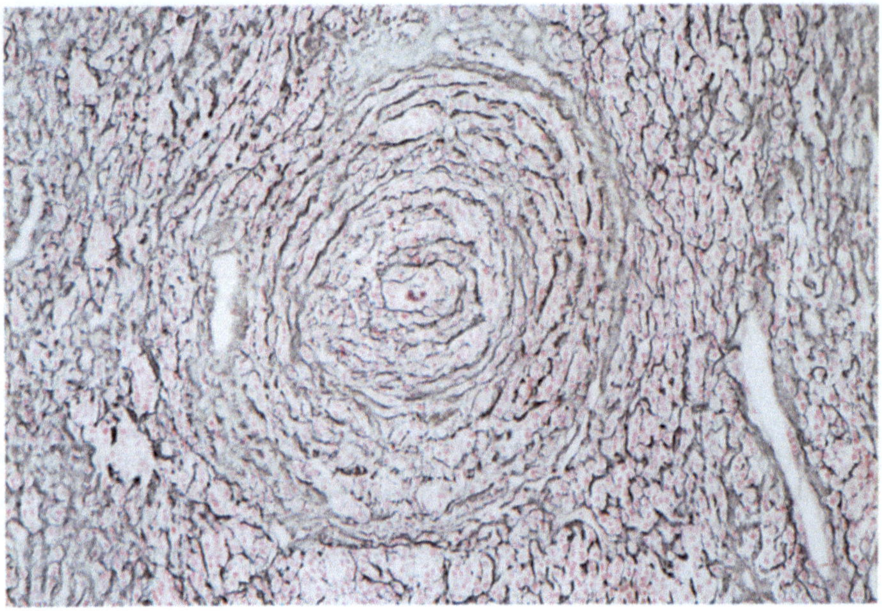

Fig. 5.41. Same view as Fig. 5.40. Silver impregnation

Differential Diagnosis

Morphologically, this type of lymphoma is indistinguishable from other peripheral T-cell lymphomas, unspecified, and specifically, the pleomorphic subtype. The detection of small foci of necrosis and many apoptotic cells may indicate a cytotoxic origin. The staining for cytotoxic granules (TIA1 and/or granzyme B) is decisive.

Primary extranodal cytotoxic NK/T-cell lymphomas have to be excluded by clinical data.

Occurrence

Primary nodal cytotoxic NK/T-cell lymphomas are exceptionally rare and are described as individual case reports; therefore, significant data are not available. The Non-Hodgkin's Lymphoma Classification Project (1997) observed only two cases out of 1,378.

Clinical Presentation and Prognosis

There is no significant lymph node predilection. The few cases described in the literature originated from cervical or inguinal lymph nodes. Most patients have a hepatosplenomegaly and bone marrow involvement. During its course, this lymphoma mostly involves extranodal sites (skin, GI-tract, gingiva, tonsils) or even becomes leukemic.

The prognosis is extremely poor. Patients do not go into complete remission under aggressive chemotherapy. Almost all patients die within 2–12 months (Takeshita et al. 1996; Ohshima et al. 1999).

5.2.2.2.2
Immunoblastic Lymphoma of T-Cell Type

Synonyms

- Kiel: Immunoblastic lymphoma of T-cell type
- REAL: Peripheral T-cell lymphoma, unspecified
- WHO: Peripheral T-cell lymphoma, unspecified

Definition

The term "T-immunoblastic lymphoma" is applied only to a tumor composed of large cells with round or oval nuclei and one large, solitary nucleolus or several medium-sized nucleoli. The cytoplasm is either markedly basophilic (dark blue), weakly basophilic (gray) or clear as water (clear cell). T-immunoblastic lymphoma may be primary, or it may develop secondarily out of various low-grade malignant T-cell lymphomas. HTLV-1-positive cases are found in endemic regions.

Morphology

The tumor is composed of fairly uniform, large cells with large (10–12 μm), round or oval nuclei. The chromatin is coarse. Usually, only one large, solitary nucleolus is found, but occasionally there are several medium-sized nucleoli (Fig. 5.42). The cytoplasm varies in

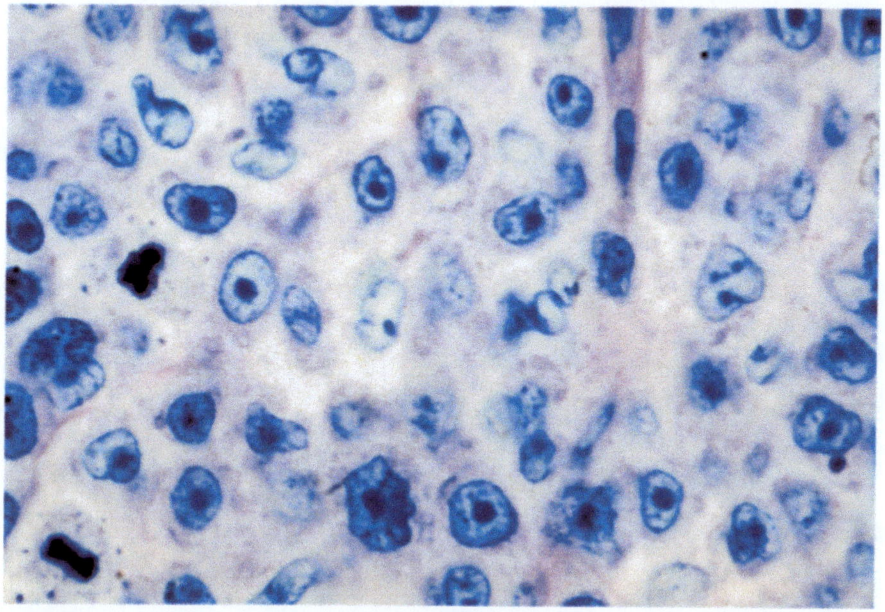

Fig. 5.42. Cytological variants of peripheral T-cell lymphoma, unspecified, immunoblastic type. Some immunoblasts show nuclear pleomorphism (Giemsa stain)

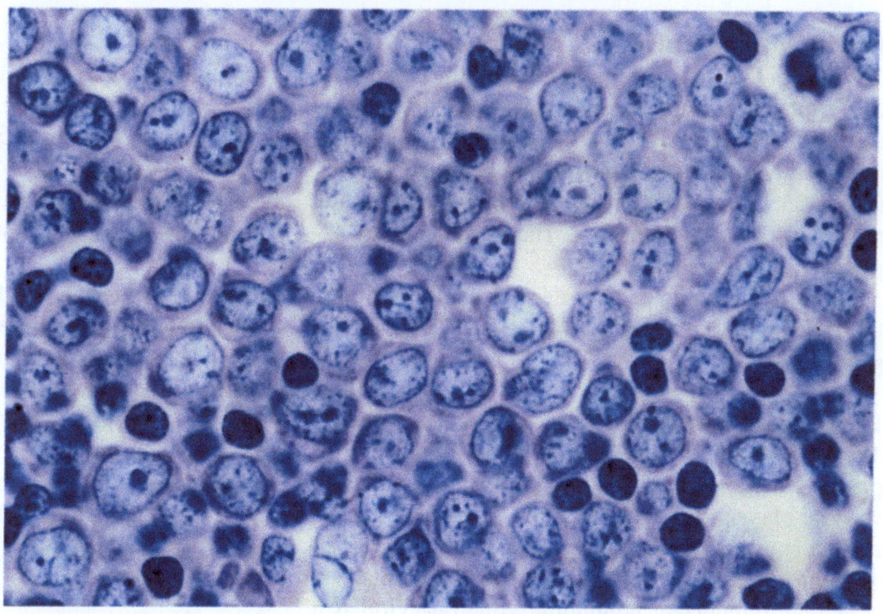

Fig. 5.43. Cytological variants of peripheral T-cell lymphoma, unspecified, immunoblastic type. Some cells resemble centroblasts with basophilic cytoplasm (Giemsa stain)

appearance: (1) It may be scanty to moderately abundant and markedly basophilic, i.e. dark blue with Giemsa staining; (2) it may be moderately abundant and gray (such tumors are sometimes CD8+, sometimes HTLV-1+; Fig. 5.43); (3) it may be abundant and clear as water (Fig. 5.44) Giant cells are rare. Sometimes the tumor cells are interspersed with eosinophils, which occasionally occur in large numbers. Mast cells are found now and again. The number of interdigitating cells is quite large in a few cases. Macrophages sometimes occur in large numbers. Clusters of epithelioid cells are seen occasionally. Mitotic activity is high. The venules do not stand out; they have flat endothelial cells and are often incompletely developed.

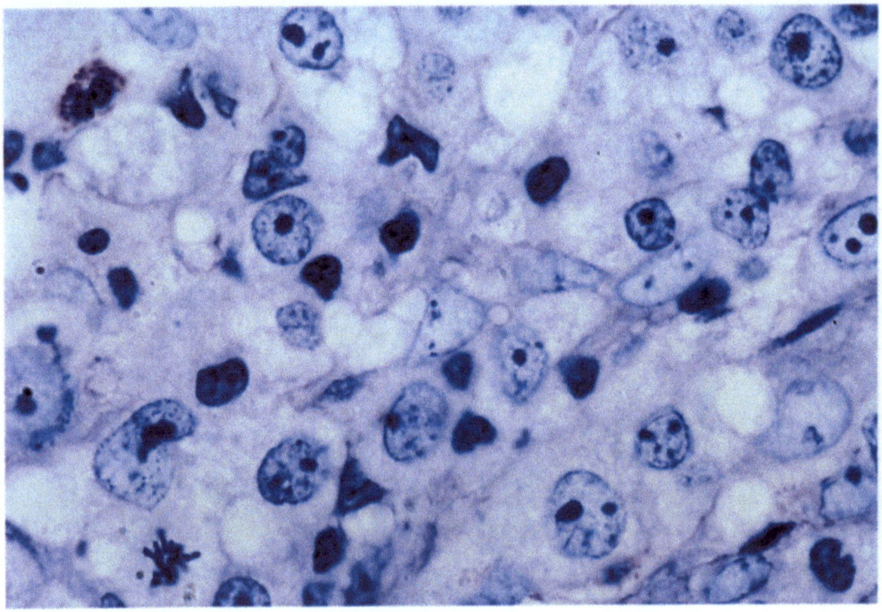

Fig. 5.44. Cytological variants of peripheral T-cell lymphoma, unspecified immunoblastic type. Cells with immunoblastic nuclei and abundant clear cytoplasm (Giemsa stain)

Immunohistochemistry

The cells of this type of lymphoma show the phenotype of peripheral T-cells. In most cases, the tumor cells express CD4, rarely CD8, but never both. T-immunoblastic lymphoma shows a partial loss of antigens (CD2, CD3, CD5, CD4 or CD8) more often than do low-grade malignant T-cell lymphomas. The number of Ki 67-positive cells is higher than 50%.

As in other types of peripheral T-cell lymphoma, there is rearrangement of the TCR-γ- and TCR-β-chain genes.

Differential Diagnosis

T-immunoblastic lymphoma with basophilic cytoplasm is isomorphic with B-immunoblastic lymphoma without plasmacytic differentiation. Therefore, immunohistochemical methods are necessary to identify an ambiguous case as a T-immunoblastic lymphoma.

A T-immunoblastic lymphoma with gray cytoplasm must be distinguished morphologically from anaplastic large-cell lymphoma (see Chap. 5.2.2.4); both types of lymphoma may be CD30-positive. The clear-cell type does not pose any problems in a differential diagnosis. Otherwise, the differential diagnosis must take into consideration the entire spectrum that was discussed in connection with B-immunoblastic lymphoma (see Chap. 4.2.2.3).

Occurrence

T-immunoblastic lymphoma is a rare disease. It makes up 1.1% of the cases in our collection, or 6.4% of the T-cell lymphomas. It can occur at any age except during the first decade of life. The youngest patient was 17 years old, the oldest was 83. A peak emerges in the seventh to eighth decade of life.

Clinical Presentation and Prognosis

A leukemic blood picture is frequently seen in the HTLV-1-positive type. This is uncommon in HTLV-1-negative cases. The tumor often develops in lymph nodes and not infrequently in the gastrointestinal tract, including the tonsils; it may also arise in other organs.

The prognosis for most patients with T-immunoblastic lymphoma is unfavorable, as shown by the survival curves presented by Suchi et al. (1987).

5.2.2.2.3 Lymphoepithelioid Lymphoma ("Lennert's Lymphoma")

In the course of a cytological investigation of Hodgkin's disease and Piringer's lymphadenitis in 1952, Lennert noticed three cases in which small focal accumulations of epithelioid cells completely destroyed the lymph node architecture and the patients died within a relatively short time. The author considered the disease to be a variant of Hodgkin's lymphoma and called it "epithelioid cellular lymphogranulomatosis" (ECLg).

In 1968, Lennert and Mestdagh studied a larger series of cases and distinguished ECLg from *Hodgkin's lymphoma with a high content of epithelioid cells.* ECLg usually contained no, or at most very few, Reed-Sternberg cells and showed small, focal accumulations of epithelioid cells. In contrast, Hodgkin's lymphoma, with a high content of epithelioid cells, exhibited moderate to large numbers of Reed-Sternberg cells and irregular, often diffuse epithelioid cell infiltrates.

Because of the frequent absence of typical Reed-Sternberg cells in ECLg, the interpretation of the lesion as Hodgkin's lymphoma was open to question. In 1973, the neutral term "lymphoepithelioid lymphoma" (LeL) was recommended, and the neoplasm was considered as a possible form of NHL (Lennert 1973).

Shortly thereafter, Dorfman and Warnke (1974) and Lukes and Tindle (1975) suggested the term "Lennert's lymphoma" and saw differential diagnostic problems with immunoblastic lymphadenopathy. Burke and Butler (1976) then published a report of 16 cases of LeL. Diebold et al. (1977) observed further cases in Europe. Since then, a lively discussion of this lymph node lesion has been conducted in the literature.

At the end of the 1970s, Noel et al. (1979, 1980) investigated the Kiel collection of cases. They found that LeL could be diagnosed in only 44.5% of the 114 cases that had been interpreted originally as ECLg or as suspicious for ECLg. In 31.5% of the cases, Noel considered the lesion to be a variant of lymphogranulomatosis X (LgX).

Immunohistochemical, cytogenetic, and molecular genetic findings obtained at the same time (Feller et al. 1986a; Gödde-Salz et al. 1986, O'Connor et al. 1986) proved that LeL is a T-cell lymphoma.

Patsouris et al. (1988, 1989a,b, 1990) had carried out morphological and immunological investigations of new cases of LeL. As shown in Table 5.3, they examined 367 cases in which the morphology of the tumors was similar to that in LeL. Only 30% of these tumors proved to be LeL. Almost as many (26.4%) were T-cell lymphomas of AILD (LgX) type with a high content of epithelioid cells. The third large group (27.0%) comprised cases of Hodgkin's lymphoma of mixed cellularity type with a high content of epithelioid cells. In addition, some tumors were lymphocyte-predominant Hodgkin's lymphoma, i.e. paragranuloma. Some 10% were immunocytoma with a high content of epithelioid cells.

Table 5.3. Differential diagnosis in 367 cases featuring a marked, focal epithelioid cell reaction that could either be interpreted as lymphoepithelioid lymphoma (LeL) or in which LeL was suspected (data from Patsouris et al. 1988)

Lymphoepithelioid lymphoma
Angioimmunoblastic T-cell lymphoma
Hodgkin's lymphoma, mixed cellularity
Nodular lymphocyte predominant Hodgkin's lymphoma (paragranuloma)
Immunocytoma
Other B-cell lymphomas
T-cell lymphoma, unspecified
Inflammation

Today we think that lymphoepithelioid Lymphoma (Lennert's lymphoma) is a very rare disease. Most of the cases are angioimmunoblastic T-cell lymphomas with a marked epithelioid cell reaction or Hodgkin's lymphomas.

Synonyms

- Kiel: Lymphoepithelioid lymphoma (Lennert's lymphoma)
- REAL: Lennert's lymphoma (provisional type)
- WHO: Peripheral T-cell lymphoma, unspecified

Definition

LeL is characterized by a focal epithelioid cell reaction. It consists chiefly of T-lymphocytes and always contains at least a few T-immunoblasts with occasional atypical large cells. There is no marked pleomorphism of the tumor cells! Typical Reed-Sternberg cells occur only exceptionally if at all. No extended network of follicular dendritic cells is found by immunohistochemistry.

Morphology

The normal structure of the lymph node is replaced by a neoplasm, which, at a low magnification, resembles Hodgkin's lymphoma more than it resembles NHL. Germinal centers or remnants of germinal centers are found only rarely. The lymph node capsule and surrounding tissue are infiltrated focally (57%), diffusely (23%), or not at all (20%).

The neoplasm consists especially of lymphocytes and epithelioid cells. The lymphocytes have round or somewhat pleomorphic nuclei (Fig. 5.45). A few LeLs show lymphocytes with abundant, pale cytoplasm (clear cells) (differential diagnosis: angioimmunoblastic T-cell lymphoma)

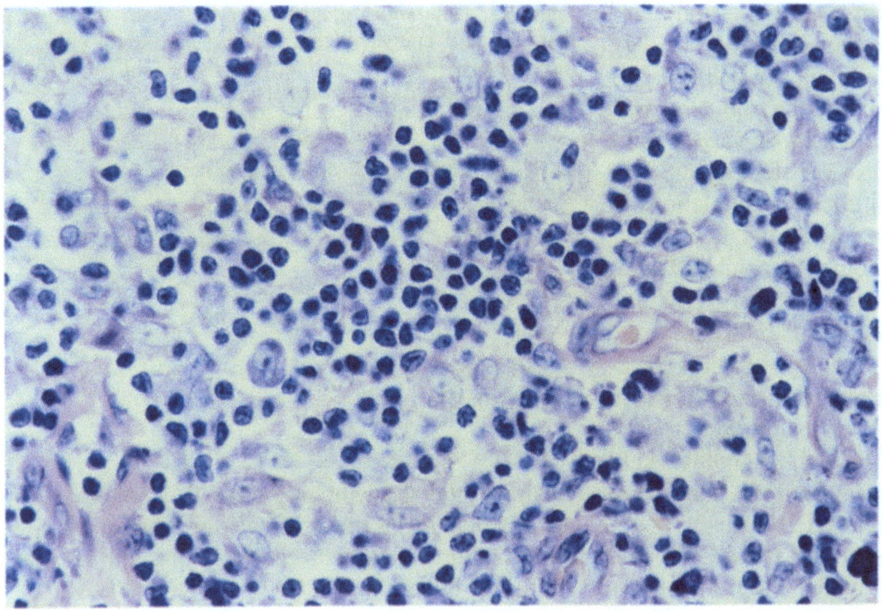

Fig. 5.45. Peripheral T-cell lymphoma, variant Lennert's lymphoma. Note the small, slightly pleomorphic lymphocytes. Blasts and epithelioid cells can also be seen (Giemsa stain)

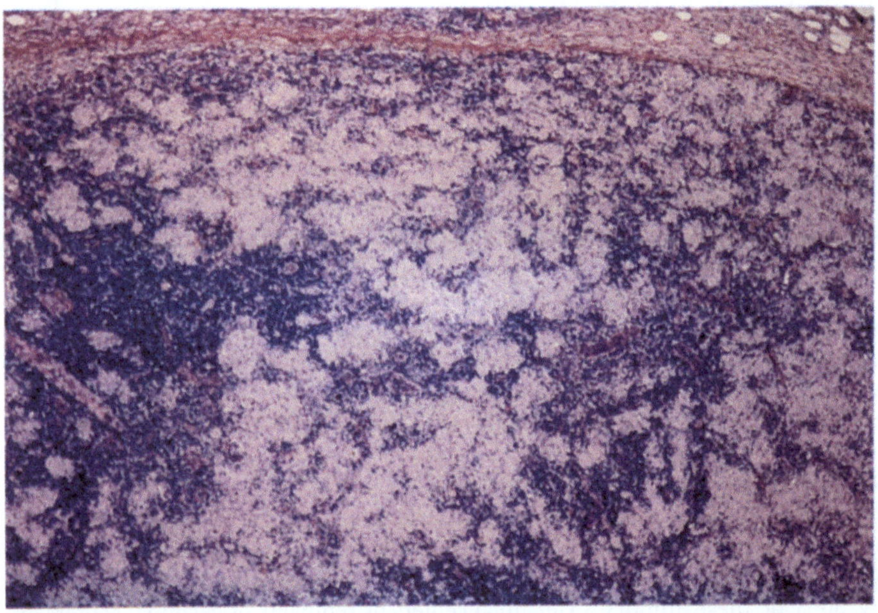

Fig. 5.46. Peripheral T-cell lymphoma, unspecified, variant Lennert's lymphoma. Small clusters of epithelioid cells are intermingled with mostly small lymphocytes, which have only slight nuclear irregularities (H and E stain)

The lymphocytes are interspersed with medium-sized lymphoid cells with round, pale nuclei, small nucleoli and scanty, weakly basophilic cytoplasm. There are also typical immunoblasts with large, solitary nucleoli and basophilic cytoplasm. These may be interpreted as T-immunoblasts, although they cannot be distinguished from B immunoblasts by morphology alone. Mitotic figures are usually sparse, but in some tumors there is moderate mitotic, or even high mitotic activity.

The epithelioid cells mostly accumulate in small foci, as in Piringer's lymphadenitis (toxoplasmosis) (Figs. 5.46, 5.47). Epithelioid cells are rarely seen in larger masses in LeL, but solitary epithelioid cells, or pairs of them, are often found among the lymphocytes. The nuclei of some epithelioid cells are oval, others are

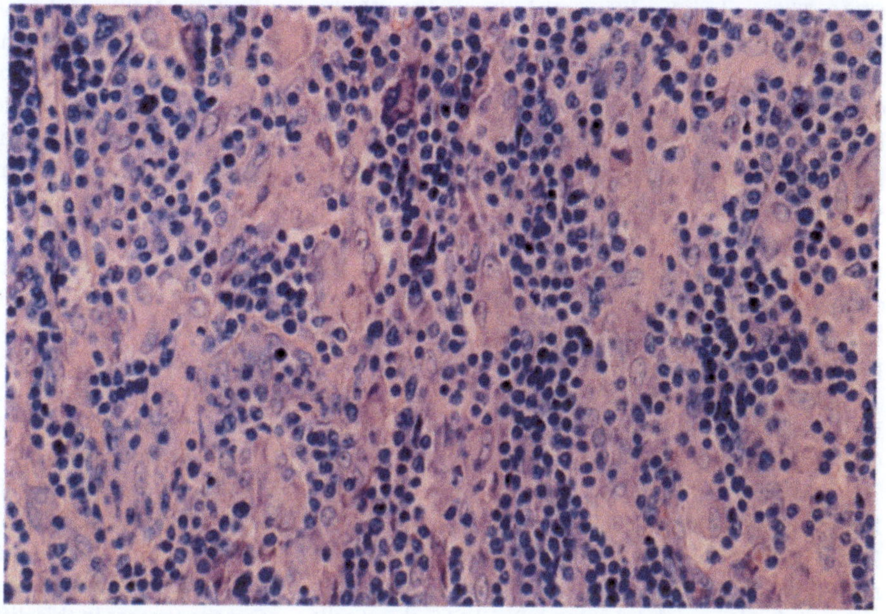

Fig. 5.47. High-power view of Fig. 5.46 (H and E stain)

elongate and arched or bent. They contain relatively large, pale reddish violet nucleoli. The chromatin is so fine that it is barely recognizable with Giemsa staining. The cytoplasm is acidophilic, but its periphery may be basophilic (violet with Giemsa staining). The epithelioid cells exhibit considerable polymorphism and may even have giant nuclei, but they rarely show mitotic activity. They are occasionally multinucleate-like Langhans' giant cells.

Besides lymphocytes and epithelioid cells, solitary, typical Reed-Sternberg cells and Hodgkin cells are seen in 2–4% of LeLs. More often, however, there are a few solitary mononuclear and multinucleate cells with a similar morphology. These cells do not correspond to classic Reed-Sternberg cells or Hodgkin cells, because their chromatin is coarser, the nucleoli are more basophilic and not as large, and the cytoplasm is more basophilic.

Plasma cells and eosinophils are usually scanty. There is hardly ever an increase in the number of neutrophil granulocytes or mast cells.

The number of epithelioid venules is modest or, at most, moderately increased. There is no significant increase in the number of fibers.

Evolution and Transformation. In 1968, Lennert and Mestdagh reported on the development of an LeL into a large-cell lymphoma. In the large series investigated by Patsouris et al. (1988), there were eight cases of large-cell T-cell lymphoma that could be classified as pleomorphic lymphoma, immunoblastic lymphoma, or anaplastic large-cell lymphoma of T-cell type. In those cases, the epithelioid cell component had almost completely disappeared. It is likely that some of these cases should not be interpreted as LeL, but rather as AIBTCL or immunocytoma with a high content of epithelioid cells. The latter two types of lymphoma can transform into B-immunoblastic lymphoma (diffuse large-B-cell lymphoma).

Immunohistochemistry

The proliferating cells (Ki-67+) have the phenotype of mature T-cells (CD2+, CD3+, CD5+). In addition, they express CD4, whereas the CD8 antigen is absent on proliferating cells (Feller et al. 1986a). However, recent publications indicate a variant in which the neoplastic cells express CD8 and are CD4-negative (Yamashita et al. 2000). Moreover, an increasing number of tumors have been described the cells of which additionally express cytotoxic granules (TIA1) (Yamashita et al. 2000).

A partial loss of antigens can occur when the lymphoma shows transformation into a high-grade malignant lymphoma.

In paraffin sections, there are relatively few plasma cells with a polytypic pattern (Patsouris et al. 1988). Giant cells corresponding or similar to Hodgkin or Reed-Sternberg cells may be positive for CD30 and

CD15. This makes the differential diagnosis to Hodgkin's disease difficult (see below).

Genetic Features

DNA analysis shows clonal rearrangement for TCR genes. Ig heavy-chain genes are in a germline configuration (compare with AIBTCL).

The cytogenetic abnormalities are almost identical to those described for AIBTCL (see Chap. 5.2.2.1). Trisomy 3 is especially frequent in LeL. Trisomy 5 is much less frequent in LeL than in AILD. Many normal metaphases are detected (Schlegelberger et al. 1994).

By PCR and in situ hybridization, the presence of EBV could be demonstrated in the majority of patients (Anagnostopoulos et al. 1994).

Diagnosis and Differential Diagnosis

LeL is characterized by a mostly focal epithelioid cell reaction against a relatively monotonous-looking lymphocytic background. In general, Reed-Sternberg cells are not found, but one or two giant cells of this type may occasionally be seen. There is no sclerosis. When the tissue specimen is skillfully embedded in a synthetic medium, the pathologist can clearly see that the neoplastic lymphocytes are larger than residual normal lymphocytes.

LeL has to be distinguished from *angioimmunoblastic T-cell lymphoma* with a high content of epithelioid cells, from *Hodgkin's lymphoma* with a high content of epithelioid cells (chiefly mixed cellularity type, sometimes paragranuloma), from very rare cases of *immunocytoma* with a high content of epithelioid cells, from other NHLs, and from focal *epithelioid cell reactions* of inflammatory type. The most important distinguishing features are summarized in Table 5.3, p. 155.

The differential diagnostic significance of *angioimmunoblastic T-cell lymphoma with a high content of epithelioid cells* (Fig. 5.48) was recognized early by Dorfman and Warnke (1974), Lukes and Tindle (1975) and Delsol et al. (1977a,b). It was confirmed by the investigations of Noel et al. (1979, 1980) and substantiated in a thorough study by Patsouris et al. (1989a).

The most important distinguishing features of AIBTCL are the cytology of the neoplastic cells, the vascularity, and the cellular background. In addition, the detection of follicular dendritic cells by immunohistochemistry is crucial. Today it has become clear that most the tumors in this differential diagnosis belong to the group of angioimmunoblastic T-cell lymphomas.

The cellular infiltrate in LeL is predominately lymphocytic and thus much less pleomorphic than in AIBTCL. Furthermore, in the latter, the vascularity is much higher in , and the vessels diffusely permeate the lymph node as well as the capsule and surrounding tissue. The vessels are largely epithelioid venules. They often have atypical features, such as sparse, flat endo-

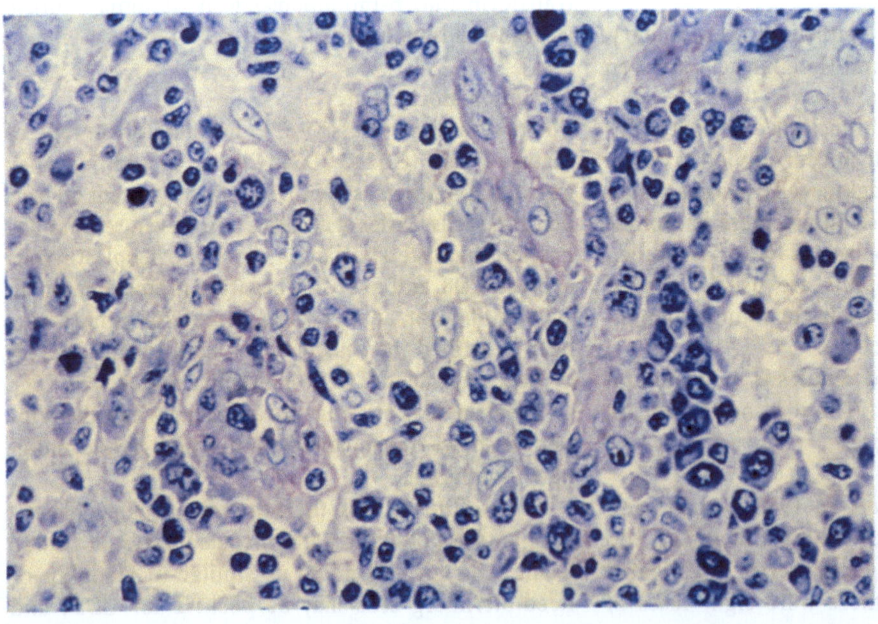

Fig. 5.48. Epithelioid-cell-rich angioimmunoblastic T-cell-lymphoma. Note the epithelioid venules and the plasmacytosis beside the lymphocytes and epithelioid cells (Giemsa stain)

thelial cells, and they are frequently branched (so-called arborizing vessels) and usually show a PAS-positive, enlarged basement membrane (see angioimmunoblastic T-cell lymphoma, Chap. 5.2.2.1). Amorphic PAS-positive material between the cells is found in about one-third of the cases of the AIBTCL, but not in LeL. Sometimes one sees so-called burnt-out germinal centers in AIBTCL; these are not present in LeL (see Fig. 5.20). With immunohistochemical staining, the follicular dendritic cells stand out, as they accumulate in large groups in AIBTCL (see Fig. 5.21). The fiber content is generally much higher, but the cell density usually appears to be much lower than that of LeL. Cytological examination of the angioimmunoblastic type reveals that, on average, there is a higher content of both plasma cells (and plasma cell precursors) and eosinophils.

There are also certain clinical differences between AIBTCL and LeL (Patsouris et al. 1989a). Pruritus, skin rashes, and bacterial infections occur much more frequently in the former. Allergic or hyperimmune reactions (autoimmune diseases, including hemolytic anemia; allergies to antibiotics or chemotherapeutics) are found almost exclusively in AIBTCL. We should like to emphasize the high incidence of carcinoma before or after manifestation of AIBTCL. The age and sex distribution of the AIBTCL is almost identical with that of LeL.

In spite of the extensive morphological and clinical differential diagnostic criteria, there are still a small number of cases that can be assigned to one of the two categories only with difficulty. This shows how closely related these two types of T-cell lymphoma are (see Cytogenetics).

Many years ago, Lennert (1953a, b) showed that focal epithelioid cell reactions are a characteristic early feature of *Hodgkin's lymphoma*, especially that of the mixed cellularity type. Such reactions are also frequently seen in the lymphocyte-predominant type. Such cases were called the "L and H type" by Lukes et al. (1966), whereby "H" stood for "histiocytic". Early stages of infiltration in Hodgkin's lymphoma of mixed cellularity type can usually be diagnosed correctly because the epithelioid cell reaction develops in the T-regions and is accompanied by a few typical Reed-Sternberg cells. Large preserved areas of the lymph node, including lymph follicles, with or without germinal centers, are still recognizable at this stage.

In contrast to LeL, epithelioid-cell-rich Hodgkin's lymphoma (mixed cellularity) always shows *numerous* typical Reed-Sternberg cells among the predominant epithelioid cells and the less prominent lymphocytes. It occasionally occurs in younger patients, but shows the same peak, in the seventh decade of life, as LeL. There is no significant difference in the sex ratio.

In nodular lymphocyte-predominant Hodgkin's lymphoma – nodular paragranuloma (Poppema et al. 1979; Lennert and Hansmann 1987) – epithelioid cells may be seen in small foci, or they may be interspersed among the lymphocytes. In nodular paragranuloma, the epithelioid cells are frequently arranged like a wreath around the nodules. Moreover, the nodularity can help the pathologist to make the correct diagnosis, since it is almost always recognizable in at least part of the lymph node; silver impregnation is especially helpful. In contrast to LeL, paragranuloma shows predominantly IgD-positive B-lymphocytes and a few giant cells of the L and H type.

Immunocytoma is one type of NHL that can be associated with a pronounced focal epithelioid cell reaction. The areas between the epithelioid cell foci contain B-lymphocytes with round nuclei *and* lymphoplasmacytoid cells or plasma cells, a few immunoblasts and centroblasts.

The most important type of *lymphadenitis* with focal epithelioid cell reactions is Piringer's lymphadenitis. This is usually the lymph node lesion seen in toxoplasmosis, but it may also occur in chronic infectious mononucleosis, leishmaniasis and brucellosis. The lymph node architecture is preserved, the follicles contain florid germinal centers, the sinuses show a sinusoidal B-cell reaction (De Almeida et al. 1984; Sheibani et al. 1984; Stein et al. 1984; van den Oord et al. 1985), and the pulp exhibits a polymorphic hyperplasia. The focal epithelioid cell reactions are seen in the pulp and in *germinal centers*. The small foci are irregularly distributed in the lymph node and are often confined to circumscribed areas of the cortex.

Another type of lymphadenitis with focal epithelioid cell reactions is seen in syphilis in stages I and II. Lymph nodes with this lesion show a toxoplasmosis-like picture and vasculitis in the septa, capsule and surrounding tissue.

Chronic miliary tuberculosis should also be considered in the differential diagnosis. The groups of epithelioid cells are somewhat larger than those found in LeL.

Finally, there were two cases in which LeL was diagnosed, but electron microscopy subsequently revealed rod-shaped bacteria, which in one case were probably pathogens of *Whipple's disease* (Kaiserling et al. 1989).

This discussion of the differential diagnosis would not be complete without noting that there will always be a few cases that cannot be identified with good morphological techniques alone. Depending on the differential diagnostic question, immunohistochemical analyses of fresh tissue, bacteriological analyses, and/or molecular genetic studies are advisable in such cases.

Occurrence

LeL is a very rare disease. It was overdiagnosed in the past especially in the differential diagnosis of AIBTCL. LeL made up 1.4% of the NHLs in the Kiel collection, which is definitely selected. Lukes et al. (1978) found six cases among 425 cases of NHL.

The GELA group identified four patients out of 288 (4%) (Gisselbrecht et al. 1998). The Non-Hodgkin's Lymphoma Study group found a similar percentage (two patients out of 96 with T-cell lymphomas)

The tumor is found chiefly in elderly patients; the age curve shows a peak between the sixth and eighth decades. There is a slight male preponderance.

Clinical Presentation and Prognosis

This discussion is based on data published by Noel et al. (1979) and Patsouris et al. (1989a,b, 1990). Generalized lymphadenopathy is found more often than localized lymphadenopathy at the time of the first clinical examination. When lymph node enlargement is localized, it is usually seen in the cervical region. Splenomegaly was reported in 43% of the patients in the Kiel series and hepatomegaly in 23%. In some cases the palatine tonsils were enlarged and infiltrated at the onset of the disease. Fever was observed in about 50% of our patients and pruritus in 18%. In contrast to patients with AILD, only 7% of those with LeL showed a skin rash. Spontaneous remission occurred in 14% of the patients.

Blood counts frequently reveal lymphopenia and, occasionally, eosinophilia or monocytosis (up to 29%). Some other clinical findings are listed in Table 5.4.

The life expectancy of the patients with LeL in the Kiel collection was relatively short. Patients presenting in stages I or II survived a median of 18 months, those in stages III or IV only 11 months (Patsouris et al. 1993). In some cases, this poorer prognosis was definitely a result of insufficiently aggressive treatment. More than 15 years ago, some of these patients were treated according to an unsuitable protocol for Hodgkin's lymphoma. If one were to treat the patients more aggressively with chemotherapy from the very beginning, better results, similar to those reported by Suchi et al. (1987), might be achieved.

5.2.2.2.4
T-Zone Lymphoma

Synonyms

- Kiel: T-zone lymphoma
- REAL: Peripheral T-cell lymphoma, unspecified
- WHO: Peripheral T-cell lymphoma, unspecified

Definition

This extremely rare lymphoma type develops in the T-zones and contains all the components of the T-zones of lymphoid tissue (analogous to follicular lymphoma,

	LeL ($n=108$) (%)	AIBTCL ($n=98$) (%)	Hodgkin's lymphoma mc ($n=99$) (%)	Immunocytoma (MALT)[a] ($n=39$) (%)
Generalized lymphadenopathy	71	84	57	73
B symptoms (Ann Arbor)	60	67	52	65
Pruritus	18	**46**	12	17
Skin rash	7	**38**	3	9
Hemolytic anemia	–	18	–	14
Sjögren's syndrome	–	–	–	31
Other autoimmune diseases	2	16	3	15
Allergies to antibiotics	5	**24**	3	4
Paraproteinemia	–	–	–	**38**
Bence-Jones proteinuria	–	–	–	**25**

[a] These data indicate that today many immunocytomas would be classified as marginal zone lymphomas

Table 5.4. Clinical features of lymphoepithelioid lymphoma (LeL) and other lymphomas with a high content of epithelioid cells (data from Patsouris et al. 1988, 1989a, b, 1990). The important differences in frequency are marked in *bold*. *LEL* Lennert's lymphoma, *AIBTCL* Angioimmunoblastic T-cell lymphoma, *mc* mixed cellularity

which contains all the components of the B-zones), i.e. T-lymphocytes, interdigitating cells, and epithelioid venules. The neoplastic T-zones are accompanied for some time by non-neoplastic B-zones (follicles with or without germinal centers). Eventually, however, the tumor loses its zonal arrangement and shows a completely diffuse pattern, although it is composed of the same tissue elements. Most of the *tumor cells are small and monomorphic or slightly pleomorphic*. There are *always* some large, transformed cells (T-immunoblasts), and clear cells are often found.

Morphology

T-zone lymphoma is characterized by a dominant proliferation of T-lymphocytes interspersed with a variable number of T-immunoblasts and all transitional forms between the two. The nuclei of the lymphocytes are usually quite monomorphic, but occasionally slightly pleomorphic, and have small nucleoli. Cytoplasm is scanty and appears pale gray with Giemsa staining (Fig. 5.49). Sometimes there are focal or larger areas of clear cells. The T-immunoblasts are usually not as basophilic as B-immunoblasts, and they show moderately abundant, gray cytoplasm. The nucleoli of T-immunoblasts are also not as basophilic as those of B-immunoblasts, but they are central, solitary and large. In addition, there are a few interdigitating cells with crumpled-looking nuclei. Foci of so-called plasmacytoid monocytes are seen occasionally. All T-zone lymphomas show a markedly increased number of *typical* epithelioid venules. Some eosinophils and a few plasma cells are often present. Occasionally, one finds mononuclear and multinucleate giant cells that may resemble Reed-Sternberg cells.

At first, the areas between the neoplastic T-zones contain relatively well-preserved (non-neoplastic) follicles with or without germinal centers (Fig. 5.50). With ongoing disease, however, the follicles begin to disappear, and eventually the whole lymph node is taken over by the T-zone neoplasm.

As the disease progresses, the tumor cells usually become larger and more anaplastic. Eventually, a tumor composed of large, uniform-appearing blast cells (T-immunoblasts) may develop.

Recently some T-zone lymphomas with a perifollicular or paracortical nodular growth pattern have been described (Rüdiger et al. 2000; Macon et al. 1995). So far they have been designated as peripheral T-cell lymphomas, unspecified. Whether they belong to the group of T-zone lymphoma is not yet clear.

Immunohistochemistry

The tumor cells have the phenotype of mature T cells (CD2+, CD3+, CD5+). Proliferating cells (Ki-67+) simultaneously express CD4. However, there are also some CD8-positive cells that evidently represent pre-

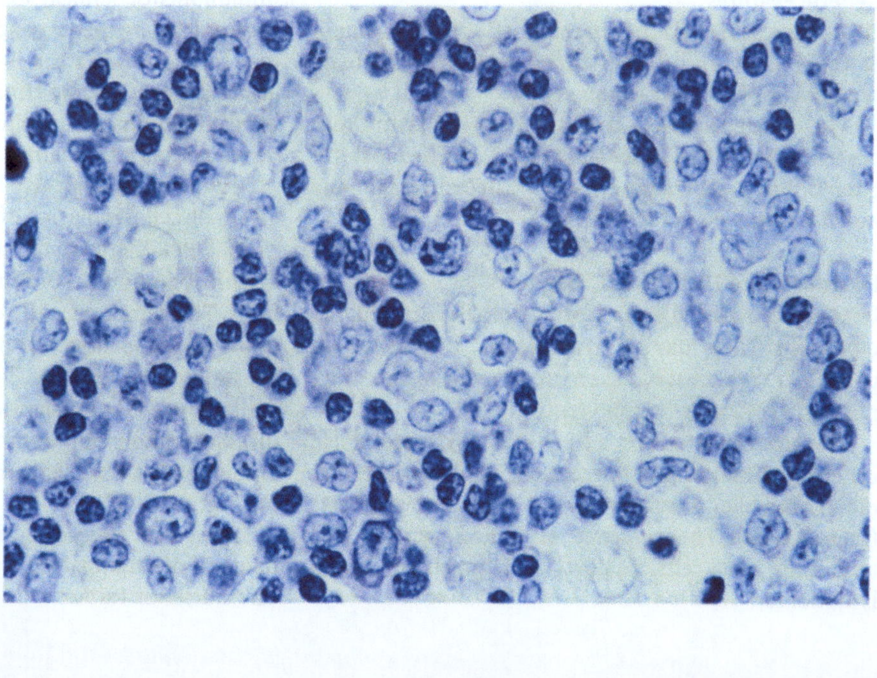

Fig. 5.49. Peripheral T-cell lymphoma, unspecified, variant T-zone-lymphoma. This type is dominated by small lymphocytes with a few blasts and histiocytes (Giemsa stain)

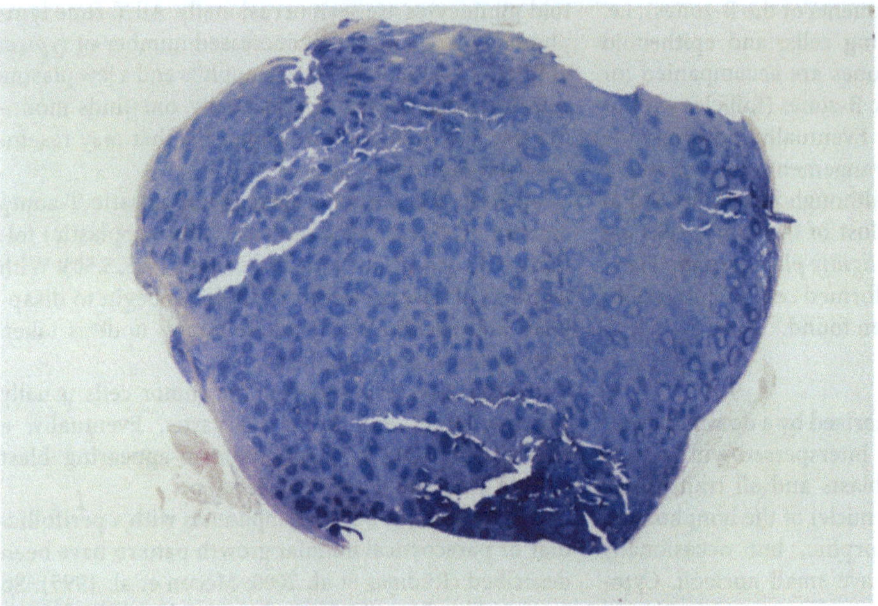

Fig. 5.50. Lymph node section (Giemsa stain) from a peripheral T-cell lymphoma, unspecified, variant T-zone-lymphoma. Note the follicular hyperplasia. The neoplastic infiltrate shows a typical interfollicular ("T-zone") growth pattern (Giemsa stain)

existent T-cells and probably do not belong to the tumor cell clone. In addition, there are a variable number of polyclonal B-cells and well-defined nodular networks of follicular dendritic cells within the B-cell follicles. An increased number of CD1a- or S100-positive interdigitating cells are seen within the T-cell infiltrates.

Genetic Features

DNA analysis reveals the characteristic rearrangement of the TCR-γ- and TCR-β-chain genes and no rearrangement of Ig heavy-chain genes.

The cytogenetic abnormalities are similar to those described for AIBTCL (see Chap. 5.2.2.1). The most frequent finding is a trisomy 3 and the detection of many normal metaphases (Schlegelberger et al. 1994).

Diagnosis and Differential Diagnosis

It is easy to make a diagnosis when follicles are still recognizable. They may be hyperplastic, in which case particular care must be taken not to make a false diagnosis of a follicular lymphoma.

The size of the tumor cells is a decisive cytological criterion. A majority of the cells are small (or intermediate), and they are interspersed with immunoblasts (mixed type). The presence of typical venules and numerous clear cells supports a diagnosis of T-zone lymphoma.

It is occasionally difficult to distinguish T-zone lymphoma from *early AIBTCL* when follicles are preserved or even hyperplastic. The venules have PAS-positive walls and look bizarre, i.e. they are not as well-developed as those of T-zone lymphoma. In AIBTCL, the tumor cells are more pleomorphic although small in these early infiltrates. AIBTCL usually shows a much larger number of eosinophils and plasma cells. On immunohistochemical analysis, a diagnosis of AIBTCL is supported by the presence of follicular dendritic cells that spread beyond the B-cell areas. Finally, there are also differences in the clinical picture. Patients with T-zone lymphoma do not show the hyperergic phenomena (including exanthema) that are typical of AIBTCL.

T-zone lymphoma also has to be distinguished from all small-cell neoplasms of the T-cell series:

In *T-PLL* there are numerous typical venules – as in T-zone lymphoma – but the cytology is more monotonous. The venules usually contain many leukemic lymphocytes, large numbers of which also migrate through the walls of the venules. There are hardly any blast cells, epithelioid cells or plasma cells. Either the follicles have disappeared, or only remnants of them are visible. In ambiguous cases, a leukemic blood picture is an obvious sign of T-CLL.

In *mycosis fungoides* and *Sézary's syndrome*, remnants of dermatopathic lymphadenitis are often seen. The nuclei of tumor cells are cerebriform, but this is recognizable only in sections of well-embedded tissue or on electron microscopy. The decisive findings are the clinical ones and the results of histological examination of a skin biopsy.

It is difficult and sometimes impossible to distinguish T-zone lymphoma from pleomorphic, small-cell T-cell lymphoma (almost always HTLV-1-positive), which is listed in the WHO classification as peripheral T-cell lymphoma, unspecified. When the neoplasm is associated with follicular hyperplasia, the possibility of pleomorphic, small-T-cell lymphoma can be excluded. The cytological picture is monotonous in both lymphoma variants, but the nuclei are more pleomorphic in the small-cell variant. Large blast cells hardly ever occur in the pleomorphic, small-cell type. There is also no admixture of plasma cells or epithelioid cells. The venules are not as prominent, and they are not as typical as those occurring in T-zone lymphoma.

T-zone lymphoma is misinterpreted most often as a B-cell lymphoma, i.e. *immunocytoma or marginal zone B-cell lymphoma of MALT.* In early stages of the development of immunocytoma, the pulp may be selectively infiltrated and sometimes has an increased number of venules. Seen at a low magnification, the well-preserved or hyperplastic follicles lead to the supposition of T-zone lymphoma. A close look at the tumor cells (admixture of plasma cells or lymphoplasmacytoid cells!) and an immunohistochemical analysis save the pathologist from such a misinterpretation.

Finally, we have observed a false diagnosis of T-zone lymphoma in children based on several lymph node biopsies that showed hyperplasia of relatively small cells in the pulp, including T-cells of atypical appearance and a small admixture of B-cells. The follicles had disappeared almost completely. In one patient, the lesion was actually caused by a protracted EBV infection. Another patient was recovering from Kawasaki syndrome. Such findings may also be associated with an autoimmune lymphoproliferative syndrome (ALPS) (van der Werff'ten Bosch et al. 1999).

Occurrence

T-zone lymphoma, as it is currently defined, is a very rare disease (< 1.0% of the NHLs in the collection). In the Non-Hodgkin's Lymphoma Classification Project (1997), 96 cases of peripheral T-cell lymphoma were collected without a single case of T-zone lymphoma . The same is true for the GELA study, in which not a single cases was observed among 288 cases (Gisselbrecht et al. 1998).

Patients range in age from 18 to 82 years, with a peak incidence in the seventh decade of life. The male-to-female ratio is about 1.5:1.

Clinical Presentation and Prognosis

The usual presentation is lymphadenopathy, which develops relatively quickly and tends to become generalized early in the course of the disease. There are some cases, however, in which the tumor is confined to one site for a relatively long period of time. Hepatomegaly and/or splenomegaly and involvement of the lungs are observed. Peripheral blood and bone marrow smears occasionally contain a few atypical lymphocytes, but a leukemic blood picture has seldom been observed (Helbron et al. 1979). HTLV-1 antibodies are not demonstrable.

Some authors report a poor prognosis (Siegert et al. 1994). According to data collected by Suchi et al. (1987), the survival rate of patients with T-zone lymphoma is significantly higher than that of patients with other malignant T-cell lymphomas. The survival curves from the Kiel collection also show a relatively favorable prognosis. However due o the rarity of the disease, no final judgment can be made.

5.2.2.3 Mycosis Fungoides[1]/Sézary's Syndrome Secondary to the Lymph Node[2] (ICD-O: 9700/3[1]; 9701/3[2])

Mycosis fungoides (reviews: Kerl and Kresbach 1979; Sterry 1985; Slater 1987) is a T-lymphocytic lymphoma with primary manifestation in the skin. Lymph nodes and other organs are involved only after a prolonged clinical course.

At first, lymph nodes show only dermatopathic lymphadenitis with a marked increase in the number of interdigitating cells, including Langerhans' cells, in T-regions (Fig. 5.51, 5.52). This stage does not allow an infiltrate to be diagnosed. Later, the specific cells of mycosis fungoides are also found in T-regions (Fig. 5.53); these cells are: (1) Lutzner cells, i.e. either small T-lymphocytes with cerebriform nuclei, which are not diagnostic on their own, as well as medium-sized and large cells, which are only found in mycosis fungoides and Sézary's syndrome. (2) The large cells are the so-called mycosis cells, having large, bizarre, in part heavily indented nucleoli. Mycosis cells have only

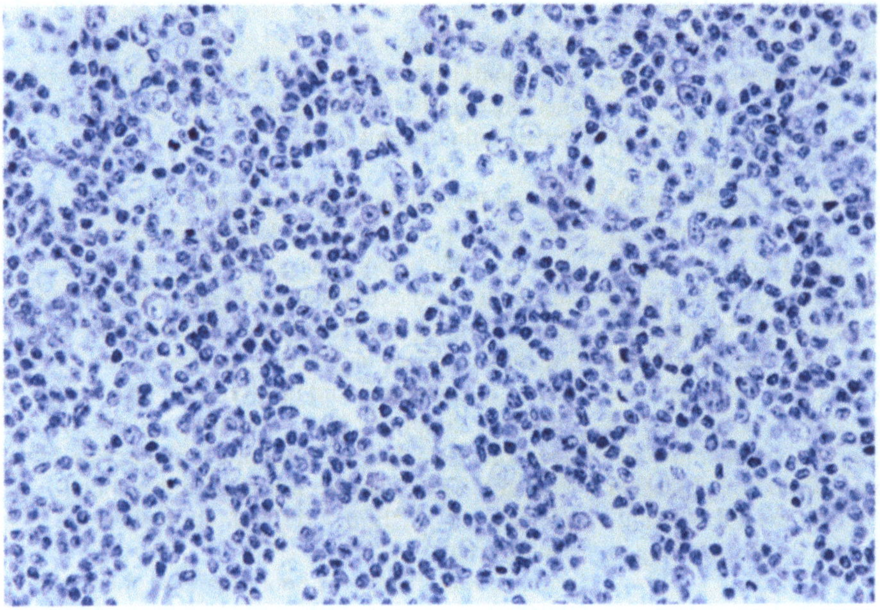

Fig. 5.51. Lymph node infiltrate in mycosis fungoides. Note the monotonous lymphocytic infiltrate intermingled with blasts and Langerhans' cells (Giemsa stain)

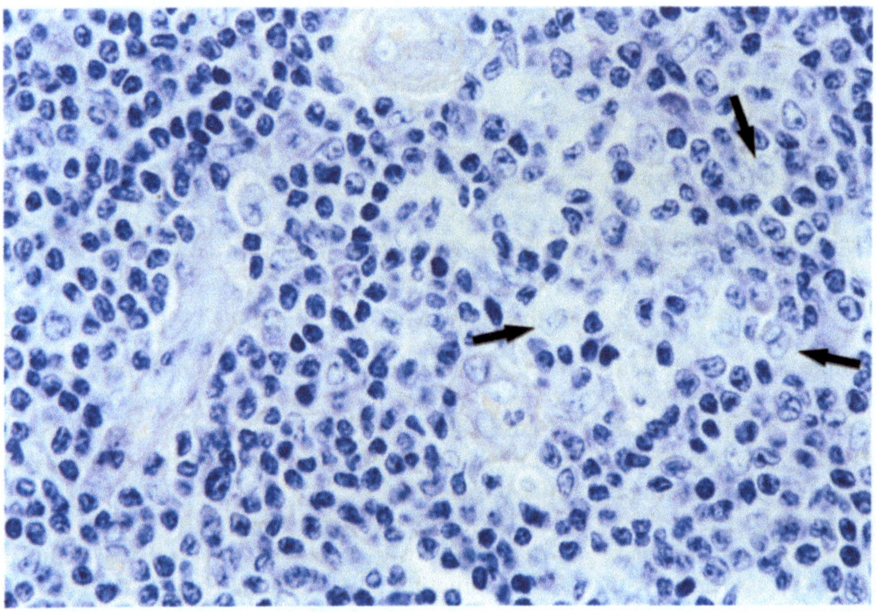

Fig. 5.52. High power view of Fig. 5.51. Note the marked nuclear pleomorphism and cerebriform nuclei. The intermingled light-appearing cells are macrophages and Langerhans' cells (→) (Giemsa stain)

a few nucleoli and slightly to intensely basophilic cytoplasm, which may be scanty or abundant. Their nucleoli are medium-sized or large, but not as large as those of typical Reed-Sternberg cells.

The infiltrate starts in the subcapsular region and interfollicular parenchyma. In general, interdigitating cells or Langerhans' cells are seen in relatively large numbers as remnants of dermatopathic lymphadenitis, even after a relatively long period of infiltration.

In the tumor phase, the tumor cells become larger, whereby all variants of malignant peripheral T-cell lymphomas may develop, i.e. medium-sized or large-cell, pleomorphic lymphoma, immunoblastic lymphoma or large-cell anaplastic lymphoma (Figs. 5.54, 5.55).

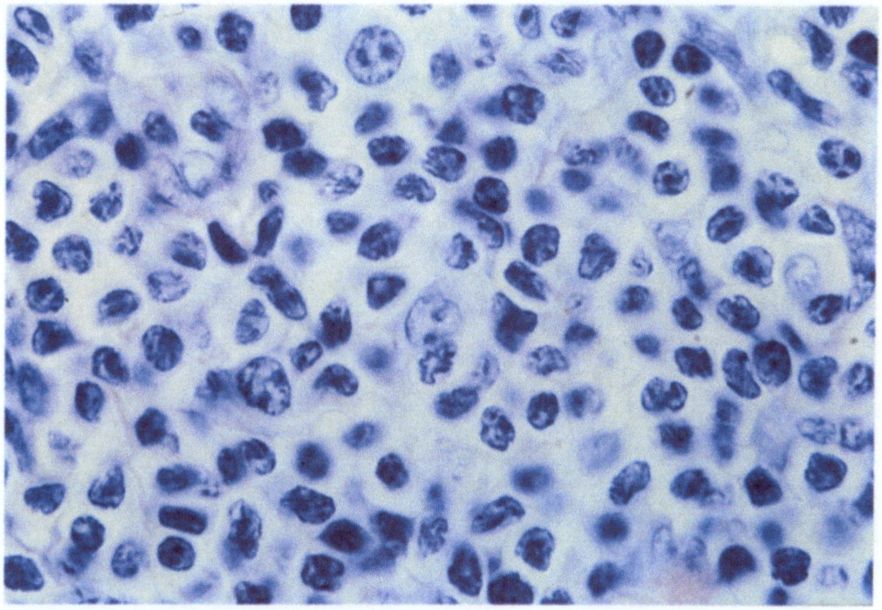

Fig. 5.53. A high-power view of Fig. 5.52. At this magnification, marked nuclear indentations are visible (Giemsa stain)

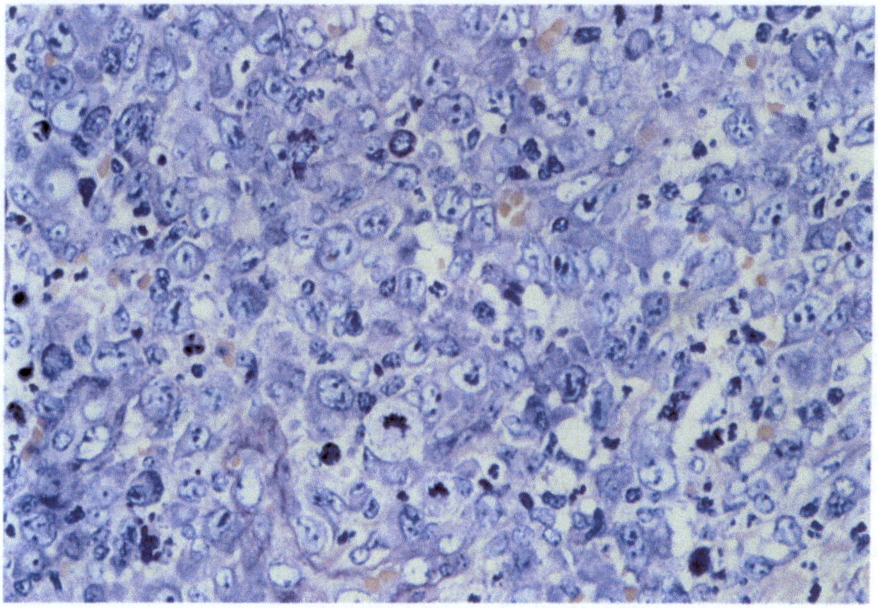

Fig. 5.54. Transformed mycosis fungoides. Note the blastic infiltrate of large, partly basophilic blasts (Giemsa stain)

In Sézary's syndrome, the skin infiltration corresponds to that of mycosis fungoides. In contrast, the lymph node is characterized by greater monotony. Evidently, a pronounced dermatopathic lymphadenitis usually does not precede the specific infiltration. Correspondingly, the T-zones are largely infiltrated by small cerebriform lymphocytes (Fig. 5.56a, b), whereas interdigitating cells are interspersed in small numbers. Since a marked increase in the number of venules is also present, the picture is reminiscent of T-CLL.

It is often extraordinarily difficult, or even impossible, to recognize infiltration of a lymph node by mycosis fungoides or Sézary's syndrome at an early stage.

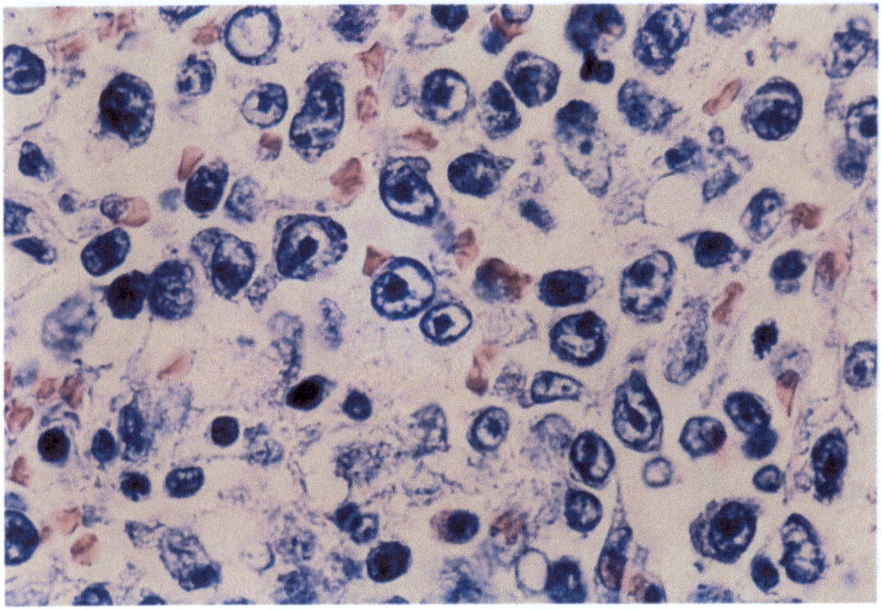

Fig. 5.55. Transformed mycosis fungoides with sheets of T-immunoblasts (Giemsa stain)

Sparse infiltrates in the large T-nodules of dermatopathic lymphadenitis are often particularly difficult to identify. Several investigators have applied quantitative methods to demonstrate neoplastic involvement of a lymph node earlier than is detectable by morphological examination. Weiss et al. (1985) analyzed DNA extracts for rearrangement of the γ-chain genes of the T-cell receptor.

Early infiltration by mycosis fungoides/Sézary's syndrome must be assumed when larger accumulations or clusters of small lymphocytes with pleomorphic nuclei are recognized histologically at the edge of T-nodules. Isolated cells with pleomorphic nuclei or abnormally large blast cells within T-nodules are not diagnostic features by themselves.

In the differential diagnosis *dermatopathic lymphadenitis, T-CLL, and peripheral T-cell lymphoma*, unspecified, pleomorphic, small-cell T-cell lymphomas have to be taken into account. The latter T cell neoplasms are more monotonous in appearance and do not show remnants of dermatopathic lymphadenitis. They also do not contain mycosis cells.

Infiltration of the lymph nodes by ATL is very much similar to the tumor stage of mycosis fungoides if it infiltrates the node. Moreover, in this stage mycosis fungoides may show giant cells that resemble Reed-Sternberg cell of *Hodgkin's lymphoma* in a background of small lymphocytes with eosinophils.

A pathologist rarely has an opportunity to examine a lymph node biopsy from a patient with mycosis fungoides or Sézary's syndrome. In 1983, 0.9% of the cases in the Kiel lymph node registry were diagnosed as mycosis fungoides or Sézary's syndrome. The patients were mostly between the ages of 50 and 90 years, and there was a slight predominance of males.

Lymph node manifestations or a tumor phase of mycosis fungoides dramatically reduces the medium survival rate to 3–6 years. The detection of a marked dermatopathic lymphadenitis already indicates progression and thus a poor prognosis, as it most probably reflects beginning progression with lymph node infiltration.

5.2.2.4 Anaplastic Large-Cell Lymphoma (T and Null Types) (ICD-O: 9714/3)

Synonyms

- Kiel: Large-cell anaplastic lymphoma of T-cell type (Ki-1)
- REAL: Anaplastic large-cell (CD30+) lymphoma (T-/null-cell type)
- WHO: Anaplastic large-cell lymphoma

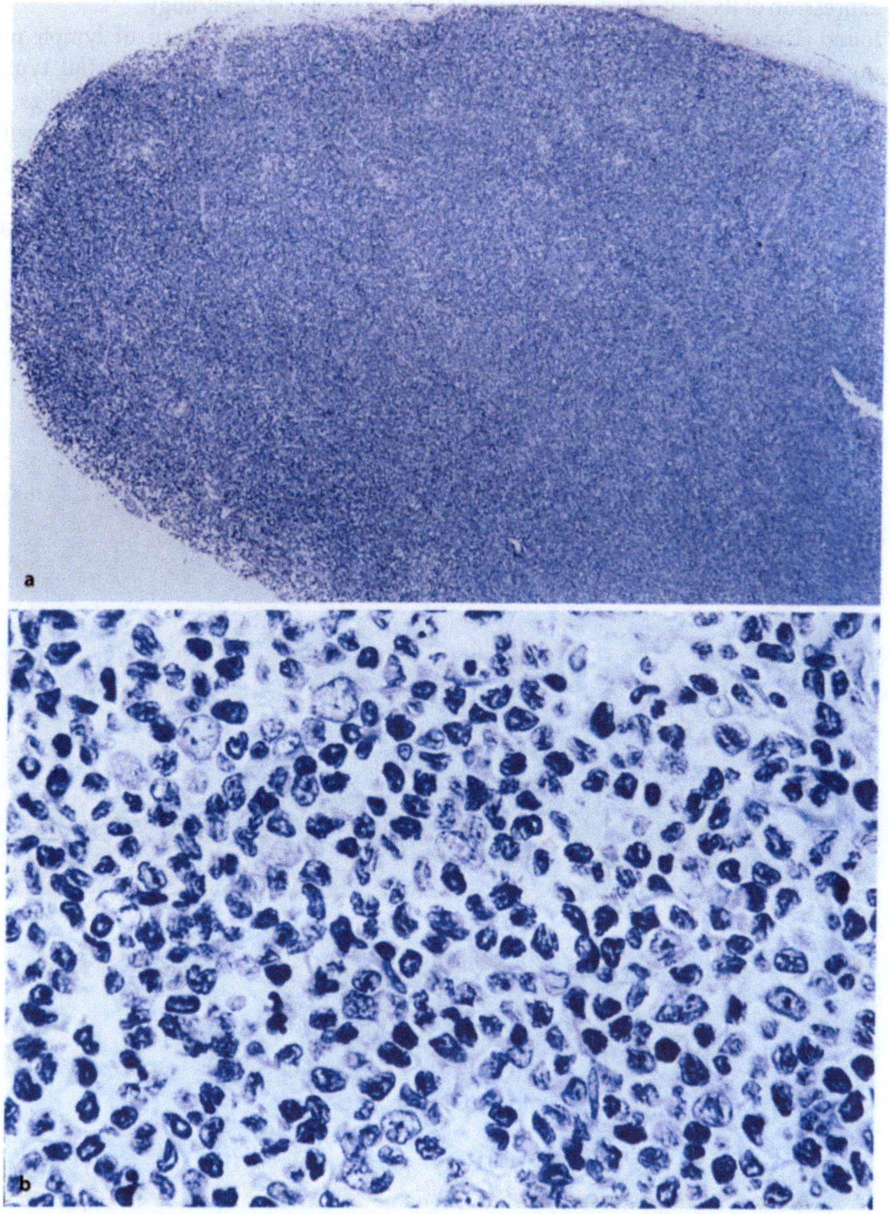

Fig. 5.56 a, b. Sézary's syndrome. Note the monotonous lymph node infiltrate. In contrast to mycosis fungoides, Langerhans' cells are absent. **a** Low-power view, **b** high-power view (Giemsa stain)

Definition

The term anaplastic large-cell lymphoma (ALCL) encompasses a heterogeneous group of subforms in terms of morphology, phenotype, cytogenetic and clinical features. ALCL was originally described as a cohesive proliferation of large pleomorphic blast cells that uniformly expressed the Ki-1/CD30 antigen and showed preferential paracortical and sinusoidal nodal involvement (Stein et al. 1985). Subsequently, the spectrum of morphological features of ALCL was broadened to include numerous morphological variants, of which the most frequent ones are the common type, the lymphohistiocytic type, and the predominant small-cell variant. In a proportion of the systemic (nodal) CD30+ ALCLs mostly affecting children and young adults, a characteristic t(2;5)(p23;q35) and expression of its related fusion protein, ALK, have been found (Drexler et al. 2000). Data accumulated indicating that ALK expression is often associated with improved clinical outcome and is thus crucial to identify favorable prognostic subsets (Gascoyne et al. 1999).

Morphology

The pattern of lymph node involvement by CD30+ ALCL may be partial, typically sinusoidal and/or paracortical, or diffuse(Figs. 5.57, 5.58). The lymphoma population exhibits a wide cytomorphological spectrum; it may be admixed with a variable number of inflammatory/reactive cells (polytypic plasma cells, eosinophil and neutrophil granulocytes). A variable

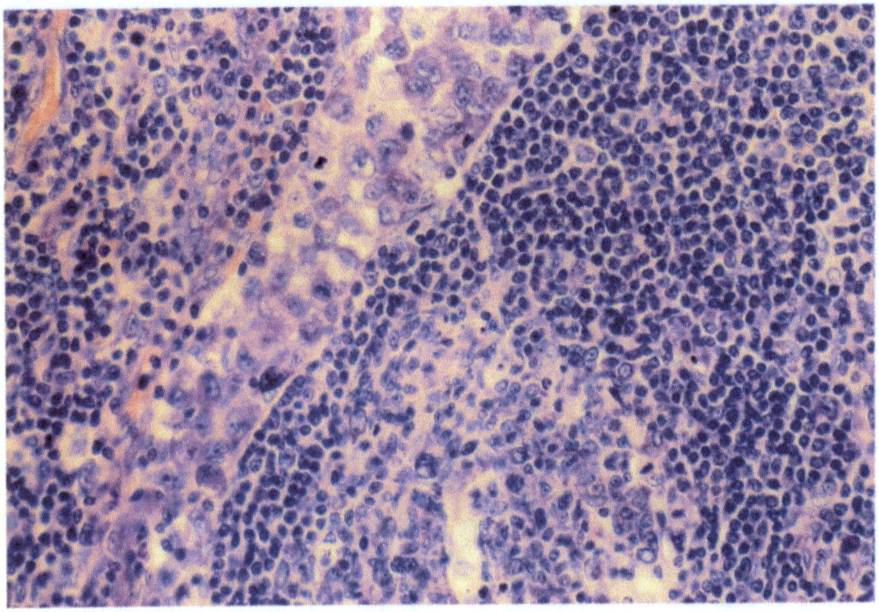

Fig. 5.57. Intrasinusoidal growth in a lymph node of an anaplastic large-cell lymphoma (Giemsa stain)

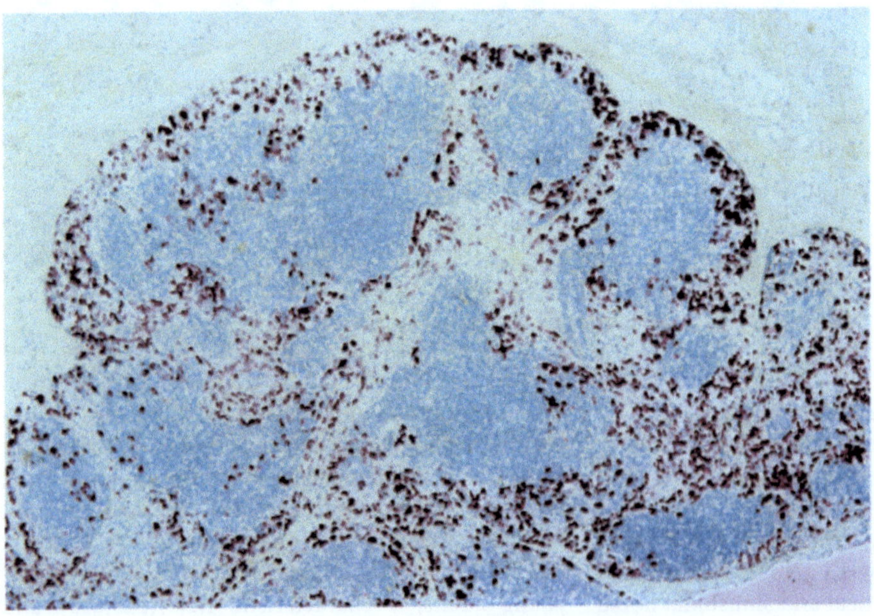

Fig. 5.58. Immunohistochemical staining for CD30 demonstrates the intrasinusoidal growth of a lymph node infiltrate of an anaplastic large-cell lymphoma (alkaline phosphatase)

amount of necrosis and fibrosis may also occur (Stein et al. 1985). The most frequent form of CD30+ALCL is the "common type", in which monomorphic and polymorphic subforms may be identified corresponding, respectively, to the cytological types I and II previously delineated by Chan et al. (1989). The monomorphic form consists of large polygonal cells with "squamoid" appearance measuring 10–30 µm in diameter, with distinct pink-stained cell membrane, pleomorphic nuclei with marked chromatin clearing, large and multiple nucleoli, and pale cytoplasm in Giemsa-stained sections (Fig. 5.59); the polymorphic form consists of round to oval cells 15–50 µm in diameter, with nuclei which are oval, lobulated, reniform or horseshoe-shaped and with multiple and prominent nucleoli (Fig. 5.60). Multinucleated wreath-like and Reed-

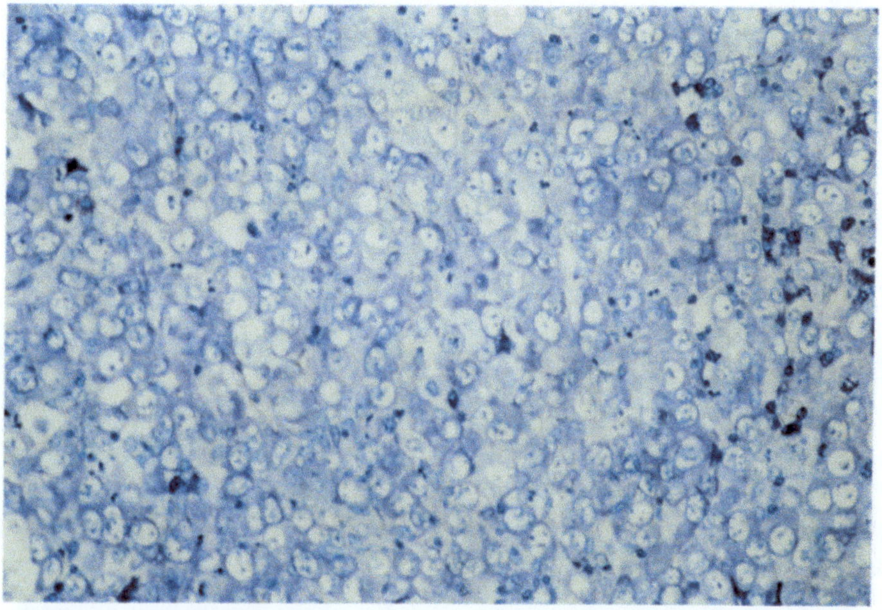

Fig. 5.59. Common type of anaplastic large-cell lymphoma. The large cells have a pale saturated cytoplasm and nuclei marked with chromatin clearing (type I) (Giemsa stain)

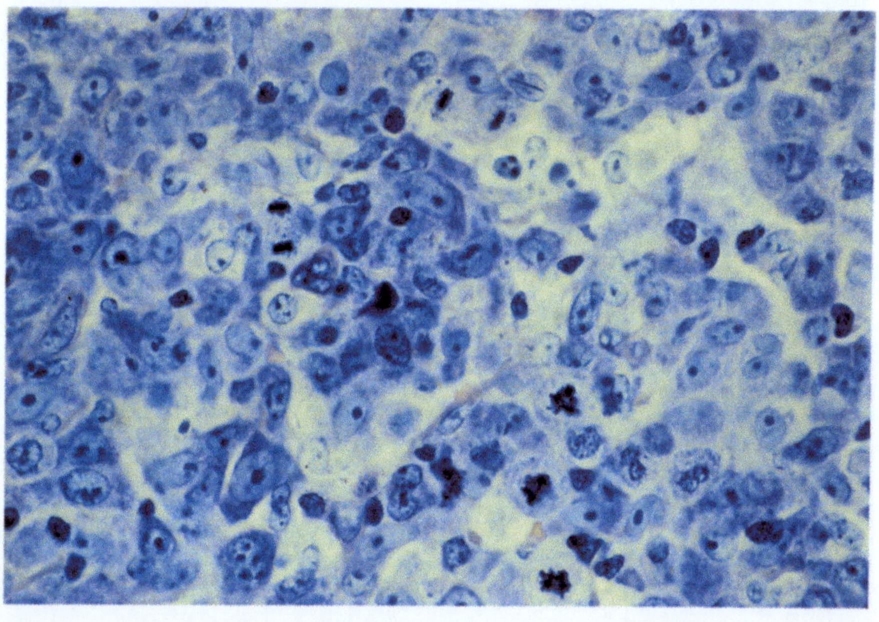

Fig. 5.60. Anaplastic large-cell lymphoma, common type, consisting mostly of round to oval cells with basophilic cytoplasm and nuclei variable in shape (type II) (Giemsa stain)

Sternberg-like cells may be observed with abundant variably basophilic cytoplasm in Giemsa-stained sections; many cells also exhibit a large pale paranuclear halo. However, the presence, of a variable admixture of monomorphic and polymorphic cells within different areas of the same tumor suggests that these two forms probably represent different morphological expressions of the same disease.

The *lymphohistiocytic variant (LH) of CD30+ ALCL*, included among the rare and ambiguous types of T-cell lymphoma in the last Kiel classification, was recognized by Pileri et al. (1990) as a peculiar histiocyte-rich form of CD30+ ALCL. It is characterized by the complete effacement of the nodal architecture by a diffuse infiltrate, composed mainly of uniform-looking histiocytes that have a broad rim of acidophilic cytoplasm

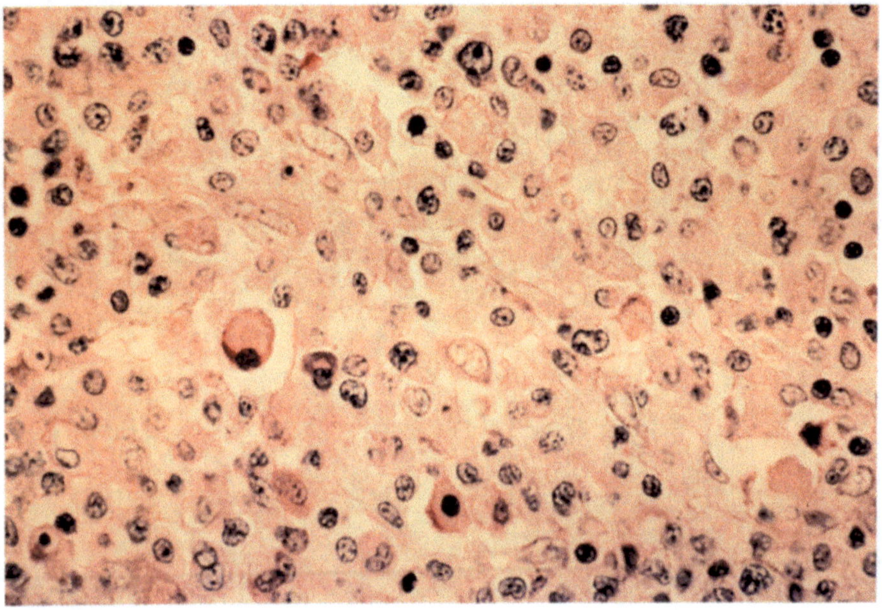

Fig. 5.61. Anaplastic large-cell lymphoma, so-called lymphohistiocytic variant. Note the small cells, histiocytes with abundant clear cytoplasm, and the presence of only a few anaplastic large cells (H and E stain)

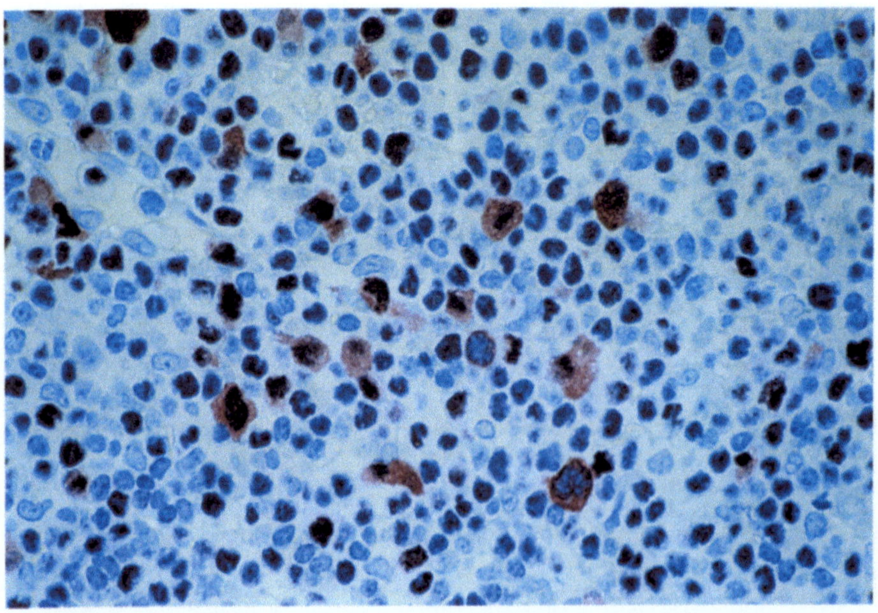

Fig. 5.62. Immunostaining for anaplastic large-cell lymphoma kinase (ALK) protein in anaplastic large-cell lymphoma, lymphohistiocytic variant. Note the mostly cytoplasmic reactivity in the large-cell component (alkaline phosphatase)

and, sometimes, a perinuclear clear-zone corresponding to the Golgi area. Among these histiocytes, a few small lymphocytes and a variable number of large cells, with typical anaplastic morphology, are present. The neoplastic cells are usually scattered among the histiocytes or arranged in clusters of a few cells but, with Giemsa staining at low power, larger foci of cohesive anaplastic cells with mitotic figures may be easily identified in most cases as dark blue areas within the pale macrophage population (Figs. 5.61, 5.62).

The *small-cell-predominant variant of ALCL*, first described by Kinney et al. (1993), contains numerous, often CD30-negative, small lymphocytes with markedly irregular, cerebriform nuclei and a minor population of large CD30+ tumor cells; the large cells are isolated or in small clusters; large tumor cells may also be found

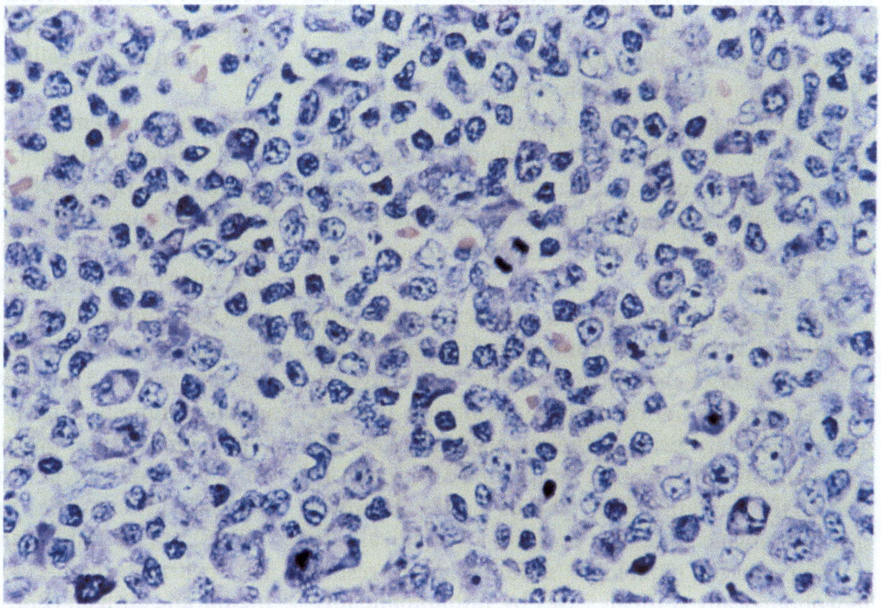

Fig. 5.63. Small-cell variant of anaplastic large-cell lymphoma. In some areas, small to medium-sized cells dominate (Giemsa stain)

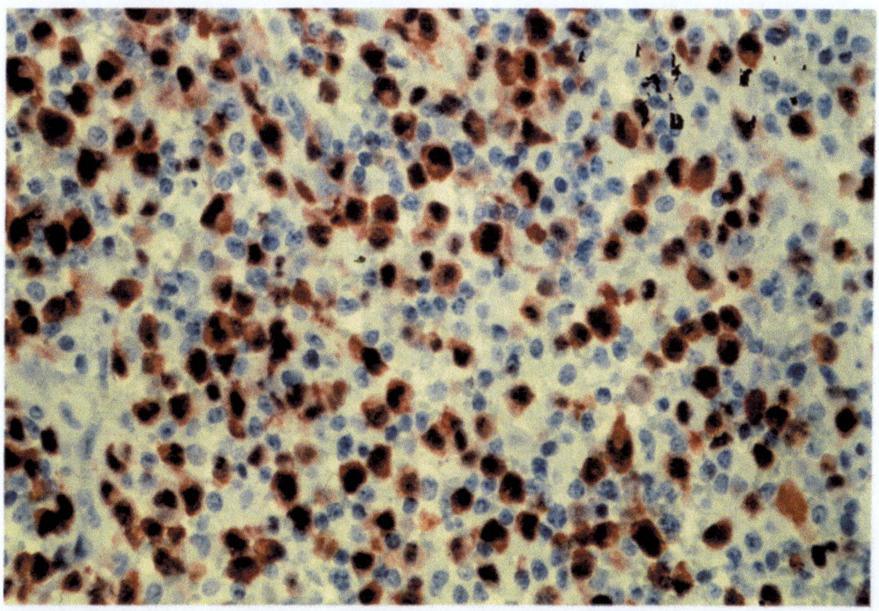

Fig. 5.64. Immunohistochemical staining for ALK-protein in small-cell type of anaplastic large-cell lymphoma (alkaline phosphatase)

in sinuses and filling small endothelial-lined spaces. A striking feature of this neoplasm is the tendency of the tumor cells to surround small vessels (perivascular cuffing). Cytologically, the large cells vary slightly in size and nuclear shape, have distinct nucleoli, and a moderate amount of clear to weakly basophilic cytoplasm (Figs. 5.63, 5.64).

Rarer Subforms. In addition to the common type, numerous other cytological variants of CD30+ ALCL have been subsequently described, including sarcomatoid (Chan et al. 1990), Hodgkin's-like (Pileri et al. 1995), neutrophil-rich (Mann et al. 1995), eosinophil-rich (McCluggage et al. 1998), giant-cell rich (Fig. 5.65) (Stein 1993), and signet-ring variants (Falini et al. 1997). However, only the lymphohistiocytic variant and the small-cell-predominant variant have been included in the recent WHO classification of hematolymphoid neoplasms.

The *sarcomatoid variant* is characterized by the spindle-cell or stellate morphology of the tumor cells, which may adopt a storiform pattern. The *Hodgkin's-like variant* has morphological similarity to Hodgkin's disease by virtue of the nodular and often syncytial growth pattern of the lymphoma cells which are frequently surrounded by fibrous bands. However, this resemblance does not indicate a biological relationship and the pathologist should strive to resolve morphologically difficult cases by immunophenotyping and, if necessary, molecular genetic studies. The *giant-cell-rich variant* can be distinguished from the common type by the presence of numerous multinucleated giant cells, often reminiscent of Reed-Sternberg cells.

In addition, it must be noted that, following chemotherapy, the tumor cells may undergo significant cytomorphological changes. In particular, a relevant reduction in size may occur so that the tumor cells ultimately resemble pleomorphic small- and medium T-cell lymphoma (peripheral nodal T-cell lymphoma, unspecified) (Lennert and Feller 1992).

Immunohistochemistry

ALCL cells are characterized by an intense immunoreactivity for the CD30 molecule, a member of the tumor necrosis factor (TNF) receptor superfamily, which is expressed by activated lymphocytes (Dürkop et al. 2000). The monoclonal antibody Ki-1 recognizes the CD30 molecule on frozen tissue, whereas BerH2 and HRS4 are suitable for paraffin section immunohistochemistry. The typical immunostaining pattern is membranous and/or paranuclear (Golgi zone) (Fig. 5.66); diffuse, cytoplasmic CD30 reactivity is of dubious significance. Other activation antigens characteristically expressed by ALCL include IL-2 receptor (CD25), transferrin receptor (CD71), HLA-DR, HLA-DR invariant chain (CD74), CDw70, and epithelial membrane antigen (EMA) (Stein et al. 1985).

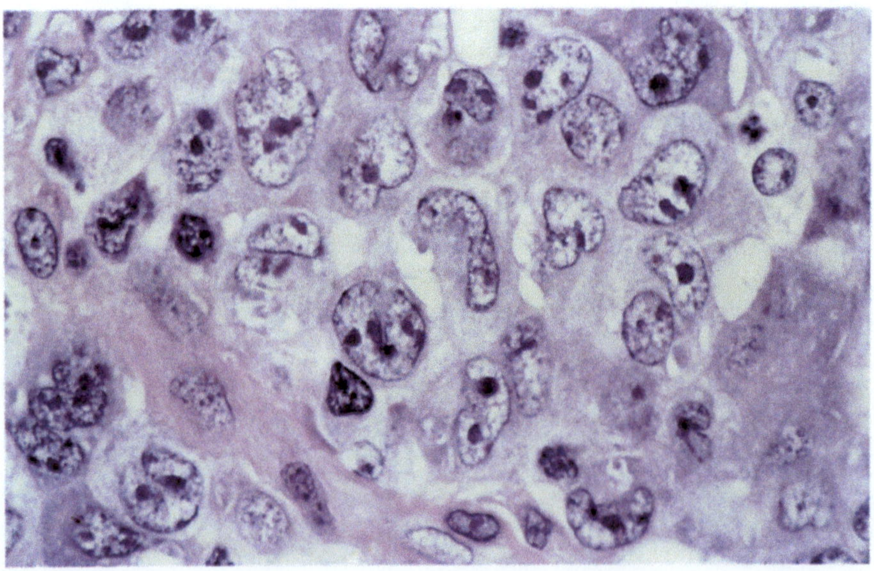

Fig. 5.65. Giant-cell variant of anaplastic large-cell lymphoma. The cells have large bizarre nuclei (Giemsa stain)

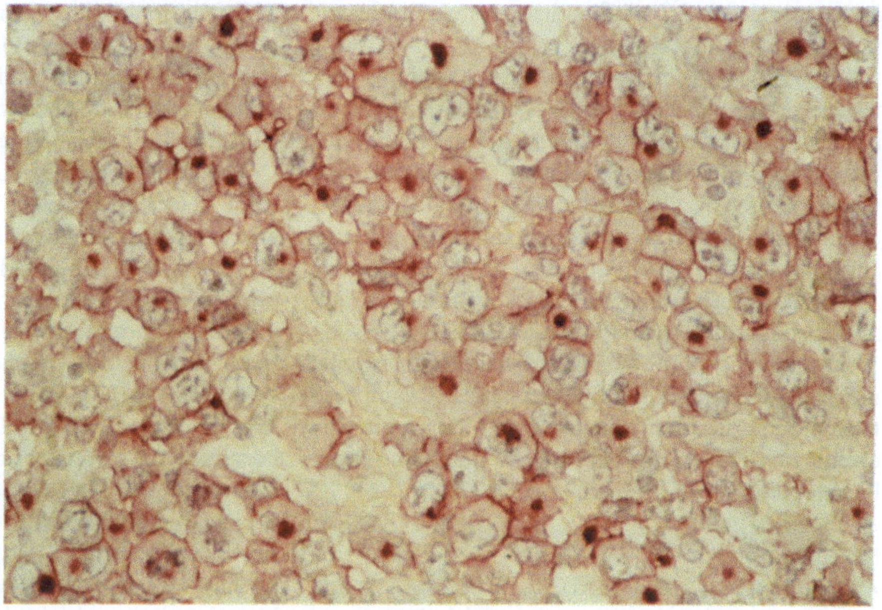

Fig. 5.66. Immunohistochemical staining for CD30 in anaplastic large-cell lymphoma. Note the typical paranuclear dot-like reactivity and faint membrane staining (alkaline phosphatase)

Up to two-thirds of ALCLs have a T-cell phenotype, 10–20% show a B-cell phenotype, the remainder expresses a null-cell phenotype (neither T- nor B-lineage markers).

Up to one-third of ALCLs lack CD45 (leukocyte common antigen, LCA) in paraffin tissue immunohistochemistry (Falini et al. 1990). This negativity, coupled with the frequent EMA expression (more than 50% of ALCLs, including primary cutaneous forms) (Delsol et al. 1988) and the reported cases of sporadic pan-cytokeratin-positive ALCL (Gustmann et al. 1991), may give an erroneous impression of carcinoma.

ALCL of T-phenotype usually exhibits a mature T-cell antigenic profile with variable expression of the CD2, CD3, CD4 or CD8 antigens; of these, CD2 is the most frequently expressed.

The revised Kiel classification includes both T/null-cell ALCL and B-cell ALCL; however, the REAL classification and the proposed WHO classification only recognize T/null-cell ALCL as a clinicopathological entity, including B-cell ALCL within all other diffuse large-B-cell lymphomas (DLBCLs).

The frequency of the null-cell types depends on the number of the tested T-cell antigens. However, it has become evident that almost all null-cell lymphomas belong to the T-cell type when the configuration of the TCR genes is investigated by molecular biology and the studies are extended to cytotoxic molecules.

Most ALCL express cytotoxic molecules including TIA1, granzyme B, and perforin, suggesting a possible cellular origin related to cytotoxic T-cells or NK-cells (Krenacs et al. 1997), as also corroborated by the sporadic expression of the CD56 NK-cell marker (Felgar et al. 1999).

Studies have reported variable frequencies (0–1%) of CD15 staining (Rosso et al. 1990); occasionally, expression of some histiocytic-related markers has been also reported in ALCL (Carbone et al. 1990), but this finding is of unclear significance.

Some systemic ALCLs, mainly those in children and young adults, are associated with a t(2;5) (Sarris et al. 1996) (see below). Using the highly specific monoclonal anti-ALK antibodies ALK1 and ALKc, both suitable for paraffin section immunohistochemistry, investigators found the expression of chimeric ALK protein to be confined to ALCL of T and null type with a frequency ranging from 53 to 89% (Benharroch et al. 1998; Pulford et al. 1997; Falini et al. 1998).

Immunohistochemical identification of ALK is useful because this protein is not detectable in normal lymphoid cells, the only other lymphoid neoplasms positive for ALK being a rare form of large-B-cell lymphoma reported by Delsol et al. (1997) and by Gascoyne et al. (1999).

In non-lymphoid tissues, ALK protein has been observed in central nervous system cells, in rhabdomyosarcomas, and in inflammatory myofibroblastic tumors and neuroblastomas.

In ALK+ ALCL, three main immunostaining patterns for the NPM-ALK protein and its fusion variants have been described depending on the subcellular distribution of the chimeric protein: cytoplasmic and nuclear (Figs. 5.62, 5.64); exclusively nuclear (more frequently observed in the predominant small-cell variant), and exclusively cytoplasmic (10–20% of cases), the latter corresponding to ALCLs harboring variant ALK fusion and 2p23 abnormalities (Falini et al. 1999b).

Detection of EBV by immunohistochemical and molecular techniques is infrequent in ALCL compared to Hodgkin's disease (Nakagawa et al. 1997) and mostly occurs in CD30+ HIV-related lymphomas of B-cell lineage (Lazzi et al. 1998).

Molecular Genetics

Approximately 80–90% of ALCLs, including most null cell types, have clonal rearrangement of the TCR-β and γ genes, as detected by PCR.

However, 10–20% of ALCLs have no PCR-detectable TCR monoclonality, possibly because the lymphoma cells originate from lymphocytes at an early stage of maturation, prior to TCR gene rearrangement (Medeiros and Carr 1999). Moreover, this TCR-negative ALCL subset may include rare cases of CD56-positive ALCLs possibly derived from NK-cells.

Cytogenetics. About one-third of systemic (nodal) forms of ALCL show a non-random t(2;5). The translocation juxtaposes the ALK (a tyrosine kinase) gene on chromosome 2p23 and the NPM (a nucleolar phosphoprotein) gene on chromosome 5q35, resulting in a novel NPM/ALK gene on the derivative 5 chromosome and to the related chimeric protein p80 (Morris et al. 1995). The NPM gene encodes an ubiquitous protein that shuttles ribosomal components between the nucleus and the cytoplasm.

The wild-type ALK protein is a 200-kDa transmembrane receptor closely related to leukocyte tyrosine kinase (LTK) and whose postnatal expression is physiologically restricted to a few cells in the nervous system (glial cells, endothelial cells and pericytes) (Pulford et al. 1997).

The 5' NPM portion of the fusion gene includes a promoter that causes ALK overexpression, which is a postulated inducer of lymphomagenesis, as ALK protein is not expressed in normal lymphoid cells (Kuefer et al. 1997). Different molecular techniques, e.g. Southern blot, reverse transcriptase (RT)-PCR, in situ hybridization, fluorescence in situ hybridization (FISH) and imunohistochemistry, have been employed to detect the NPM-ALK translocation and the related chimeric protein.

The t(2;5) frequency varies between different series from 12 to 80% as determined by molecular analysis, and is lower in adult patients and higher in children and young adults (Skinnider et al. 1999).

Variant translocations involving fusion of the ALK-gene with other partner genes have been also reported: TPM3 (tropomyosin III gene) in t(1;2)(q25;p23) (Lamant et al. 1999); TGF (TRK fused gene) in t(2;3)(p23;q21) (Hernandez et al. 1999); ATIC (5-aminoimidazole-4-carboxamide-1-β-D-ribonucleotide transphorylase/inosine monophosphate cyclohydrolase) in inv(2)(p23;q35) (Colleoni et al. 2000); CLTCL (clathrin heavy-polypeptide-like gene) in t(2;22)(p23;q11.2) (Touriol et al. 2000).

These variant translocations result in ALK immunohistochemical positivity being confined to the cytoplasm. In addition, two ALK-fusion proteins (CTCL-ALK and moesin-ALK) have been recently described to have a peculiar immunohistochemical staining pattern which is a granular cytoplasmic and a membrane bound one (Falini and Mason 2002). Sporadically, other cytogenetic abnormalities have been observed in ALCL, such as complex hyperdiploid karyotypes as well as (17)t (1;7) (q11,p11) (Ishii et al. 2000).

Differential Diagnosis

Other than in Reed-Sternberg cells and in most ALCLs (sporadic CD30-negative ALCL may occur), CD30 antigen has also been detected in normal lymphoid tissues, various types of NHL, and non-lymphoid tumors. Thus, ALCL must be differentiated from other lymphoid malignancies as well as from non-hematolymphoid neoplasms.

Lymphoid Malignancies. In nodal and tonsil lymphoid tissue, CD30 is expressed by activated lymphoid cells usually located in perifollicular areas. Thus, some reactive lymphoid hyperplasias (i.e. subacute necrotizing lymphadenitis, abscess-forming lymphadenitis, dermatopathic lymphadenitis, infectious mononucleosis, etc) may be misdiagnosed as ALCL and thus require careful evaluation of morphofunctional findings and clinical data.

Immunoblastic and *pleomorphic T-cell NHL* of medium- and large-cell type may contain a variable number of CD30-positive cells, as may the group of peripheral T-cell NHL defined as low-grade in the updated Kiel classification, in which CD30 expression may be found in a minority of large cells.

CD30 is also the hallmark of a wide spectrum of primary *cutaneous T-cell lymphoproliferative disorders* including *lymphomatoid papulosis* (see Chap. 6.14.2) (Paulli et al. 1995).

Even though it is expressed with lower frequency and less intensity than in T-cell tumors, the CD30 antigen may be expressed in B-cell NHLs, including immunoblastic, centroblastic, and, more rarely, Burkitt-type lymphoma and low grade subtypes, particularly immunocytoma and plasmocytoma (Pallesen 1990).

Although the typical growth pattern and cytomorphology of the lymphoma cells remain the clue for ALCL identification, immunohistochemistry is crucial to corroborate the diagnosis. The possibility of ALCL also cannot be dismissed after a negative LCA reaction (Falini et al. 1990); instead, a wider immunohistochemical panel, including, besides CD30, anti-ALK protein coupled with T- and B-cell markers, is required.

Distinction between ALCL and *Hodgkin's disease*, especially the syncytial variant of the nodular sclerosis and lymphocyte depletion types, can be difficult.

In the early 1990s, the term ALCL-HD-like was introduced (Pileri et al. 1995), reflecting the tendency to believe that most of these "gray zone" lymphomas were ALCL mimicking Hodgkin's disease. However, nowadays data have emerged favoring the opinion that ALCL-HD-like is a tumor-cell-rich variant of classic Hodgkin's disease and not a true ALCL.

In some difficult cases, immunohistochemistry may reveal of some aid. ALCL usual phenotypic profile is CD30+; CD15–; CD45+/–; CD2+; CD20–; ALK+/–, in contrast with the usual HD phenotype CD30+, CD15+, CD45–, T–, B–, ALK–; CD20–/+

Finally, the distinction between ALCL and malignant histiocytosis, nowadays is less relevant as almost all cases of malignant histiocytosis have been proven to be ALCL. However, individual cases of true malignant histiocytosis do exist, most of which are CD30-negative.

Non-lymphoid Tumors. For obvious morphological reasons (i.e. the sinusoidal growth pattern), various non-lymphoid neoplasias (metastatic carcinoma, melanoma, embryonal carcinoma, seminoma and, occasionally, mesenchymal tumors) may be considered in the differential diagnosis of ALCL.

The CD30 antigen may be sporadically detected in various epithelial carcinomas(e.g. pancreas, salivary glands, lung, and mesothelioma) and non-epithelial tumors including malignant fibrous histiocytoma, melanoma and germ-cell tumors (embryonal carcinoma, embryonal component of mixed germ-cell tumors, yolk-sac tumors and seminomas).

However, the Ber-H2 immunostaining pattern may be helpful in the differential diagnosis, providing in most of the above-mentioned tumors a diffuse cytoplasmic positivity related to its cross-reactivity with an epitope of an antigen other than CD30, altered by formaldehyde (Piris et al. 1990). On the other hand, the vast majority of ALCLs show a typical membrane and/or paranuclear "dot-like" reactivity.

The presence or absence of additional immune markers may be therefore of further help in the differential diagnosis.

LCA positivity excludes embryonal carcinoma or any other non-hematopoietic tumor but its absence by no means rules out ALCL since a proportion of them are CD45-negative. EMA is of no practical value in distinguishing an epithelial tumor from an ALCL, usually EMA-positive. The antibody to placental alkaline phosphatase (PLAP) labels embryonal carcinoma but not ALCL; LCA and other leukocyte-specific antigens (e.g. CD2, CD4) may be positive in ALCL but not in embryonal carcinoma. Cytokeratins may be detected in both neoplasias. Thus, if a PLAP positivity is recorded in an anaplastic tumor simultaneously with cytokeratin and CD30 antigen, the diagnosis of an embryonal carcinoma will be favored.

Occurrence

Systemic (nodal) ALCL accounts for about 7% of all adult NHLs (The Non-Hodgkin's Lymphoma Classification Project 1997) and approximately 20–30% of large-cell lymphomas in children (Mora et al. 2000). ALCL has a bimodal age distribution, with a larger peak in the second and third decades, and a smaller one in the sixth and seventh decades. Male gender predominates (ratio 1.6:1).

Clinical Features

Three major clinical profiles relevant to outcome are described: primary systemic (nodal) ALCL, secondary ALCL (arising as a progression of other lymphomas), and primary extranodal (cutaneous) ALCL. In addition, rare cases of ALCL may occur in immunodeficiency conditions such as HIV infection and iatrogenically induced immunosuppression.

Primary Systemic (Nodal) ALCL. This form accounts for about 7% of all adult NHLs and approximately 20–30% of large-cell lymphomas in children. ALCL has a bimodal age distribution (Fig. 5.57), with a larger peak in the second and third decades, and a smaller one in the sixth and seventh decades. Male gender predominates (ratio 1.6:1).

The clinical features and outcomes of systemic ALCL varied in different studies probably due to differences in the adopted diagnostic criteria, the age distribution of patients, and the inclusion, in clinical trials, of provisional categories such as ALCL-HD like, ALCL of B-cell phenotype, and primary cutaneous ALCL.

In most systemic ALCLs, about 70% of patients have generalized lymphadenopathy and half of them present with B-symptoms and advanced stage disease (Ann Arbor stage III or IV). Extranodal presentation may frequently occur, involving preferentially skin, bone, lung, gastrointestinal tract and soft-tissues; mediastinal involvement is rare. Bone marrow involvement is uncommon, but some authors report a higher rate by analyzing trephine biopsies with immunohistochemistry (Stein et al. 2000). Within primary ALCL clinico-prognostic subgroups have been recently identified based on the expression of the ALK protein. It has been reported that ALK-positive ALCL, mostly occurring in children and young adults (median age 16–30 years), has a significantly improved 5-year overall survival rate (71–93%) compared to the ALK-negative group (30–37%) (Shiota et al. 1995). Two studies that used multivariate analysis showed ALK to be an independent prognostic marker, along with the IPI and serum LDH levels (Falini et al. 1999a). In a Japanese study on a large series of patients, the results of a multivariate analysis did not identify ALK expression as an independent prognostic factor (Suzuki et al. 2000). However, this does not contradict the fact that ALK-positive ALCL is a distinct subtype, because the expression of ALK closely correlates with age and IPI. It is therefore not fruitful to discuss whether age or ALK expression is more prognostically significantly for ALCL, since these two factors are interrelated and have the same impact on the prognosis for ALCL.

A matter of debate regards B-cell ALCL. Some data indicate that true B-cell ALCLs may exist, and that they may have features distinct from those of conventional DLBCL. By morphological criteria, a recent study found that B-cell ALCL had a better prognosis than conventional DLBCL, but other investigators have suggested that ALCL of B-cell lineage does not have distinctive clinicobiological features compared with the usual DLBCL forms (Tilly et al. 1997). For this reason, proper clinicopathological correlations with this postulated B-cell variant have not been established yet. Thus, their prognostic significance and implications for treatment, other than as for DLBCL, are unrecognized, and the biological distinction from T/null-cell ALCL remains to be determined.

Primary Extranodal (Cutaneous) ALCL. In accordance with the criteria of the E.O.R.T.C. Cutaneous Lymphoma Study Group (a 6-month cut-off adopted to identify true primary cutaneous lymphoma), primary cutaneous ALCL must be restricted to skin-limited lesions for at least 6 months from the time of diagnosis (Willemze et al. 1997).

In the recent WHO lymphoma classification, primary cutaneous ALCL (9% of all cutaneous NHLs) characteristically lacking the t(2;5), has been considered a separate clinicopathological entity with a significantly better survival than systemic ALCL (Beljaards et al. 1993).

The clinicopathological features of primary cutaneous ALCL will be discussed in detail in a further chapter of this volume (see Chap. 6.14.2.3).

Immunodeficiency-Related ALCL. ALCL has been reported in HIV-positive patients and, sporadically (personal observations), in drug-induced imunosuppressed organ transplant recipients.

In HIV-positive patients, true ALCL, especially the form bearing chimeric ALK protein, is rare. Most of these tumors have a B-cell phenotype and are frequently EBV-positive (Tirelli et al. 1995), thus being more probably related to the anaplastic variant of DLBCL. In our series of 765 transplant recipients (heart, lung, heart/lung) there were three patients with ALK-negative CD30+ ALCL: two with systemic (one with B-phenotype, the other with T-cell lineage) and one with primary T-cell cutaneous form. Two of these patients harbored EBV infections as determined by both immunohistochemistry for LMP-1 and in situ hybridization for Epstein-Barr-virus-encoded RNA (EBER). Presently, limited data are available on the outcome of immunodeficiency-related ALCL, which seems to be largely linked to the general status of the patient.

Table 5.5. Diagnosis in 95 cases of CD30-positive non-Hodgkin's lymphoma (NHL) (data from Engelhard et al. 1991)

NHL	(*n*)
Anaplastic large-cell lymphoma T cell	72
Primary	52
Secondary	20
In T-cell lymphoma	17
Mycosis fungoides	3
Angioimmunoblastic	3
Lymphoepithelioid lymphoma	1
T-zone lymphoma	5
Peripheral T-cell lymphoma, unspecified	5
In Hodgkin's lymphoma	3
CD30-positive diffuse large B-cell lymphoma	11
Centroblastic	5
Immunoblastic	3
Unclassified	3

Secondary ALCL. Secondary ALCL, usually ALK - 1 neg., occurs in older adults and may arise in the progression of other lymphomas (mycosis fungoides, peripheral T-cell NHL, Hodgkin's disease, or lymphomatoid papulosis) (Salhany et al. 1988) (Table 5.5). The treatment approaches are similar to those for primary systemic ALCL, but, although there is little definitive management information, the prognosis is usually poor. Thus, in such cases, the appearance of CD30 expression in a previously CD30– lymphoma (most frequently indolent primary cutaneous T-cell lymphomas) may represent an unfavorable prognostic marker.

In addition, it has been recently reported that, in the predominant small-cell variant of ALCL, the lymphoma population may transform to large anaplastic cells of the common type. This switch is likely to be predictive of a rapid clinical course, a finding that awaits confirmation by a study on a larger series (Hodges et al. 1999).

Prognosis

The morphological heterogeneity of ALCL has little predictive value with respect to clinical presentation and prognosis (Skinnider et al. 1999).

Despite the anaplastic cytology, ALCL is not necessarily aggressive. Several studies revealed that patients with ALCL have a better outcome than those with other aggressive NHLs (5-year overall survival range of 81–83%) (The Non-Hodgkin's Lymphoma classification Project 1997). As previously mentioned, there are significant differences between ALK-positive and ALK-negative systemic ALCL that may have a bearing on treatment and prognosis (Gascoyne et al. 1999).

The prognosis of ALK-positive ALCL with adriamycin-based combination chemotherapy is superior to that of peripheral T-cell lymphoma of equivalent prognostic parameter distribution, with reported 5-year survival rates in excess of 70%. Children and young patients appear to respond to treatment particularly well: the reported 5-year survival rate is greater than 80%, even including those patients with advanced stage disease (Mora et al. 2000). By contrast, ALK-negative ALCL is at the most unfavorable end of the spectrum of NHLs (30–40% 5-year survival) and a strong case can be made for early intensification of therapeutic protocols with or without autologous stem cell support.

Recently, Falini et al. (1999a) and later Gascoyne et al. (1999) demonstrated that, within the good prognostic group of chimeric ALK+ cases, the 5-year survival was 94%±5% for the low- and intermediate-risk group (age-adjusted IPI=0–1) and 41%±12% for the high- and intermediate-risk group (age-adjusted IPI≥=2). These findings contrast with the data of the Non-Hodgkin's Lymphoma Classification Project (1997) in which no significant difference was observed between ALCL patients with a low or a high IPI. However, this result was obtained in a more heterogeneous group of patients, often not tested with anti-ALK antibodies.

Therefore, it must be stressed that the identification of different clinical subgroups of ALCLs requires a combined clinicopathological approach in which immunohistochemical labeling techniques are crucial to identify those ALCLs having a good prognosis (ALK+ lymphomas) in view of optimal therapeutic strategies.

References

Abruzzo LV, Schmidt K, Weiss LM, Jaffe ES, Medeiros J, Sander CA, Raffeld M (1993) B-cell lymphoma after angioimmunoblastic lymphadenopathy: a case with oligoclonal gene rearrangements associated with Epstein-Barr virus. Blood 82:241–246

Anagnostopoulos I, Hummel M, Finn T, Tiemann M, Korbjuhn P, Dimmler C, Gatter K, Dallenbach F, Parwaresch MR, Stein H (1992) Heterogeneous Epstein-Barr virus infection patterns in peripheral T-cell lymphoma of angioimmunoblastic lymphadenopathy type. Blood 80:1804–1812

Anagnostopoulos I, Hummel M, Tiemann M, Korbjuhn P, Parwaresch MR, Stein H (1994) Frequent presence of latent Epstein-Barr virus infection in lymphoepithelioid cell lymphoma (Lennert's lymphoma). Histopathology 25:331–337

Anderson JR, Wilson JF, Jenkin RD, Meadows AT, Kersey J, Chilcote RR, Coccia P, Exelby P, Kushner J, Siegel S, Hammon D (1983) Childhood Non-Hodgkin's lymphoma: the results of a randomized therapeutic trial comparing a 4-drug regimen (COMP) with a 10-drug regimen (LSA_2-L_2). N Engl J Med 308:559–565

Attygalle A, Al-Jehani R, Diss TC, Munson P, Liu H, Du MQ, Isaacson PG, Dogan A (2002) Neoplastic T cells in angioimmunoblastic T-cell lymphoma express CD10. Blood 99:627–33

Beljaards RC, Kaudewitz P, Berti E, Gianotti R, Neumann C, Rosso R, Paulli M, Meijer CJ, Willemze R (1993) Primary cutaneous CD30-positive large cell lymphoma: definition of a new type of cutaneous lymphoma with a favorable prognosis. Cancer 71:2097–2104

Benharroch D, Meguerian-Bedoyan Z, Lamant L, Amin C, Brugières L, Terrier-Lacombe MJ, Haralambieva E, Pulford K, Pileri S, Morris SW, Mason DY, Delsol G (1998) ALK-positive lymphoma: a single disease with a broad spectrum of morphology. Blood 91:2076–2084

Blattner WA, Kalyanaraman VS, Robert-Guroff M, Lister TA, Galton DAG, Sarin PS, Craw-ford MH, Catovsky D, Greaves M, Gallo RC (1982) The human type-C retrovirus. HTLV in Blacks from the Caribbean region, and relationship to adult T-cell leukemia/lymphoma. Int J Cancer 30:257–264

Brittinger G, Bartels H, Common H, Dühmke E, Fülle HH, Gunzer U, Gyenes T, Heinz R, König E, Meusers P et al (1984) Clinical and prognostic relevance of the Kiel classification of non-Hodgkin lymphomas results of aprospective multicenter study by the Kiel Lymphoma Study Group. Hematol Oncol 2:269–306

Burke JS, Butler JJ (1976) Malignant lymphoma with a high content of epithelioid histiocytes (Lennert's lymphoma). Am J Clin Pathol 66:1–9

Carbone A, Gloghini A, De Re V, Tamaro P, Boiocchi M, Volpe R (1990) Histopathologic, immunophenotypic, and genotypic analysis of Ki-1 anaplastic large cell lymphomas that express histiocyte-associated antigens. Cancer 66:2547–2556

Catovsky D, Greaves MF, Rose M, Galton DAG, Goolden AWG, McCluskey DR, White JM, Lampert I, Bourikas G, Ireland R, Brownell AI, Bridges JM, Blattner WA, Gallo RC (1982) Adult T-cell lymphoma-leukemia in Blacks from the West Indies. Lancet i:639–643

Chan JKC, Ng CS, Hui PK, Leung TW, Lo ESF, Lau WH, McGuire LJ (1989) Anaplastic large cell Ki-1 lymphoma. Delineation of two morphological types. Histopathology 15:11–34

Chan JKC, Buchanan R, Fletcher CDM (1990) Sarcomatoid variant of anaplastic large cell Ki-1 lymphoma. Am J Surg Pathol 14:983–988

Chen W, Cheng JT, Tsai LH, Schneider N, Buchanan G, Carroll A, Crist W, Ozanne B, Siciliano MJ, Baer R (1990) The tal-gene undergoes chromosome translocation in T cell leukemia and potentially encodes a helix-loop-helix protein. EMBO 9:415–424

Colleoni GW, Bridge JA, Garicochea B, Liu J, Filippa DA, Ladany M (2000) ATIC-ALK: a novel variant ALK gene fusion in anaplastic large cell lymphoma resulting from recurrent cryptic chromosomal inversion, inv(2)(p23q35). Am J Pathol 156:781–789

Conde-Sterlin DA, Aguilera NSI, Nandedkar MA, Abbondanzo SL (2000) Immunoperoxidase detection of CD10 in precursor T-lymphoblastic lymphoma/leukemia. A clinicopathologic study of 24 cases. Arch Pathol Lab Med 124:704–708

De Almeida PC, Harris NL, Bhan AK (1984) Characterization of immature sinus histiocytes (monocytoid cells) in reactive lymph nodes by use of monoclonal antibodies. Hum Pathol 15:330–335

Dellagi K, Brouet J-C, Seligmann M (1984) Antivimentin autoantibodies in angioimmunoblastic lymphadenopathy. N Engl J Med 310:215–218

Delsol G, Al Saati T, Gatter KC, Gerdes J, Schwarting R, Caveriviere P, Rigal-Huguet F, Robert A, Stein H, Mason DY (1988) Coexpression of epithelial membrane antigen (EMA), Ki-1, and interleukin-2 receptor by anaplastic large cell lymphomas. Diagnostic value in so-called malignant histiocytosis. Am J Pathol 130:59–70

Delsol G, Familiades J, Voigt JJ, Gorguet B, Pris J, Laurent G, Fabre J (1977a) Les adenopathies dysimmunitaires et pseudo-lymphomateuses. I. Lymphadenopathies immunoblastiques et plasmocytaires. Ann Anat Pathol (Paris) 22:41–60

Delsol G, Familiades J, Voigt JJ, Gorguet B, Pris J, Lauent G, Fabre J (1977b) Les adenopathies dysimmunitaires et pseudo-lymphomateuses. II. Lymphadenopathies riches en cellules epithelioides. Ann Anat Pathol (Paris) 22:61–74

Delsol G, Lamant L, Mariame B, Pulford K, Dastugue N, Drousset P, Rigal-Huguet F, Al Saati T, Cerretti DP, Morris SW, Mason DY (1997) A new sub-type of large B-cell lymphoma expressing the ALK-kinase and lacking the 2;5 translocation. Blood 89:1483–1490

Diebold J, Reynes M, Tricot G. James J-M, Zittoun R, Bilski Pasquier G (1977) Lymphome malin lympho-epithelioide (lymphome de Lennert). Nouv Presse Med 6:2145–215

Dorfman RF, Warnke R (1974) Lymphadenopathy simulating the malignant lymphomas. Hum Pathol 5:519–550

Drexler HG, Gignac SM, von Wasielewski R, Werner M, Dirks WG (2000) Pathobiology of NPM-ALK and variant fusion genes in anaplastic large cell lymphoma and other lymphomas. Leukemia 14:1533–1559

Dürkop H, Foss HD, Eitelbach F, Anagnostopoulos I, Latza U, Pileri S, Stein H (2000) Expression of the CD30 antigen in non-lymphoid tissues and cells. J Pathol 190:613–618

Eden OB, Hann I, Imeson J, Cotterill S, Gerrard M, Pinkerton CR (1992) Treatment of advanced stage T cell lymphoblastic lymphoma: results of the United Kingdom Children's Cancer Study Group (UKCCSG)

Falini B, Mason DY (2002) Proteins encoded by genes involved in chromosomal alterations in lymphoma and leukemia: clinical value of their detection by immunocytochemistry. Blood 99:409–426

Falini B, Pileri S, Stein H, Dieneman D, Dallenbach F, Delsol G, Minelli O, Poggi S, Martelli MF, Pallesen G et al (1990) Variable expression of leucocyte-common (CD45) antigen in CD30 (Ki1)-positive anaplastic large cell lymphoma: implications for the differential diagnosis between lymphoid and nonlymphoid malignancies. Hum Pathol 21:624–629

Falini B, Liso A, Pasqualucci L, Flenghi L, Ascani S, Pileri S, Bucciarelli E (1997) CD30+ anaplastic large-cell lymphoma, null type, with signet-ring appearance. Histopathol 30:90–92

Falini B, Bigerna B, Fizzotti M, Pulford K, Pileri SA, Delsol G, Carbone A, Paulli M, Magrini U, Menestrina F, Giardini R, Pilotti S, Mezzelani A, Ugolini B, Billi M, Pucciarini A, Pacini R, Pelicci PG, Flenghi L (1998) ALK expression defines a distinct group of T/null lymphomas ("ALK lymphomas") with a wide morphological spectrum. Am J Pathol 153:875–886

Falini B, Pileri S, Zinzani PL, Carbone A, Zagonel V, Wolf-Peeters C, Verhoef G, Menestrina F, Todeschini G, Paulli M, Lazzarino M, Giardini R, Aiello A, Foss HD, Araujo I, Fizzotti M, Pelicci PG, Flenghi L, Martelli MF, Santucci A (1999a) ALK+ lymphoma: clinico-pathological findings and outcome. Blood 93:2697–2706

Falini B, Pulford K, Pucciarini A, Carbone A, De Wolf-Peeters C, Cordell J, Fizzotti M, Santucci A, Pelicci PG, Pileri S; Campo E, Ott G, Delsol G, Mason DY (1999b) Lymphomas expressing ALK fusion protein(s) other than NPM-ALK. Blood 94:3509–3515

Felgar RE, Salhany KE, Macon WR, Pietra GG, Kinney MC (1999) The expression of TIA-1+ cytolytic-type granules and other cytolytic lymphocyte-associated markers in CD30+ anaplastic large cell lymphomas (ALCL): correlation with morphology, immunophenotype, ultrastructure, and clinical features. Hum Pathol 30:228–236

Feller AC, Griesser GH, Mak TW, Lennert K (1986a) Lymphoepithelioid lymphoma (Lennert's lymphoma) is a monoclonal proliferation of helper/inducer T cells. Blood 68:663–666

Feller AC, Parwaresch MR, Stein H, Ziegler A, Herbst H, Lennert K (1986b) Immunophenotyping of T-lymphoblastic lymphoma/leukemia: correlation with normal T-cell maturation. Leuk Res 10:1025–1031

Feller AC, Griesser H, von Schilling C, Wacker HH, Dallenbach F, Bartels H, Kruse R, Mak TW, Lennert K (1988) Clonal gene rearrangement patterns correlate with immunophenotype and clinical parameters in patients with angioimmunoblastic lymphadenopathy. Am J Pathol 133:549–557

Frizzera G, Moran EM, Rappaport H (1974) Angio-immunoblastic lymphadenopathy with dysproteinaemia. Lancet i:1070–1073

Gascoyne RD, Aoun P, Wu D, Chhanabhai M, Skinnider BF, Greiner TC, Morris SW, Connors JM, Vose JM, Viswanatha DS, Coldman A, Weisenburger DD (1999) Prognostic significance of anaplastic lymphoma kinase (ALK) protein expression in adults with anaplastic large cell lymphoma. Blood 93:3913–3921

Gisselbrecht C, Gaulard P, Lepage E, Coiffier B, Briere J, Haioun C, Cazals-Hatem D, Bosly A, Xerri L, Tilly H, Berger F, Bouhabdallah R, Diebold J (1998) Prognostic significance of T-cell phenotype in aggressive non-Hodgkin's lymphomas. Groupe d'Etudes des Lymphomes de l'Adulte (GELA). Blood 92:76–82

Gödde-Salz E, Feller AC, Lennert K (1986) Cytogenetic and immunohistochemical analysis of lymphoepithelioid cell lymphoma (Lennert's lymphoma): further substantiation of its T-cell nature. Leuk Res 10:313–323

Greenberg JM, Quertermous T, Seidman JG, Kersey JH (1986) Human T cell γ-chain gene rearrangements in acute lymphoid and nonlymphoid leukemia: comparison with the T cell receptor β-chain gene. J Immunol 137:2043–2049

Grossman B, Schechter GP. Horton JE, Pierce L, Jaffe E, Wahl L (1981) Hypercalcemia associated with T-cell lymphoma-leukemia. J Clin Pathol 75:149–155

Gustmann C, Altmannsberger M, Osborn M, Criesser H, Feller AC (1991) Cytokeratin expression and vimentin content in large cell anaplastic lymphomas and other non-Hodgkin's lymphomas. Am J Pathol 138:1413–1422

Hanaoka M (1984) Adult T cell leukemia and Sézary-Syndrome. Leuk Rev Int 2:17–44

Hara J, Benedict SH, Champagne E, Mak TW, Minden M, Gelfand EW (1988) Comparison of T cell receptor α, β, and γ gene rearrangement and expression in T cell acute lymphoblastic leukemia. J Clin Invest 81:989–996

Hast R, Jacobsson B, Petrescu A, Hjalmar V (1999) Successful treatment with fludarabine in two cases of angioimmunoblastic lymphadenopathy with dysproteinemia. Leuk Lymph 34:597–601

Helbron D, Brittinger G, Lennert K (1979) T-Zonen-Lymphom. Klinisches Bild, Therapie und Prognose. Blut 39:117–131

Hernandez L, Pinyol M, Hernandez S, Bea S, Pulford K, Rosenwald A, Lamant L, Falini B, Ott G, Mason DY, Delsol G, Campo E (1999) TRK-fused gene (TFG) is a new partner of ALK in anaplastic large cell lymphoma producing two structurally different TFG-ALK translocations. Blood 94:3265–3268

Hodges KB, Collins RD, Greer JP, Kadin ME, Kinney MC (1999) Transformation of the small cell variant Ki-1+ lymphoma to anaplastic large cell lymphoma: pathologic and clinical features. Am J Surg Pathol 23:49–58

Ichinohasama R, Endoh K, Ishizawa KI, Okuda M, Kameoka JI, Meguro K, Myers J, Kadin ME, Mori S, Sawai T (1996) Thymic lymphoblastic lymphoma of committed natural killer cell precursor origin. Cancer 77:2592–2603

Ishii E, Honda K, Nakagawa A, Urago K, Oshima K (2000) Primary CD30/Ki-1 positive anaplastic large cell lymphoma of skeletal muscle with der(17)t(1;17)(q11;p11). Cancer Genet Cytogenet 122:116–120

Jaffe ES (1996) Classification of natural killer (NK) cell and NK-like T-cell malignancies. Blood 87:1207–1210

Jaffe ES, Chan JKC, Su IJ, Frizzera G, Mori S, Feller AC, Ho FCS (1996) Report of the workshop on nasal and related extranodal angiocentric T/natural killer cell lymphomas. Am J Surg Pathol 20:103–111

Kadin ME, Kamoun M (1982) Nonendemic adult T-cell leukemia/lymphoma. Hum Pathol 13:691–693

Kaiserling E, Patsouris E, Müller-Hermelink HK, Wichterich D, Lennert K (1989) Bacterial lymphadenitis with the picture of a lymphoepithelioid cell lymphoma (Lennert's lymphoma). Histopathology 14:161–178

Kaneko Y, Frizzera G, Shikano T, Kobayashi H, Maseki N, Sakurai M (1989) Chromosomal and immunophenotypic patterns in T cell acute lymphoblastic leukemia (T ALL) and lymphoblastic lymphoma (LBL). Leukemia 3:886–892

Kerl H, Kresbach H (1979) Lymphoreticuläre Hyperplasien und Neoplasien der Haut. In: Schnyder UW (ed) Histopathologie der Haut, 2nd edn, part 2. Stoffwechselkrankheiten und Tumoren. Springer, Berlin Heidelberg New York, pp 351–480 (Spezielle pathologische Anatomie, vol 7, part 2)

Khalidi HS, Chang KL, Medeiros LJ, Brynes RK, Slovak ML,

Murata-Collins JL, Arber DA (1999) Acute lymphoblastic leukemia. Survey of immunophenotype, French-American-British classification, frequency of myeloid antigen expression, and karyotypic abnormalities in 210 pediatric and adult cases. Am J Clin Pathol 111:467–476

Kikuchi M, Mitsui T, Takeshita M, Okamura H, Naitoh H, Eimoto T (1986) Virus associated adult T-cell leukemia (ATL) in Japan: clinical, histological and immunological studies. Hematol Oncol 4:67–81

Kinney MC, Collins RD, Greer JP, Whitlock JA, Sioutos N, Kadin ME (1993) A small-cell-predominant variant of primary Ki-1 (CD30)+ T-cell lymphoma. Am J Surg Pathol 17:859–868

Knecht H, Lennert K (1981a) Vorgeschichte und klinisches Bild der Lymphogranulomatosis X (einschließlich [angio]immunoblastischer Lymphadenopathie). Schweiz Med Wochenschr 111:1108–1121

Knecht H, Lennert K (1981b) Verlauf, Therapie und maligne Transformation der Lymphogranulomatosis X (einschließlich [angio]immunoblastischer Lymphadenopathie). Schweiz Med Wochenschr 111:1122–1130

Knecht H, Lennert K (1981c) Ultrastructural findings in lymphogranulomatosis X ([angio]immunoblastic lymphadenopathy). Virchows Arch [B] 37:29–47

Knecht H, Schwarze E-W, Lennert K (1985) Histological, immunological and autopsy findings in lymphogranulomatosis X (including angio-immunoblastic lymphadenopathy). Virchows Arch [A] 406:105–124

Knowles DM (1988) Phenotypic markers and gene rearrangement analysis in T-cell neoplasia. Am J Surg Pathol 12:160–163

Koita H, Suzumiya J, Ahshima K, Takeshita M, Kimura N, Kikuchi M, Doono M (1997) Lymphoblastic lymphoma expressing natural killer cell phenotype with involvement of the mediastinum and nasal cavity. Am J Surg Pathol 21:242–248

Kojima M, Nakamura S, Itoh H, Motoori T, Sugihara S, Shinkai H, Masawa N (2001a) Angioimmunoblastic T-cell lymphoma with hyperplastic germinal centers: aclinicopathological and immunohistochemical study of 10 cases. APMIS 109:699–706

Kojima M, Nakamura S, Oyama T, Motoori T, Itoh H, Yoshida K, Suchi T, Masawa N (2001b) Autoimmune disease-associated lymphadenopathy with histological appearance of T-zone dysplasia with hyperplastic follicles. A clinicopathological analysis of nine cases. Pathol Res Pract 197:237–44

Krenacs L, Wellmann A, Sorbara L, Himmelmann AW, Bagdi E, Jaffe ES, Raffeld M (1997) Cytotoxic cell antigen expression in anaplastic large cell lymphomas of T- and null-cell type and Hodgkin's disease: evidence for distinct cellular origin. Blood 89:980–989

Kuefer MU, Look AT, Pulford K, Behm FG, Pattengale PK, Mason DY, Morris SW (1997) Retrovirus-mediated gene ALCL transfer of NPM-ALK causes lymphoid malignancy in mice. Blood 90:2901–2910

Lamant L, Dastugue N, Pulford K, Delsol G, Mariame B (1999) A new fusion gene TPM3-ALK in anaplastic large cell lymphoma created by a (1;2)(q25;p23) translocation. Blood 93:3088–3095

Lazzi S, Ferrari F, Palummo N, De Milito A, Zazzi M, Leoncini l, Luzzi P, Tosi P (1998) HIV-associated malignant lymphomas in Kenya (Equatorial Africa). Hum Pathol 29:1285–1289

Lennert K (1952) Zur histologischen Diagnose der Lymphogranulomatose. Habilitationsschrift, Frankfurt/Main

Lennert K (1953a) Histologische Studie zur Lymphogranulomatose. I. Die Cytologie der Lymphogranulomzellen. Frankf Z Pathol 64:209–234

Lennert K (1953b) Studien zur Histologie der Lymphogranulomatose. II. Die diagnostische Bedeutung der einzelnen Zellelemente. Frankf Z Pathol 64:343–356

Lennert K (1973) Pathologisch-histologische Klassifizierung der malignen Lymphome. In: Stacher A (ed) Leukämien und maligne Lymphome. Urban and Schwarzenberg, Munich, pp 181–194

Lennert K, Feller AC (1992) Histopathology of non-Hodgkin's lymphomas, second edition. Springer, Berlin Heidelberg New York

Lennert K, Hansmann ML (1987) Progressive transformation of germinal centers: clinical significance and lymphocytic predominance Hodgkin's disease – the Kiel experience (abstract). Am J Surg Pathol 11:149–150

Lennert K, Mestdagh J (1968) Lymphogranulomatosen mit konstant hohem Epitheloidzellgehalt. Virchows Arch [A] 344: 1–20

Lennert K, Kikuchi M, Sato E, Suchi T, Stansfeld AG, Feller AC, Hansmann M-L, Müller-Hermelink HK, Gödde-Salz E (1985) HTLV-positive and -negative T-cell lymphomas. Morphological and immunohistochemical differences between European and HTLV-positive Japanese T-cell lymphomas. Int J Cancer 35:65–72

Liao KT, Rosai J, Daneshbod K (1972) Malignant histiocytosis with cutaneous involvement and eosinophilia. Am J Clin Pathol 57:438–448

Lukes RJ, Tindle BH (1973) Immunoblastic lymphadenopathy: presented at the Pathology Panel for Clinical Trials, NCI, 26–28 Jan

Lukes RJ, Tindle BH (1975) Immunoblastic lymphadenopathy. A hyperimmune entity resembling Hodgkin's disease. N Engl J Med 292

Lukes RJ, Butler JJ, Hicks EB (1966) Natural history of Hodgkin's disease as related to its pathologic picture. Cancer 19:317–344

Lukes RJ, Parker JW, Taylor CR, Tindle BH, Gramer AD. Lincoln TL (1978) Immunologic approach to non-Hodgkin lymphomas and related leukemias. Analysis of the results of multiparameter studies of 425 cases. Semin Hematol 15:322–351

Lukes RJ, Taylor CR, Parker JW. Lincoln TL, Pattengale PK, Tindle BH (1978) A morphologic and immunologic surface marker study of 299 cases of non-Hodgkin lymphomas and related leukemias. Am J Pathol 90:461–486

Macon WR, Williams ME, Greer JP, Cousar JB (1995) Paracortical nodular T-cell lymphoma. Identification of an unusual variant of peripheral T-cell lymphoma. Am J Surg Pathol 19:297–303

Mann KP, Hall B, Kamino H, Borowitz MJ, Ratech H (1995) Neutrophil-rich, Ki-1-positive anaplastic large-cell malignant lymphoma. Am J Surg Pathol 19:407–416

Manns A, Hisada M, La Grenade L (1999) Human T-lymphotropic virus Type I infection. Lancet 353:1951–1958

McCluggage WG, Walsh MY, Bharucha H (1998) Anaplastic large cell malignant lymphoma with extensive eosinophilic or neutrophilic infiltration. Histopathol 32:110–115

Medeiros LJ, Carr J (1999) Overview of the role of molecular methods in the diagnosis of malignant lymphomas. Arch Pathol Lab Med 123:1189–1207

Mora J, Filippa DA, Thaler HAT, Polyak T, Cranor ML, Wollner N (2000) Large cell non-Hodgkin's lymphoma of childhood: analysis of 78 consecutive patients enrolled in 2 consecutive protocols at the Memorial Sloan-Kettering Cancer Center. Cancer 88:186–197

Morris SW, Kirstein MN, Valentine MB, Dittmer K, Shapiro DN, Look AT, Saltman DL (1995) Fusion of a kinase gene, ALK, to a nucleolar protein gene, NPM, in non-Hodgkin's lymphoma. Science 267:316–317

Müller-Hermelink HK, Zettl A, Pfeifer W, Ott G (2001) Pathology of lymphoma progression. Histopathology 38:285–306

Nakagawa A, Nakamura S, Ito M, Shiota M, Mori S, Suchi T (1997) CD30-positive anaplastic large cell lymphoma in childhood: expression of p80npm/alk and absence of Epstein-Barr virus. Mod Pathol 10:210–215

Nakamura S, Koshikawa T, Yatabe Y, Suchi T (1998) Lymphoblastic lymphoma expressing CD56 and TdT (letter to the editor). Am J Surg Pathol 22:135–137

Noel H, Helbron D, Lennert K (1979) Die epitheloidzellige Lymphogranulomatose (so genanntes "Lennert's lymphoma"). In: Stacher A, Höcker P (eds) Lymphknotentumoren. Urban and Schwarzenberg, Munich, pp 40–45

Noel H, Helbron D, Lennert K (1980) Epithelioid cellular lymphogranulomatosis (lymphoepithelioid cell lymphoma). Histologie and clinical observations. In: Van den Tweel JG (ed) Malignant lymphoproliferative diseases. Leiden Univ Press, The Hague, pp 433–445 (Boerhaave series for postgraduale medical education, vol 17)

O'Connor NTJ, Feller AC, Wainscoat JS, Gatter KC, Pallesen G, Stein H, Lennert K, Mason DY (1986) T-cell origin of Lennert's lymphoma. Br J Haematol 64:521–528

Ohshima K, Suzumiya J, Kato A, Tashiro K, Kikuchi M (1997) Clonal HTLV-I-infected CD4+ T-lymphocytes and non-clonal non-HTLV-infected giant cells in incipient ATLL with Hodgkin-like histologic features. Int J Cancer 72:592–598

Ohshima K, Suzumiya J, Sugihara M, Kanda M, Shimazaki K, Kawasaki C, Haraoka S, Kikuchi M (1999) Clinical, immunohistochemical and phenotypic features of aggressive nodal cytotoxic lymphomas, including α/β, γ/δ T-cell and natural killer cell types. Virchows Arch 435:92–100

Ohshima K, Suzumiya J, Kikuchi M (2002) The World Health Organization classification of malignant lymphoma: incidence and clinical prognosis in HTLV-1-endemic area of Fukuoka. Pathol Int 52:1–12

Pallesen G (1990) The diagnostic significance of the CD30 (Ki-1) antigen. Histopathology 16:409–413

Patsouris E, Noel H, Lennert K (1988) Histological and immunohistological findings in lymphoepithelioid cell lymphoma (Lennert's lymphoma). Am J Surg Pathol 12:341–350

Patsouris E, Noel H, Lennert K (1989a) Angioimmunoblastic lymphadenopathy-type of T-cell lymphoma with a high content of epithelioid cells. Histopathology and comparison with lymphoepithelioid cell lymphoma. Am J Surg Pathol 13:262–275

Patsouris E, Noel H, Lennert K (1989b) Cytohistologic and immunohistochemical findings in Hodgkin's disease, mixed cellularity type, with a high content of epithelioid cells. Am J Surg Pathol 13:1014–1022

Patsouris E, Noel H, Lennert K (1990) Lymphoplasmacytic/lymphoplasmacytoid immunocytoma with a high content of epithelioid cells. Histologic and immunohistochemical findings. Am J Surg Pathol 14:660–670

Patsouris E, Engelhard M, Zwingers T, Lennert K (1993) Lymphoepithelioid cell lymphoma (Lennert's lymphoma): clinical features derived from analysis of 108 cases. Br J Haematol 84:346-348

Paulli M, Berti E, Rosso R, Boveri E, Kindl S, Klersy C, Lazzarino M, Borroni G, Menestrina F, Santucci M, Gambini C, Vassallo G, Magrini U, Sterry W, Burg G, Geerts ML, Meijer CJLM, Willemze R, Feller AC, Müller-Hermelink HK, Kadin ME (1995) CD30/Ki-1-positive lymphoproliferative disorders of the skin. Clinicopathologic correlation and statistical analysis of 86 cases: a multicentric study from the European Organization for Research and Treatment of Cancer Cutaneous Lymphoma Project Group. J Clin Oncol 13:1343–1354

Pautier P, Devidas A, Delmer A, Dombret H, Sutton L, Zini JM, Nedelec G, Molina T, Marolleau JP, Brice P (1999) Angioimmunoblastic-like T-cell non Hodgkin's lymphoma: outcome after chemotherapy in 33 patients and review of the literature. Leuk Lymph 32:545–552

Pelicci PG, Knowles DM, Favera RD (1985) Lymphoid tumors displaying rearrangements of both immunoglobulin and T cell receptor genes. J Exp Med 162:1015–1024

Petkovic I, Josip K, Nakic M, Kastelan J (1996) Cytogenetic, cytomorphologic, and immunologic analysis in 55 children with acute lymphoblastic leukemia. Cancer Genet Cytogenet 88:57–65

Pileri S, Falini B, Delsol G, Stein H, Baglioni P, Poggi S, Martelli MF, Rivano MT, Mason DY, Stansfeld AG (1990) Lymphohistiocytic T-cell lymphoma (anaplastic large cell lymphoma CD30+/Ki-1+ with a high content of reactive histiocytes). Histopathology 16:383–391

Pileri SA, Piccaluga A, Poggi S, Sabattini E, Piccaluga PP, De Vivo A, Falini B, Stein H (1995) Anaplastic large cell lymphoma: update of findings. Leuk Lymph 18:17–25

Pilozzi E, Müller-Hermelink HK, Falini B, De Wolf-Peeters C, Fidler C, Gatter K, Wainscoat J (1999) Gene rearrangements in T-cell lymphoblastic lymphoma. J Pathol 188:267–270

Piris M, Brown DC, Gatter KC, Mason DY (1990) CD30 expression in non-Hodgkin's lymphoma. Histopathology 17:211–218

Poiesz BJ, Ruscetti FW, Gazdar AF, Bunn PA, Minna JD, Gallo RC (1980) Detection and Isolation of type C retrovirus articles from fresh and cultured lymphocytes of a patient with cutaneous T-cell lymphoma. Proc Natl Acad Sci USA 77:7415–7419

Poppema S, Kaiserling E, Lennert K (1979) Nodular paragranuloma and progressively transformed germinal centers. Ultrastructural and immunohistologic findings. Virchows Arch [B] 31:211–225

Pui CH, Rubnitz JE, Hancock ML, Downing JR, Raimondi SC, Rivera GK, Sandlund JT, Ribeiro RC, Head DR, Relling MV, Evans WE, Behm FG (1998) Reappraisal of the clinical and biologic significance of myeloid-associated antigen expression in childhood acute lymphoblastic leukemia. J Clin Oncol 16:3768–3773

Pulford K, Lamant L, Morris SW, Butler LH, Wood KM, Stroud D, Delsol G, Mason DY (1997) Detection of anaplastic lymphoma kinase (ALK) and nucleolar protein nucleophosmin (NPM)-ALK proteins in normal and neoplastic cells with the monoclonal antibody ALK1. Blood 89:1394–1404

Reiter A, Schrappe M, Parwaresch R, Henze G, Müller-Weihrich S, Sauter S, Sykora K-W, Ludwig W-D, Gadner H, Riehm H (1995) Non-Hodgkin's lymphomas of childhood and adolescence: results of a treatment stratified for biologic subtypes and stage: a report of the Berlin-Frankfurt-Münster Group. J Clin Oncol 13:359–372

Reiter A, Schrappe M, Ludwig WD, Tiemann M, Parwaresch R, Zimmermann M, Schirg E, Henze G, Schellong G, Gadner H, Riehm H (2000) Intensive ALL-type therapy without local radiotherapy provides a 90% event-free survival for children with T-cell lymphoblastic lymphoma: a BFM group report. Blood 95:416–421

Rosso R, Paulli M, Magrini U, Kindl S, Boveri E, Volpato G, Poggi S, Baglioni P, Pileri S (1990) Anaplastic large cell lymphoma, CD30/Ki-1 positive, expressing the CD15/Leu-M1 antigen. Immunohistochemical and morphological relationships to Hodgkin's disease. Virchows Arch A Pathol Anat 416:229–235

Rüdiger T, Ichinohasama R, Ott MM, Muller-Deubert S, Miura I, Ott G, Muller-Hermelink HK (2000) Peripheral T-cell lymphoma with distinct perifollicular growth pattern: a distinct subtype of T-cell lymphoma? Am J Surg Pathol 24:117–122

Rüdiger T, Weisenburger DD, Anderson JR, Armitage JO, Diebold J, MacLennan KA, Nathwani BN, Ullrich F, Müller-Hermelink HK (2002) Peripheral T-cell lymphoma (excluding anaplastic large-cell lymphoma): results from the Non-Hodgkin's Lymphoma Classification Project. Ann Oncol 13:140–149

Salhany KE, Cousar JB, Greer JP, Casey TT, Fields JP, Collins RD (1988) Transformation of cutaneous T-cell lymphoma to large cell lymphoma: a clinicopathologic and immunologic study. Am J Pathol 132:265–277

Sarris AH, Luthra R, Papadimitracopoulou V, Waasdorp M, Dimopoulos MA, MacBride JJ, Cabanillas F, Duvic M, Deisseroth A, Morris SW, Pugh WC (1996) Amplification of genomic DNA demonstrates the presence of the t(2;5)(p23;q35) in anaplastic large cell lymphoma, but not in other non-Hodgkin's lymphomas, Hodgkin's disease, or lymphomatoid papulosis. Blood 88:1771–1779

Schlegelberger B, Himmler A, Gödde E, Grote W, Feller AC, Lennert K (1994) Cytogenetic findings in peripheral T-cell lymphomas as a basis for distinguishing low-grade and high-grade lymphomas. Blood 83:505–511

Schlegelberger B, Zwingers T, Hohenadel K, Henne-Bruns D, Schmitz N, Haferlach T, Tirier C, Bartels H, Sonnen R, Kuse R, Grote W (1996) Significance of cytogenetic findings for the clinical outcome in patients with T-cell lymphoma of angioimmunoblastic lymphadenopathy type. J Clin Oncol 14:593–599

Sheibani K, Winberg C, Burke J, Rappaport H (1984) Monocytoid cells in reactive follicular hyperplasia with and without multifocal histiocytic reactions: an immunohistochemical study of 21 cases including suspected cases of toxoplasmic lymphadenitis. Lab Invest 50:53A–54A

Shimoyama M, Minato K, Saito H, Takenaka T, Watanabe S, Nagatani T, Naruto M (1979) Immunoblastic lymphadenopathy (IBL)-like T-cell lymphoma. Jpn J Clin Oncol 9 [Suppl]:347–356

Shiota M, Nakamura S, Ichinohasama R, Abe M, Akagi T, Takeshita M, Mori N, Fujimoto J, Miyauchi J, Mikata A et al (1995) Anaplastic large cell lymphomas expressing the chimeric protein p80 NPM/ALK: a distinct clinico-pathologic entity. Blood 86:1954–1960

Siegel R, Gartenhaus R, Kuzel T (2001) HTLV-I associated leukemia/lymphoma: epidemiology, biology, and treatment. Cancer Treat Res 104:75–88

Siegert W, Nerl C, Meuthen I, Zahn T, Brack N, Lennert K, Huhn D (1991) Recombinant human interferon-α in the treatment of angioimmunoblastic lymphadenopathy. Results in 12 patients. Leukemia 5:892–895

Siegert W, Agthe A, Griesser H, Schwerdtfeger R, Brittinger G, Engelhard M, Kruse R, Tiemann M, Lennert K, Huhn D (1992) Treatment of angioimmunoblastic lymphadenopathy (AILD) type T-cell lymphoma using prednisone with or without the COPBLAM/IMVP-16 regimen. A multicenter study. Kiel Lymphoma Study Group. Ann Intern Med 117:364–70

Siegert W, Nerl C, Engelhard M, Brittinger G, Tiemann M, Parwaresch R, Heinz R, Huhn D (1994) Peripheral T-cell non-Hodgkin's lymphomas of low malignancy: prospective study of 25 patients with pleomorphic small cell lymphoma, lymphoepitheloid cell (Lennert's) lymphoma and T-zone lymphoma. The Kiel Lymphoma Study Group. Br J Haematol 87:529–534

Siegert W, Nerl C, Agthe A, Engelhard M, Brittinger G, Tiemann M, Lennert K, Huhn D (1995) Angioimmunoblastic lymphadenopathy (AILD)-type T-cell lymphoma: prognostic impact of clinical observations and laboratory findings at presentation. Ann Oncol 6:659–664

Skinnider BF, Connors JM, Sutcliffe SB, Gascoyne RD (1999) Anaplastic large cell lymphoma: a clinicopathologic analysis. Hematol Oncol 17:137–148

Slater DN (1987) Recent developments in cutaneous lymphoproliferative disorders. J Pathol 153:5–1

Stein H (1993) Ki-1-anaplastic large cell lymphoma: is it a discrete entity? Leuk Lymph 10:81–84

Stein H, Lennert K, Mason DY, Liangru S, Ziegler A (1984) Immature sinus histiocytes. Their identification as a novel B-cell population. Am J Pathol 117:44–52

Stein H, Mason DY, Gerdes J, O'Connor N, Wainscoat J, Pallesen G, Gatter K, Falini B, Delsol G, Lemke H et al (1985) The expression of the Hodgkin's disease associated antigen Ki-1 in reactive and neoplastic lymphoid tissue: evidence that Reed-Sternberg cells and histiocytic malignancies are derived from activated lymphoid cells. Blood 66:848–858

Stein H, Foss HD, Durkop H, Marafioti T, Delsol G, Pulford K, Pileri S, Falini B (2000) CD30+ anaplastic large cell lymphoma: a review of its histopathologic, genetic, and clinical features. Blood 96:3681–3695

Sterry W (1985) Mycosis fungoides. Curr Top Pathol 74:167–223

Suchi T, Lennert K, Tu LY, Kikuchi M, Sato E, Stansfeld AG, Feller AC (1987) Histopathology and immunohistochemistry of peripheral T-cell lymphomas: a proposal for their classification. J Clin Pathol 40:995–1015

Suzuki R, Kagami Y, Takeuchi K, Kami M, Okamoto M, Ichinohasama R, Mori N, Kojima M, Yoshino T, Yamabe H, Shiota M, Mori S, Ogura M, Hamajima N, Seto M, Suchi T, Morishima Y, Nakamura S (2000) Prognostic significance of CD56 expression for ALK-positive and ALK-negative anaplastic large-cell lymphoma of T/null cell phenotype. Blood 96:2993–3000

Tajima K, Kuroishi T (1985) Estimation of rate of incidence of ATL among ATLV (HTLV-I) carriers in Kyushu, Japan. Jpn J Clin Oncol 15:423–430

Tajima K, Tominaga S, Suchi T (1986) Malignant lymphomas in Japan: epidemiological analysis on adult T-cell leukemia, lymphoma. Hematol Oncol 4:31–44

Takatsuki K, Uchiyama T, Sagawa K, Yodoi J (1976) Adult T cell leukemia in Japan. Excerpta Medica Int Congr Ser 415:73–77

Takeshita M, Akamatsu M, Ohshima K, Suzumiya J, Kikuchi M, Kimura N, Uike N, Okamura T (1996) Agiocentric immunoproliferative lesions of the lymph node. Am J Clin Pathol 106:69–77

Tawa A, Benedict SH, Hara J, Hozumi N, Gelfand EW (1987) Rearrangement of the T cell receptor γ-chain gene in childhood acute lymphoblastic leukemia. Blood 70:1933–1939

The Non-Hodgkin's Lymphoma Classification Project (1997) A clinical evaluation of the International Lymphoma Study Group classification of non-Hodgkin's lymphoma. The Non-Hodgkin's Lymphoma Classification Project. Blood 89:3909–3918

Tilly H, Gaulard P, Lepage E, Dumontet C, Diebold J, Plantier I, Berger F, Symann M, Petrella T, Lederlin P, Briere J (1997) Primary anaplastic large-cell lymphoma in adults: clinical presentation, immunophenotype, and outcome. Blood 90:3727–3734

Tirelli U, Vaccher E, Zagonel V, Talamini R, Bernardi D, Tavio M, Gloghini A, Merola MC, Monfardini S; Carbone A (1995) CD30 (Ki-1)-positive anaplastic large-cell lymphomas in 13 patients with and 27 patients without human immunodeficiency virus infection: the first comparative clinicopathologic study from a single institution that also includes 80 patients with other human immunodeficiency virus-related systemic lymphomas. J Clin Oncol 13:373–380

Touriol C, Greenland C, Lamant L, Pulford K, Bernard F, Rousset T, Mason DY, Delsol G (2000) Further demonstration of the diversity of chromosomal changes involving 2p23 in ALK-positive lymphoma: two cases expressing ALK kinase fused to CTLC (clathrin chain polypeptide-like). Blood 95:3204–3207

Trinkler B, Mustroph D, Hagenah H, Mönch H, von Heyden HW (1989) Alpha-interferon for the treatment of angioimmunoblastic lymphadenopathy and B-cell prolymphocytic leukemia. Mol Biother 1 [Suppl]: abstract 93

Tsukasaki K, Koeffler P, Tomonage M (2000) Human T-lymphotropic virus type 1 infection. Baillieres Best Pract Res Haematol 13:231–243

Tubergen DG, Krailo MD, Meadows AT, Rosenstock J, Kadin M, Morse M, King D, Steinherz PG, Kersey JH (1995) Comparison of treatment regimens for pediatric lymphoblastic Non-Hodgkin's lymphoma: a Childrens Cancer Group study. J Clin Oncol 13:1368–1376

Van den Oord JJ, de Wolf-Peeters C, de Vos R, Desmet VJ (1985) Immature sinus histiocytosis. Light- and electron-microscopic features, immunologic phenotype, and relationship with marginal zone lymphocytes. Am J Pathol 118:266–277

van der Werff' ten Bosch J, Delabie J, Bohler T, Verschuere J, Thielemans K (1999) Revision of the diagnosis of T-zone lymphoma in the father of a patient with autoimmune lymphoproliferative syndrome type II. Br J Haematol 106:1045–1048

Vyth-Dreese FA, de Vries JE (1982) Human T-cell leukemia virus in lymphocytes from T-cell leukemia patient originating from Surinam (letter). Lancet ii:993

Weisenburger DD, Nathwani BN, Forman SJ, Rappaport H (1982) Noncutaneous peripheral T-cell lymphoma histologically resembling mycosis fungoides. Cancer 49:1839–1847

Weiss LM, Hu E, Wood GS, Moulds C, Cleary ML, Warnke R, Sklar J (1985) Clonal rearrangements of T-cell receptor genes in mycosis fungoides and dermatopathic lymph-adenopathy. N Engl J Med 313:539–544

Willemze R, Kerl H, Sterry W, Berti E, Cerroni L, Chimenti S, Diaz-Perez JL, Geerts ML, Goos M, Knobler R, Ralfkiaer E, Santucci M, Smith N, Wechsler J, van Vloten WA, Meijer CJ (1997) EORTC classification for primary cutaneous lymphomas: a proposal from the Cutaneous Lymphoma Study Group of the European Organization for Research and Treatment of Cancer. Blood 90:354–371

Willenbrock K, Roers A, Seidl C, Wacker HH, Kuppers R, Hansmann ML (2001) Analysis of T-cell subpopulations in T-cell non-Hodgkin's lymphoma of angioimmunoblastic lymphadenopathy with dysproteinemia type by single targetgene amplification of T cell receptor-beta gene rearrangements. Am J Pathol 158:1851–1857

Yamamura M, Honda M, Yamada Y, Itoyama T, Sohda H, Yubashi T, Momita S, Kamihira S, Ohmoto Y, Tomonaga M (1996) Increased levels of interleukin-6 (IL-6) in serum and spontaneous in vitro production of IL-6 by lymph node mononuclear cells of patients with angio-immunoblastic lymphadenopathy with dysproteinemia (AILD), and clinical effectiveness of cyclosporin A. Leukemia 10:1504–1508

Yamashita Y, Nakamura S, Kagami Y, Hasegawa Y, Kojima H, Nagasawa T, Mori N (2000) Lennert's lymphoma: a variant of cytotoxic T-cell lymphoma? Am J Surg Pathol 24:1627–1633

Zettl A, Lee SS, Rudiger T, Starostik P, Marino M, Kirchner T, Ott M, Müller-Hermelink HK, Ott G (2002) Epstein-Barr virus-associated B-cell lymphoproliferative disorders in angioimmunoblastic T-cell lymphoma and peripheral T-cell lymphoma, unspecified. Am J Clin Pathol 117:368–379

Further Reading

Lymphoblastic T

Amylon MD, Shuster J, Pullen J, Berard C, Link MP, Wharam M, Katz J, Yu A, Laver J, Ravindranath Y, Kurtzberg J, Desai S, Camitta B, Murphy SB (1999) Intensive high-dose asparaginase consolidation improves survival for pediatric patients with T cell acute lymphoblastic leukemia and advanced stage lymphoblastic lymphoma: a Pediatric Oncology Group study. Leukemia 13:335–342

Bernard A, Boumsell L, Reinherz EL, Nadler LM, Ritz J, Coppin H, Richard Y, Valensi F, Dausset J, Flandrin G, Lemerle J,

Schlossman SF (1981) Cell surface characterization of malignant T cells from lymphoblastic lymphoma using monoclonal antibodies: evidence for phenotypic differences between malignant T cells from patients with acute lymphoblastic leukemia and lymphoblastic lymphoma. Blood 57:1105–1110

Brumpt C, Delabesse E, Beldjord K, Davi F, Gayuela JM, Millien C, Villarese P, Quartier P, Buzyn A, Valensi F, Macintyre E (2000) The incidence of clonal T-cell receptor rearrangements in B-cell precursor acute lymphoblastic leukemia varies with age and genotype. Blood 96:2254–2261

Felix CA, Wright JJ, Poplack DG, Reaman GH, Cole D, Goldman P, Korsmeyer SJ (1987) T cell receptor α-, β-, and γ-genes in T cell and pre-B cell acute lymphoblastic leukemia. J Clin Invest 80:545–556

Kersey J, Abramson C, Perry G, Goldman A, Nesbit M, Gajl-Peczalska K, LeBien T (1982) Clinical usefulness of monoclonal-antibody phenotyping in childhood acute lymphoblastic leukemia. Lancet ii:1419–1423

Knowles DM (1986) The human T-cell leukemias: clinical, cytomorphologic, immunophenotypic, and genotypic characteristics. Hum Pathol 17:14–33

Korsmeyer SJ, Arnold A, Bakhshi A, Ravetch JV, Siebenlist U, Hieter PA; Sharrow SO, LeBien TW, Kersey JH, Poplack DG, Leder P, Waldmann TA (1983) Immunoglobulin gene rearrangement and cell surface antigen expression in acute lymphocytic leukemias of T cell and B cell precursor origins. J Clin Invest 71:301–313

Laver J, Amylon M, Desai S, Link M, Schwenn M, Mahmoud H, Shuster J (1998) Randomized trial of r-metHu granulocyte Colony-stimulating factor in an intensive treatment for T-cell leukemia and advanced-stage lymphoblastic lymphoma of childhood: a Pediatric Oncology Group pilot study. J Clin Oncol 16:522–526

Look AT, Roberson PK, Williams DL, Rivera G, Bowman WP, Pui CH, Ochs J, Abromowitch M, Kalwinsky D, Dahl GV, George S, Murphy SB (1985) Prognostic importance of blast cell DNA content in childhood acute lymphoblastic leukemia. Blood 65:1079–1086

Rosenquist R, Lindh J, Roos G, Holmberg D (1997) Immunoglobulin V_H gene replacements in a T-cell lymphoblastic lymphoma. Mol Immunol 34:305–313

Sano K, Goji J, Kosaka Y, Nakamura H, Nakamura F, Tatsumi E (1998) Translocation (10;12)(q24;q15) in a T-cell lymphoblastic lymphoma with myeloid hyperplasia. Cancer Genet Cytogenet 105:168–171

Uckun FM, Sensel MG, Sun L, Steinherz PG, Trigg ME, Heerema NA, Sather HN, Reaman GH, Gaynon PS (1998) Biology and treatment of childhood T-lineage acute lymphoblastic leukemia. Blood 91:735–746

Wan TSK, Ma SK, Chan GCF, Ching LM, Ha SY, Chan LC (2000) Complex cytogenetic abnormalities in T-lymphoblastic lymphoma: resolution by spectral karyotyping. Cancer Genet Cytogenet 118:24–27

Weiss LM, Bindl JM, Picozzi VJ, Link MP, Warnke RA (1986) Lymphoblastic lymphoma: an immunophenotype study of 26 cases with comparison to T cell acute lymphoblastic leukemia. Blood 67:474–478

Lymphoblastic T+B

Amor DJ, Algar EM, Slater HR, Smith PJ (1998) High frequency of t(12;21) in childhood acute lymphoblastic leukemia detected by RT-PCR. Pathology 30:381–385

Berger R (1997) Acute lymphoblastic leukemia and chromosome 21. Cancer Genet Cytogenet 94:8–12

Bollum FJ (1979) Terminal deoxynucleotidyl transferase as a hematopoietic cell marker. Blood 54:1203–1215

Chimenti S, Fink-Puches R, Peris K, Pescarmona E, Pütz B, Kerl H, Cerroni L (1999) Cutaneous involvement in lymphoblastic lymphoma. J Cutan Pathol 26:379–385

Greaves MF, Chan LC, Furley AJW, Watt SM, Molgaard HV (1986) Lineage promiscuity in hemopoietic differentiation and leukemia. Blood 67:1–11

Hoelzer D, Thiel E, Löffler H, Bodenstein H, Plaumann L, Büchner T, Urbanitz D, Koch P, Heimpel H, Engelhardt R, Müller U, Wendt F-C, Sodomann H, Rühl H, Herrmann F, Kaboth W, Dietzfelbinger H, Pralle H, Lunschen C, Hellriegel K-P, Spors S, Nowrousian RM, Fischer J, Fülle H, Mitrous PS, Pfreundschuh M, Görg C, Emmerich B, Queisser W, Meyer P, Labedzki L, Essers U, König H, Mainzer K, Herrmann R, Messerer D, Zwingers T (1984) Intensified therapy in acute lymphoblastic and acute undifferentiated leukemia in adults. Blood 64:38–47

Horibe K, Hara J, Yagi K, Tawa A, Komada Y, Oda M, Nishimura SI, Ishikawa Y, Kudoh T, Ueda K (2000) Prognostic factors in childhood acute lymphoblastic leukemia in Japan. Int J Hematol 72:61–68

Kaiser U, Uebelacker I, Havemann K (1999) Non-Hodgkin's lymphoma protocols in the treatment of patients with Burkitt's lymphoma and lymphoblastic lymphoma: a report on 58 patients. Leuk Lymph 36:101–108

Kjeldsberg CR, Wilson JF, Berard CW (1983) Non-Hodgkin's lymphoma in children. Hum Pathol 14:612–627

Knowles DM (2001) Lymphoblastic lymphoma. In: Knowles DM (ed) Neoplastic hematopathology. Lippincott Williams and Wilkins, Philadelphia, pp 915–951

Kung PC, Long JC, McCaffrey RP, Ratliff RL, Harrison TA, Baltimore D (1978) Terminal deoxynucleotidyl transferase in the diagnosis of leukemia and malignant lymphoma. Am J Med 64:788–794

Mittelman F (1981) The 3rd international workshop on chromosomes in leukemia. Lund, Sweden, 21–25 July 1980. Introduction. Cancer Genet Cytogenet 4:96–98

Nakamura F, Tatsumi E, Kawano S, Tani A, Kumagai S (1997) Acute lymphoblastic leukemia/lymphoblastic lymphoma of natural killer (NK) lineage: quest for another NK-lineage neoplasm (letter to the editor). Blood 89:4665–4666

Nathwani BN, Diamond LW, Winberg CD, Kim H, Bearman RM, Glick JH, Jones SE, Gams RA, Nissen NI, Rappaport H (1981) Lymphoblastic lymphoma: a clinicopathologic study of 95 patients. Cancer 48:2347–2357

Pui CH (1995) Childhood leukemias. N Engl J Med 332:1618–1630

Raimondi SC (1993) Current status of cytogenetic research in childhood acute lymphoblastic leukemia. Blood 81:2237–2251

Sheibani K, Nathwani BN, Winberg CD, Burke JS, Swartz WG, Blayney D, van de Velde S, Hill LR, Rappaport H (1987) Antigenically defined subgroups of lymphoblastic lymphoma.

Relationship to clinical presentation and biologic behavior. Cancer 60:183–190
Sobol RE, Mick R, Royston I, Davey FR, Ellison RR, Newman R, Cuttner J, Griffin JD, Collins H, Nelson DA, Bloomfield CD (1987) Clinical importance of myeloid antigen expression in adult acute lymphoblastic leukemia. N Engl J Med 316:1111–1117
Soslow RA, Bhargava V, Warnke RA (1997) MIC2, TdT, bcl-2, and CD34 expression in paraffin-embedded high-grade lymphoma/acute lymphoblastic leukemia distinguishes between distinct clinicopathologic entities. Hum Pathol 28:1158–1165
Suryanarayan K, Hunger SP, Kohler S, Carroll AJ, Crist W, Link MP, Cleary ML (1991) Consistent involvement of the BCR gene by 9;22 breakpoints in pediatric acute leukemias. Blood 77:324–330
Tawa A, Hozumi N, Minden M, Mak TW, Gelfand EW (1985) Rearrangement of the T-cell receptor β-chain gene in non-T-cell, non-B-cell acute lymphoblastic leukemia of childhood. N Engl J Med 313:1033–1037
Thomas X, Archimbaud E, Charrin C, Magaud JP, Fiere D (1995) CD34 expression is associated with major adverse prognostic factors in adult acute lymphoblastic leukemia. Leukemia 9:249–253
Vannier JP, Bene MC, Faure GC, Bastard C, Garand R, Bernard A (1989) Investigation of the CD10 (cALLA) negative acute lymphoblastic leukemia: further description of a group with a poor prognosis. Br J Haematol 72:156–160
Williams DL, Tsiatis A, Brodeur GM, Look AT, Melvin SL, Bowman WP, Kalwinsky DK, Rivera G, Dahl GV (1982) Prognostic importance of chromosome number in 136 untreated children with acute lymphoblastic leukemia. Blood 60:864–871
Zinzani PL, Bendandi M, Visani G, Gherlinzoni F, Frezza G, Merla E, Manfroi S, Gozzetti A, Tura S (1996) Adult lymphoblastic lymphoma: clinical features and prognostic factors in 53 patients. Leuk Lymph 23:577–582

Angioimmunoblastic T-Cell Lymphoma

Lukes RJ, Tindle BH (1975) Immunoblastic lymphadenopathy: a hyperimmune entity resembling Hodgkin's disease. N Engl J Med 292:1–8
Lukes RJ, Tindle BH (1978) Immunoblastic lymphadenopathy: a prelymphomatous state of immunoblastic sarcoma. Rec Res Cancer Res 64:241–246
Nathwani BN, Rappaort H, Moran EM, Pangalis GA, Kim H (1978) Evolution of immunoblastic lymphoma in angioimmunoblastic lymphadenopathy. Rec Res Cancer Res 64:235–240
Radaszkiewicz T, Lennert K (1975) Lymphogranulomatosis X. Klinisches Bild, Therapie und Prognose. Dtsch Med Wochenschr 100:1157–1163
Radaszkiewicz T, Hansmann M-L, Lennert K (1989) Monoclonality and polyclonality of plasma cells in Castleman's disease of the plasma cell variant. Histopathology 14:11–24
Shimoyama M, Tobiani K, Minato K, Watanabe S (1987) Immunoblastic lymphadenopathy (IBL)-like T cell lymphoma. Rec Adv RES Res 23:161–170

6 Extranodal Lymphoma

6.1 Introduction

About 30–40% of all malignant lymphomas arise primarily at extranodal sites. The incidence of extranodal lymphomas in different countries parallels that of nodal lymphomas, indicating that a high frequency of nodal lymphomas implies a high frequency of extranodal lymphomas as well (Newton et al. 1997). Beyond that, a dramatic increase of extranodal lymphomas has been observed due to AIDS. The most frequent sites of extranodal lymphomas in general are the gastrointestinal tract and the skin.

However, the definition of a primary extranodal lymphoma (PENL) is to some extent still an artificial one. Today, it is more or less agreed that lymphomas which at one time have had their major tumor mass at an extranodal site are defined as being extranodal. However, nodal and extranodal lymphomas which have disseminated may be difficult to classify correctly in terms of their primary origin. This is especially true as the morphology and the immunophenotype of some extranodal lymphomas can be identical to those of nodal ones.

On the other hand, it has become clear, especially with the current concept of the mucosa-associated lymphoid tissue (MALT) systems and its lymphomas, that some extranodal lymphomas have their own biology, morphology, and even immunophenotype. Thus it is possible to define some clinical pathological entities.

In principle, all organ sites may be site of origin of a PENL (Table 6.1). The most common sites which are involved are also indicated.

Table 6.1. Organ localization of extranodal non-Hodgkin's lymphomas

Gastrointestinal tract
Upper aerodigestive tract
Salivary glands
Eye, lacrimal glands and orbit
Mediastinum
Lung
Pleura
Heart
Spleen
Liver
Reproductive and urinary system
Endocrine organs
Skin
Soft tissue
Bone
Central nervous system
Intravascular lymphoma

Those lymphoma types which today represent distinct clinicopathological entities will be described in detail. Those which are morphologically and immunophenotypically identical to their nodal counterparts are simply indicated, and the reader is referred to the chapter on nodal lymphomas. It is clear that the main distinction between B- and T-cell lymphomas, which was first introduced by the Kiel classification in 1988 for nodal lymphomas, is also valid and important for extranodal lymphomas. Therefore this distinction is also used in this chapter.

Moreover, it is clear that nearly all nodal lymphoma types can disseminate secondarily from a nodal to extranodal sites. These types are described in the chapter on nodal lymphomas and are mentioned here only with respect to their frequency of occurrence. Each section is preceded by a table of the secondary extranodal lymphomas.

6.2 Gastrointestinal Lymphoma

The GI-tract is the most frequent site of extranodal lymphomas. Virtually almost all these neoplasms are non-Hodgkin's lymphomas, indicating that the diagnosis of a primary Hodgkin's lymphoma in the GI-tract is a suspicious one. The total incidence for the GI-tract is around one case/100,000 inhabitants. These tumors account for 30–40% of all extranodal lymphomas (d'Amore et al. 1992). The primary site within the GI-tract is the stomach (60–70%) followed by the small bowel and, finally, the large bowel.

It is of major importance that the GI-tract is frequently (40–70%) involved in widespread lymphomas, which also indicates a high frequency of secondary GI-tract lymphomas. These have to be strictly distinguished from primary ones (Fischbach et al. 1992).

6.2.1 B-Cell Lymphoma

6.2.1.1 Extranodal Marginal Zone B-Cell Lymphoma of MALT (ICD-O: 9699/3)

Extranodal marginal zone B-cell lymphoma of MALT occurs in numerous organs. This MALT system consists of highly specialized epithelium and lymphoid tissue and is found mostly at sites of mucous membranes. It fulfills the duties of a mucosal immune system. Lymphomas from this system may occur at the site of a preexisting hyperplastic lymphoid system in which lymphoid tissue assembles secondarily due to the presence of a preceding inflammatory agent, the most prominent of which is *Helicobacter pylori*, or associated with certain autoimmune diseases. The various sites at which low-grade malignant lymphoma of MALT have been found are listed in Table 6.2. The most common location is undoubtedly the stomach. Other important sites are the intestine, lungs, orbit and salivary gland. Common features of all these lymphomas are the development of lymphoepithelial lesions and the occurrence of polytypic germinal centers (Isaacson 1999a).

In this section, the lymphomas of the gastrointestinal tract will be described. Other sites of MALT lymphomas will be described in the sections dealing with the different organs.

Table 6.2. Various sites of development of extranodal marginal zone lymphoma of mucosa-associated lymphoid tissue (MALT)

Conjunctiva, including the orbit
Salivary glands
Waldeyer's ring
Thyroid gland
Breast
Larynx
Lung
Stomach
Small and large intestines
Rectum
Prostate gland
Skin

Synonyms

- Kiel: Low-grade malignant B-cell lymphoma of MALT type
- REAL: Marginal zone B-cell lymphoma, extranodal
- WHO: Extranodal marginal zone B-cell lymphoma of MALT

Definition

The tumor developing in MALT predominately comprises small to medium-sized cells that have centrocyte-like (irregularly shaped) nuclei. The tumor cells may also have monocytoid or round – lymphocytic – nuclei. Basophilic blasts are always intermingled. A monotypic plasma cell component is frequently observed. The histological hallmark is the formation of lymphoepithelial lesions infiltrating and destroying the glandular epithelium. Frequently, the neoplastic cells surround reactive follicles, which are progressively colonized.

The normal cell counterpart of MALT lymphoma cells in the GI-tract is thought to be the marginal zone B-cells surrounding the follicles.

Morphology

MALT lymphoma is characterized by a typical growth pattern as well as a typical cytological appearance. The tumor cells are small to medium-sized and thus slightly larger than lymphocytes, with centrocyte-like nuclei. The cytoplasm is moderate to abundant and light or clear in Giemsa stain (Figs. 6.1, 6.2). Beside these characteristic cells, this lymphoma can cover a quite broad cytological spectrum, with monocytoid cells (bean-shaped nuclei) (Fig. 6.3) or lymphocytes with or without lymphoplasmacytoid/cytic differentiation (this latter type covers immunocytoma of the Kiel classifica-

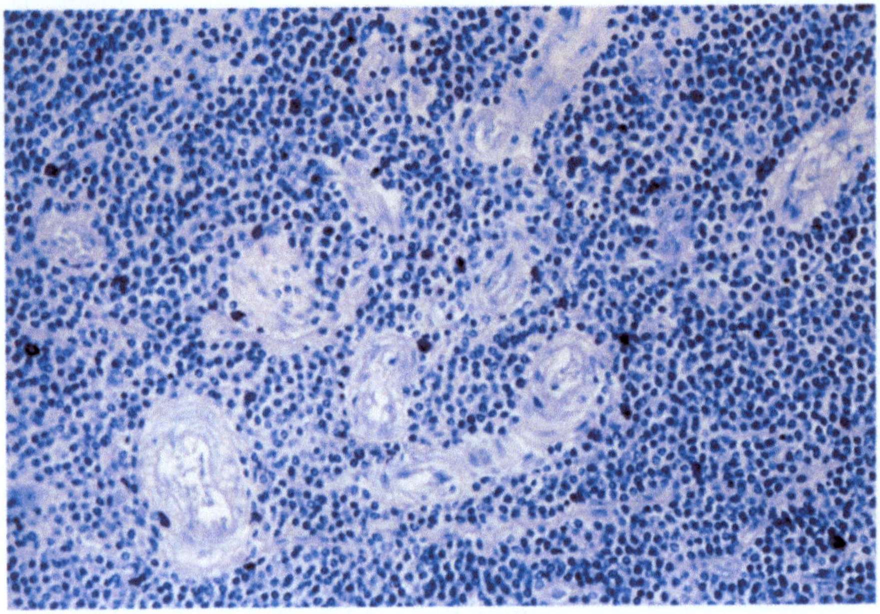

Fig. 6.1. Low-power view of a mucosa-associated lymphoid tissue (MALT) lymphoma. Diffuse infiltrate of small to medium-sized cells with an increased number of mast cells (Giemsa stain)

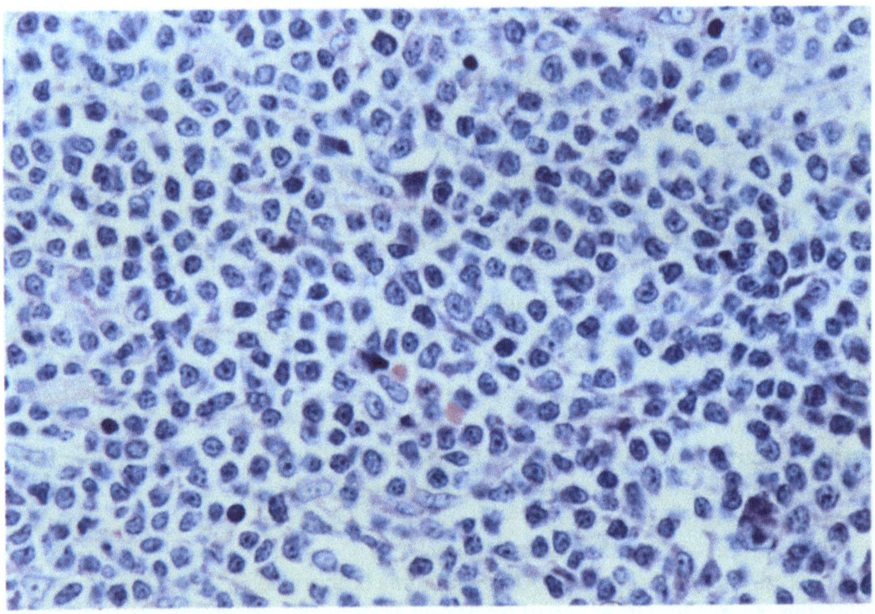

Fig. 6.2. MALT lymphoma. Note the homogeneous area of neoplastic cells and the typical centrocyte-like appearance of the nuclei (Giemsa stain)

tion). The different cell types can be intermingled with each other, or only one cell type predominates. These tumor cells are, as a rule, interspersed with large, basophilic blast cells, usually of the immunoblast type. One-third of MALT lymphomas show a plasma cell differentiation; however, it is difficult to morphologically distinguish these neoplastic plasma cells from reactive lamina propria plasma cells (Fig. 6.4).

The early infiltration pattern closely follows the structure of Peyer's patches. The lymphoma starts in the marginal zone surrounding reactive follicles (Figs. 6.5, 6.6). From this marginal zone area, the lymphoma spreads diffusely into the surrounding lamina propria and muscularis mucosae, and into the follicles. This latter phenomenon is called follicular colonization (Isaacson et al. 1991) (Fig. 6.7). If follicular coloni-

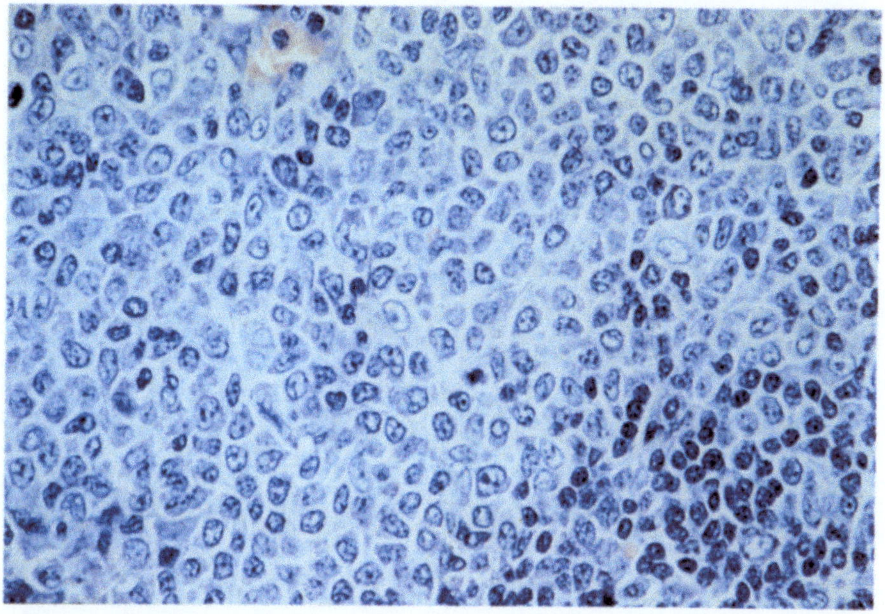

Fig. 6.3. MALT-lymphoma with an area of medium-sized cells. Note the light chromatin pattern characteristic of monocytoid B-cells (Giemsa stain)

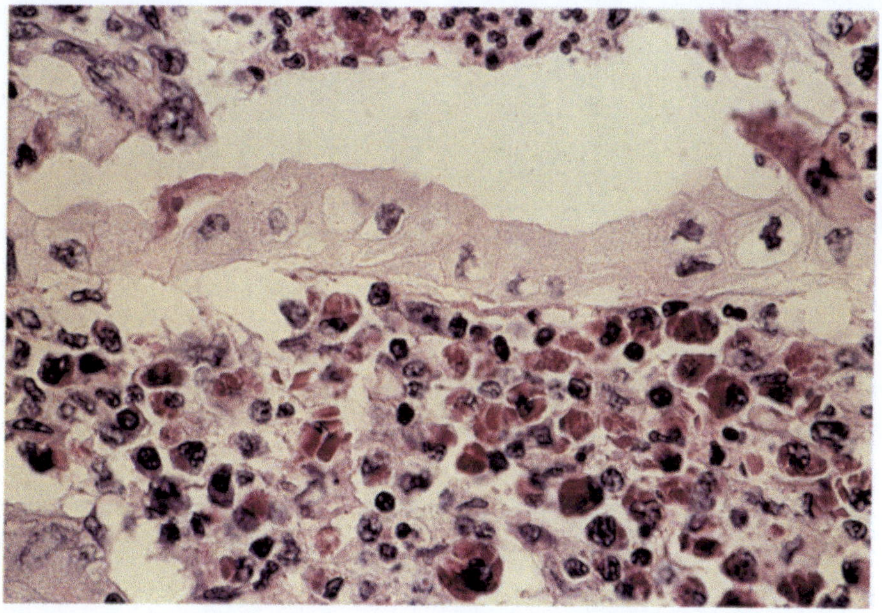

Fig. 6.4. MALT-lymphoma with multiple Dutcher bodies in a tumor with plasmacellular differentiation. (PAS stain)

zation predominates, MALT lymphoma may mimic follicular lymphoma of the stomach. The germinal centers eventually lose all centroblasts and centrocytes and are finally recognizable only from the network of follicular dendritic cells. There are also networks of follicular dendritic cells, however, that contain no other germinal center cells and may never have done so previously. Such networks are seen especially in the outermost ramifications of the tumor. Quite frequently, follicular colonization is accompanied by a marked plasma cell differentiation. This can be so prominent that one gets the impression of a plasmacytoma. Primarily, the neoplastic plasma cells are found beneath the luminal epithelium.

A hallmark of MALT lymphoma is the development of lymphoepithelial lesions (Figs. 6.8, 6.9). These are an invasion of small clusters (at least 3–5 cells) of neo-

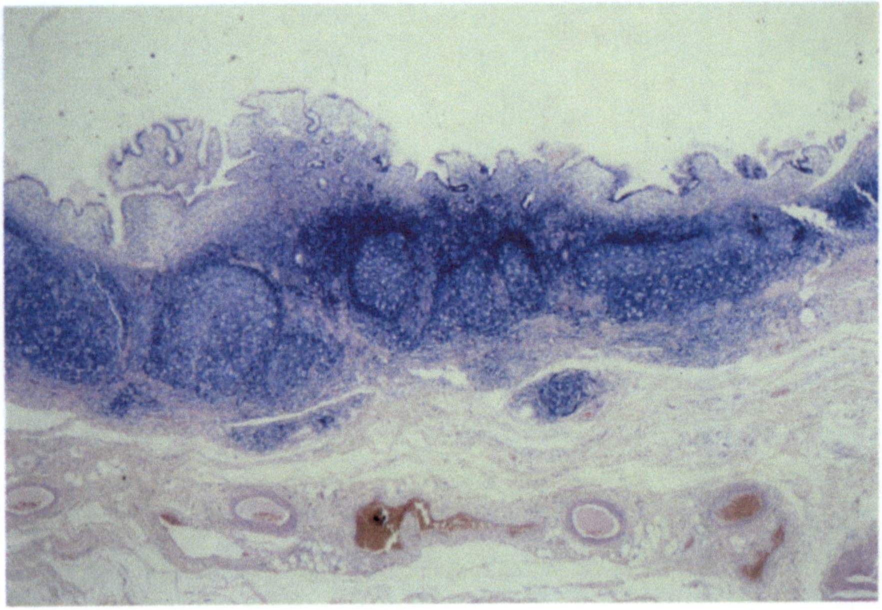

Fig. 6.5. Low-power view of an early infiltrate of a MALT-lymphoma in the stomach. Note the prominent reactive follicles surrounded by the early infiltrate (Giemsa stain)

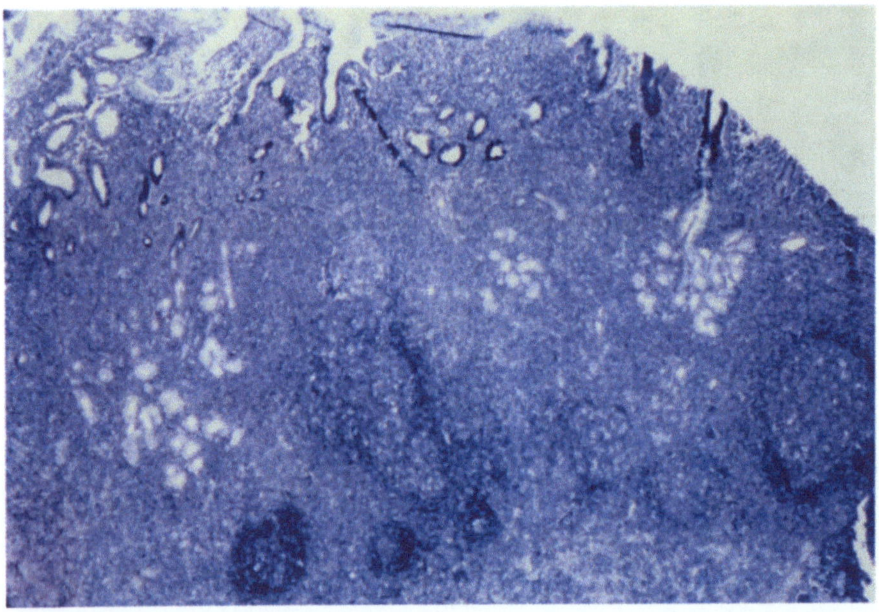

Fig. 6.6. A more diffuse infiltrate of a MALT lymphoma, with some remnants of reactive follicles (Giemsa stain)

plastic B-cells with partial or, finally, complete destruction of mucosal glands and/or crypts. Although this is a leading diagnostic hallmark, it has to be kept in mind that invasion of mucosal glands mostly without destruction may also be observed in active chronic gastritis, mostly associated with a *H. pylori* infection, and, much less frequently, in other small cell B-cell lymphomas, such as mantle cell lymphoma and follicular lymphoma. As MALT lymphoma may be multifocal, especially in the stomach, reactive-appearing follicles outside the main tumor have to be carefully studied for follicular colonization and for individual lymphoepithelial lesions in the adjacent tissue.

This possible multifocal appearance of MALT lymphoma could be explained by the coexistence of MALT lymphoma and *H. pylori* infection. The normal gastric

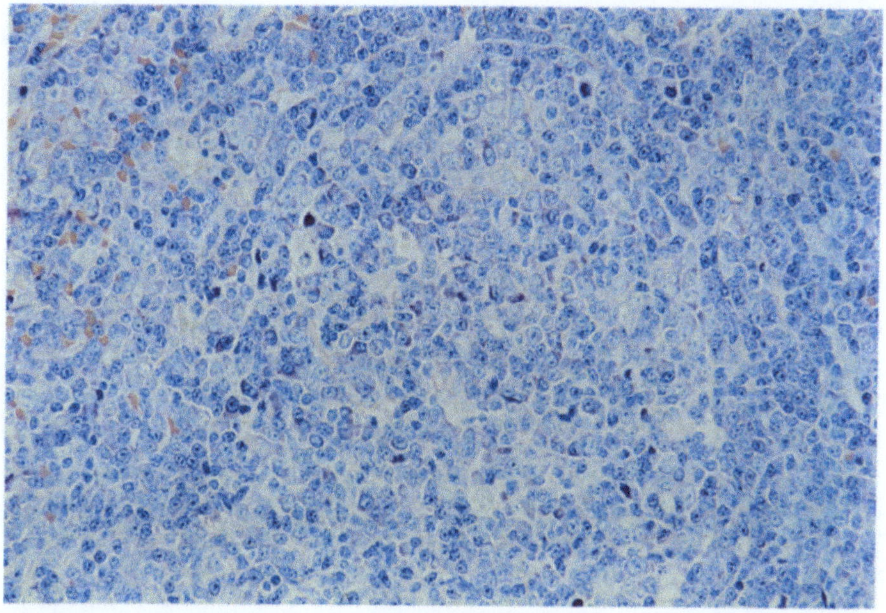

Fig. 6.7. Giemsa stain of a marginal zone B-cell lymphoma with follicular colonization. In the center, note the plasmacellular differentiation of monoclonal plasma cells (Giemsa stain)

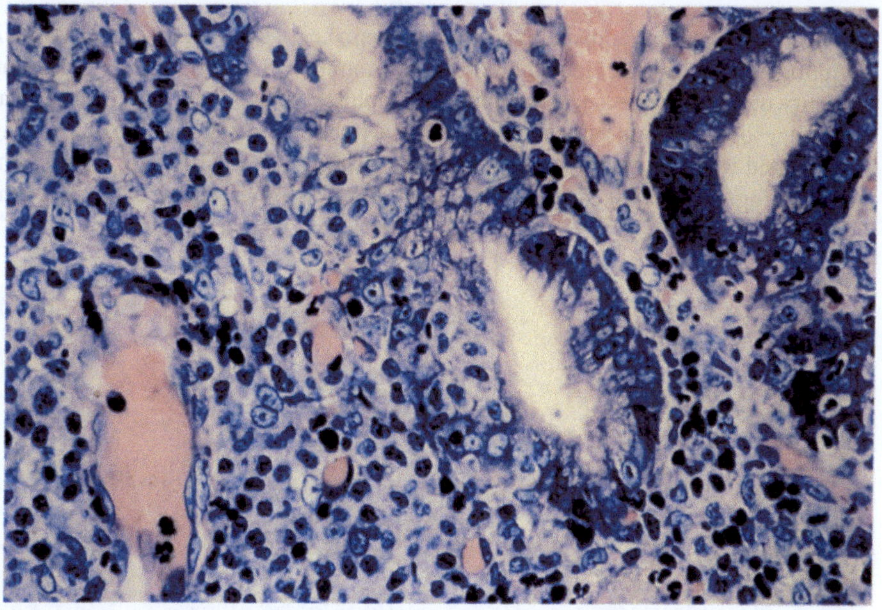

Fig. 6.8. MALT lymphoma with typical lymphoepithelial lesions (Giemsa-stain)

mucosa does not contain lymphoid tissue. Thus, reactive lymphoid tissue in this location is acquired due to longstanding infection with *H. pylori*. Therefore it is not surprising that an *H. pylori* infection can be detected in more than 90% of MALT lymphomas.

There is increasing evidence that early infiltrates of MALT lymphoma can be eradicated by antibiotic treatment. However, this is restricted to tumors confined to the mucosa. It can thus not be definitively excluded that such cases represent extreme variants of a chronic *H. pylori*-associated gastritis, especially as a continuous spectrum from chronic gastritis to early MALT lymphoma does exist. Regardless of how such cases are designated, biopsies from patients with so-called early MALT lymphoma infiltrates and a subsequent eradication therapy have to be carefully evaluated. In the pri-

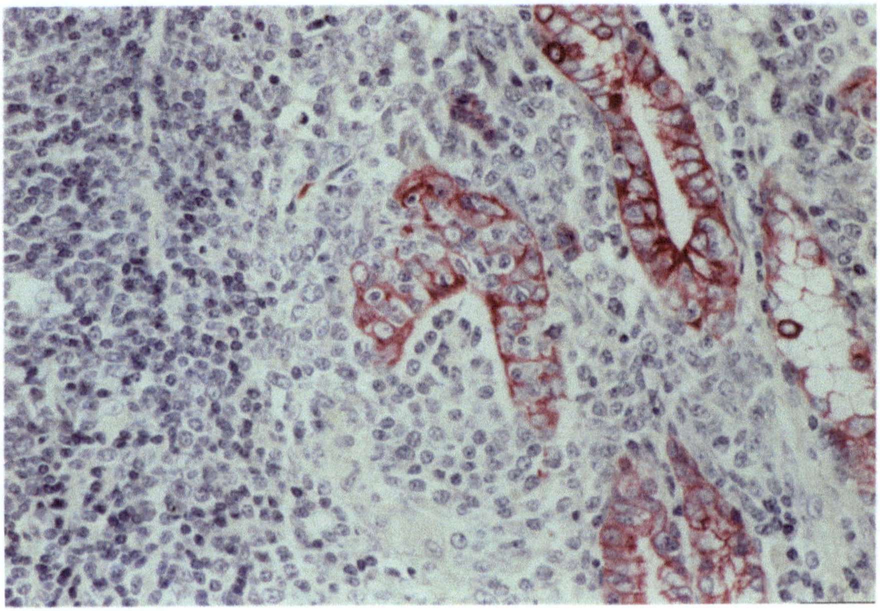

Fig. 6.9. Cytokeratin staining (KL1) demonstrates the lymphoepithelial lesions of the negative infiltrating B-cells (immunohistochemistry, alkaline phosphatase)

mary diagnosis, all prerequisites have to be present, i.e. lymphoepithelial lesions, reactive follicles, and monoclonality of the infiltrate as detected by immunohistochemistry or PCR. Subsequent biopsies have to be investigated with the identical methods to confirm or exclude progression of the disease.

Large-Cell Gastric MALT Lymphoma (Figs. 6.10, 6.11). This lymphoma represents a simultaneous or subsequent development from a small-cell MALT lymphoma and should thus be distinguished from a primary diffuse large-B-cell lymphoma (DLBCL). Whereas the former entity comprises small-cell components or was preceded by a "low grade" MALT lymphoma, the latter

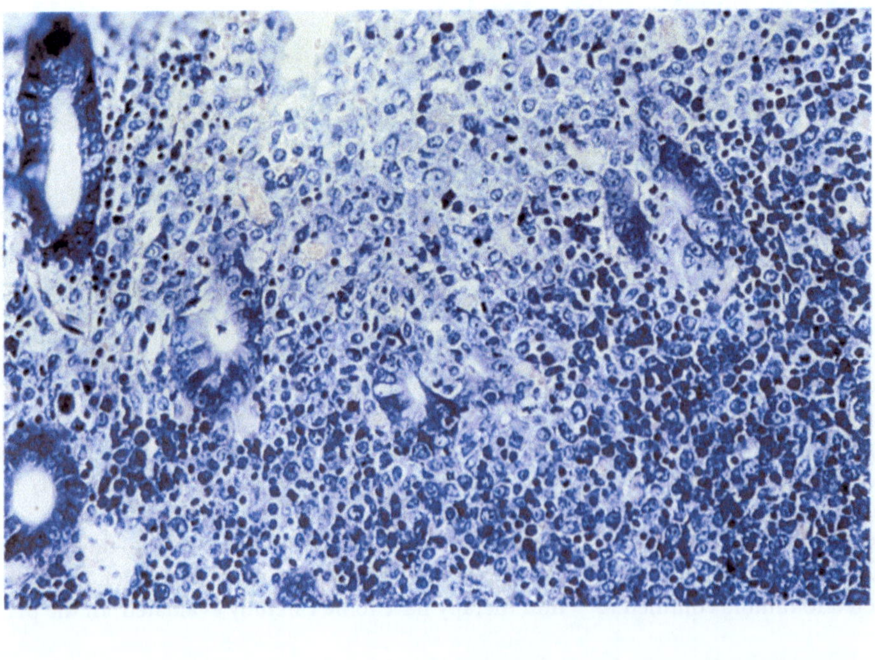

Fig. 6.10. MALT lymphoma demonstrating transformation into a diffuse large-B-cell lymphoma. Some lymphocytic infiltrates have formed lymphoepithelial lesions and are destroying the epithelial glands (Giemsa stain)

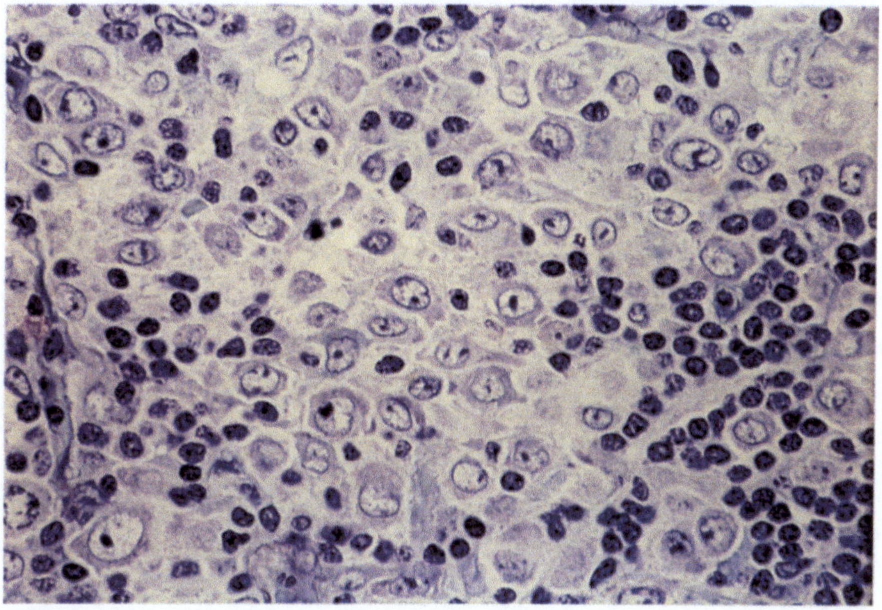

Fig. 6.11. High-power view of blasts in a MALT lymphoma that transformed into a diffuse large-B-cell lymphoma (Giemsa stain)

entity is a DLBCL de novo and thus does not comprise a small-cell component. It is still a matter of discussion whether also primary DLBCLs of the stomach belong to MALT lymphomas, as lymphoepithelial lesions can be detected and a bcl-2 rearrangement has not been found. However, the prognosis and clinical presentation seems to be different for these two types (Yoshino et al. 2000b). Irrespective of this ongoing discussion, a large-cell or blastic MALT lymphoma or a transformation can be diagnosed if confluent clusters or sheets of large blasts are detected. Cytologically, the cells may have the appearance of centroblasts, blasts with coarser chromatin, and a basophilic cytoplasm in Giemsa stain, or they may show an immunoblastic/plasmablastic differentiation. Lymphoepithelial lesions of the large-cell component are rarely seen.

Different criteria or scoring systems that can aid in the differential diagnosis (Wotherspoon et al. 1991) and in predicting prognosis are available.

De Jong et al. (1997) defined three groups of MALT lymphoma, each described by its amount of blasts within a small-cell infiltrate. Type A is defined by occasional blasts not exceeding 1 % of the total infiltrate and not forming clusters of more than five blasts. Type B allows up to 10 % blasts and occasional blasts with up to 20 cells, not forming larger sheets. If a larger amount or larger clusters are found, the infiltrate is designated as a "high-grade" lesion. This model was used to predict the outcome of patients with MALT lymphoma after disease eradication. Complete regression was achieved in 56 % of the patients. Histological grading was highly predictive in early stages (IE1) with complete remission in ten out of 12 patients in group A and one out of eight patients in group B (de Jong et al. 2001).

Lymph Node Involvement. Gastric lymph nodes are involved in 20–30 % of patients, which is equivalent to stage IIE1 (Montalban et al. 1995; Thieblemont et al. 2000). This leads to a primary interfollicular or perifollicular growth pattern, which is similar to an infiltrate in the marginal zone of the spleen. This infiltrate may be accompanied by follicular colonization. These cases have to be distinguished from follicular lymphomas. More advanced lymph node infiltrates finally completely destroy the lymph node architecture resulting in a diffuse infiltrate. The cellular composition is identical to that of the primary infiltrate. Importantly, in some cases of GI-tract MALT lymphoma, one may find an enlargement of the outer follicular mantle in the regional lymph nodes. However, this can be a reactive enlargement (Fig. 6.12) and must be thoroughly investigated by immunohistochemistry, proving or excluding monoclonality.

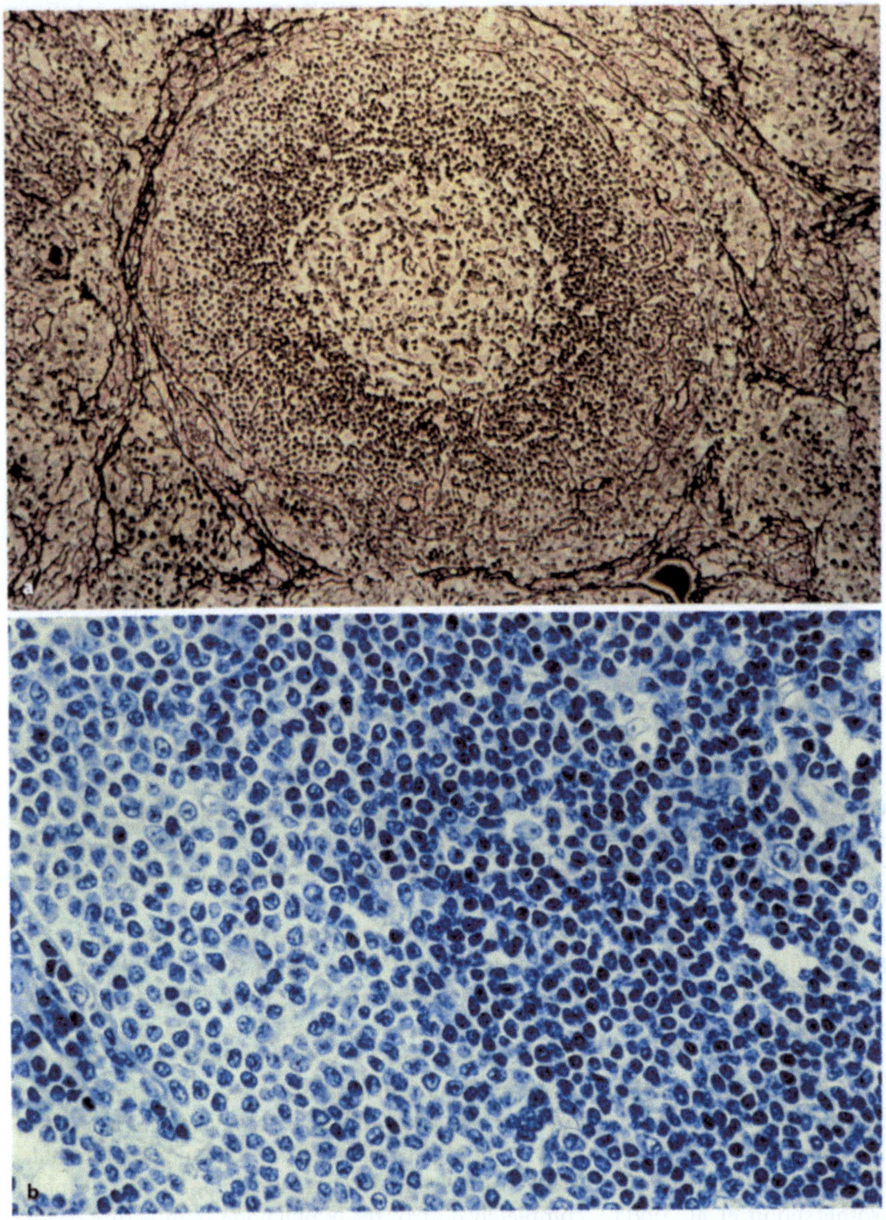

Fig. 6.12 a, b. Reactive enlargement of the marginal zone in mesenteric lymph nodes of a patient with MALT lymphoma. **a** Silver impregnation shows the enlarged marginal zone above the follicular mantle. The B cells are polyclonal. **b** High-power view of **a**: the enlarged polyclonal marginal zone appears as a light band of lymphoid cells compared to the follicular mantle (Giemsa stain)

Evolution and Transformation (Figs. 6.10, 6.11). MALT lymphoma can transform into large-B-cell lymphoma. In many cases, both components occur simultaneously. The frequency of a simultaneous large-cell or blastic component strongly depends on the number of investigated specimens (Chan et al. 1990; Hoshida et al. 1997). If up to 50 specimens are investigated, about 30% may exhibit a simultaneous large-cell or blastic component in which both components derive from the same B-cell clone (Du et al. 2000). These observations explain why there is a marked difference in detecting a high-grade component in biopsies or in resection specimens. In an additional 15–20% of the resection specimens, a high-grade component was not previously detected. The value of a detailed description of the number of blasts within a typical MALT lymphoma has been detailed by de Jong et al. (2001).

If MALT lymphoma is progressing or disseminating, it primarily involves other mucosal sites and/or the bone marrow. Generally. about 30 % of patients have disseminated disease (Thieblemont et al. 2000). If MALT lymphoma disseminates to the spleen, it homes within the marginal zone (Du et al. 1997). This has to be distinguished from primary splenic marginal zone B-cell lymphoma (MZBCL) as primary spleen involvement is associated with a favorable prognosis (Berger et al. 2000).

The association between *H. pylori* infection, ongoing chronic gastritis, and evolving MALT lymphoma is well-documented. Thus *H. pylori* is detected in more than 90 % of the gastric MALT lymphoma biopsies. Recently, it has been reported that 50 % of patients with MALT lymphoma carry anti-hepatitis-C-virus (HCV) antibodies and have detectable HCV sequences on the RNA level. Thus, HCV might be another trigger for developing MALT lymphoma (Luppi et al. 1996).

Immunohistochemistry

The tumor cells express surface immunoglobulins, mostly IgM, in addition to the B-cell antigen CD20. If a marked plasma cell differentiation is found, these cells can be stained by CD79α and CD38. With CD20 and cytokeratin KL1, lymphoepithelial lesions are readily detected. The plasma cell component has to be investigated for monotypic light-chain restriction. The neoplastic plasma cells show a prevalence of cIgM expression whereas reactive plasma cells more frequently express IgA or IgG. The tumor cells typically lack CD5, CD23 and cyclin D1 (bcl-1).

MALT lymphomas at extra-gastrointestinal sites may coexpress CD5. This immunophenotype might be associated with a tendency for dissemination to the bone marrow and other organs (Ferry et al. 1996). Such cases have been described in the Kiel classification as immunocytomas.

The follicles can be highlighted by immunohistochemical staining for follicular dendritic cells (CD23, CD35, KiM4p). The staining pattern depends on the extent of follicular colonization. Reactive follicles have preserved networks of follicular dendritic cells and contain a few polyclonal plasma cells. The reaction for bcl2 is negative, except on T cells. CD10 is weakly positive in reactive follicles. With increasing colonization, monotypic plasma cells can be detected. The network of follicular dendritic cells is reduced and less dense. The infiltrating tumor cells are bcl2-positive, and the follicle becomes CD10-negative if it is completely colonized. With increasing colonization, the number of proliferating cells (Ki-67) strongly decreases.

CD43 can be found in about 30 % of MALT lymphomas whereas it is described to be consistently negative in chronic gastritis (Arends et al. 1999).

Genetic Features

About 60 % of MALT lymphomas carry a trisomy 3 (Wotherspoon et al. 1995) whereas it occurs in about one-third of splenic MZBCLs . Other, much less frequent trisomies have been described involving chromosomes 7, 12, and 18.

No rearrangement of bcl-1, bcl-2, or bcl-6 has been detected. Translocations t(1;14) (bcl-10) (Wotherspoon et al. 1992) and t(11;18) (Griffin et al. 1992) have been reported. The bcl-2 and bcl-6 mutations are indicative of tumors that will fail to respond to eradication therapy; such patients were studied in a multicenter analysis (Wotherspoon 2000). Subsequent reports have substantiated this observation.

Immunoglobulin heavy- and light-chain rearrangements can be detected in up to 85 % of MALT lymphomas. Using PCR, single or dominant bands have been described in chronic gastritis with lymphoid hyperplasia (Torlakovic et al. 1997). However, there is some doubt as to the validity of this observation and whether such cases can be designated as gastritis. PCR results have to be carefully evaluated, but today they are without a doubt a necessity in histologically questionable cases (review Wotherspoon 1998).

By contrast, PCR-based clonality analysis is a reliable diagnostic tool as it may detect clonality in patients whose disease cannot be morphologically diagnosed as lymphoma but in whom relapses developed after tumor eradication (Aiello et al. 1999).

Moreover, a clone-specific analysis has documented that MALT lymphoma may be much more disseminated than can be detected by pure morphology or immunohistochemistry (Du et al. 2000). It was shown that clone-specific neoplastic B-cells can be detected even in histologically non-neoplastic lymphocytic infiltrates as well as in the resection margins.

Differential Diagnosis

The first disease to consider in establishing a differential diagnosis, especially based on biopsy specimens, is *chronic gastritis with marked lymphoid hyperplasia.* The leading feature is a follicular hyperplasia, having well-formed germinal centers and a more- or less-developed follicular mantle. The outer follicular zone or marginal zone is small and inconspicuous. There is a tendency of lymphocytes to infiltrate the epithelium either as single cells or as small clusters; however, this phenomenon is less pronounced than in MALT lymphoma and there is less tendency of a destruction of the glands or crypts. Nevertheless, the border between these two diseases is not sharp but covers a continuous spectrum. Such cases frequently need repeated biopsies to be additionally studied by both immunohistochemistry and molecular techniques.

In order to overcome this problem in the differential diagnosis Wotherspoon et al. suggested a scoring system (1993b). In Table 6.3 the detailed criteria are given. Several studies have shown the applicability and value of this system (Savio et al. 1996).

Table 6.3. Histological scoring for the diagnosis of MALT lymphoma. *CCL* Centrocyte-like, LEL, lymphoepithelial lesion. Data from Wotherspoon et al. (1991)

Grade	Description	Histological features
0	Normal	Scattered plasma cells in the lamina propria. No lymphoid follicles.
1	Chronic active gastritis	Small clusters of lymphocytes in the lamina propria. No lymphoid follicles. No LELs.
2	Chronic active gastritis with florid lymphoid follicle formation	Prominent lymphoid follicles with surrounding mantle zone and plasma cells. No LELs.
3	Suspicious lymphoid infiltrate in the lamina propria, probably reactive	Lymphoid follicles surrounded by small lymphocytes that infiltrate diffusely in the lamina propria and occasionally into epithelium
4	Suspicious lymphoid infiltrate in the lamina propria, probably lymphoma	Lymphoid follicles surrounded by CCL cells that infiltrate diffusely in the lamina propria and into the epithelium in small groups
5	Low-grade B-cell lymphoma of MALT	Presence of dense diffuse infiltrate of CCL in lamina propria with prominent LELs

If there is a marked follicular colonization or early infiltrates with many follicles and a less-developed infiltrate in the marginal zone, then follicular lymphomas grade 1 must be included in the differential diagnosis. This can best be done by immunohistochemistry (see Immunohistochemistry).

Some cases of *chronic peptic ulcers* may be accompanied by a marked follicular hyperplasia. The follicles are well-developed with typical germinal centers and a follicular mantle. The marginal zone is inconspicuous. Such ulcers are frequently surrounded by prominent scarring including into the muscularis propria.

Individual cases with the endoscopic impression of a *lymphomatoid polyposis* as in mantle cell lymphoma have been described (Breslin et al. 1999). However, typical mantle cell lymphoma has a more monotonous infiltrate lacking blasts, a follicular hyperplasia is mostly absent, and the tumor cells should be CD5-positive and express cyclin D1.

A *secondary involvement of the stomach* either by a small-cell lymphoma or by a nodal DLBCL, e.g. centroblastic or immunoblastic, has to be excluded. *Lymphocytic lymphomas* mostly have a clinical history, typical lymphoepithelial lesions are absent, and they are mostly CD5- and CD23-positive. If the stomach is infiltrated by a *large-cell lymphoma* without a small-cell component, a secondary involvement of the stomach from a nodal lymphoma has to be excluded by clinical investigation. On a purely morphological basis this is usually not possible.

Occurrence

Extranodal lymphomas comprise about 30 – 35 % of all NHLs. Gastric MALT lymphomas make up about 8 – 10 % of all NHLs, and thus 25 – 30 % of all extranodal lymphomas. The frequency varies greatly between different countries. There is a high prevalence in some areas of Italy, with an incidence of about 13/100,000 per year, whereas the overall incidence in Europe is around 1 – 3/100,000 per year (Ulrich et al. 2002). There are some indications of a continuous increase in frequency during the past 10 years.

More than half of patients with gastric lymphoma present with either primary or secondary large-cell lymphoma (Montalban et al. 1995; Cogliatti et al. 1991; Johnsson et al. 1992), about two-thirds of these patients have a primary large-B-cell lymphoma.

Clinical Presentation and Prognosis

Gastric MALT lymphomas primarily occur in older patients, with a peak between 60 and 65 years. Patients with a high-grade component tend to be 70–75 years old. The disease affects both sexes, with some reports of a slight male preponderance. More than 80% of the patients present in stage I. B symptoms are absent (90%), the performance status is 0 in more than 80% of patients. Thus, most patients have an indolent course of disease. The 5-year survival is around 90–95% for stage I and around 80% for stage II. Whether disease dissemination in small-cell MALT lymphoma influences overall prognosis is not yet clear (Montalban et al. 1995), although it has recently been reported that such patients respond as well to therapy as do patients with localized disease (Thieblemont et al. 2000). Dissemination is more frequently found associated with large-cell gastric lymphomas (Koch et al. 1997). A successful treatment with antibiotics for *H. pylori* eradication has been reported. However, after a 6-year follow-up, 50% of the patients had relapses (Isaacson et al. 1999).

It became clear that eradication of *H. pylori* is definitely able to induce long-term remission, especially in patients with limited stage and superficial infiltrates (Wotherspoon et al. 1993; Wotherspoon 2000). This remission is not always associated with complete eradication of the infiltrate and of detectable clonal proliferation, as shown by PCR analysis (Savio et al. 1996; for review, see Wotherspoon 2000).

Further Reading

De Jong D, Aleman BM, Taal BG, Boot H (1999) Controversies and consensus in the diagnosis, work-up and treatment of gastric lymphoma: an international survey. Ann Oncol 10:275–280

De Jong D, Boot H, Taal B (2000) Histological grading with clinical relevance in gastric mucosa-associated lymphoid tissue (MALT) lymphoma. Recent Results Cancer Res 156: 27–32

Isaacson PG, Norton AJ (1994) Low-grade B-cell gastric lymphoma of MALT. In: Isaacson PG, Norton AJ (eds) Extranodal lymphomas. Churchill Livingstone, Edingburgh, pp 18–45

Koch P, Hiddemann W (1999) Therapy of gastric lymphoma of MALT, including antibiotics. In: Mason DY, Harris NL (eds) Human lymphomas: clinical implications of the REAL classification. Springer, Berlin Heidelberg New York, chap 20

Koch P, Berdel WE, Willich N, Tieman M (2000) Grading in marginal-zone lymphomas (letter to the editor). J Clin Oncol 18:2788

Montalban C, Santon A, Boixeda D, Redondo C, Alvarez I, Calleja JL, de Argila CM, Bellas C (2001) Treatment of low grade gastric mucosa-associated lymphoid tissue lymphoma in stage I with Helicobacter pylori eradication. Long-term results after sequential histologic and molecular follow-up. Haematologica 86:609–617

Wotherspoon AC, Dogan A, Du MQ (2002) Mucosa-associated lymphoid tissue lymphoma. Curr Opin Hematol 9:50–55

6.2.1.2 Intestinal Follicular Lymphoma (ICD-O: 9690/3)

Primary intestinal follicular lymphoma is an extremely rare disease. It has been described in the small bowel, especially in the duodenum, the ileocecal region, and the stomach. Follicular lymphomas make up about 4% of all primary GI-tract lymphomas (Yoshino et al. 2000a).

The tumors may present as small polyps or diffuse infiltrates (Fig. 6.13). The lesion are unifocal in about 60–70% (Damaj et al. 2003). Morphologically, they comprise typical neoplastic follicles as described for nodal lymphomas, giving the impression of a nodular infiltrate similar to that seen in mantle cell lymphoma and some cases of MALT lymphoma (Isaacson and Norton 1994) (Fig. 6.14). Centrocytes dominate intermingled with a few centroblasts. The morphology of the neoplastic follicles is almost identical to that of nodal follicular lymphomas. They are predominately follicular lymphomas grade 1. The detection of lymphoepithelial lesions does not exclude the diagnosis of a follicular lymphoma. Sclerosis may accompany the neoplastic infiltrate, which is primarily localized in the mucosa.

The major differential diagnostic problem is mantle cell lymphoma. At the macroscopic level, follicular lymphoma can present with multiple polyposis. For that reason, some authors propose reserving the term multiple polyposis for the macroscopy of some lymphomas, knowing that this pattern can be observed either in mantle cell lymphoma or in follicular lymphoma (Moynihan et al. 1996). At the microscopic level, the nodular pattern and the possible predominance of small centrocytes may be cause difficulties in distinguishing follicular lymphoma from mantle cell lymphoma or even from marginal zone lymphoma of MALT. Immunohistochemistry is thus mandatory.

The immunophenotype and the cytogenetic abnormalities are identical to those in nodal follicular lymphomas (Freeman et al. 1997).

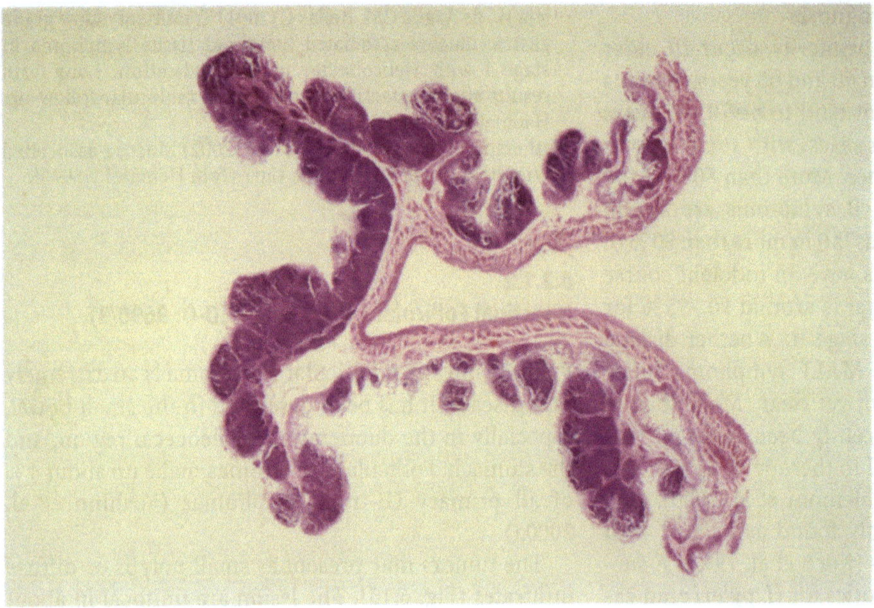

Fig. 6.13. Section of a follicular lymphoma in the small intestinal tract presenting as small polyps. The morphology resembles that of an intestinal mantle cell lymphoma (lymphomatous polyposis) (H and E stain)

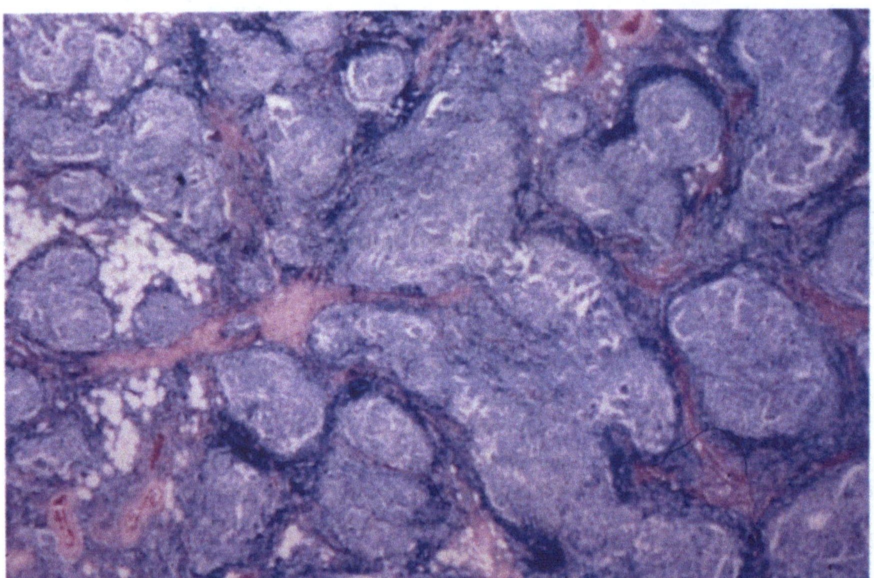

Fig. 6.14. Typical follicular growth pattern of a follicular lymphoma in the stomach (Giemsa stain)

The medium age of patients with intestinal follicular lymphoma is between 50 and 60 years. There is a female predominance of 2.0:1.0. The patients present with abdominal pain and, less frequently, intestinal obstruction (Damaj et al, 2003). The clinical follow-up indicates a quite indolent behavior of this lymphoma type.

6.2.1.3
Multiple Lymphomatous Polyposis – Intestinal Mantle Cell Lymphoma (ICD-O: 9673/3)

Synonyms

- Kiel: Centrocytic lymphoma/mantle cell lymphoma
- REAL: Mantle cell lymphoma
- WHO: Mantle cell lymphoma

Definition

The lymphatic infiltrate produces multiple polyps consisting of a monotonous infiltrate of medium-sized cells with deeply indented nuclei (centrocytes) and a nodular growth pattern.

Morphology

Macroscopically, multiple (up to 100) polyps are found predominately in the small and large bowel. They measure from 0.2 cm to 1.0 cm sometimes producing large tumor masses (Fig. 6.15).

Histologically, a nodular growth pattern is dominant (Fig. 6.16). The nodules appear as a dense infiltrate of medium-sized cells with deeply indented nuclei, which are thus identical to the nodules in nodal mantle cell lymphoma (Fig. 6.17). Sometimes remnants of germinal centers are mirror the mantle zone growth pattern. Finally, the germinal centers are completely colonized by the neoplastic infiltrate. Blasts should only be found as remnants of germinal centers. Usually, several small nodules form small polyps having a tendency to grow upwards towards the intestinal lumen. Sometimes lymphoepithelial lesions can be observed and are thus not exclusive for MALT lymphomas (Isaacson and Norton 1994; Lavergne et al. 1994; Fraga et al. 1995).

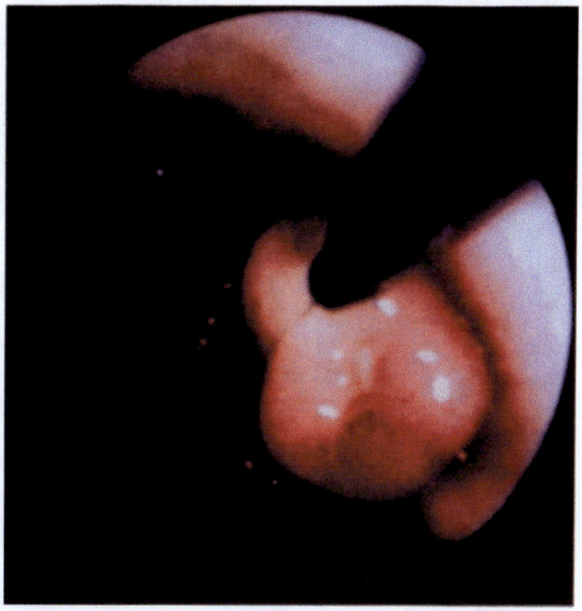

Fig. 6.15. Macroscopy of a polypous mass of a mantle cell lymphoma (lymphomatous polyposis)

Immunohistochemistry

The immunophenotype is identical to that of nodal mantle cell lymphoma (see Chap 4.2.1.7), i.e. CD20+, CD5+, CD10–, cyclinD1+.

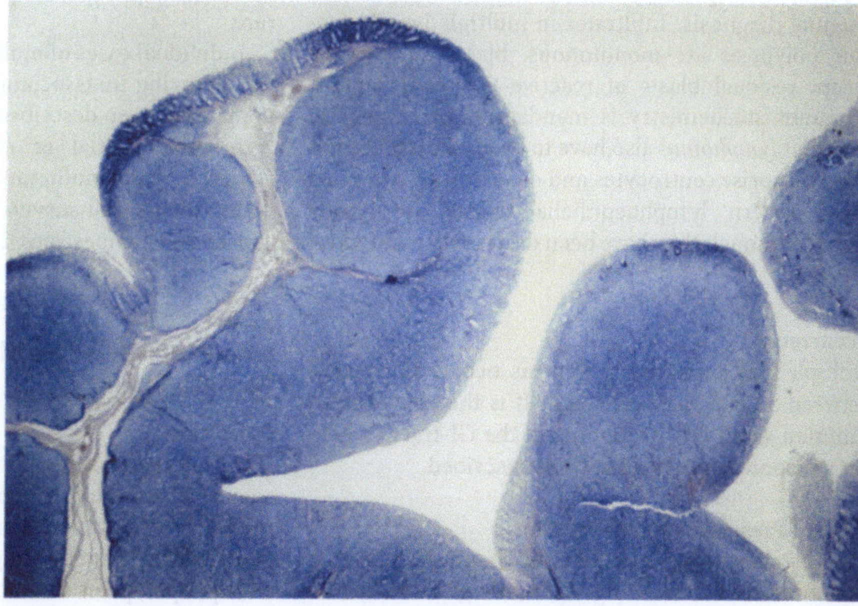

Fig. 6.16. Polypous nodular growth pattern of a mantle cell lymphoma in the intestinal tract (Giemsa stain)

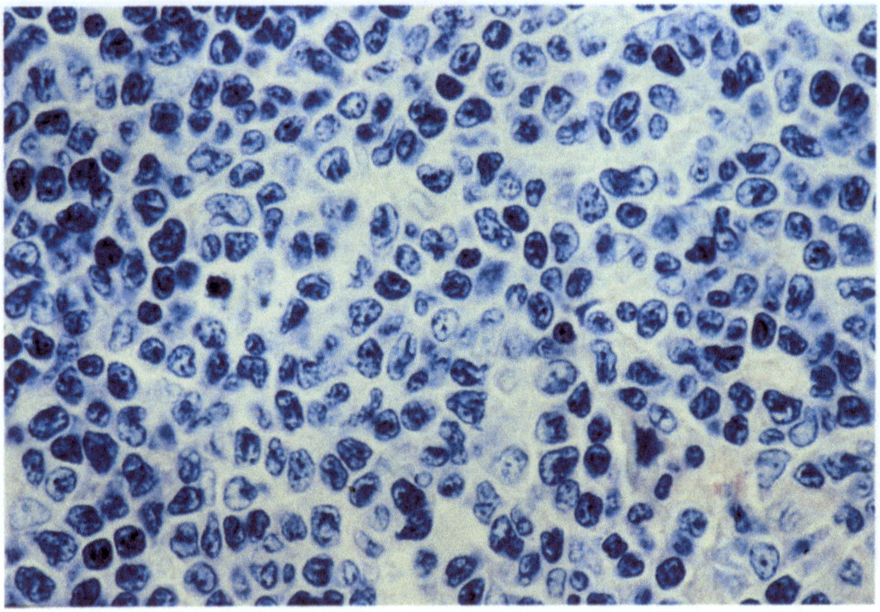

Fig. 6.17. Typical neoplastic centrocytes in an intestinal mantle cell lymphoma (lymphomatous polyposis) (Giemsa stain)

Genetic Features

Ig heavy- and light-chain genes are rearranged. In 30–40% of the tumors, the translocation t(11;14) is found (Kumar et al. 1996).

Differential Diagnosis

The endoscopic aspect greatly resembles *familial adenomatous polyposis.* On the basis of histology, *MZBCL of MALT* is the primary disease to consider in the differential diagnosis. Infiltrates in multiple lymphomatous polyposis are monotonous, blasts are missing except residual blasts of reactive germinal centers. Immunohistochemistry is mandatory. Rare types of *follicular lymphomas* also have to be excluded. The follicles comprise centrocytes and centroblasts without a zonal pattern, lymphoepithelial lesions are mostly absent, although they have been described in individual cases.

Occurrence

Multiple lymphomatous polyposis occurs in patients between 50 and 70 years of age. It is the second most common small-cell lymphoma in the GI-tract. A gender preponderance has not been described.

Clinical Presentation and Prognosis

Patients present with abdominal pain, diarrhea, or sometimes rectal bleeding. Thus, weight loss can be observed. The intestinal tract may be the primary manifestation of mantle cell lymphoma; however, this lymphoma type frequently disseminates from a primary nodal site secondary to the intestinal tract. It is predominately localized in the ileocecal region and in the colon in primary GI-cases but frequently disseminates throughout the small and large bowel. Mesenteric lymph nodes are mostly involved, particularly Waldeyer's ring. A primary manifestation in the stomach is rare.

Individual cases of multiple lymphomatous polyposis occurring in association with colonic adenocarcinoma have been described (Kanehira et al. 2001).

A good partial or complete remission can be achieved by chemotherapy; however, relapses are frequent, the overall survival after 5 years is below 50% (Ruskone-Fourmestraux 2000; Hashimoto et al. 1999).

6.2.1.4 Diffuse-Large-B-Cell Lymphoma of Gastrointestinal Tract (ICD-O: 9680/3)

Definition

Diffuse large-B-cell lymphoma can develop in the GI-tract as a secondary tumor. It may be associated with primary marginal zone lymphoma of MALT or, less frequently, with mantle zone cell lymphoma presenting as multiple polyposis or with α-heavy-chain disease (see

Chap. 7.3.4). When components of both small-B-cell and large-B-cell lymphomas are present, a transformation from primary small-B-cell to large-B-cell lymphoma can be suspected.

DLBCL can also occur secondarily as an extension of a lymphoma developing in adjacent tissues, e.g. spleen, liver, ovary, or kidney. Clinical presentation allows this condition to be easily recognized.

Other DLBCL arise in the GI-tract without any recognizable associated small-B-cell lymphoma of MALT. These DLBCLs have been included in the classification proposed by Isaacson et al. (1988) under the term "high-grade MALT lymphoma" only because they develop from MALT tissue. This opinion is not accepted by all pathologists. It has been proposed that DLBCL showing lymphoepithelial lesions made up of large cells, which could represent high-grade MALT lymphoma, be distinguished from DLBCL without such lesions. But again, this proposal is currently not fully accepted. This led D. Wright (1994) to state "high-grade MALT lymphoma currently cannot be identified except in the presence of residual low-grade tumor".

DLBCL without the morphological criteria for a MALT origin are perhaps equivalent to DLBCL arising in a lymph node from post-germinal-center cells of an origin other than marginal zone cells.

Morphology

Common to all DLBCL sites is the presence of tumorous masses made of whitish or brownish tissue with areas of necrosis and hemorrhages often extending throughout the layers of the digestive tract and associated with nodal involvement.

In the stomach, there is a marked mucosal nodularity due to multiple tumor masses often with extensive ulceration, distinctive invasion of the muscularis propria and sometimes perforation (Fig. 6.18) (Levison and Shepherd 1986; Morson and Dawson 1990; Lewin et al. 1978; Lewin and Appelman 1995).

In the small intestine, often the main involved site is the terminal ileum, with extension to the cecum. The tumor protrudes into the lumen as a bulky, sometimes polypoid mass with secondary mucosal ulceration. Infiltration of the muscle coat is responsible for annular or plaque-like thickenings. Sometimes multiple localizations along the ileum can be observed. Fissuring ulceration mimicking that seen in Crohn's disease, sometimes leading to perforation, have been observed (Lewin et al. 1978; Shepherd et al. 1988; Morson and Dawson 1990).

In the large intestine, with or without regional lymph node involvement, three main pattern are found (Lewin et al. 1978; Shepherd et al. 1988; Morson and Dawson 1990). The most common is an annular or plaque-like thickening. The second is a bulky protuber-

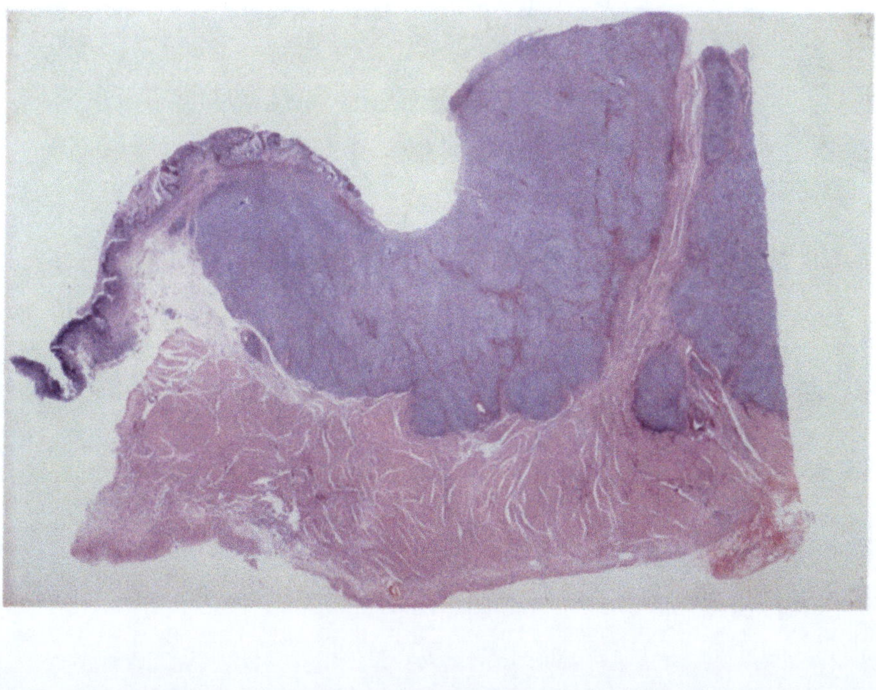

Fig. 6.18. Gastric infiltration of a diffuse large-B-cell lymphoma, infiltrating into the muscularis propria. The infiltrate exhibits a slight nodularity without being a follicular lymphoma (Giemsa stain)

ant growth reducing the size of the lumen, often with ulceration. Rarely, a thickening of the bowel wall is associated with aneurysmal dilatation.

The cecum is involved in 60% of patients and is often associated with involvement of the terminal ileum. The rectum is involved in 20% of the patients. In the other 20%, various sites along the colon are involved.

Some colorectal lymphomas may complicate longstanding ulcerative colitis or Crohn's disease.

Histopathology

In primary digestive tract lymphoma, different types of DLBCL can be observed. The most frequent are subtypes of centroblastic lymphomas, often the polymorphic subtype (Figs. 6.19, 6.20). Less frequently immu-

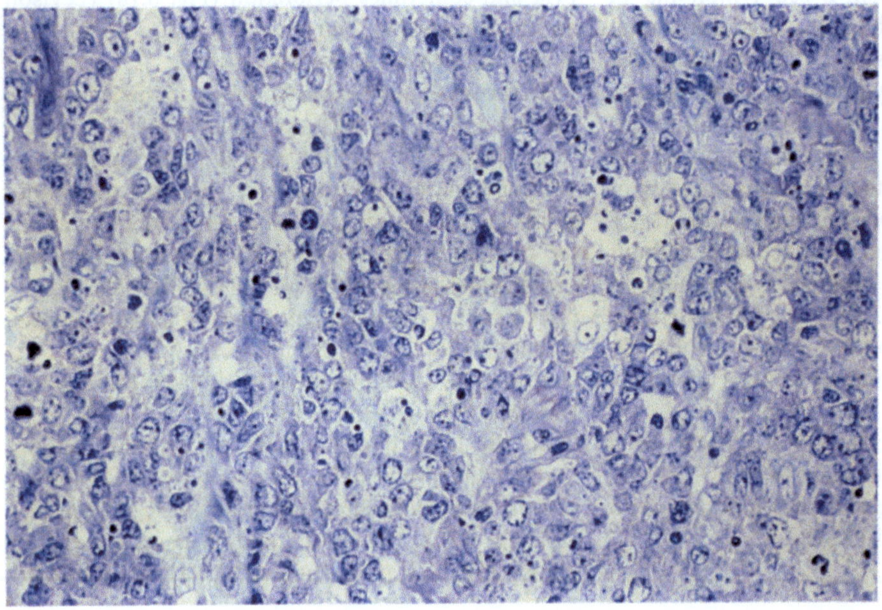

Fig. 6.19. A typical polymorphic centroblastic lymphoma in the stomach (Giemsa stain)

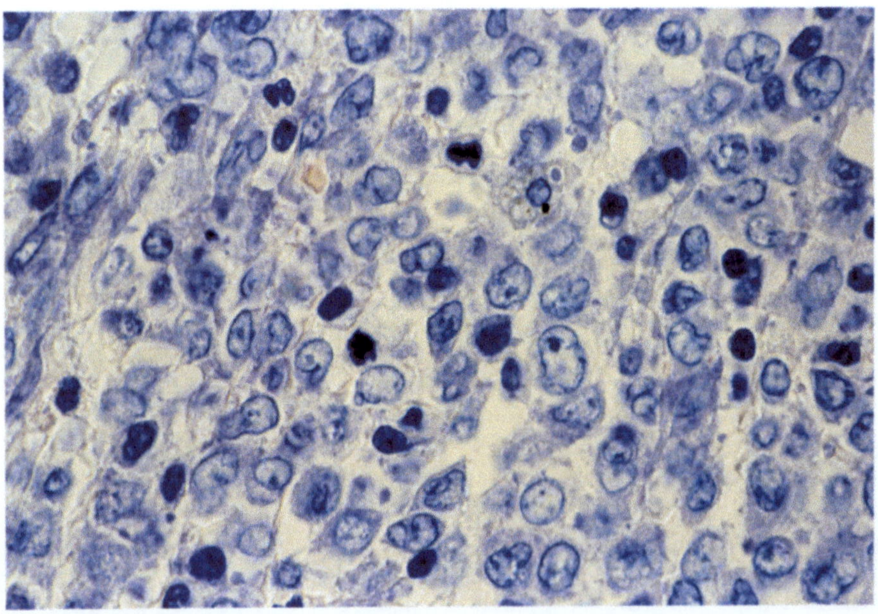

Fig. 6.20. Diffuse large-B-cell lymphoma of the stomach. Note the multilobated centroblasts (Giemsa stain)

noblastic lymphoma, usually with a plasmablastic differentiation, is found. There have been a few cases of anaplastic large-B-cell lymphoma, but T-cell-rich B-cell lymphoma seems to be rare.

The cytology is frequently highly polymorphic, perhaps even with Reed-Sternberg-like cells (Lewin and Appelman 1995). Reactive lymphocytes, plasma cells, histiocytes, and eosinophils are often present (Lewin et al. 1978).

Secondary DLBCL is associated with MALT marginal zone cell lymphomas, or, rarely, with mantle zone cell lymphoma, and even more rarely with α-heavy-chain disease (see Chap. 7).

Immunohistochemistry

This technique is useful for the diagnosis of DLBCL. The results are quite similar to those reported for the different types of nodal DLBCL (see Chap. 4.2.2). Intracytoplasmic immunoglobulins are demonstrated in one third of the tumors (Van Krieken et al. 1992).

Two important points should be stressed:

1. DLBCL with an immunoblastic morphology can be negative for CD20 and even CD79 in tumors exhibiting a plasmacytoid differentiation. Often these cells do not express sIg.
2. Immunoblastic lymphomas with a plasmablastic or plasmacytic differentiation express epithelial membrane antigen (EMA). A few tumors may lack expression of CD45 but show intracytoplasmic positivity for different types of cytokeratins (de Mascarel et al. 1989). To avoid an incorrect diagnosis of undifferentiated carcinoma, morphology plays an important role. A triangular-shaped cytoplasm and an eccentric nucleus, amphophilia on H and E staining and basophilia with Giemsa staining, the presence of a large Golgi apparatus, as well as the demonstration of intracytoplasmic monotypic immunoglobulins are all features of DLBCL.

Genetic Features

Clonal rearrangement of immunoglobulin heavy-chain is disclosed by PCR. Clonal rearrangement of the bcl-6 gene has been reported in 17% of primary nodal DLBCLs and in 48% of primary gastric lymphomas in a series of 39 Chinese patients from Hong Kong (Liang et al. 1997a). Thus, bcl-6 gene rearrangement seems to play a role in the development of primary gastric lymphoma. Hypermutations of the bcl-6 gene at the E1.11 segment were detectable in 73% primary gastric and 22% primary nodal lymphomas. Three out of 22 patients with primary gastric lymphoma also had mutations at segment E1.12. The proportion of hypermutations in the group with bcl-6 gene rearrangement was similar to that in the germ-line group (70% vs 75%) (Liang et al. 1997b).

Differential Diagnosis

In a few cases, DLBCL of the GI-tract can be difficult to distinguish from poorly differentiated or *undifferentiated carcinoma* or *metastatic melanotic melanoma*, particularly in small biopsies or when large areas of necrosis modify the morphology of the cells. Reactive cells, such as lymphocytes, histiocytes, and plasma cells, may be very numerous in some cases of so-called medullary carcinoma of the stomach and may overshadow the carcinoma cells, mimicking a lymphoma (Morson and Dawson 1990). Immunohistochemistry is then very useful: cytokeratins, CD45 and CD20 expression is indicative and can be demonstrated even in areas of necrosis.

The most important and difficult diagnosis is represented by *reactive immunoblastic hyperplasia*, in which there is diffuse infiltration of the entire wall of the terminal ileum by large cells with an immunoblastic morphology associated with a variable number of plasma cells and lymphocytes, and sometimes follicular hyperplasia. These immunoblasts express B-cell markers but are Epstein-Barr virus (EBV)-negative. It is not possible to demonstrate a monotypic population either by immunohistochemistry or by PCR. The morphology is not that of a DLBCL but more that of an immunoblastic hyperplasia. The etiology is unknown. The evolution is characterized by a spontaneous regression (Isaacson et al. 1988).

Occurrence

DLBCL represents the majority of lymphomas developing primarily in the digestive tract, for example, in the stomach they comprise 40–60% of all gastric lymphomas (Lewin et al. 1978; Levison and Shepherd 1986; Van Krieken et al. 1989). DLBCLs mostly occur in older patients with an average age of about 60 years. Gastric, ileocecal, and rectal primary lymphoma are frequent in patients with immunodeficiencies, particularly AIDS (see Chap. 8.2.1).

Clinical Features

DLBCL patients commonly present with weight loss, fever, and anemia.

In primary lymphoma of the stomach, patients complain of epigastric pain, nausea, and vomiting. A palpable epigastric mass may be present. Patients often present with advanced disease that has an aggressive course, with spreading beyond the stomach to the adjacent soft tissues, to the draining lymph node (perigastric, para-aortic), and to other abdominal viscera, in 40–60% of the cases (Lewin et al. 1978; Jones et al. 1988; Cogliatti et al. 1991; Lewin and Appelman 1995). There is also spreading to extra-abdominal organs, including lymph nodes, lung, brain, and meninges, in up to 50% of the patients (Lewin et al. 1978; Lewin and Appelman 1995).

The majority of the patients relapse 1 year after the diagnosis and most of them die within 1 year of relapse (Lewin and Appelman 1995). The size of the tumor and the stage according to the Ann Arbor system, as revised by Musshoff, have prognostic value (Jones et al. 1988; Lewin and Appelman 1995). A 5-year overall survival is seen in about 40–55% of patients (Van Krieken et al. 1989; Cogliatti et al. 1991; Lewin and Appelman 1995) which is similar to that for patients with nodal DLBCL (Salles et al. 1991).

In a group of patients with primary gastric lymphoma from Hong Kong, significantly more patients in the germline bcl-6 gene group had advanced stage (II, III or IV) disease (Liang et al. 1997a). Complete remission rates following primary therapy appeared to be higher for the positive rearrangement group (70% vs 30%) but this was not statistically significant. Patients with a rearranged bcl-6 gene also appeared to have better survival at 5 years, 58% vs 36%, but again this was not statistically significant. Patients classified as being at low risk of relapse according to the International Prognostic Index had significantly better survival at 5 years (89% vs 9%, $p=0.0001$) (Liang et al. 1997a). Hypermutations of the bcl-6 gene did not appear to carry any prognostic significance clinically (Liang et al. 1997b).

In small and large bowel, the presence of an abdominal tumor mass, peritonitis due to perforation, obstruction syndrome, and intussusception are the most frequent clinical features. The evolution and prognostic factors are more or less similar to those of DLBCL of the stomach.

6.2.1.5 Burkitt's Lymphoma of the Gastrointestinal Tract (ICD-O: 9687/3)

Definition

Burkitt's lymphoma can occur primarily in the ileocecal region or, more rarely, in the stomach (Lewin et al. 1978; Levine et al. 1982).

Morphology

Macroscopy. The lesions are often advanced at the time of diagnosis. There is extensive involvement of all layers of the ileocecum or stomach wall with small mucosal ulcerations.

Recurrence is often associated with widespread peritoneal dissemination.

Histology. The histopathological features are identical to those of classic Burkitt's lymphoma, or sometimes to the plasmacytoid variant, or even to atypical Burkitt's lymphoma, as described in the lymph nodes (see Chap. 4.2.3).

Immunohistochemistry and Genetics

These are similar to what was described for nodal Burkitt's lymphoma (see Chap. 4.2.3).

Differential Diagnosis

The only problem is the distinction between some Burkitt's lymphomas and some DLBCLs of monomorphic centroblastic type. The differential diagnosis can be particularly difficult in the presence of necrosis. EBV latent infection favors a diagnosis of Burkitt's lymphoma.

Occurrence

Ileocecal involvement is frequently the initial site of abdominal development of Burkitt's lymphoma, particularly the non-endemic form of Burkitt's. But the number of cases of ileocecal involvement seems to be increasing even in endemic Burkitt's. Burkitt's lymphoma occurring in immunodeficiencies may also involve the digestive tract. Children are more often affected than adults.

Clinical Features

Burkitt's lymphoma of the GI-tract is identical to other lymphomas of the ileocecal or gastric area. The evolution and prognosis are similar to what was described for other sites of involvement.

6.2.2 Primary Gastrointestinal T-Cell Lymphoma

Gastrointestinal T-cell lymphomas (GITCL) have a long history and in the past were ascribed to different cell systems. In 1978, Isaacson and Wright (1978) described patients with lymphomas of the small intestinal tract associated with villous atrophy and a history of malabsorption, although an association between malabsorption and lymphoma had already been recognized by Fairley in 1937. These neoplasms were interpreted by Isaacson and Wright as malignant histiocytosis. The same authors recognized some years later that such tumors had a T-cell immunophenotype and they interpreted them as being T-cell lymphomas (Isaacson et al. 1985). Anaplastic large-cell lymphoma of the intestine had a similar history, initially described by Isaacson et al. as malignant histiocytosis and years later as CD30 anaplastic large-cell lymphomas (Isaacson et al. 1988). The observation of an association between intestinal T-cell lymphomas, villous atrophy, and an enteropathy with preceding malabsorption led to the designation of enteropathy-type T-cell lymphoma (ETTCL) (O'Farelly et al. 1986). The immunophenotype, especially the detection of CD103 in normal intestinal intraepithelial lymphocytes, and ETTCL led to the hypothesis that these lymphomas arise from intraepithelial T-lymphocytes. The additional detection of CD56-positive lymphomas in the GI-tract further enlarged the group of GITCLs.

Today, we are thus faced with four major groups: (1) enteropathy-type T-cell lymphoma (CD103+), which might be enteropathy-associated or not, and includes the group of CD56+ GITCLs; (2) peripheral T-cell lymphomas, unspecified; and (3) anaplastic large-cell lymphomas (CD30+) of T-cell type; (4) individual cases of natural killer (NK)/T-cell lymphomas, nasal type, have been described.

T-cell lymphomas make up about one -third of all small intestinal lymphomas (Domizio et al. 1993).

6.2.2.1 Enteropathy-Type T-Cell Lymphoma (ICD-O: 9717/3)

Synonyms

- Kiel: Pleomorphic small-cell, pleomorphic medium-and large-cell (in part)
- REAL: Intestinal T-cell lymphoma (± enteropathy-associated)
- WHO: Enteropathy-type T-cell lymphoma

Definition

These lymphomas are a common complication of celiac disease, evolving from intraepithelial T-lymphocytes. The cytology is highly variable, from small pleomorphic to large anaplastic cells. They are mostly localized in the jejunum and frequently associated with villous atrophy.

Morphology

Most of these lymphomas are characterized by villous atrophy with crypt hyperplasia, increased intraepithelial lymphocytes, fissured or ulcerating lesions, and a cytologically variable neoplastic infiltrate associated with a heavy inflammatory component of histiocytes, plasma cells, and eosinophils. The neoplastic cells are variable in their morphology, ranging from small pleomorphic to medium and large cells, to large immunoblastic or anaplastic, as well as cells that have round nuclei, are medium-sized, and resemble lymphoblasts or myeloblasts (Figs. 6.21–6.23). They predominately infiltrate the mucosa, heavily invading and partly destroying the epithelium. Some tumors have a more patchy appearance and may invade the entire mucosa and submucosa (Fig. 6.24). Others show a band-like infiltrate (Chott et al. 1992). Ulcerations are frequently found. In somewhat preserved areas, there is only a marked epitheliotropism. The number of intraepithelial lymphocytes – sometimes appearing as normal, slightly pleomorphic lymphocytes – is highly variable. In some cases they may be extremely dense, partially or completely destroying the epithelial layering or crypts. The intestinal tract frequently exhibits multiple lesions, especially in the jejunum. Lymph nodes in the mesentery are mostly involved. Enteropathy-type T-cell lymphoma characteristically shows villous atrophy with an increase of intraepithelial lymphocytes also in uninvolved areas. In some cases only intraepithelial lymphocytes are increased, without villous atrophy.

The associated eosinophilia may be so prominent that it appears as the dominating feature at first glance.

A few patients may present with disease very much resembling multiple lymphomatous polyposis (Figs. 6.25, 6.26, 6.27a, b) (Hirakawa et al. 1996; Ogawa et al. 2000).

In Figs. 6.28a, b, examples of peripheral T-cell lymphomas, unspecified, occurring primarily in the stomach and without expression of CD103 or CD56 are shown. Such cases are mostly localized tumors without enteropathy.

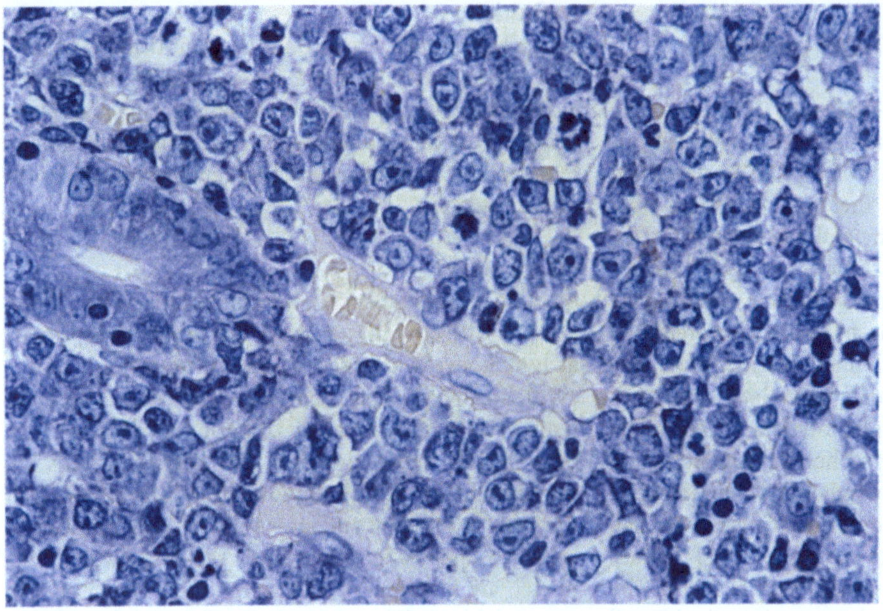

Fig. 6.21. Cytological variant of enteropathy-associated gastrointestinal T-cell-lymphoma: blastic/immunoblastic T-cell-lymphoma (Giemsa stain)

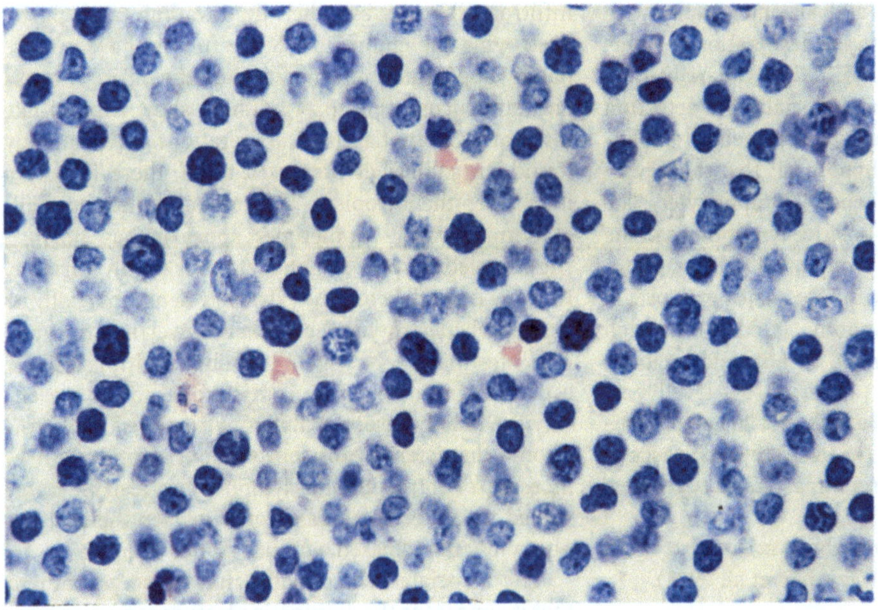

Fig. 6.22. Cytological variant of enteropathy-associated gastrointestinal T-cell-lymphoma: medium sized slightly pleomorphic neoplastic T-cells (Giemsa stain)

Immunohistochemistry

Most typical ETTCLs have a phenotype of CD3+, CD5–, CD7+, CD4– and CD8– (Fig. 6.27a). Almost all of these tumors express CD103, which, as of this writing, can only be detected on frozen section. Most of the tumors are also positive for cytotoxic granules (TIA-1) (Chott et al. 1992; Chan et al. 1999) (Fig. 6.27b) while a smaller group is CD56-positive and then coexpress CD8 (Chott et al. 1998). CD30 is expressed to a variable degree. If a strong, complete positivity is recognized (i.e., all lymphoma cells are positive), a primary anaplastic large-cell lymphoma (ALCL) has to be taken into account. The intraepithelial lymphocytes, even those outside the tumor infiltrate, show a typical phenotype with expression of cCD3 and negativity for CD5, CD4 and CD8.

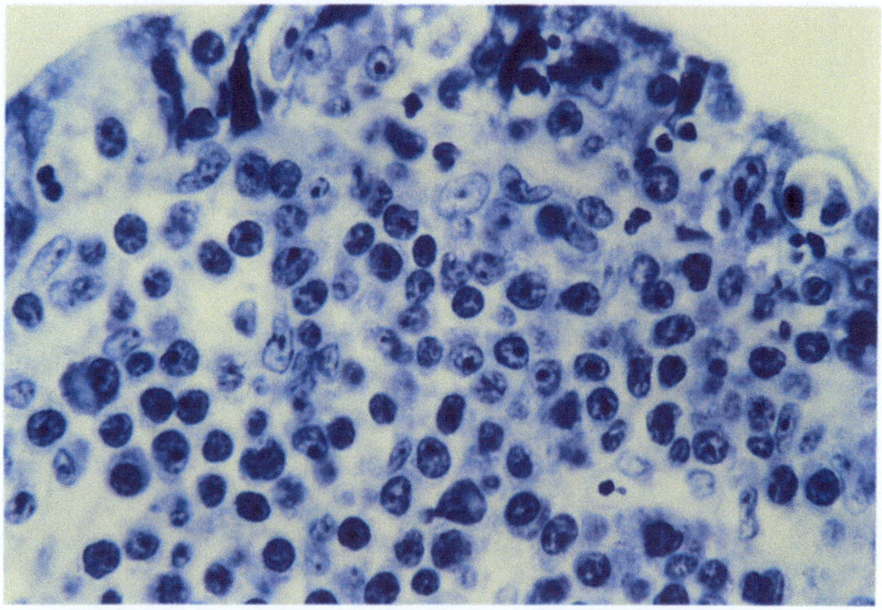

Fig. 6.23. Cytological variant of enteropathy-type gastrointestinal T-cell-lymphoma: small- to medium-sized blasts. This lymphoma additionally expressed NK-cell-antigens (CD56) (Giemsa stain)

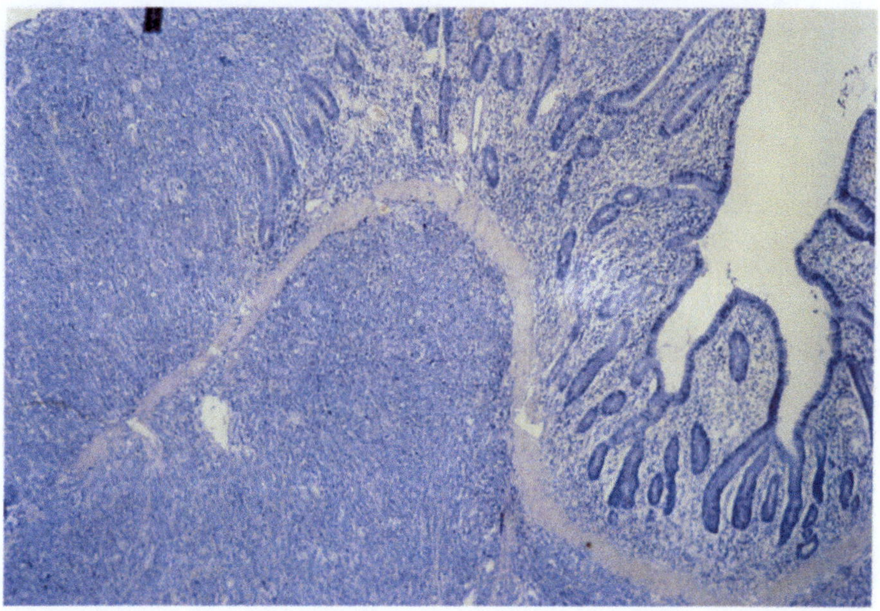

Fig. 6.24. Mucosal and submucosal intestinal infiltrate of an enteropathy-associated T-cell-lymphoma (Giemsa stain)

A low or absent expression of HLA-ABC and HLA-DR (Ashton-Key et al. 1996) is described.

Recently, there have been three cases reported with coexpression of CD4 and CD8, and a high apoptotic rate localized in the stomach (Barth et al. 2000).

It could also be shown that refractory sprue is different from celiac disease. The former is characterized by an abnormal phenotype of the intraepithelial lymphocytes (cCD3+, CD8–) and rearranged T-cell receptor (TcR) genes (Cellier et al. 2000; Patey-Mariaud et al. 2000). Patients whose intraepithelial lymphocytes have a normal phenotype may recover with proper diet and respond to steroid therapy. This is of importance, as in these studies lymphomas only developed in patients with refractory sprue.

There might be a more frequent association of

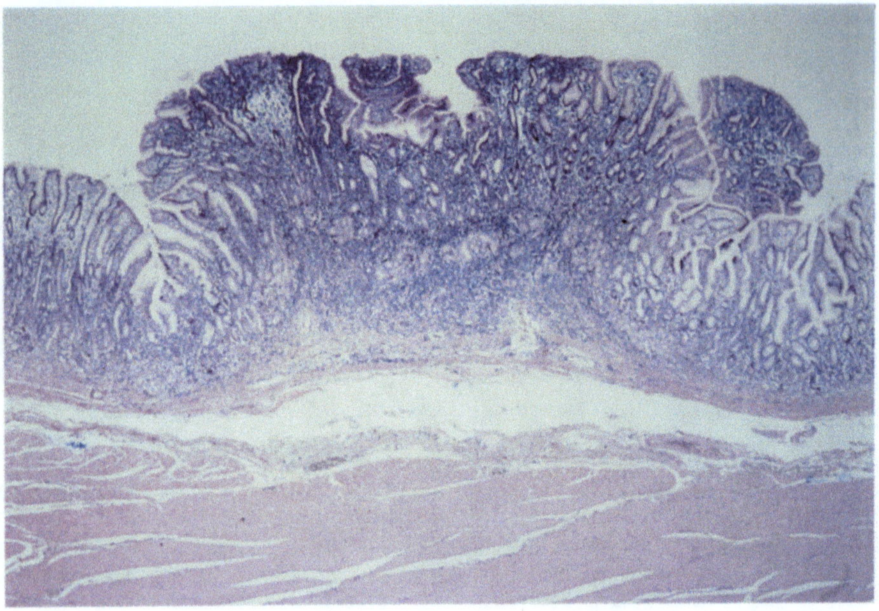

Fig. 6.25. Small polypous mass of an intestinal T-cell-lymphoma with NK/T-cell phenotype (Giemsa stain)

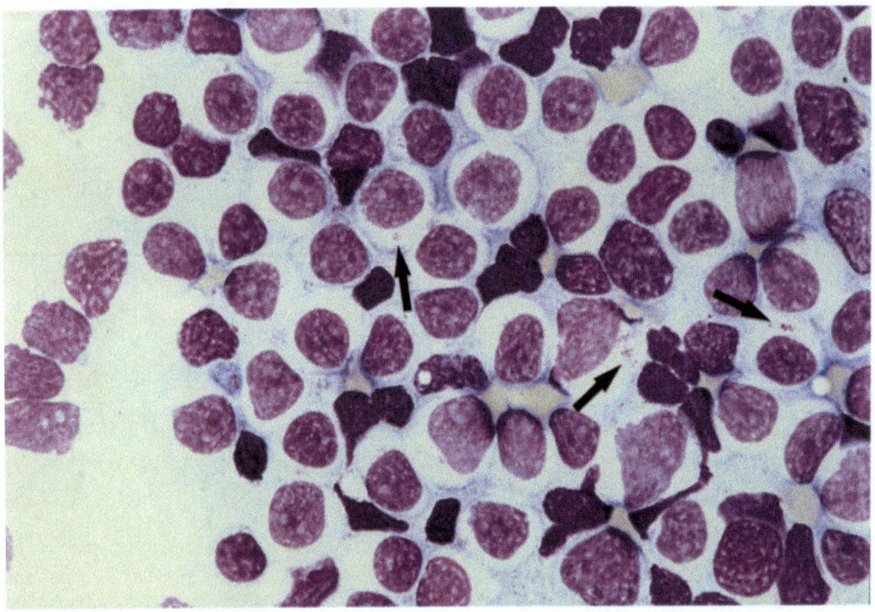

Fig. 6.26. Imprint of the intestinal T-cell-lymphoma in Fig. 6.25. The cells exhibit a clear cytoplasm with some azurophilic granules (→) (Pappenheim stain)

ETTCL with EBV in Japan (Katoh et al. 2000). A high frequency is also found in Mexican patients (see Genetic Features).

In individual cases of ETTCL, tumor cells may express CD79α (CD20-negative) together with cCD3; these cases should not be misinterpreted as B-cell lymphomas (Blakolmer et al. 2000).

Genetic Features

All ETTCLs have clonally rearranged TCR genes. The same is true if uninvolved tissue with an increase of intraepithelial lymphocytes is investigated, indicating that these cells are the precursor lesions of the apparent lymphoma.

Recently, it became clear that ulcerative jejunitis and refractory sprue are closely related to or may evolve

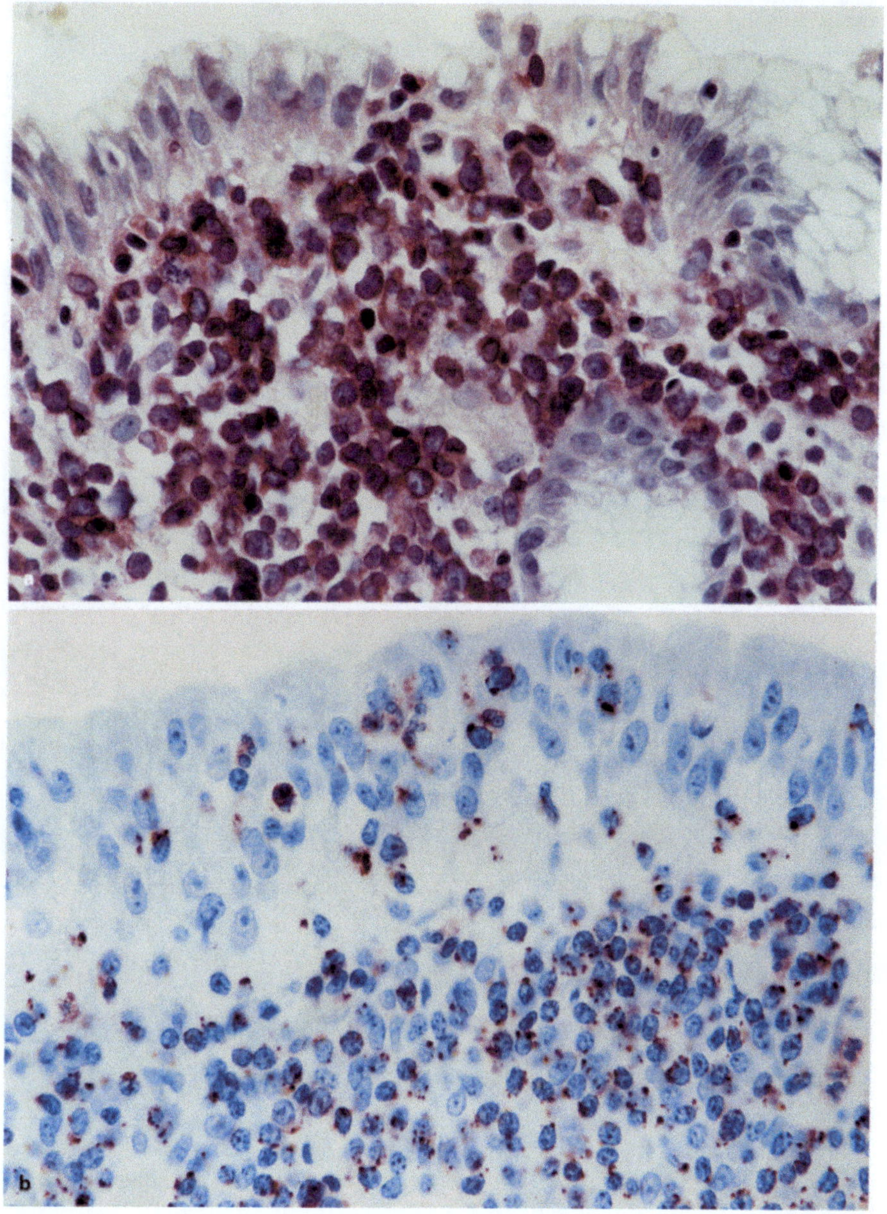

Fig. 6.27a, b. Same case as Fig. 6.25. Immunohistochemical staining for CD3 (**a**) and cytotoxic granules (TIA1) (**b**) (alkaline phosphatase)

into ETTCL. Interestingly both of these diseases are frequently associated with the detection of a T-cell clone, whereas in patients with celiac disease with sensitivity to a gluten-free diet there is almost always a polyclonal rearrangement pattern for TcR. Thus patients with therapy-resistant enteropathy with villous atrophy have to be carefully searched for monoclonal T-cells as the disease possibly evolves into ETTCL (Ashton-Key et al. 1997; Carbonnel et al. 1998; Bagdi et al. 1999; Daum et al. 2001).

Recently, gains on chromosome 9q have been described in 58% of ETTCLs. Less frequently, aberrations on chromosomes 7, 5, and 1 were found (Zettl et al. 2002).

Whereas almost all patients in Europe and the USA are EBV-negative, there is convincing evidence that

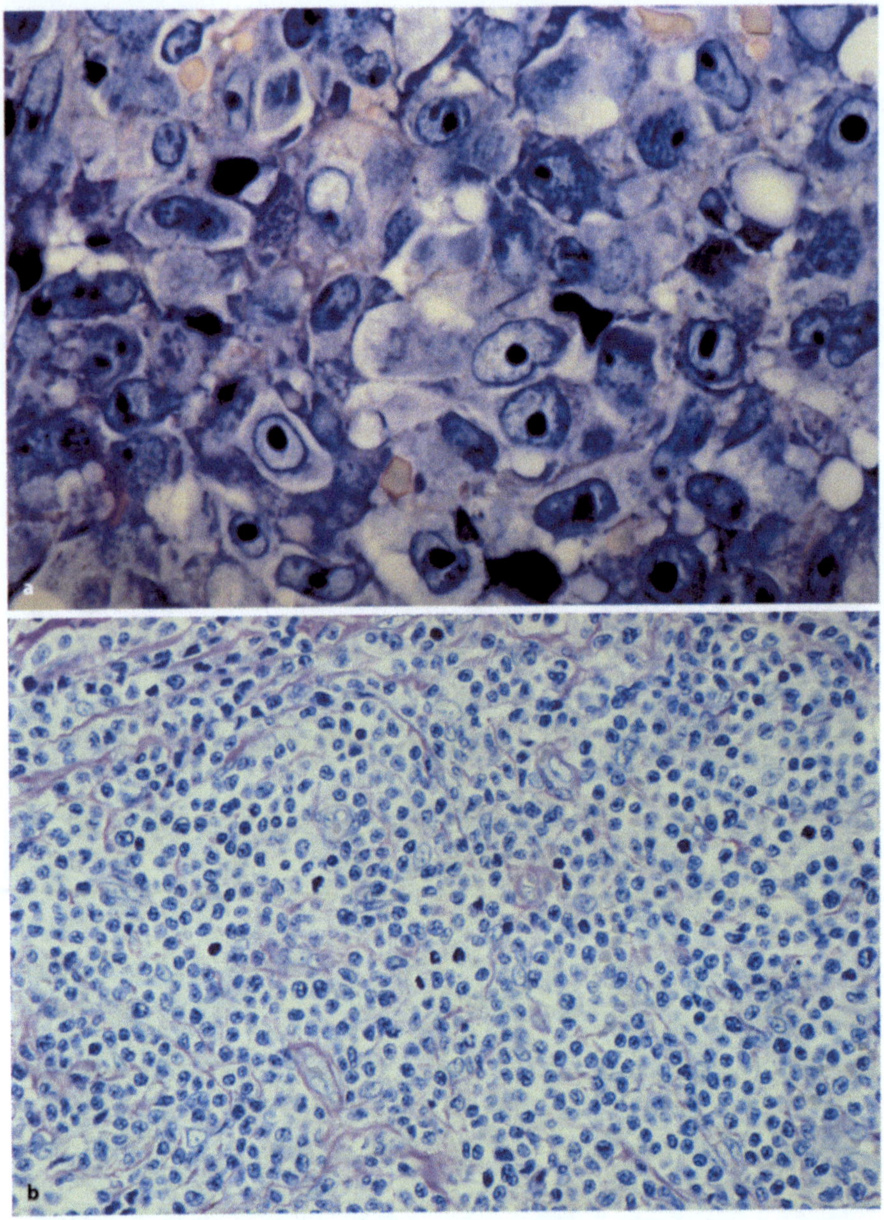

Fig. 6.28 a, b. Cytological variants of gastrointestinal T-cell-lymphoma, unspecified type. **a** T-immunoblastic; **b** medium sized pleomorphic (Giemsa stain)

there is a prevalence in other areas. Quintanilla-Martinez (1997) found LMP-1 and EBER in seven out of seven Mexican ETTCL patients. Interestingly, the median age of these patients was markedly different than that of European patients (24 vs 63 years).

Differential Diagnosis

- NK/T-cell lymphoma, nasal type
- DLBCL
- Ulcerative jejunitis: complication of celiac disease, with non-specific inflammatory mucosal ulcer; patients have increasing resistance to a gluten-free diet and some may develop ETTCL.
- Refractory sprue: loss of response to gluten-free diet
- Celiac disease
- Hodgkin's disease (Kumar et al. 2000)

Occurrence

The median patient age is around 60 years with a slight male preponderance (for review, see Isaacson et al. 1999). ETTCLs make up about 2–3 % of all gastrointestinal lymphomas. In the small intestine, they account for more than one-third of all lymphomas. The overall frequency among NHLs is below 1 % (Koh et al. 2001; The Non-Hodgkin's Lymphoma Classification Project 1997). Patients in areas endemic for HTLV-1 may be positive, which influences neither the histological nor the clinical picture.

Clinical Presentation and Prognosis

Most patients present with abdominal pain frequently evolving into acute abdominal symptoms with perforation or obstruction. Rapid weight loss before onset of acute signs is recognized. The majority of the patients have a history of celiac disease mostly of short duration

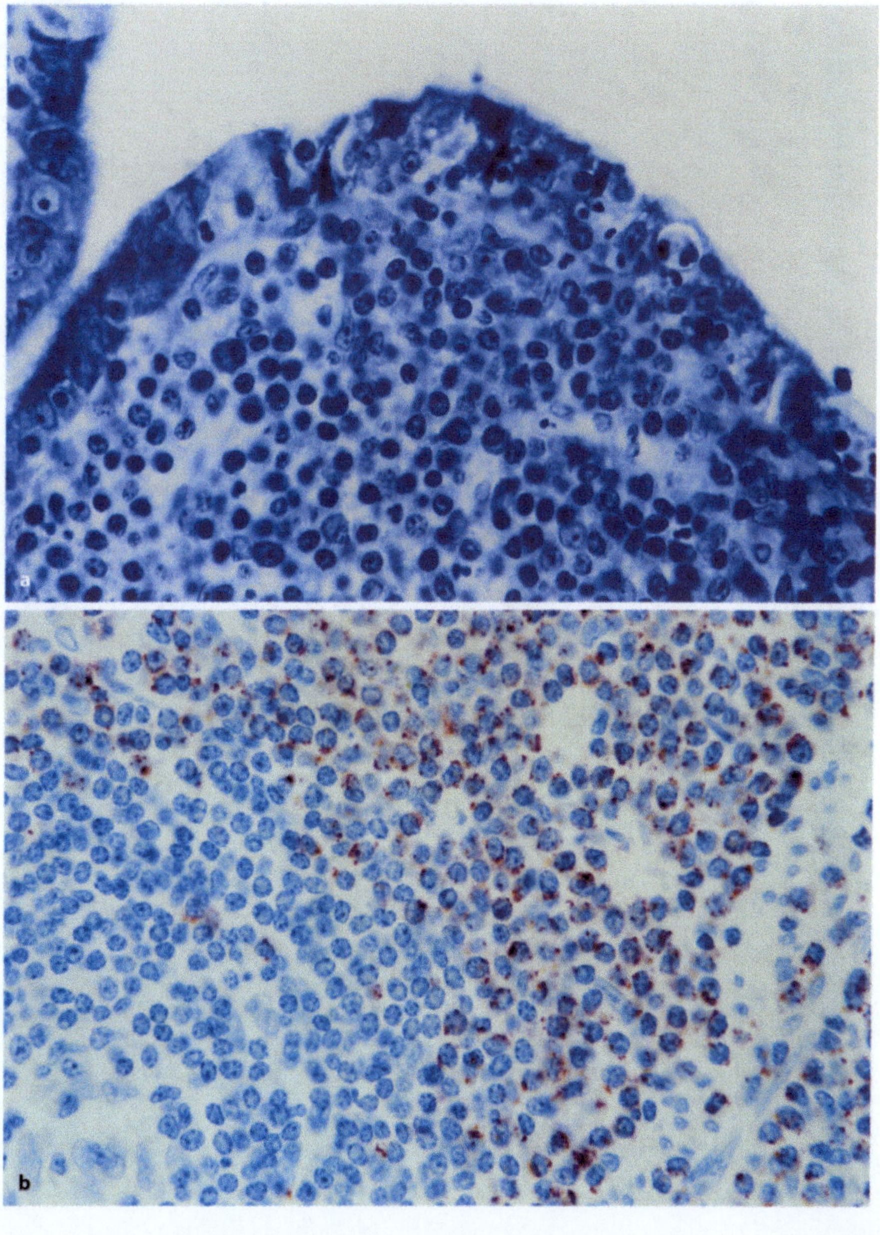

Fig. 6.29. Intestinal NK/T-cell lymphoma. The neoplastic cells infiltrate the epithelial layer (Giemsa stain) (**a**) and stain positive in a granular pattern for cytotoxic granules (TIA1) (**b**) (alkaline phosphatase)

and with signs of malabsorption. Only about one-third have a disease history of years (Gale et al. 2000).

Patients with celiac disease may have a HLA-DR/DQ-associated phenotype, which can indicate an increased risk of developing ETTCL. Most lymphomas are localized in the jejunum followed by the ileum. Other sites of the GI-tract are mostly involved when the lymphoma is disseminated. Frequently, multiple lesion are observed. In a few patients there is dissemination to other organs (Chott et al. 1992).

Despite surgery and chemotherapy, the overall prognosis is poor (Chott et al. 1992). The patients have frequent relapses. The failure-free survival for 1 year and 5 years is 19 % and 3 %, respectively (Gale et al. 2000).

6.2.2.2 NK/T-Cell Lymphoma, Nasal Type (ICD-O: 9719/3)

This subtype has been described predominately in the intestinal tract and, rarely, in the stomach (Fig. 6.29). It

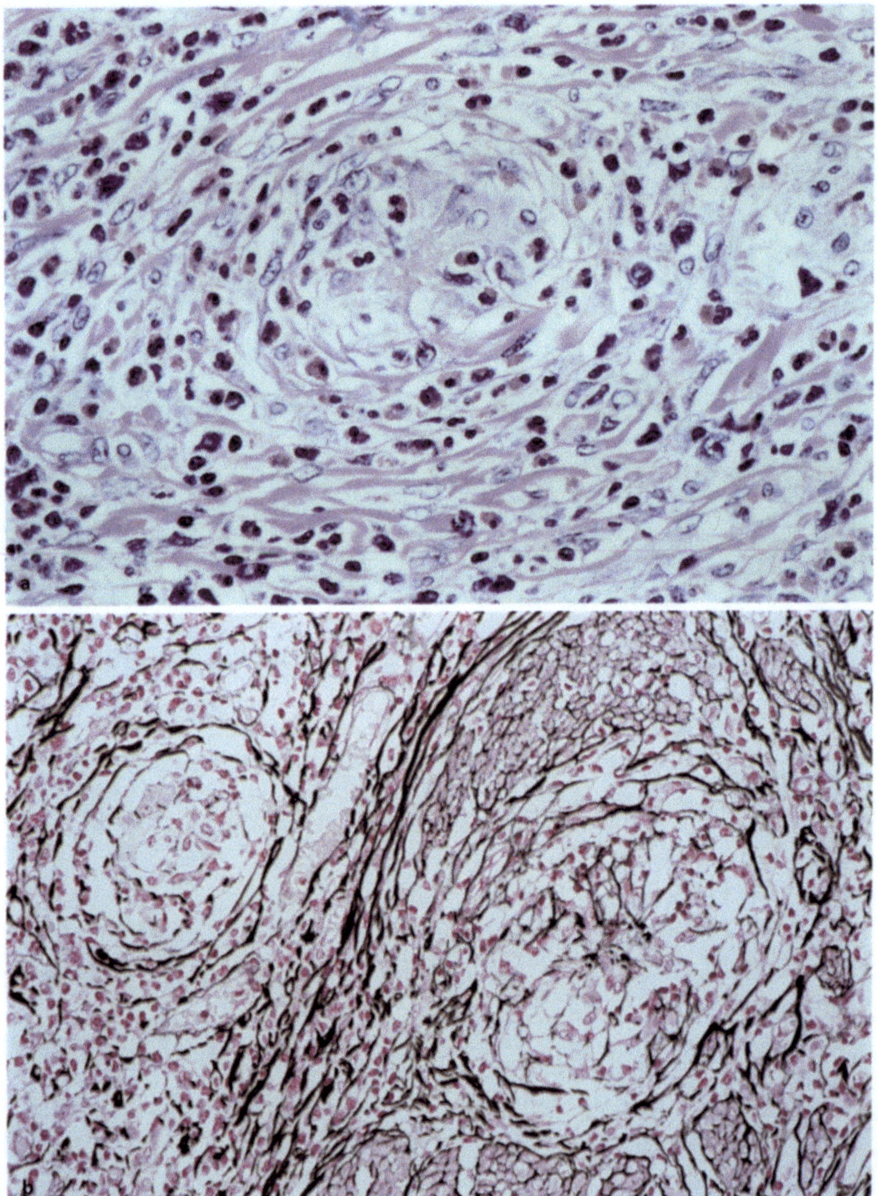

Fig. 6.30 a, b. Intestinal T-cell-lymphoma with angiocentricity. **a** NK/T-cell-lymphoma, nasal type (Giemsa-stain); **b** silver impregnation

cannot be distinguished from ETTCL based on cytological features; however, a marked epitheliotropism is absent, angiocentricity and angioinvasion are regularly found in larger specimens (Figs. 6.30a, b). and they more frequently infiltrate as a tumor mass. NK/T-cell lymphoma, nasal type, is negative for CD103 and usually EBV-positive. This subtype may also be accompanied by eosinophilia (Hsiao et al. 1996; Lavergne et al. 1998; Drut and Drut 2001). Other specific features are described in Chap. 6.3.3.2.

6.2.2.3
Anaplastic Large-Cell Lymphoma

Individual cases of ALCL have been described, especially in the stomach. However, it is a matter of debate weather it constitutes a separate entity or whether it belongs to the group of ETTCLs. The expression of CD30 is by no means enough to separate these lymphomas, as many cases of ETTCL express CD30 to a variable extent. Therefore, T-cell-type ALCL of the GI-tract should show the typical morphology, not be associated with villous atrophy, and be completely and strongly positive for CD30. Such tumors may coexpress CD68.

That true ALCL does exist in this location is documented by the more favorable survival of these patients than those with ETTCL (Ross et al. 1992; Mori et al. 1994). ALCL should also be differentiated from very rare cases of true malignant histiocytosis, in which expression of CD68 and lysozyme are found (Copie-Bergman et al. 1998). Whether CD30 is coexpressed remains a matter of debate.

6.3
Lymphoma of the Upper Aerodigestive Tract

Three main types of lymphomas occur in this area: MZBCL of MALT, DLBCL, and NK/T-cell lymphoma with a cytotoxic phenotype.

As the aerodigestive tract is in close contact to exogenous/infectious agents, it is of interest that predominately those entities occur which are in part known to be associated with bacterial (MALT lymphoma) and viral (NK/T cell cytotoxic lymphoma) infection .

In principal, the different localizations can be divided into three major groups based on the prevalence of the different lymphoma types.

Oral cavity, Waldeyer's ring and pharynx

- Small-B-cell lymphoma
  Marginal zone B-cell lymphoma of MALT
  Mantle cell lymphoma
  Follicular lymphoma
  Extramedullary plasmacytoma
- Diffuse-large-B-cell lymphoma
- Peripheral NK/T-cell lymphoma, nasal type (secondary extension)

Nasal cavity and paranasal sinuses

- Small-B-cell lymphoma
  Lymphocytic lymphoma
  Follicular lymphoma
  Mantle cell lymphoma
  Marginal zone B-cell lymphoma of MALT (monocytoid B-cell)
  Extramedullary plasmacytoma
- Diffuse large-B-cell lymphoma
- Burkitt's lymphoma
- NK/T-cell lymphoma, nasal type

Larynx and trachea

- Small-B-cell lymphoma
  Marginal zone B-cell lymphoma of MALT
  Extramedullary plasmacytoma
- Diffuse-large-B-cell lymphoma

6.3.1
Lymphoma of the Oral Cavity

Definition

Lymphomas arising in the oral cavity, excluding Waldeyer's ring lymphoma, are rare. Some develop as primary tumors. Other are secondary to the extension of lymphomas of Waldeyer's ring or, more often, of NK/T-cell lymphomas from the nose.

Morphology

1. Diffuse-large-B-cell lymphomas (centroblastic or immunoblastic) are the most frequent type of primary lymphoma (Mills et al. 2000; Solomides et al, 2002). Plasmablastic lymphoma often occurs in the gingiva in HIV-positive patients (see Chap. 8.2.1).
2. A few cases of MZBCL of MALT that showed lymphoepithelial lesions have been reported in accessory salivary glands (Takahashi et al. 1993).
3. Follicular lymphomas are extremely rare (Mills et al. 2000).

4. Extramedullary plasmacytoma has been observed (see Chap. 7.2).
5. Rarely, peripheral NK/T-cell lymphoma may develop in the mouth. Most NK/T-cell lymphomas of nasal type secondarily involve the palate, demonstrating typical midline lymphoma (lethal midline granuloma; see Chap. 6.3.3).

Differential Diagnosis

DLBCL should be distinguished from undifferentiated carcinoma (by cytokeratin demonstration) and from myeloid (granulocytic) sarcoma. Peripheral T-cell lymphoma should be distinguished from the exceptional cases of NK/T-cell lymphoproliferative diseases extending to the mouth from the digestive tract mucosa; these have been reported to regress after a long period (up to 17 years) (Egawa et al. 1995).

Occurrence

These lymphomas are localized mostly in the palate and gingiva, less frequently in the tongue, buccal mucosa, floor of the mouth, and lip (Takahashi et al. 1993). In the largest published study (Takahashi et al. 1993), the median age was 53 years with twice as many males as females. Extramedullary plasmacytomas have been described but are rare, involving the palate (2% of tumors of the upper aerodigestive tract), the tongue and the gingiva (1% each) (Mills et al. 2000).

Clinical Presentation

Patients complain of swelling of the oral tissue, without pain and mostly without any general symptoms. There is a female predominance of 2.0 : 1.0.

Survival after radiotherapy and chemotherapy depends on the histopathological type and the stage. In Asia, patients with peripheral NK/T-cell lymphoma of the nose extending to the oral cavity have a poor prognosis (see Chap. 6.3.3.2).

6.3.2 Lymphoma of Waldeyer's Ring and the Pharynx

Definition

Waldeyer's ring comprises the palatine and pharyngeal tonsils and lymphoid tissue of the base of the tongue (Chan et al. 1987a).

These lymphoid tissues and the pharynx have the characteristics of mucosa-associated lymphoid tissue: no sinusoids but the presence of a marginal zone, direct contact with an epithelium, and intraepithelial B-lymphocytes (Wright 1994). Waldeyer's ring lymphoid tissue has an intermediate place between MALT and nodal lymphoid tissue (Wright 1994). Menarguez et al. (1994) have shown some peculiar features that are common to Waldeyer's ring lymphoma and MALT lymphoma of the digestive tract but in contrast to marginal zone nodal lymphomas. These differences have justified the inclusion of Waldeyer ring lymphomas, particularly involving the tonsils, into the group of extranodal lymphomas.

Lymphomas developing in Waldeyer's ring are regarded as primary when the tumor predominates in this area, when there are no tumor masses at a distance, and no bone marrow involvement (Menarguez et al. 1994).

Morphology

The most frequent primary lymphomas are DLBCL (about 85%), mostly of *centroblastic type* and sometimes with a partially follicular growth pattern. A few patients present with *immunoblastic lymphoma* (Barton et al. 1984; Albada et al. 1985; Saul and Kapadia 1985; Shirato et al. 1986; Menarguez et al. 1994). DLBCL secondary to MALT lymphoma does occur; however, it is necessary to recognize a small-cell component in such cases. Although this phenomenon was missing in their series, Menarguez et al. (1994) interpreted many DLBCLs as secondary MALT lymphomas due to differences existing between their cases and nodal DLBCL, i.e. lower incidence of bcl-2 expression, lower clinical stage, and better survival. Paulsen and Lennert (1994) showed areas of DLBCL in two of their twelve cases of MALT lymphomas.

Individual cases of *T-cell-rich/histiocyte-rich B-cell lymphomas*, *anaplastic large B-cell lymphomas*, and a few typical *non-endemic Burkitt's lymphomas* have been observed (Menarguez et al. 1994).

Despite the fact that the lymphoid tissue of Waldeyer's ring belongs to the MALT system, *marginal zone cell lymphomas of MALT* are rare, representing about 3.6% of the lymphomas (Wright 1994). In a review of 329 cases of low-grade lymphomas of Waldeyer's ring, Paulsen and Lennert (1994) identified only 12 cases, two secondary to a primary gastric lymphoma, a condition described before (Ree et al. 1980), and the other ten cases apparently primary.

In the series of Menarguez et al. (1994), three cases were interpreted as monocytoid B-cell lymphomas and only one case was tentatively classified as MALT lymphoma.

Wright (1994) stressed the difficulty of the diagnosis in the presence of a non-pathological heavy infiltration of B-cells into the epithelium thus making it difficult to recognize typical lymphoepithelial lesions.

Other types of *small-B-cell lymphomas* can be observed: *follicular lymphomas* are most frequent in the tonsils, whereas *mantle cell lymphomas* (Fig. 6.31a, b, 6.32) are more frequent in the nasopharynx (Albada et al. 1985). *Gamma-heavy-chain disease* should also be mentioned here, even if no cases has been reported in the published series (see Chap. 7.3.4).

A few number of *extramedullary plasmacytomas* have been described (see Chap. 7.2).

Rare cases of *peripheral NK/T-cell lymphomas* have also been observed (Menarguez et al. 1994), particularly in Asian patients with tumor angiocentricity, corresponding to the entity now called *NK/T-cell lymphomas, nasal type* (Kojima et al. 1993). One case of *anaplastic large T-cell lymphoma* has been recognized (Menarguez et al. 1994).

Differential Diagnosis

Viral diseases, and particularly infectious mononucleosis, can mimic, in some cases, a DLBCL. The presence of many cells of different size with a plasmacytoid morphology, polytypic immunoglobulin synthesis and the presence of immunoblasts of B- and T-cell type, the latter expressing CD8, favor the diagnosis of infectious mononucleosis. This can be confirmed by the expression of Epstein-Barr virus nuclear antigen 2 (EBNA2), LMP-1, and the presence of EBER-1 in the B-cells.

In the differential diagnosis of the different types of small-B-cell lymphoma, we want to stress, in addition to the morphology, the value of CD5 (Wright 1994) and cyclin D1 to differentiate mantle cell lymphoma from MZBCL of MALT, and the importance of CD10 in the diagnosis of follicular lymphoma.

Occurrence

Waldeyer's ring lymphoma represents 10–15% of all extranodal lymphomas and 60–70% of all extranodal lymphomas of head and neck (Freeman et al. 1972; Saul and Kapadia 1985; Isaacson and Norton 1994). Thus, it is the second most frequent site of extranodal lymphomas after the GI-tract. The incidence of NHLs of Waldeyer's ring at presentation is 7–16%, representing

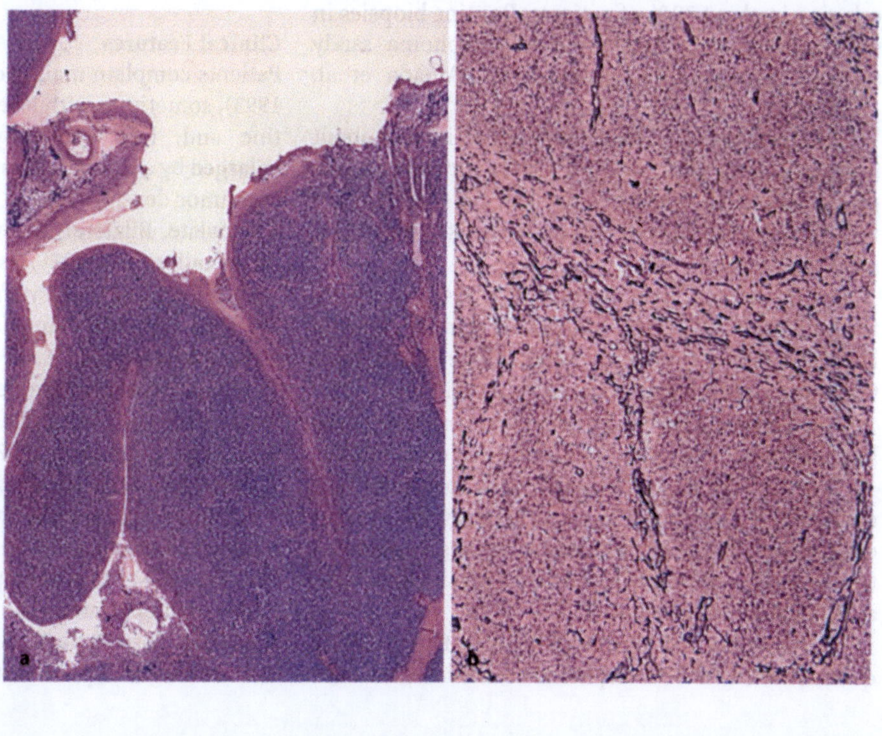

Fig. 6.31 a, b. Mantle cell lymphoma of the tonsil. **a** Massive infiltrate of the tonsil with a vague nodularity (H and E stain). **b** Gomori silver impregnation underlines the presence of nodules

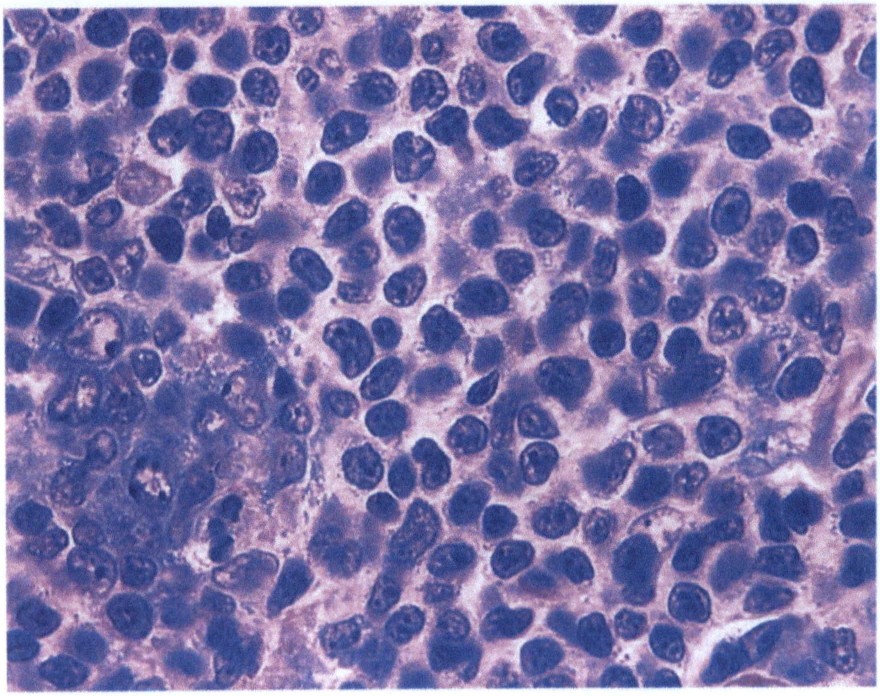

Fig. 6.32. Same patient as in Fig. 6.31. The neoplastic cells are small to medium-sized lymphoid cells with an irregular nucleus. Notice to the *left*, the large cells representing remnants of a reactive germinal center (Giemsa stain)

one-third of all extranodal lymphomas (Freeman et al. 1972; Hoppe et al. 1978; Albada et al. 1985). Disseminated NHL clinically shows an involvement of Waldeyer's ring in about 30 % of patients. Routine biopsies in patients without clinical signs of lymphoma rarely show a manifestation histologically (Albada et al. 1985).

The incidence of MALT lymphoma is low, about 3.6 % (Paulsen and Lennert 1994). Extramedullary plasmacytomas have been described; 7 % of this type of tumor occurring in head and neck arise from the tonsils (Mills et al. 2000).

In the series of Menarguez et al. (1994), the age of the patients ranged from 4 to 88 years (mean 54.9). In DLBCL, there is a broader range of age distribution than observed in small-B-cell lymphoma.

In the different series, a slight female predominance has been found (Barton et al. 1984; Chan et al. 1987a).

The predominance of B-cell lymphomas is even observed in Asian patients, contrasting with the predominance of T-cell lymphomas of the nasopharynx in this geographical area (Chan et al. 1987a, b; Shibuya et al. 1987; Kojima et al. 1993).

Nasopharynx and tonsil represent the two most frequent sites for the development of the rare follicular lymphoma in children. These lymphomas are bcl-2-negative and often show a plasmacytoid differentiation.

Clinical Features

Patients complain mainly of sore throat (Kojima et al. 1993), sometimes with fever and weight loss. The palatine and, less frequently, pharyngeal tonsils are enlarged by a tumor that is often ulcerated. Sometimes the tumor develops on the base of the tongue or on the soft palate. Bilateral involvement can be observed at presentation (10 – 20 %) as well as an involvement of multiple sites of Waldeyer's ring (10 – 20 %) (Barton et al. 1984; Saul and Kapadia 1985; Shirato et al. 1986; Kojima et al. 1993).

About 70 % of all Waldeyer's ring lymphomas were localized (stage I or II). (Menarguez et al. 1994; Barton et al. 1985; Chan et al. 1987a; Kojima et al. 1993).

About 10 – 20 % of patients with primary Waldeyer's ring lymphoma relapse into the gastrointestinal tract (Saul and Kapadia 1985; Shirato et al. 1986; Paulsen and Lennert 1994). Regarding prognosis, Menarguez et al. (1994) demonstrated that an advanced clinical stage and a high histological grade (Kiel classification) were associated with a poor survival probability.

The size of the tumoral mass also has prognostic value. The 5-year survival rate in patients with a palatine tonsil mass of more than 4 cm or with cervical adenopathy of more than 5 cm was 31 %, contrasting with 63 % survival in patients with smaller tumors (Shirato et al. 1986). Association with cervical adenopathy does not seem to have prognostic value.

Follicular lymphoma occurring in children and remaining localized to the tonsils or the pharynx has a favorable prognosis.

6.3.3 Lymphoma of the Nasal Cavity and Paranasal Sinuses

Definition

Lymphomas arising in the nasal cavity and/or in the paranasal sinuses can be of B- and T-cell type. There is a difference in the incidence depending on the geography. These lymphomas appear mostly as primary tumors.

6.3.3.1 B-Cell Lymphoma

Morphology

DLBCL represents the most frequent type of B-cell lymphoma (Frierson et al. 1984; Fellbaum et al. 1989; Abbondanzo and Wenig 1995), and Burkitt's lymphoma the second most frequent.

Small-B-cell lymphomas are less frequent than DLBCL and comprise *follicular lymphoma*, *small lymphocytic lymphoma*, and, less frequently, *lymphoplasmacytic lymphoma* and *marginal zone B cell lymphoma of MALT.*

Extramedullary plasmacytomas have also been reported. *B-lymphoblastic* and *mantle cell lymphomas* seem to be extremely rare (Mills et al. 2000).

All these lymphomas have in common sheets of tumor cells infiltrating the subepithelial tissue, extending to the soft tissue and destroying the bone. However, in contrast to NK/T-cell lymphoma, there is no fibrosis, no necrosis, no angiocentric angiodestructive infiltration, and no inflammatory cell infiltrate.

In Japan, about half of the DLBCLs have been reported to express LMP-1, thus indicating that the patients are chronically infected with EBV.

Differential Diagnosis

DLBCL should be distinguished from undifferentiated carcinoma, which can be associated with EBV, melanoma, olfactory neuroblastoma, rhabdomyosarcoma, and myeloid sarcoma. Morphology is often able to aid in the correct diagnosis. Immunohistochemistry may be useful.

The difference between some extramedullary plasmacytomas and extension from multiple myeloma can be difficult, as can the diagnosis of anaplastic plasmacytoma or myeloma vs immunoblastic lymphomas with plasmablastic differentiation. Clinical data are then mandatory (HIV serology, bone marrow biopsy).

Occurrence

B-cell lymphomas are more frequent than T-cell lymphomas in the sinonasal tract in patients in Western countries (Fellbaum et al. 1989; Abbondanzo and Wenig 1995).

Lymphomas of the sinonasal tract represent about 6 % of all sinonasal tumors. In a series published in 1984 (Frierson et al.), lymphomas arising in this location represented only 1.5 % of all NHLs. In the Kiel lymph node registry (Fellbaum et al. 1989), only 0.17 lymphomas out of 33,402 developed primarily in the sinonasal tract and only 0.44 % of the extranodal lymphomas were sinonasal.

B-cell lymphomas are less frequently restricted to the nasal cavity than NK/T-cell lymphomas, but they are more often confined to a paranasal sinus (Abbondanzo and Wenig 1995). In fact, often multiple sinuses can be involved, particularly the maxillary antrum and ethmoid sinus (Cleary and Batsakis 1994).

The sixth decade represents the median age (ranging from 3 to 94 years) with a male predominance (Frierson et al. 1984; Abbondanzo and Wenig 1995).

Clinical Presentation

Patients present with signs of nasal obstruction, a nasal tumor mass with facial swelling and discharge, epistaxis, and pain. They may also have associated headaches and visual disturbances. General symptoms such as weight loss, fever, anorexia, and malaise are mostly observed in patients with regional tumor extension.

B-cell lymphoma of the sinonasal tract may spread to the nasopharynx, palate, cheek or orbit.

Data concerning the outcome of this type of lymphoma are scarce (Mills et al. 2000). Histopathological type and tumor stage are important factors regarding prognosis (Mills et al. 2000).

6.3.3.2 Extranodal NK/T-Cell Lymphoma – Nasal Type (ICD-O: 9719/3)

Synonyms

- Kiel: Pleomorphic T-cell lymphoma
- REAL: (In part) angiocentric lymphoma
- Other: Malignant midline reticulosis, lethal midline granuloma, polymorphic reticulosis
- WHO: Extra nodal NK/T-cell lymphoma nasal type

Definition

This extranodal disease mostly presents in the nasal area, midline facial structures, GI-tract, and skin. It frequently shows angiocentric growth with angiodestruction and subsequent necrosis. The cellular infiltrate is variable, with mostly medium- and large-cell pleomorphic but sometimes also round, lymphoblastic-like cells. Thus the morphology is not decisive. The tumor cells are CD56-positive and carry EBV genome in the atypical cells.

The postulated normal cell counterpart is either activated NK cell or, less frequently, cytotoxic T cells (Chan et al. 2001).

Morphology

The major primary characteristic is the extranodal growth in the nasopharyngeal region. The infiltrate is diffuse or patchy and, under low-power magnification, sometimes gives the impression of an inflammatory infiltrate. Necrosis is a very frequent feature and occurs in a zonal pattern (Fig. 6.33). It is usually accompanied by angiocentric tumor growth, i.e. angioinvasion and angiodestruction (Fig. 6.34). Angiocentricity should thus only be diagnosed when both of these are present. Furthermore, angiocentricity has to be differentiated from perivascular growth, which is a frequent finding in other malignant and benign lymphoproliferations. Angiocentric growth can best be detected by silver impregnation.

The neoplastic infiltrate is variable. Mostly the cells have pleomorphic nuclei that range in size from small, to medium to large (Fig. 6.35). A minority of tumors have a more homogeneous picture, with medium-sized round cells similar to lymphoblasts but mostly with a lighter chromatin pattern (Fig. 6.36). These tumors may lack necrosis and are EBV-negative. (see Differential Diagnosis). Alternatively, the large blastic cells similar to immunoblasts dominate. Sometimes large, bizarre, anaplastic tumor cells are intermingled. The

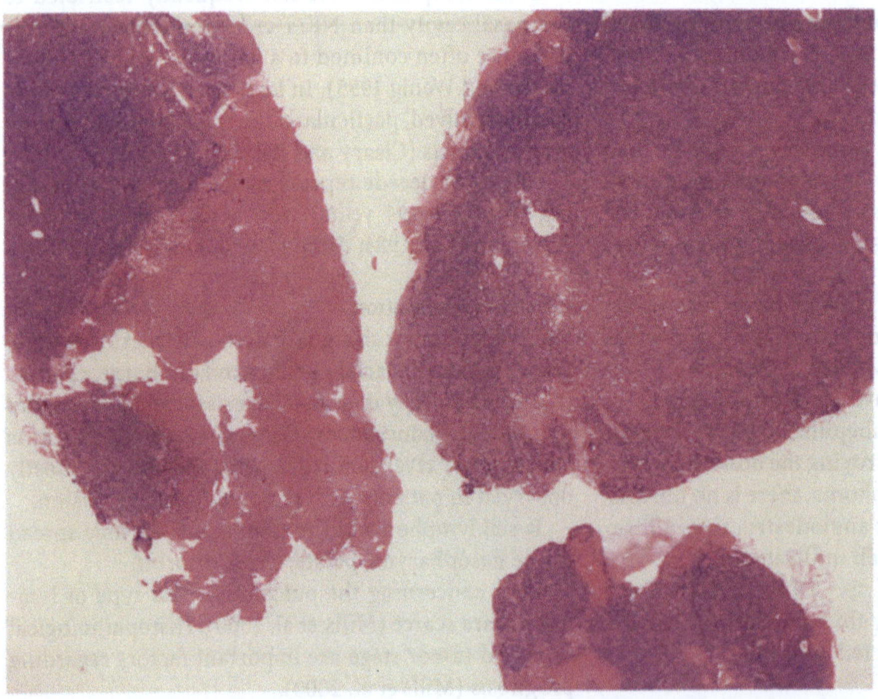

Fig. 6.33. NK/T-cell lymphoma, nasal type. The lymphoma shows large necrotic areas (H and E stain)

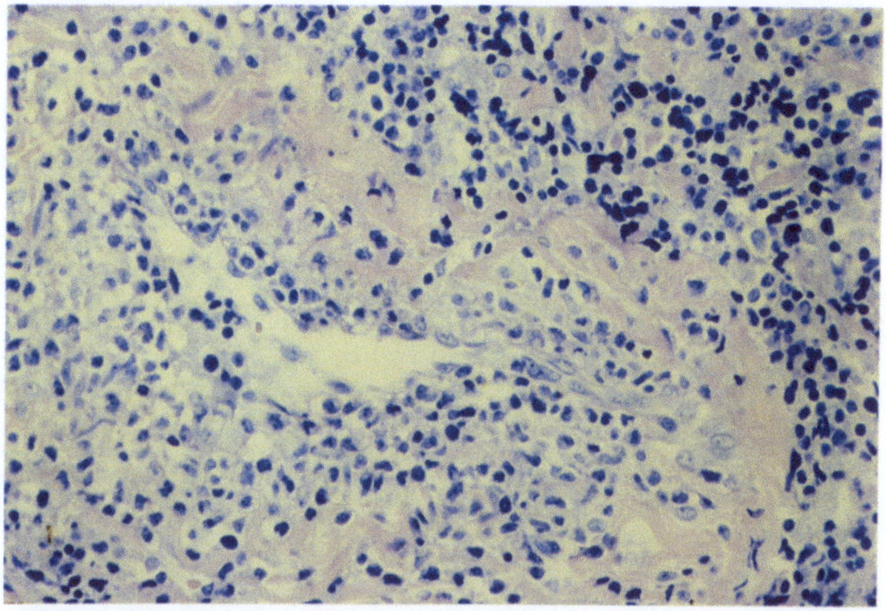

Fig. 6.34. NK/T-cell lymphoma, nasal type. Lymphomatous infiltrate with perivascular growth pattern (angiocentricity). The infiltrate has invaded the vascular wall resulting in angiodestruction (Giemsa stain)

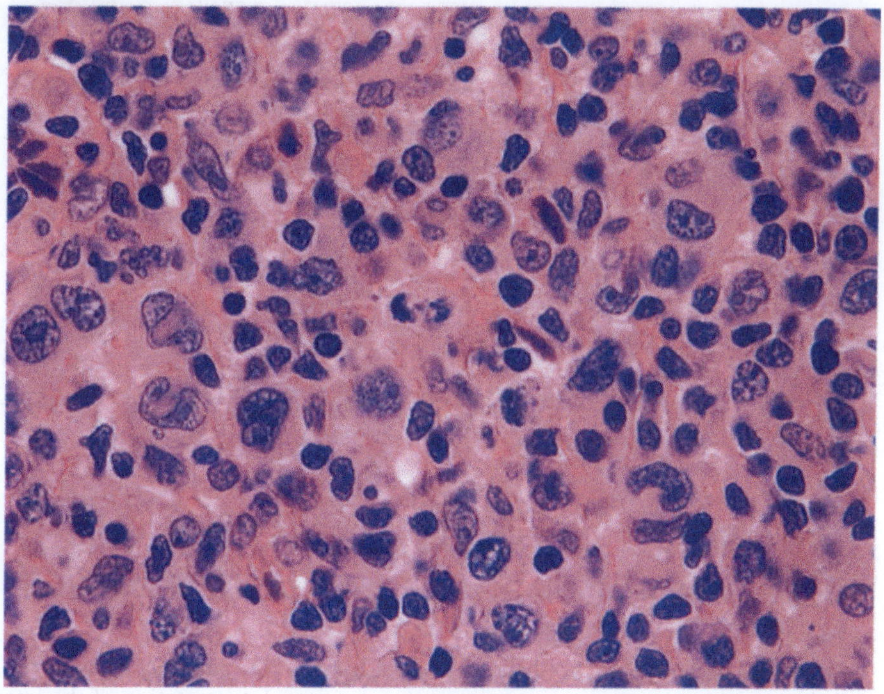

Fig. 6.35. NK/T-cell lymphoma, nasal type. The medium-sized and large lymphoma cells are highly pleomorphic with irregular nuclei (H and E stain)

mitotic activity is usually high; apoptosis is a prominent finding.

The neoplastic infiltrate is regularly accompanied by an inflammatory infiltrate of histiocytes, plasma cells, and eosinophils. In some cases, this infiltrate may dominate which makes detection of the lymphoma difficult. This has to be taken into account especially in small biopsies! The inflammatory infiltrate is frequently dense directly beneath the epithelial mucosa and the tumor infiltrate can only be found in a

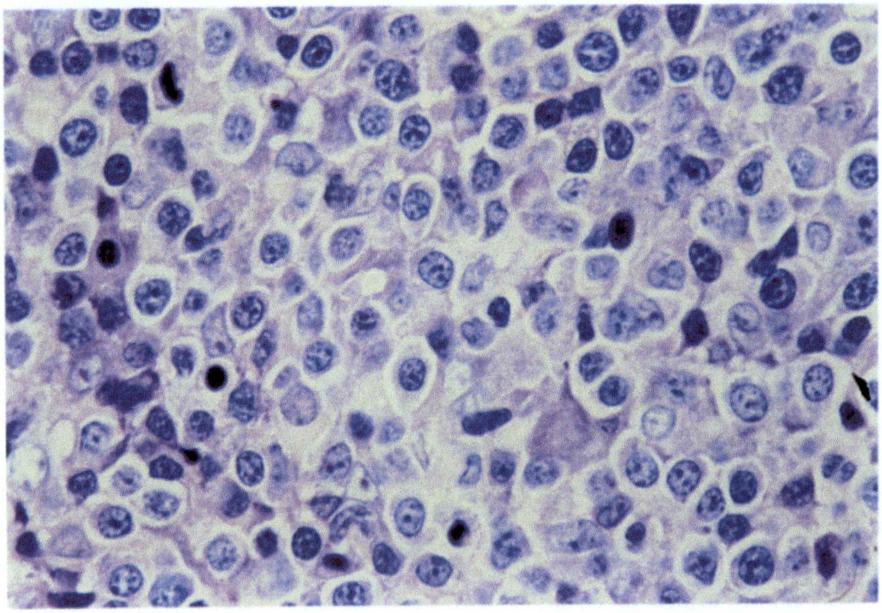

Fig. 6.36. NK/T-cell lymphoma, nasal type. In this case, the nuclei of the lymphoma cells are less irregular. Note the clear cytoplasm (Giemsa stain)

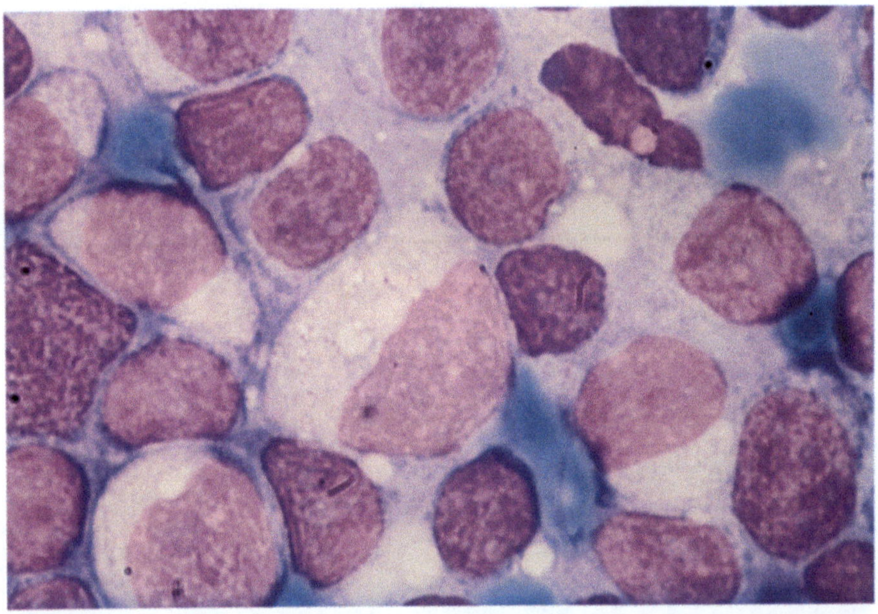

Fig. 6.37. NK/T-cell lymphoma, nasal type. On imprint, the lymphoma cells range in size and have a large pale cytoplasm with azurophilic granules (Pappenheim stain)

deeper layer of the biopsy. Epitheliotropism of tumor cells is rare.

The borders of the ulceration may present as an intense epithelial hyperplasia, which can be misdiagnosed as carcinoma.

Only in touch imprints can the typical and frequently occurring azurophilic granules be seen (Fig. 6.37) (Wong et al. 1992).

Immunohistochemistry

Interpretation of the immunohistochemistry findings is sometimes difficult due to extensive necrosis and a prominent inflammatory background. However, the phenotype is distinctive (Wong et al. 1992). By definition CD56 is expressed mostly together with CD2, CD45RO, TIA1 and, less frequently, granzyme B/perforin. Moreover, cCD3 is found. Only some tumors express sCD3, but this is difficult to distinguish from cCD3 on paraffin sections. CD57 is usually negative, as are CD5 and βF1.

Recently, the expression of CD95/CD95L has been described in 70–90% of tumors. This system is thought to play an important role in triggering apoptosis (Ng et al. 1999).

Almost all tumors express EBV, which is best documented by LMP-1 staining and EBER-1 in situ hybridization (Petrella et al. 1996; Elenitoba-Johnson et al. 1998; Jaffe 1999).

Finally, one can try to distinguish between NK/T-cell lymphomas and true NK-cell lymphomas on the basis of the immunophenotype and the genotype. True NK-cell lymphomas should either stain for TcR-δ1 (TcR-γ/δ cells) (only applicable on frozen sections), or should be at least negative for βF1 and have no TCR gene rearrangement. All other cases are designated as NK/T-cell lymphomas.

Genetic Features

Specific chromosomal abnormalities have not yet been described (Wong et al. 1999).

NK/T-cell lymphomas show TCR gene rearrangement, whereas true NK-cell lymphomas are in germline configuration for TCR. An Ig heavy-chain gene rearrangement is not detected.

Differential Diagnosis

The clinical presentation, morphology, and immunophenotype are so peculiar that the diagnosis is usually evident. The most important point is not to miss the diagnosis of lymphoma due to the *inflammatory reaction* with necrosis. Small biopsies, superficial biopsies, and crushed material may lead to such a misdiagnosis. A good clinicopathological correlation is needed and new biopsies should be performed in cases of disagreement.

Other inflammatory disorders demonstrating such an intense granulomatous pattern and tissue destruction are very rare. *Wegener's granulomatosis* is one of them; however, giant cells are often present and the clinical presentation is completely different, as the patient has renal dysfunction.

Rarely, the epithelial hyperplasia at the border of ulceration of the mucosae may lead to a false diagnosis of *squamous cell carcinoma.*

Some B-cell lymphomas may present with a destructive and inflammatory reaction, for example, some *MALT lymphomas* or *DLBCLs.* The morphology of the cells and their immunophenotype allow the correct diagnosis.

Lymphomatoid granulomatosis is currently interpreted as a completely different disorder that should not be confused with this type of lymphoma (see Chap. 6.7.1.4).

Finally, the different NK/T-cell lymphomas like *blastic/lymphoblastic NK-cell lymphoma, aggressive NK-cell leukemia, NK/T-cell lymphoma* in immunocompromised patients, and peripheral T-cell lymphoma, unspecified (pleomorphic T-cell lymphoma), have to be differentiated. This is best done by immunohistochemistry.

Occurrence

While NK-cell lymphomas are extremely rare in Europe and the USA, they nonetheless represent the largest single group of lymphomas primarily presenting in the nose. These lymphomas are much more frequent in Asia and South America. The largest series are from Hong Kong, Taiwan, and Japan. The frequency in these countries is between 2% and 10% of all NHLs. In Western countries the frequency is below 1%. The above-described geographical distribution might indicate the importance of racial factors that predispose for this disease (Chan et al. 1987, 2001; Arber et al. 1993; Van Gorp et al. 1994; Cheung et al. 1998; Quintanilla-Martinez et al. 1999).The median age is around 45–50 years with a range from 20 to 80 years. There is a clear male preponderance with a male to female ratio of 1.5–3:1 (Chan et al. 2001).

Clinical Presentation and Prognosis

The majority of the patients, more than 80%, present with a localized disease stages I and II. Mostly, the nose is the primary site of the disease followed by additional involvement of the nasopharynx. Clinically, many patients present with midfacial destructive disease, described earlier as lethal midline granuloma or polymorphic reticulosis. These terms describe a locally aggressive, destructive, growing tumor in midline facial structures invading the surrounding organs by continuous growth.

Only about 15% of the patients have B symptoms (Kanavaros et al. 1993; Chan et al. 1986; Kwong et al. 1997; Cheung et al. 1998). Rarely, these lymphomas have secondary spreading to the lung, GI-tract, testis, and, most frequently, to the skin.

Data on randomized trials are not available. In patients from Hong Kong, it was shown that limited stage was the only favorable prognostic finding (Shibuya et al. 1987). In these early stages, there was no significant therapeutic difference between local radiation with or without chemotherapy.

In a recent study (Cheung et al. 1998), the 5-year overall survival was around 30%, the median overall survival 12 months. A complete remission was achieved by 50% of the patients; 20% had a local relapse, but lymph node involvement in relapse was exceptional.

6.3.4 Lymphoma of the Larynx and Trachea

Definition

These lymphomas develop in the larynx and trachea. Some are primary and are mostly localized. Others may extend from lymphomas of the upper aerodigestive tract (for example, nose or nasopharynx). A few represent secondary involvement during dissemination of lymphomas from other sites.

Morphology

Marginal zone B-cell lymphoma of MALT, *plasmacytoma*, and *diffuse large-B-cell lymphoma* are probably the most frequent types of lymphoma observed in the larynx (Diebold et al. 1990; Fidias et al. 1996) and in the trachea (Kaplan et al. 1992).

In MALT lymphomas, a diffuse infiltration by small centrocyte-like cells is associated with follicles showing either reactive or colonized germinal centers (Fig. 6.38a). At the periphery of this diffuse infiltrate, sheets of monocytoid B-cells or sometimes a lymphoplasmacytic component can be recognized (Fig. 6.38b) (Diebold et al. 1990). Lymphoepithelial lesions may be seen but are often absent. Most of the so-called pseudolymphomas in the past were in fact MALT lymphomas.

Other B-cell lymphomas have been described but in older publications it is not easy to identify the precise diagnosis. For example, what were previously described as small cleaved and lymphoplasmacytic lymphomas may instead be MZBCLs of MALT.

In extramedullary plasmacytoma, sheets of plasma cells infiltrate the supraglottic portion of the larynx, particularly the epiglottis, while the subglottic portion is involved in less than 10% of patients (Mills et al. 2000). In the majority of the cases, the tumor cells are

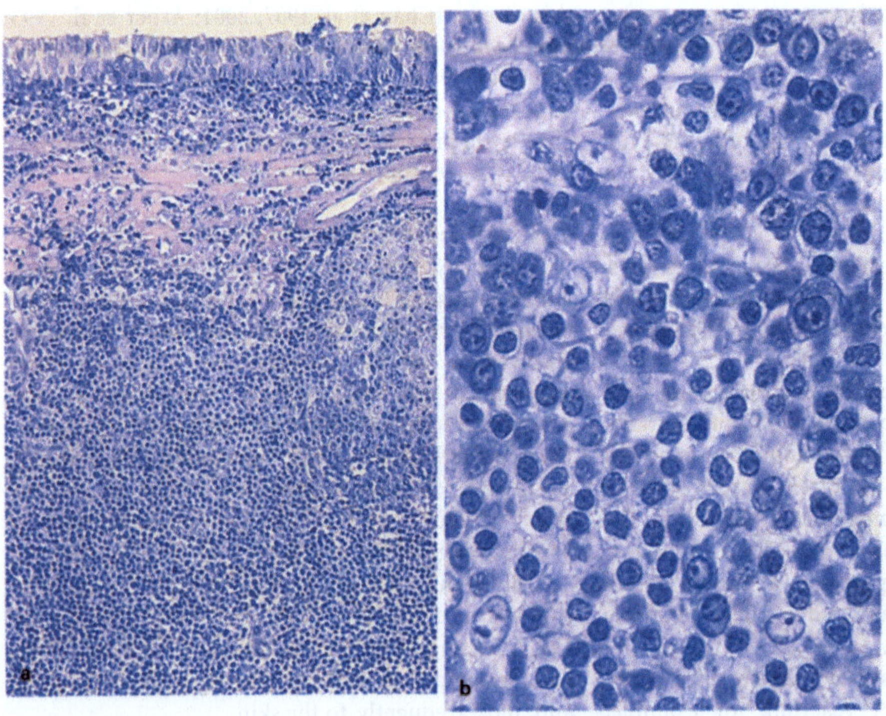

Fig. 6.38 a, b. Primary laryngeal marginal zone lymphoma of MALT. **a** Diffuse infiltrate of the mucosae with reactive germinal center to the *right* and at the *top*; the epithelium is of respiratory type without typical lymphoepithelial lesions. **b** The neoplastic cells exhibit the morphology of monocytoid B-cells and mature plasma cells (both Giemsa stain). This latter cell population produces an intracytoplasmic, monotypic, IgM κ immunoglobulin (not shown)

mature plasma cells, but large cells (plasmablasts, immunoblasts) or even anaplastic cells may be present. In some cases there are associated amyloid deposits.

Burkitt's lymphomas are rare.

NK/T-cell lymphoma, EBV-related, can involve the larynx primarily but is mostly secondary to the extension of a sinonasal tract lymphoma.

Differential Diagnosis

The differential diagnosis includes several different types of lesions:

1. Non-hematopoietic tumors: *undifferentiated carcinoma, olfactory neuroblastoma, melanoma*
2. *Myeloid sarcoma*
3. *Reactive plasmacytosis* (immunohistochemistry is decisive)

The so-called pseudolymphomas of the larynx are in fact *MALT lymphomas.*

Finally, the distinction between immunoblastic lymphomas with plasmablastic differentiation and the anaplastic variant of extramedullary plasmacytoma can be extremely difficult and the diagnosis is almost arbitrary.

Occurrence

Lymphoma involving only the larynx is a very rare condition (Morgan et al. 1989; Shima et al. 1990; Diebold et al. 1990; Horny and Kaiserling 1995; Fidias et al. 1996) accounting for less than 1 % of all laryngeal neoplasias. Considering extranodal lymphomas of the head and neck, the larynx was involved in 4 % of the cases (Shima et al. 1990). The male to female ratio is 1.3 : 1. The median age is about 58 years, ranging from 4 to 90 years.

Primary tracheal lymphomas are even more rare (Kaplan et al. 1992). Compression and displacement of the trachea by adenopathies with narrowing of the lumen are most frequent (Mills et al. 2000). The age range is from 52 to 81 years.

Mills et al. (2000) showed that 8 % of plasmacytomas arose in the larynx and 1 % in the trachea. This type of lymphoma seems to be one of the most frequent lymphomas of the larynx. A total of 90 cases were reported in 1995 (Horny and Kaiserling), in contrast to 65 cases of other types of lymphoma. There is a wide age range with most patients being in the fifth to seventh decades of life. About 80 % of the patients are men (Mills et al. 2000).

Clinical Presentation

Patients complain of hoarseness, dysphonia, stridor, cough, and dysphagia in case of larynx involvement, or dyspnea, stridor, and wheezing in case of tracheal involvement, sometimes with weight loss. Lymphomas of the larynx involve the supraglottic area, particularly the epiglottis and aryepiglottic folds. The glottic or subglottic regions are more rarely involved.

Localized laryngeal and tracheal lymphomas may completely respond to radiotherapy. A good long-term survival can be expected.

MZBCL of MALT has a good prognosis. During the course of the disease, another location may be involved (lung, orbit, eye, thyroid, etc.).

Patients with extramedullary plasmacytoma have no bone marrow involvement and serum and urine proteins are in the normal range. Radiation therapy is the best treatment. In the absence of amyloid deposits, total regression is obtained in 3 months. In cases with amyloidosis, regression after radiotherapy is not completed and surgical excision is recommended. The 5-year overall survival is mostly good, but dissemination can occur in 35–50 % of the patients, even several decades later (Mills et al. 2000).

6.4 Malignant Lymphoma of the Major Salivary Glands

- Small-B-cell lymphoma
  - Marginal zone B-cell of MALT/immunocytoma
  - Follicular lymphoma
  - Mantle cell lymphoma
  - Extraosseous plasmacytoma
- Diffuse large-B-cell lymphoma
- Peripheral NK/T-cell lymphoma

Definition

These tumors are defined as a malignant, localized neoplastic proliferation of lymphoid cells in which major salivary gland involvement is usually the first clinical manifestation of the disease. If at clinical staging other, non-contiguous sites are found to be involved (stage III or IV), then these lymphomas are regarded as secondary rather than primary (Ellis and Auclair 1996).

Primary lymphomas are closely linked to so-called myoepithelial sialadenitis (Schmid et al. 1989), also known as "benign lymphoepithelial lesion", which develops often, but not always, in patients with Sjögren's disease (Ellis and Auclair 1996).

Morphology

Macroscopy. The involved gland presents as a firm, solid, sometimes polycyclic mass consisting of a homogeneous whitish tissue.

Histology. Marginal zone cell lymphoma of MALT is the most frequent type of lymphoma involving the major salivary glands (Isaacson and Wright 1984; Isaacson and Spencer 1987). The normal architecture is destroyed and replaced by diffuse sheets of small to medium-sized centrocyte-like cells (Isaacson and Wright 1984; Takahashi et al. 1992). Follicles either with a reactive or a colonized germinal center are observed (Fig. 6.39). Areas of monocytoid B-cells are

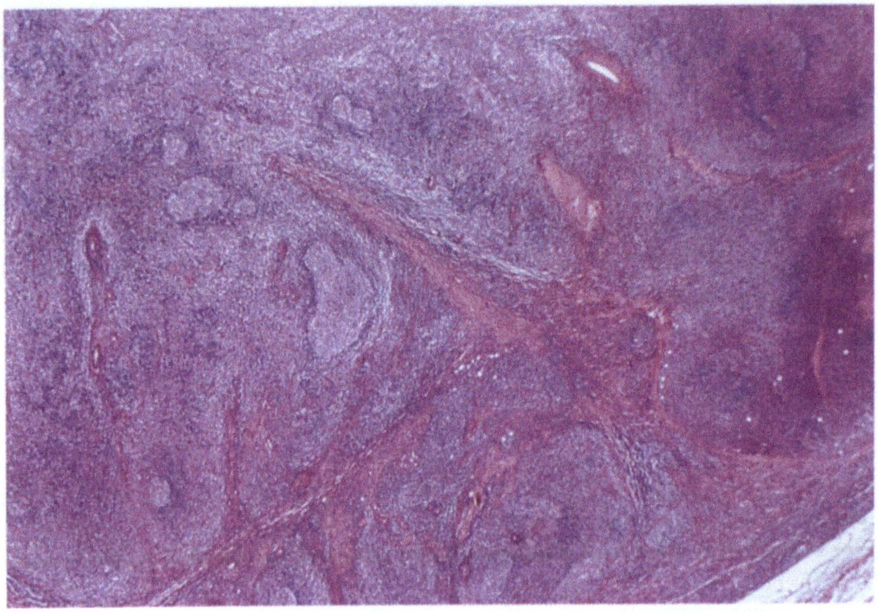

Fig. 6.39. Primary marginal zone lymphoma of MALT in the salivary gland. Coalescent sheets of lymphoid cells have destroyed the normal architecture. Note the presence of reactive germinal centers (H and E stain)

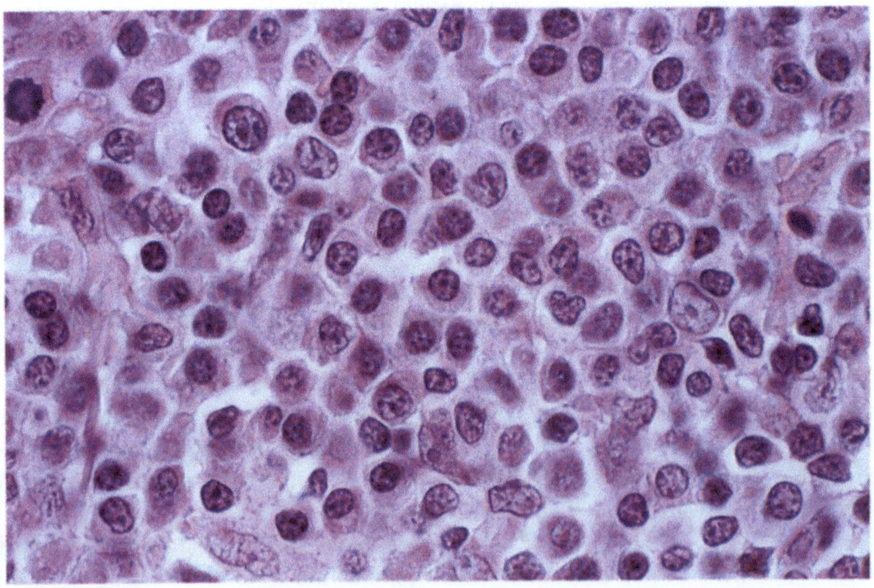

Fig. 6.40. Same patient as in Fig. 6.39. The diffuse infiltrate consists of numerous monocytoid B-cells and plasma cells (producing a monotypic, IgM-κ immunoglobulin; not shown) (H and E stain)

associated, usually surrounding ductal structures (Fig. 6.40). Both types of cells often surround and invade myoepithelial complexes (Schmid et al. 1982a, b). Sheets of plasma cells sometimes showing Dutcher-Fahey bodies are frequently seen (Fig. 6.40). Rarely, lymphoepithelial lesions are disclosed in the epithelium of larger ducts. The lymphoma extend into the capsule, as well as the trabecular and the fat tissue surrounding the salivary gland. At a distance from the major tumor mass, multiple distinct foci develop separated by normal gland parenchyma.

Lymphoplasmacytic lymphomas were reported frequently in the past. Today, at least most if not all of these are regarded as MALT lymphomas with a predominant lymphoplasmacytic component.

Other *small-B-cell lymphomas* can be observed, particularly *follicular lymphoma* or less frequently *mantle cell lymphoma.* Sometimes these lymphomas involve the intraparotid lymph nodes without extension into the glandular tissue.

Some *follicular lymphomas* may occur in association with cystadenolymphoma (Whartin tumor). *Extraosseous plasmacytoma* may be found primarily in the major salivary glands, sometimes associated with amyloidosis (Figs. 6.41, 6.42).

Diffuse large-B-cell lymphomas are also observed; they are classified as one of the subtypes of the updated Kiel classification. Some are secondary to MALT lymphoma (Schmid et al. 1982a; Isaacson and Wright 1984).

Rarely, *peripheral NK/T-cell type lymphoma* has been reported.

Immunohistochemistry and Genetic Features

Some MZBCLs/immunocytomas coexpress CD5. It is not yet clear whether this subset constitutes a separate entity and should be designated as true immunocytomas or whether they are a variant of MALT lymphomas.

Demonstration of light-chain restriction in the B-cell population in "myoepithelial sialadenitis" (MESA) is a good argument in favor of a lymphoma arising from Sjögren's syndrome (Schmid et al. 1982b, 1989; Lennert and Schmid 1983). The same is true for the demonstration by a variety of methods, including PCR, of Ig heavy-chain gene rearrangement, which seems to be observed in the majority of cases of MESA (Isaacson and Norton 1994). The cells of the myoepithelial complexes are cytokeratin-positive (Fig. 6.43).

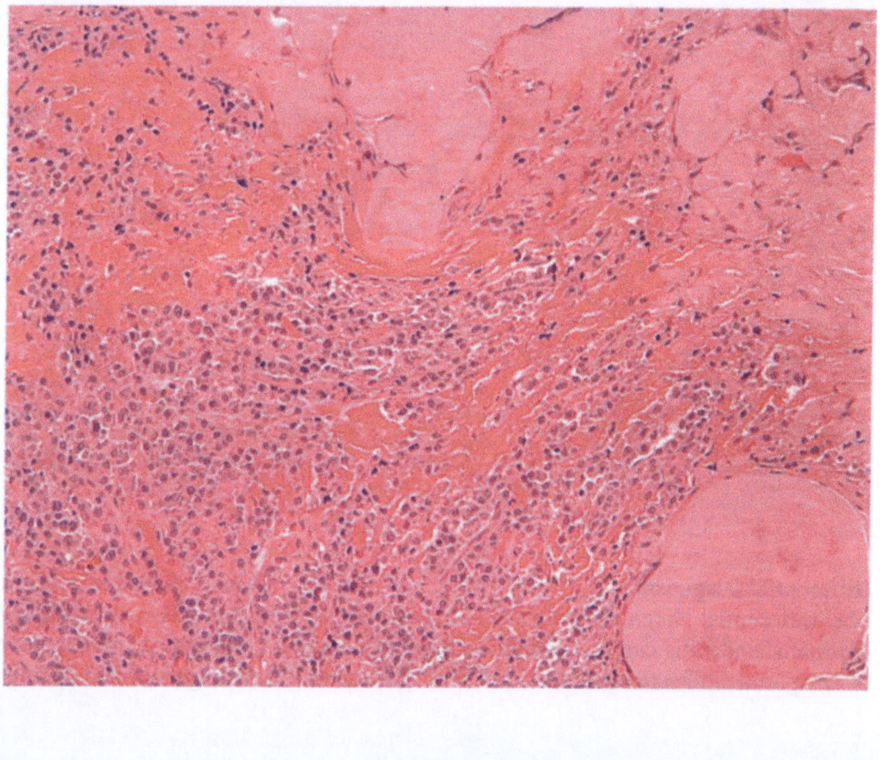

Fig. 6.41. Primary plasmacytoma of the salivary gland, associated with amyloidosis. The diffuse infiltrate has destroyed the gland; note the large eosinophilic amyloid deposits (H and E stain)

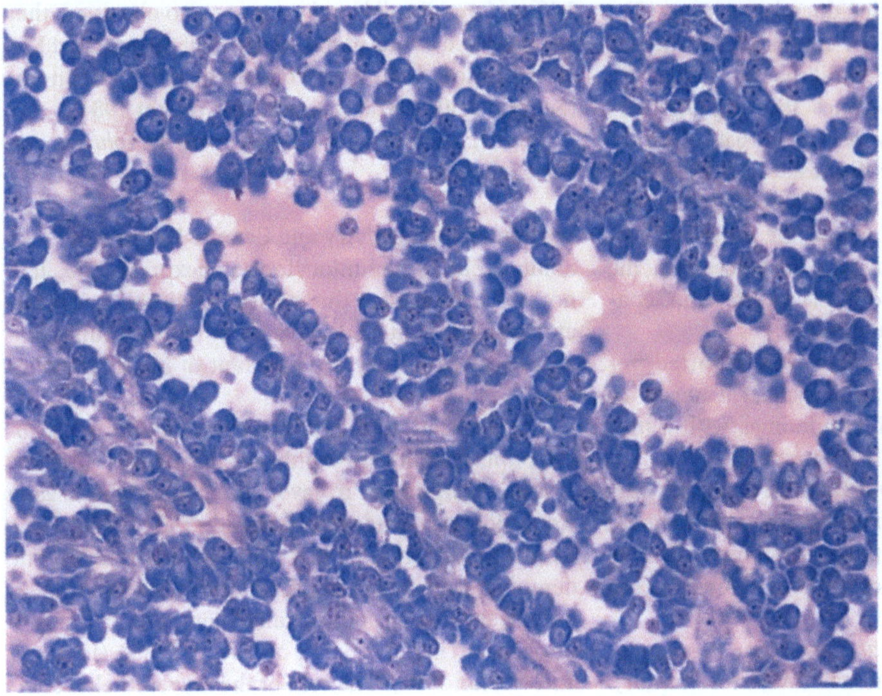

Fig. 6.42. Same patient as in Fig. 6.41. The diffuse infiltrate is made up of mature plasma cells. Note the pseudoangiomatous pattern, which is often seen in this type of lymphoma (Giemsa stain)

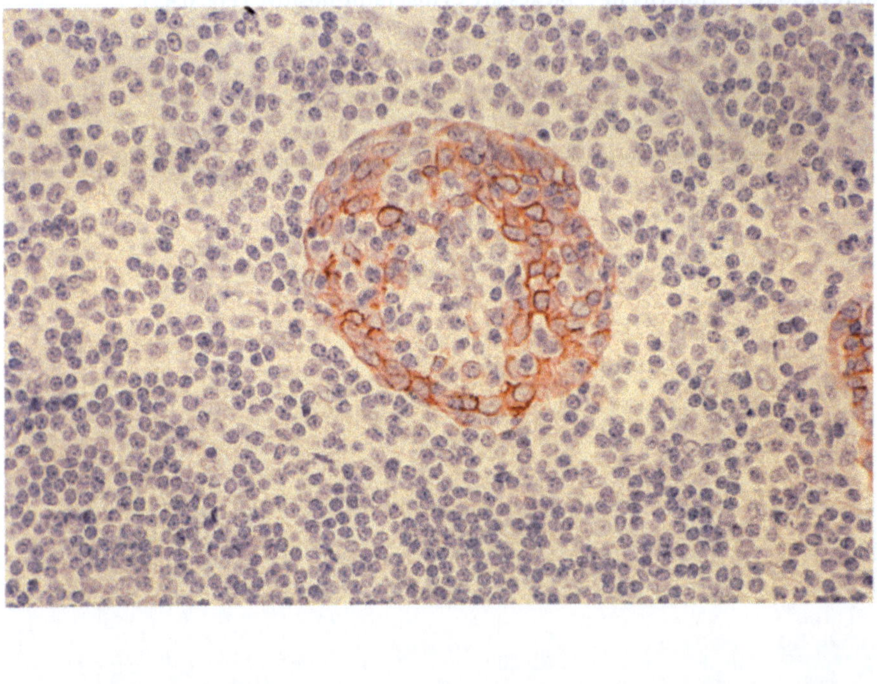

Fig. 6.43. Same patient as in Figs. 6.39 and 6.40. Immunohistochemistry. Demonstration of cytokeratin (KL1) allows recognition of myoepithelial complexes (alkaline phosphatase)

Differential Diagnosis

The differential diagnosis to rule out non-specific chronic sialadenitis can be difficult. A predominance of lymphoid infiltrates around ducts with periductal fibrosis, ductal ectasia, and malpighian metaplasia are arguments against MESA/MALT.

The most important consideration in the differential diagnosis is to distinguish between MESA associated with Sjögren's syndrome and marginal zone cell lymphoma of MALT. Both lesions comprise myoepithelial complexes and follicular hyperplasia. In MESA, numerous T-lymphocytes surround and infiltrate the myoepithelial complexes in association with B-lymphocytes. Plasma cells are polytypic.

In MALT lymphoma, myoepithelial complexes are surrounded by sheets of B-cells with the morphology of centrocyte-like cells and/or monocytoid B-cells. The majority of the cells infiltrating the myoepithelial complexes are B-centrocyte-like lymphocytes. These small lymphocytes may colonize and obscure the follicles.

Intermediate stages between the two disorders have been recognized. Currently, demonstration of a monotypic B-cell population and/or monotypic plasma cells is regarded as an argument in favor of MALT lymphoma (Schmid et al. 1982a,b, 1989; Lennert and Schmid 1983; Janin et al. 1992).

There is probably a close relationship between MESA and MALT lymphoma, since the genes coding for immunoglobulin heavy- or light-chains are rearranged in almost all cases of MESA.

Finally, a bilateral parotid swelling can occur as an initial clinical manifestation in HIV-positive patients. This swelling is due to follicular hyperplasia with follicular lysis and a diffuse infiltrate of CD8-positive lymphocytes and should be distinguished from MZBCL of MALT.

Occurrence

Lymphomas of major salivary glands are rare, representing about 5% of all non-Hodgkin's lymphomas (Gleeson et al. 1986).

The majority of MZBCLs of MALT develop in preexisting MESA (Schmid et al. 1982b, 1989; Lennert and Schmid 1983; Janin et al. 1992; Ellis and Auclair 1996; Gleeson et al. 1986). Symptoms of a preexisting Sjögren's syndrome are observed in only 10% of patients presenting salivary gland primary lymphoma (Gleeson et al. 1986).

Large-B-cell lymphomas of the salivary glands are rare. Some are secondary to MALT lymphoma.

Other *small-B-cell lymphomas* and *T/NK-cell lymphomas* remain extremely rare (Isaacson and Norton 1994).

There is no sex predominance in patients without Sjögren's syndrome. Of the patients with Sjögren's syndrome, 80–90% are women. Most of the patients are elderly, with a mean age of 63 years. The range is from 4 to 96 years (Ellis and Auclair 1996).

Clinical Presentation

Patients present with a tumor mass either in the parotid (70% of the cases) or the submaxillary (30%) gland. Unilateral cervical adenopathy can be disclosed. Radiology is not able to discriminate between lymphoma or pleomorphic adenoma. Surgical resection allows diagnosis.

The majority of the patients present with a stage IE or IIE (86% in Gleeson et al. 1986). Disseminated lymphomas may lead to secondary salivary gland involvement.

About 10% of the patients present with symptoms of Sjögren's syndrome: keratoconjunctivitis sicca, xerostomia, episodic or chronic bilateral enlargement of major salivary glands (Ellis and Auclair 1996).

Relapse-free survival occurs in about 60–70% of the patients at 5 years after surgery and radiotherapy. Overall survival is estimated between 52 and 61% at 5 years (Gleeson et al. 1986).

6.5 Lymphoma of the Eye, Lachrymal Glands, and Orbit

6.5.1 Lymphoma of the Conjunctiva, Eyelids, Lachrymal Glands, and Orbit

- Small-B-cell lymphoma
  - Marginal zone cell lymphoma of MALT
  - Lymphoplasmacytic
  - Follicular lymphoma
  - Mantle cell lymphoma
- Diffuse large-B-cell lymphoma (eyelid)
- Burkitt's lymphoma
- Peripheral NK/T-cell lymphoma

6.5.2 Lymphoma of the Uvea and Retina (Similar to CNS Lymphoma)

- Diffuse large-B-cell lymphoma
- Burkitt's lymphoma

Definition

Tissues of conjunctiva, the eyelids (Ellis et al. 1985; Jenkins et al. 2000; Leff et al. 1985; Medeiros and Harris 1989; Knowles et al. 1990; Petrella et al. 1991; Wotherspoon et al. 1993; Akpek et al. 1999a), lachrymal glands

(Ellis et al. 1985), and orbit (Medeiros and Harris 1989) are in contact with the exterior environment and are thus equipped with lymphoid tissue similar or identical to that of the MALT system. Therefore, MZBCLs predominate. Often, these lymphomas are associated with a lymphoid infiltrate secondary to allergic disease (follicular conjunctiva) or autoimmune diseases such as Sjögren's syndrome (lachrymal glands).

On the other hand, intraocular lymphomas in the vitreous chamber, the uveal tract, the retina, or the optic nerve (Trudeau et al. 1988; Whitcup et al. 1993) are related to the CNS. Thus DLBCL dominates.

The same sites can be involved secondarily by different types of nodal and extranodal lymphomas (Bairey et al. 1994).

6.5.3 Primary Lymphoma of the Eye, Lachrymal Glands, and Orbit

Morphology

Macroscopy. The macroscopy of these lymphomas can be grouped as follows:

1. Conjunctival lymphoma presents as a small, indolent, red-colored nodule of the epibulbar conjunctiva. It is often associated and even preceded by chronic conjunctivitis with a diffuse eye redness.
2. Lymphomas of the eyelids present as a nodule bulging under the skin which appears normal or may be reddish. Ulceration is seen only after a long evolution.
3. In lachrymal gland involvement, the gland is swollen and firm. Dryness of the eye is frequent.
4. Lymphomas in the orbit present as a tumor mass consisting of firm, fish-flesh-like whitish tissue that occupies a variable part of the orbit with infiltration of the oculomotor muscles and compression of the optic nerve and the bulbus.
5. Uveal or retinal lymphomas are mostly recognized by an increasing loss of vision.

Histology. A recent report of 108 patients demonstrated that, using the REAL classification, four main types of lymphomas can be recognized: marginal zone, lymphoplasmacytic, follicular, and DLBCL (Jenkins et al. 2000).

Marginal zone B-cell lymphoma of MALT is the most frequently observed type (Petrella et al. 1991; Wotherspoon et al. 1993; Isaacson and Norton 1994; Jenkins et al. 2000; Coupland et al, 2002). In the conjunctiva and eyelids, there is a diffuse infiltrate beneath the epithelium or epidermis with lymphoepithelial lesions (Fig. 6.44). Small ulcerations may be present. This infiltrate comprises centrocyte-like cells, sometimes with sheets of monocytoid B-cells at the periphery of the

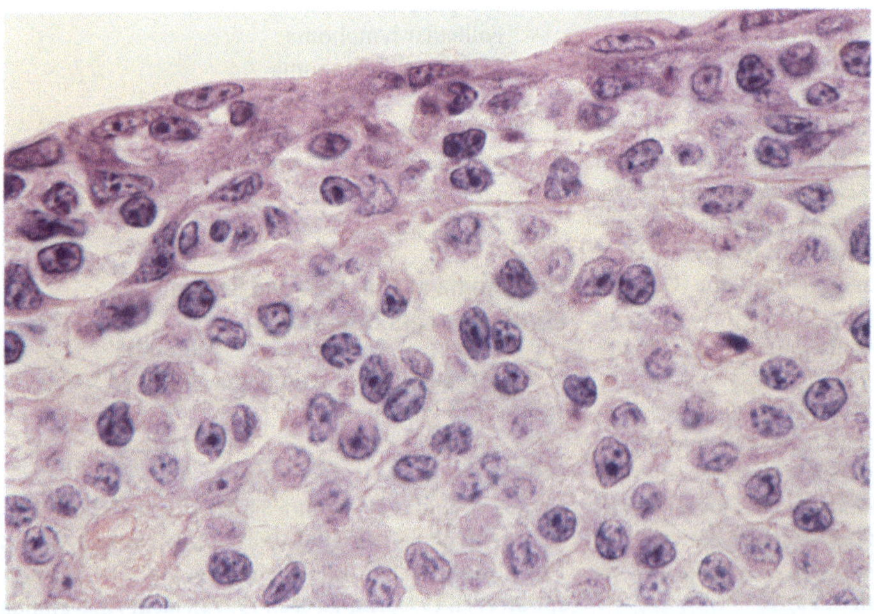

Fig. 6.44. Primary conjunctival marginal zone lymphoma of MALT. There is a diffuse infiltrate beneath the epithelium, which shows lymphoepithelial lesions. Reactive germinal centers were present deeper in the infiltrate (Giemsa stain)

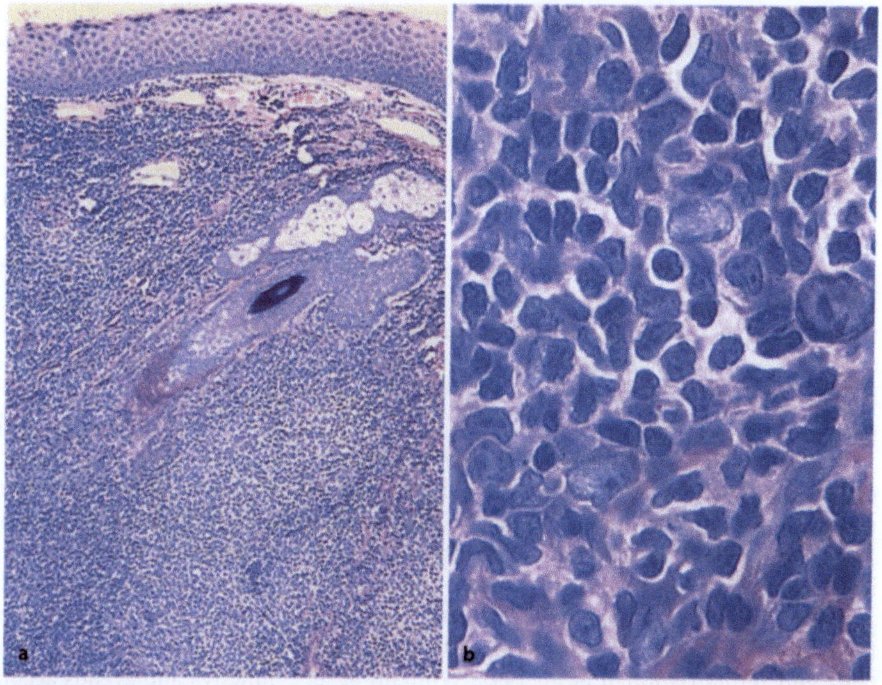

Fig. 6.45 a, b. Primary conjunctival follicular lymphoma. **a** Neoplastic follicles invading the connective tissue of the eyelid (Giemsa stain). **b** The neoplastic follicles comprise mostly centrocytes with a few centroblasts (grade 1) (Giemsa stain)

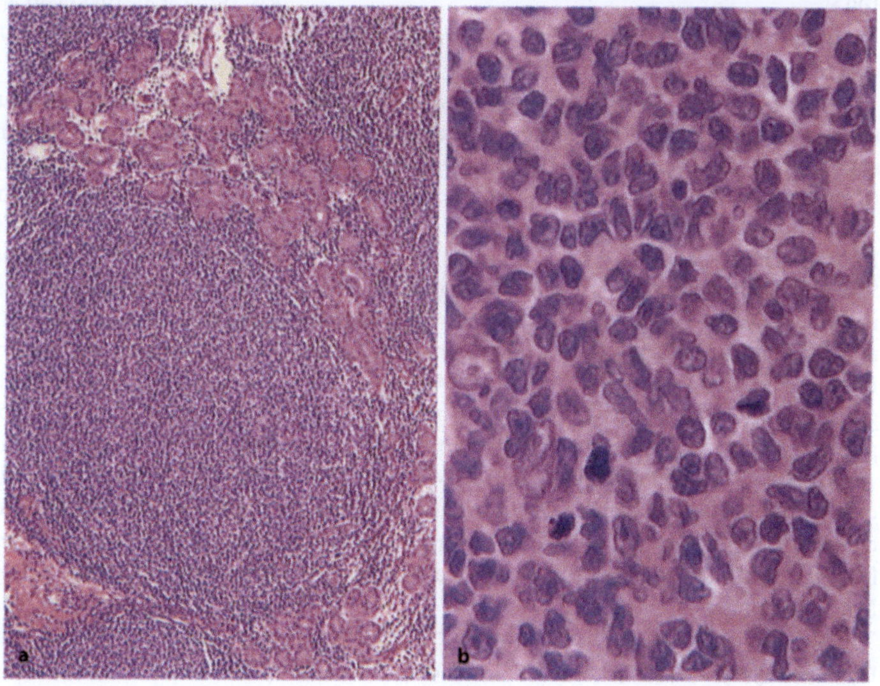

Fig. 6.46 a, b. Primary follicular lymphoma of the lachrymal gland. **a** Neoplastic follicles have destroyed the normal architecture of the lachrymal gland (H and E stain). **b** At higher magnification, a predominance of centrocytes (grade 1) is seen. Note the pale nuclei of follicular dendritic cells near the *top* (H and E stain)

tumor. A few large-B-cells are dispersed throughout. In many cases, plasma cells with an Ig light-chain restriction are present, either dispersed or in clusters. In the diffuse infiltrate, follicles can be recognized either with a more or less active germinal center or with colonization obscuring the germinal center. Lymphoepithelial lesions are not found in the lachrymal glands but sometimes in the duct epithelium.

Lymphoplasmacytic lymphoma was described by Lazzarino et al. (1985) and is sometimes associated with monoclonal serum gammopathy. Currently, most of these cases are interpreted as marginal zone cell lymphoma of MALT type with an important lymphoplasmacytic component.

Sometimes *follicular lymphoma* or *mantle cell lymphoma* can develop in the conjunctiva (Fig. 6.45) or in other sites, for example, the lachrymal glands (Fig. 6.46) (Reiser et al. 2001). *Plasmacytomas* are very infrequent but occur only on the eyelids.

Diffuse large-B-cell lymphomas develop mostly in the orbit (Leff et al. 1985), on the eyelids, and in the uvea and retina (Hofman et al. 1992; Whitcup et al. 1993).

Individual cases of *Burkitt's lymphoma* have been described in the orbit.

Peripheral NK/T-cell lymphomas have been reported (Leidenix et al. 1993), but remain extremely rare. In a small series of seven cases, only two were primary (Coupland et al. 1999).

Differential Diagnosis

Small-B-cell lymphomas should be distinguished from reactive lesions. *Allergic follicular conjunctivitis* should not be confused with MZBCL or follicular lymphoma. In the orbit, this type of lymphoma has to be distinguished from follicular hyperplasia. A diffuse infiltrate predominately made up of B-cells, which occurs in *Sjögren's syndrome*, should not be confused with small-B-cell lymphoma in the lachrymal gland. There may be a continuous spectrum between reactive and malignant lesions similar to what was described for salivary gland MALT lymphomas.

The structure of the follicles, immunohistochemistry showing a polytypic population, and the absence of monoclonal rearrangement of Ig heavy-chain are useful characterizing features.

Other tumors with medium or large cells must also be considered. *Myeloid sarcomas* often occur in the orbit. Rhabdomyosarcoma or other soft-tissue tumors is another possibility. In children, dissemination of neuroblastic tumors can lead to difficulties in the diagnosis.

Melanoma, particularly in the conjunctiva or in the uvea, must also be ruled out; however, the diagnosis can be very difficult.

Finally, it may be problematic to distinguish extension from a myeloma involving facial bones from lymphomas with a plasmacytic differentiation.

Occurrence

Primary lymphomas of the eye and ocular adnexa represent about 1.5% of non-Hodgkin's lymphomas.

These lymphomas can be observed at any age, with a predominance in older patients (>50 years), with extremes in age ranging from 17 to 93 years (Isaacson and Norton 1994). There is a female predominance (Lazzarino et al. 1985).

The vast majority of these tumors are B-cell lymphomas. The orbit is the most frequent location, representing 64% of case (Knowles et al. 1988) while conjunctiva and eyelids account respectively for 28% and 8% (Ellis et al. 1985; Leff et al. 1985; Medeiros and Harris 1989; Petrella et al. 1991; Wotherspoon et al. 1993; Akpek et al. 1999a).

DLBCLs are more frequent in the eyelids and orbit than in the conjunctiva and lachrymal glands. These lymphomas are often associated with a chronic lymphoid infiltrate due to an allergic reaction (chronic conjunctivitis) or Sjögren's syndrome. They represent the majority of the intraocular lymphomas (Whitcup et al. 1993) that are often associated with CNS lymphoma. These lymphomas can be diagnosed by cytological examination of the cerebrospinal fluid.

Primary B-cell lymphoma of the eye or ocular adnexa in HIV-positive patients has been observed, but is very rare. Some of these lymphomas were in the orbit. There were two patients with Burkitt's lymphoma (Brooks et al. 1984), and one with a DLBCL with cerebral extension (De Girolami et al. 1989). Hofman et al. (1992) described a large-B-cell lymphoma with an initial involvement restricted to the uveal tract but with large neoplastic B-cells in the pleura and pericardium.

Clinical Presentation

The majority of the lymphomas are of the MALT and have a long indolent evolution. Patients present with symptoms of chronic conjunctivitis (Akpek et al. 1999a) and progressive development of a small tumor of the conjunctiva or eyelids. The lesions are often bilateral. In patients with MALT lymphoma, a monoclonal gammopathy may be detected, often with cryoglobulinemia type II or cold agglutinin (Lazzarino et al. 1985; Bairey et al. 1994).The lymphoma remains localized, corresponding to stage IE when unilateral or stage IIE when bilateral.

Patients with lymphoma in the orbit complain of pain with exophthalmos or paresis of the oculomotor muscles. Radiography and CT scan disclose the orbital tumor. The tumor should be immediately removed after a staging procedure showing that is localized (stage IE).

Lachrymal gland lymphomas are often associated with dryness of the eye.

Uveal involvement presents as uveitis which can be followed by blindness.

Intraocular lymphomas are DLBCLs that occur in the uvea and retina and are often associated with a cerebral localization. In a series published by Trudeau et al. (1988), 60 % of patients had initial isolated intraocular involvement but 80 % showed multivisceral dissemination during the evolution (Trudeau et al. 1988). In another series (Whitcup et al. 1993), all cases were associated with CNS lymphomas.

In the majority of patients, particularly those with small-B-cell lymphomas, the tumor remains localized (stage IE or IIE) with possible bilateral involvement in conjunctival localizations. Radiotherapy is the most common type of treatment and can lead to complete remission.

Whatever the site, the 10-year survival rate is about 60–75 % (Knowles et al. 1988; Reiser et al. 2001).

During the evolution of MZBCL of MALT, about 10 % of the patients develop other extranodal lymphomas in MALT tissue (lung, thyroid, stomach, salivary glands, etc.) (Isaacson and Norton 1994).

In a study of 108 patients, the ocular adnexal lymphomas were reclassified according to the REAL classification (Jenkins et al. 2000). The frequency of previous or concurrent extraorbital disease increased from marginal zone lymphoma, diffuse lymphoplasmacytic lymphoma, follicle center lymphoma, DLBCL to other histological lymphoma variants. During disease evolution, the proportion of patients with at least one extraorbital recurrence after 5 years was 47 % for marginal zone lymphoma, 48 % for lymphoplasmacytic lymphoma, 64 % for follicle center lymphoma, 81 % for DLBCL and 95% for others lymphoma variants. The corresponding estimated rates of 5-years lymphoma-related mortality were 12 %, 19 %, 22 %, 48 % and 53 %, respectively (Jenkins et al. 2000).

Evolution depends on staging. Knowles et al. (1988) reported that 86 % of patients in their series with a unilateral or bilateral stage IE lymphoma were alive and free of disease during a median follow-up period of 51 months, contrasting with 20 % of patients with a past or concurrent extraocular localization. Due to this possibility, patients need a complete staging of their disease by a hematologist/oncologist (Reiser et al. 2001).

6.6 Lymphoma of the Mediastinum

- Marginal zone B-cell lymphoma of the thymus
- Mediastinal (thymic) large-B-cell lymphoma
- Burkitt's lymphoma
- Precursor T- or B-lymphoblastic lymphoma

Lymphomas of the mediastinum predominately consist of three types: mediastinal large-B-cell lymphoma, MZBCL of MALT, and precursor B- and T-lymphoblastic lymphoma. All of these are of thymic origin. Exceptional cases arise primarily from the regional lymph nodes (Burkitt's lymphoma). Secondary involvement of lymph nodes can be seen in all lymphoma types (refer to the respective sections).

6.6.1 Mediastinal (Thymic) Large-B-Cell Lymphoma (ICD-O: 9679/3)

Synonyms

- Kiel: Large-cell, sclerosing B-cell lymphoma of the mediastinum
- REAL: Primary mediastinal(thymic) large-B-cell lymphoma
- WHO: Mediastinal (thymic) large-B-cell lymphoma

Definition

Mediastinal large-B-cell lymphoma (MLBCL) is a tumor located in the mediastinum, specifically, in the upper anterior region. It is made up of large-B-cells and is associated with sclerosis. This lymphoma has distinct sites of dissemination.

The lymphoma arises in the thymus from B-cells present around vessels between the thymic cortex and medulla (Isaacson et al. 1987; Joos et al. 1996). Some immunophenotypic characteristics of the tumor cells have been interpreted as reflecting terminal steps of B-cell differentiation (Möller et al. 1986, 1987). Lymph nodes are secondarily infiltrated by the perinodal tumor. Hence, strictly speaking, MLBCL is an extranodal subtype of DLBCL, albeit with some unique characteristics (Barth et al. 2001).

Morphology

This diffusely growing tumor is composed of large cells which vary in size and nuclear shape as well as in cytoplasmic features (Fig. 6.47) (Addis and Isaacson 1986; Möller et al. 1986; Paulli et al. 1999). In many instances, there is a similarity to monomorphic and polymorphic centroblastic lymphoma (Fig. 6.47) (Cazals-Hatem et al. 1996; Paulli et al. 1999) with even some multilobate nuclei. Most investigators have morphologically related the lymphoma cells to germinal center cells (centrocytes and centroblasts) with slightly or moderately basophilic cytoplasm (Fig. 6.48) (Cazals-Hatem et al. 1996). In some cases, a variable number of tumor cells exhibit a more abundant, clear or pale cytoplasm (Möller et al. 1986; Cazals-Hatem et al. 1996). A complete "clear-cell lymphoma" can be observed (Fig. 6.49) but is rare (Möller et al. 1986, 1987; Cazals-Hatem et al. 1996). Sporadically, giant cells mimicking Reed-Sternberg cells have been found (Chadburn and Frizzera 1999).

Between these large cells, there are medium-sized cells resembling centrocytes. In addition, band-like accumulations of lymphocytes, with or without plasma cells and with or without eosinophils, have been recognized. There is associated sclerosis in the majority of cases (Möller et al. 1986, 1987; Cazals-Hatem et al. 1996). Strands of collagen fibers intertwine around or enclose the tumor cells (Fig. 6.47). The fibrosis compartmentalizes the cells, which sometimes appear to be organized in lobules, thus mimicking carcinoma, or organized in annular bands, as in nodular sclerosing Hodgkin's lymphoma. The type and extension of the fibrosis varies from one part of the tumor to the other. Remnants of thymic tissue may be present, and is more or less easily recognizable.

The diagnosis often has to be made based on small tissue fragments obtained by mediastinoscopy; crush artifacts can lead to great difficulties.

Association with typical nodular sclerosing Hodgkin's lymphoma has been reported (Jaffe et al. 1992).

Immunohistochemistry

In more than 70% of the cases, the tumor cells express the B-cell antigen CD20 together with CD79α (Möller et al. 1986, 1987; Cazals-Hatem ct al. 1996).

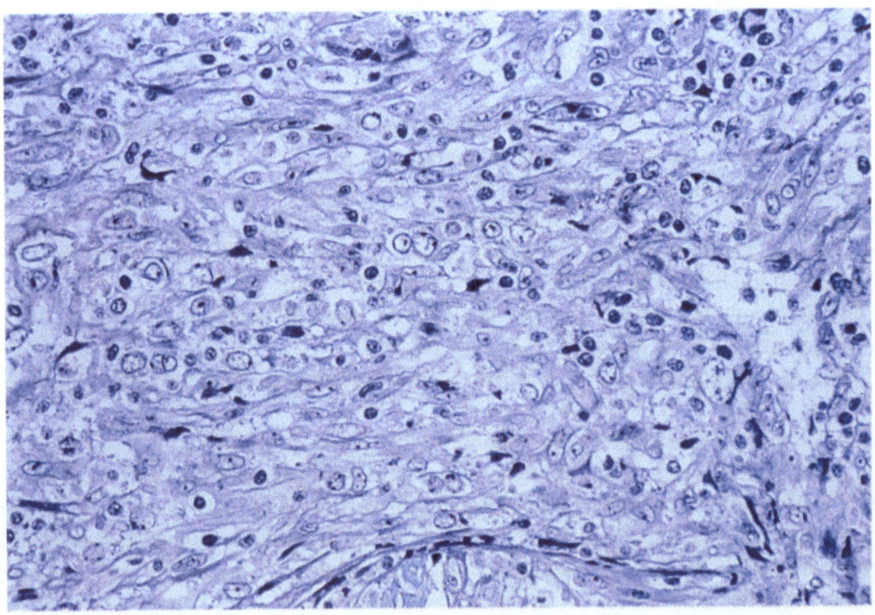

Fig. 6.47. Mediastinal large-B-cell lymphoma. The tumor cells resemble centroblasts and are associated with collagenous fibrosis and a few reactive (mostly T-) lymphocytes (Giemsa stain)

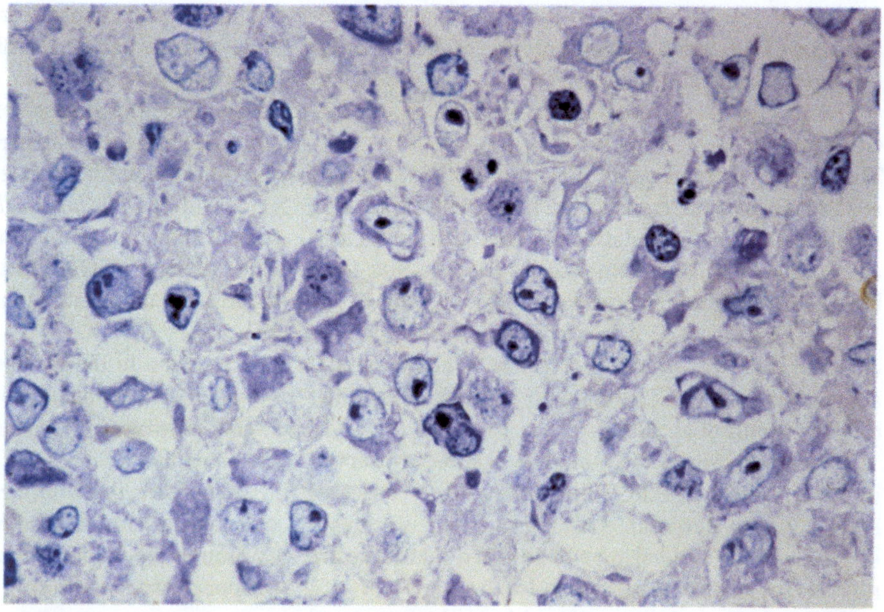

Fig. 6.48. Mediastinal large-B-cell lymphoma. This tumor is difficult to classify due to the highly variable morphology of the lymphoma cells (Giemsa stain)

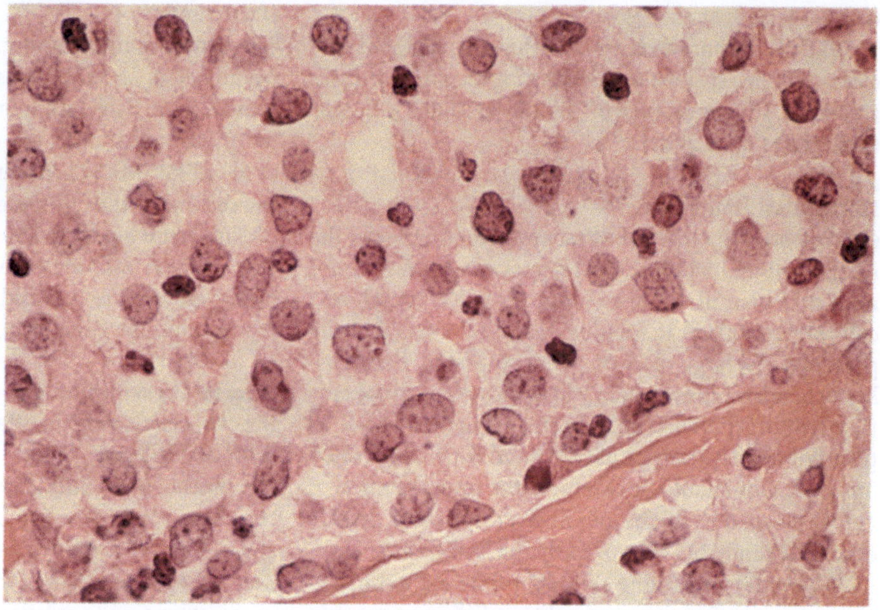

Fig. 6.49. Mediastinal large-B-cell lymphoma. The majority of the tumor cells have an abundant pale cytoplasm (H and E stain)

Another characteristic of this lymphoma is the consistent absence of cIg expression. sIg is detected only in exceptional cases, whereas common leukocyte antigen (CD45)is regularly found. Expression of HLA class II and I antigens is lacking in about 30% of the cases. CD11c and CD23 may be expressed (Möller et al. 1987). CD5, CD10, and CD21 are generally negative. By contrast, CD30 is expressed in approximately 70% of the cases but expression is weaker than in Hodgkin's and anaplastic large-cell lymphomas (Falini et al. 1995; Higgins and Warnke 1999). Aberrant expression of β-HCG has been observed in one patient (Fraternali et al. 1999). LMP-1 is negative in the vast majority of cases (Cazals-Hatem et al. 1996).

A recent paper (de Leval et al. 2001) analyzed the expression of bcl-6 and CD10 in 19 tumors and showed that all were positive for the bcl-6 protein and one-third for CD10, results which are interpreted as favoring a germinal center B-cell origin.

Genetics

The Ig genes are rearranged (Brandter et al. 1989; Tsang et al. 1996), contrasting with the absence of expression of sIg, with somatic mutations in the variable regions as in other DLBCLs. Abnormalities in the c-myc gene have been observed in some young adults (Scarpa et al. 1991). The karyotype is hyperdiploid, with a gain in chromosome 9p, which represents a characteristic aberration for MLBCL along with amplification of the rel gene (Bentz et al. 2001).

Overexpression of the mal gene has been observed in some cases of MLBCL but not in other types of DLBCL (Copie-Bergman et al. 1999). c-myc is variably rearranged. It should also be mentioned that there are no rearrangements of bcl-2 or bcl-6.

EBV sequences have not been demonstrated (Cazals-Hatem et al. 1996).

MLBCL is characterized by a heavily mutated and class-switched Ig gene and is thought to originate from a specific subpopulation of thymic medullary B-cells (Leithäuser et al. 2001).

Differential Diagnosis

Carcinoma of thymus and other epithelial tumors of the mediastinum, including dysgerminomas and seminomas, may be difficult to rule out when the lymphoma cells are organized in lobules due to sclerosis and the presence of a large clear or pale cytoplasm. Immunohistochemistry is mandatory to demonstrate cytokeratins and/or epithelial membrane antigen, as well as positivity and negativity of CD45 and B-cell associated antigens. One should be careful in the interpretation of cytokeratins due to the possible presence of thymic epithelial remnants colonized by the lymphoma.

In samples containing abundant fibrosis, some *soft-tissue tumors*, for example, solitary fibrous tumor of the mediastinum, should be discussed; however, this remains a rare condition.

Hodgkin's lymphoma represents the most difficult diagnosis in some cases (Chadburn and Frizzera 1999), particularly when only small biopsy fragments are available. Some Hodgkin's lymphomas can be rich in large "Hodgkin's cells" mimicking large-B-cells, some of them showing a B-cell immunophenotype. On the other hand, some MLBCLs may have Reed-Sternberg like-cells, with expression of CD30, the presence of thick fibrotic bands as well as plasma cells and eosinophils. The expression of CD45 and CD20 by all the tumor cells, the absence of CD15, and the demonstration of a monoclonal rearrangement of Ig genes allows the differential diagnosis to be clarified.

The *anaplastic large-cell lymphoma* comprises larger cells that are negative for B-cell-associated antigens. They express CD30, EMA, and in about 50% of the tumors the anaplastic lymphoma kinase (ALK)-1 protein.

Extension to the mediastinum of *diffuse large-B-cell lymphoma, lymphoblastic or Burkitt's lymphoma* is mostly easy to recognize based on morphology and immunohistochemistry. Fibrosis is lacking in these cases.

Metastatic amelanotic melanoma may be very difficult to differentiate from MLBCL. Again, morphology, immunohistochemistry, and clinical data allow the proper diagnosis.

Occurrence

The tumor is uncommon, but not extremely rare: the frequency is about 2 cases out of 1,000 of nodal lymphoma in the Kiel lymphoma registry. In a large series, it represented about 2.4% of all lymphomas (Armitage et al. 1998). MLBCL occurs in young patients during the second or third decade of life.

The mean age is 36–39 years. The youngest patient was 10 years old, the oldest 63. Women show a lower mean age but are affected about 2.5 times as often as men (Armitage et al. 1998).

Clinical Presentation and Prognosis

Masses developing in the anterior mediastinum are responsible for shortness of breath, cough, and pain in the breast, neck and arms. Subsequently, a superior vena cava syndrome can occur. Patients are usually in stage IE or IIE with extension to pleura, lung, pericardium, heart, and large mediastinal vessels. In rare cases, extension to subclavicular areas or nodes is possible.

This type of lymphoma has a very peculiar dissemination to extranodal sites, starting on the opposite side of the diaphragm (kidney, adrenal), disseminating to the liver and brain (Bishop et al. 1999). Even skin localizations have been reported.

MLBCL can be brought to remission with chemotherapy associated with or without radiotherapy (Cazals-Hatem et al. 1996; Lazzarino et al. 1997).

In a series of 141 patients (Cazals-Hatem et al. 1996), 79% achieved a complete remission while only 68% with non-mediastinal DLBCL treated by the same protocol achieved complete remission ($p=0.01$). The 3-year survival rates were, respectively, 66% and 61% ($p=0.05$) and disease-free survival 64% and 61%.

A 5-year survival rate of about 50% is obtained with polychemotherapy combined with radiotherapy (Armitage et al. 1998).

Favorable prognostic factors are the patient's age (older than 25 years at the time of diagnosis), the limited stage (Ie or IIe), and a good response to initial therapy.

Disease extending into adjacent thoracic viscera has a poor prognosis, and spreading to infradiaphragmatic viscera is even worse (Möller et al. 1986; Isaacson et al. 1987; Cazals-Hatem et al. 1996; Paulli et al. 1999).

6.6.2 Extranodal Marginal Zone B-Cell Lymphoma of the Thymus

Definition

A small-B-cell lymphoma occurring primarily in the thymus and presenting all the morphological and evolutionary criteria of MALT lymphoma as defined by Isaacson and Spencer (1987). It is the predominant type among small-B-cell lymphomas of the thymus (Lorsbach et al. 2000).

Morphology

Macroscopy. The lymphoma consists of encapsulated masses 9–12 cm in diameter. The cut surface is homogeneous and pale, with numerous cysts containing serous fluid. Extension to the pericardium can be observed.

Histology (Isaacson et al. 1990; Takagi et al. 1992; Shimosato and Mukai 1997). A diffuse lymphoid infiltrate obscures the normal architecture but Hassall's corpuscles can still be recognized. The infiltrate comprises small to medium-sized lymphocytes with a more or less irregular, cleaved nucleus (centrocyte-like) and an abundant clear cytoplasm. A monocytoid B-cell component can be observed (Lorsbach et al. 2000). A few large cells with the morphology of centroblasts or immunoblasts are present, dispersed, and never organized in sheets. Follicles with germinal centers are also present, showing a variable degree of colonization. The cysts are lined by a flattened epithelium. Lymphoepithelial lesions can be observed in thymic epithelial cell cords, in the epithelium of the cysts and in Hassall's corpuscles. Sometimes, there is a plasma cell component (Lorsbach et al. 2000).

Differential Diagnosis

The two diseases which should first be discussed are *follicular lymphoid hyperplasia of the thymus* and *Castleman's disease* developing in regional nodes and extending to the thymus. Morphology is often sufficient for the diagnosis. The absence of a monoclonal B-cell component and the absence of immunoglobulin heavy- and light-chain gene rearrangements allow these reactive non-neoplastic diseases to be recognized. It should be noted that exceptional cases of Castleman's disease may have a monoclonal plasma cell component. *Teratomas* should also be discussed, particularly when there are many cysts.

Clinical Presentation

The evolution of this lymphoma is silent and indolent. The tumor is mainly discovered on systematic chest X-rays, in the anterosuperior part of the mediastinum. Extension to regional or to axillary nodes has been observed (Takagi et al. 1992). Some patients present with Sjögren's syndrome or other autoimmune diseases (Lorsbach et al. 2000). Surgical resection without or with radiotherapy may cure the lymphoma (Isaacson et al. 1990; Takagi et al. 1992).

6.6.3 Mediastinal Involvement in Precursor T- or B-Cell Lymphoblastic Lymphoma

Some of these lymphoblastic lymphomas may present with a predominant mediastinal tumor due to a thymic infiltrate, with no or only minimal peripheral blood or bone marrow involvement (see Chap. 4.1.5.1).

A diffuse infiltration extends throughout the thymic parenchyma, often mimicking a lymphocyte-rich thymoma. Hassall's corpuscles can persist. Infiltration extends into the fibrous trabeculae, the vessel walls, and the thymic capsule. The lymphoid cells are medium-sized, with pale cytoplasm and a nucleus with dispersed chromatin and an inconspicuous nucleolus. The nuclei are round or oval, often with deep infolding, giving the nuclei a lobulated (convoluted) pattern. About

80 % of lymphoblastic lymphomas have cells with such convoluted nuclei (Knowles 1992). The mitotic index is high. A starry-sky pattern can be present.

Mediastinal nodes may be involved. The infiltrate begins in the perifollicular areas and extends progressively to all the surfaces of the lymph nodes.

The cellular origin has to be determined by immunohistochemistry.

Clinical Presentation

Patients present with a huge mediastinal mass and acute respiratory distress. Thus the diagnosis has to be treated as an emergency. Often, soon after initial presentation, leukemia or other sites of involvement are disclosed, as well as bone marrow involvement. Extension to the gonads and central nervous system are frequent. The evolution is the same as in lymphoblastic lymphoma of other sites.

6.6.4 Mediastinal Involvement in Small-B-Cell Lymphoma

B-cell chronic lymphocytic leukemia (*B-CLL*), *mantle cell lymphoma*, and *follicular lymphoma* (see Chap. 4.2.1) can be responsible for this type of extension. Morphology, immunohistochemistry, and genetics, as well as clinical features, support a correct final diagnosis.

6.6.5 Mediastinal Involvement in Large-B-Cell Lymphoma Other Than Primary Mediastinal Large-B-Cell Lymphoma and Burkitt's Lymphoma

Mediastinal involvement in all these lymphomas is secondary to other localizations. Again, clinical presentation, morphology, immunohistochemistry, genetics, and molecular biology allow these extensions to be distinguished from primary large-B-cell lymphomas.

6.6.6 Mediastinal Involvement in NK/T-Cell Lymphoma

Until now, a predominant involvement of the thymus and/or the mediastinum by peripheral T-cell lymphoma of any type has not been observed.

6.7 Lymphoma of the Lung

6.7.1 Primary Lymphoma of the Lung

Primary lymphomas of the lung are rare. They present mostly as a lymphoma with predominant involvement of bronchi and/or pulmonary parenchyma without any extrapulmonary localization at presentation and within 3 months after onset (Addis et al. 1988; Isaacson and Norton 1994).

These lymphomas account for 0.4 % of NHLs, 3.6 % of extranodal lymphomas (Berkman et al. 1996), and 0.5 – 1 % of all primary neoplasms of the lung (L'Hoste et al. 1984; Isaacson and Norton 1994). They occur mostly in adults over 40 years of age with a mean age of 55 years (L'Hoste et al. 1984) or 58.4 years (Fiche et al. 1995), without sex predominance.

Primary lung lymphomas seem to be frequently associated with immune disorders, particularly those arising from Sjögren's syndrome.

About 70 % of the lymphomas are MZBCLs of MALT, whereas other small-B-cell lymphomas are rare, e.g. follicular and mantle cell lymphomas. The same is true for Burkitt's lymphoma. The second most frequent lymphoma of the lung is DLBCL (10 – 20 %). T-cell lymphomas are exceptional (Li et al. 1990; Fiche et al. 1995).

6.7.1.1 Extranodal Marginal Zone B-Cell Lymphoma of MALT

Definition

This lymphoma has the same histological characteristics as digestive tract MALT lymphoma (Peterson et al. 1985; Addis et al. 1988; Li et al. 1990; Isaacson and Norton 1994; Fiche et al. 1995; Nicholson et al. 1995). In the past, these lymphomas were classified as either pseudo-lymphoma (Marchevsky et al. 1983; Kennedy et al. 1985; Koss et al. 1985), due to the presence of follicles with reactive germinal centers and a long non-aggressive evolution, or as small-B-cell lymphoma (small lymphocytic, centrocytic or lymphoplasmacytic lymphoma using the up-dated Kiel classification) (Le Tourneau et al. 1983) before the description of MALT lymphoma (Isaacson and Wright 1984).

Such lymphomas develop from preexisting reactive lymphoid tissue. The so-called "bronchus associated lymphoid tissue" (BALT) was described in the lung of rabbits (Bienenstock 1973; Bienenstock and Johnston 1976). BALT consists of follicles developing in close contact to a flattened non-ciliated epithelium and include a large marginal zone (Sminia and van deer Brugge-Gamelkoorn 1989). In animals, the development of BALT is stimulated by bacterial infections (Delventhal et al. 1992). The presence and functional role of BALT in humans is still controversial (Daniele 1990; Stockley et al. 1990). Well-developed BALT has been observed in humans with undefined pulmonary infections (Pabst 1992) and in a few patients (8 %) with severe chronic bronchitis and bronchiectasis (Delventhal et al. 1992) (see Chap. 6.2.1.1). Sjögren's syndrome has been described in patients with primary lung lymphoma of MALT.

Morphology

Macroscopy. The disease most often starts with multiple, small whitish nodules sometimes evolving to masses with a polycyclic outline in one or the other pulmonary lobes (unilateral or bilateral). There may be associated pleural effusion. Dissection of the resected lobe or lung often shows bronchial involvement with protrusion into the lumen. Peribronchial or mediastinal lymph nodes may be involved.

Histology. The lung parenchyma is densely infiltrated (Fig. 6.50a) by a uniform cell population with the morphology of small lymphoid cells having a more or less irregular nucleus (centrocyte-like) with sometimes a clear cytoplasm. A vague nodularity can be observed (Fig. 6.50a). Active germinal centers may be present but they are often more or less colonized by the small lymphoid cells (Fig. 6.50b). The cells at the periphery of the nodules may present a monocytoid B-cell morphology (Fig. 6.51). In addition, in some cases, a plasmacytic population is observed, explaining why, in the past, such lymphomas were diagnosed as lymphoplasmacytic lymphomas. A few large cells are dispersed in the small-cell population. At the periphery of the mass, a lymphoid infiltrate extends into the alveolar walls (interstitial infiltrate). The walls of the large and medium-sized bronchi are infiltrated, often with erosion of cartilage. The neoplastic infiltrate protrudes into the lumen of the bronchi.

Typical lymphoepithelial lesions are seen in the bronchial epithelium (Fig. 6.52). Some bronchioles are completely destroyed.

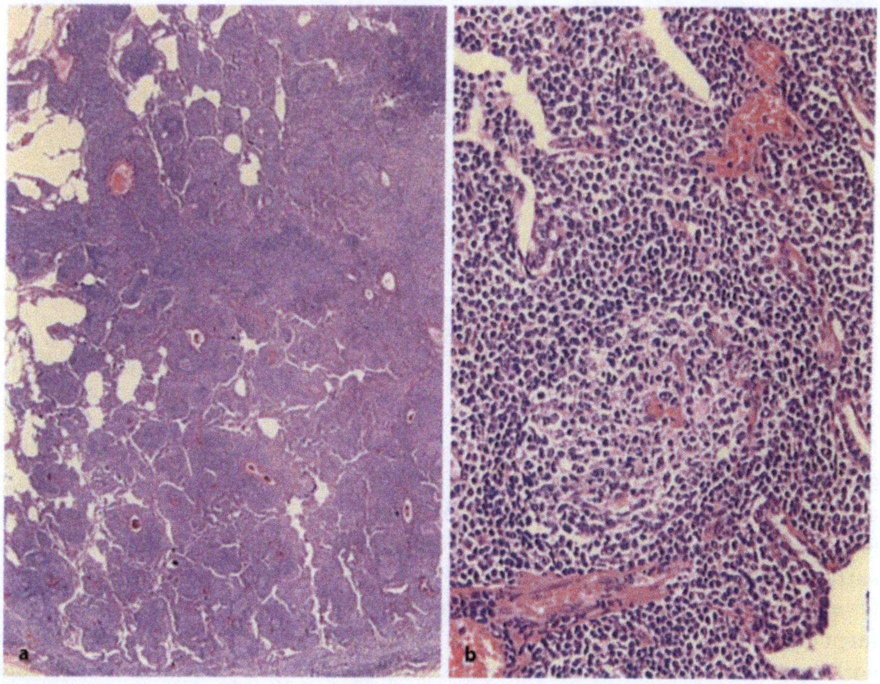

Fig. 6.50. Primary lung marginal zone lymphoma of MALT. **a** Massive infiltrate of the lung parenchyma with a nodular pattern. Note the extension to the pleura (*bottom right*) and along the bronchovascular complexes at the periphery of the tumor (*upper left*) (H and E stain). **b** A reactive germinal center in a diffuse infiltrate of centrocyte-like cells, with extension into the small bronchi (H and E stain)

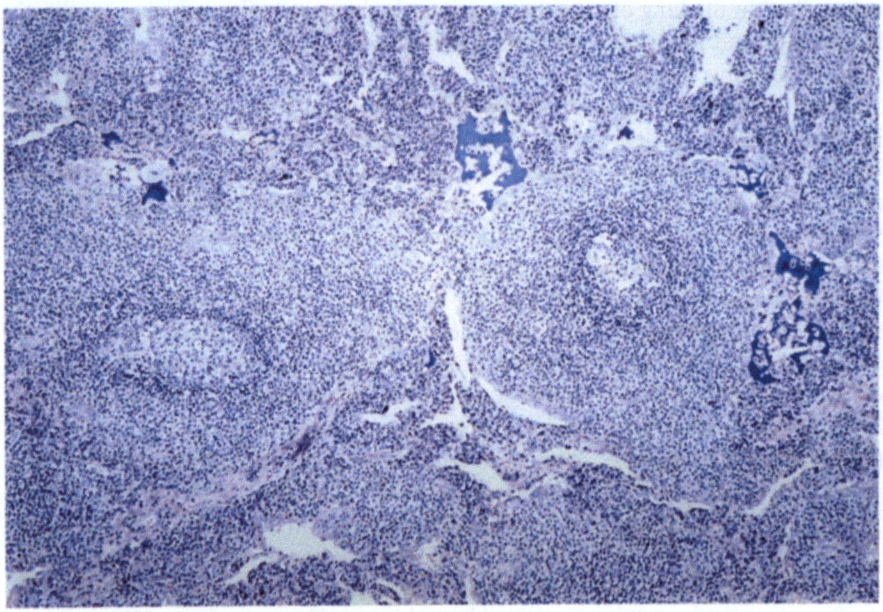

Fig. 6.51. Primary lung marginal zone lymphoma of MALT. A marginal zone pattern consisting of monocytoid B-cells is clearly recognized (Giemsa stain)

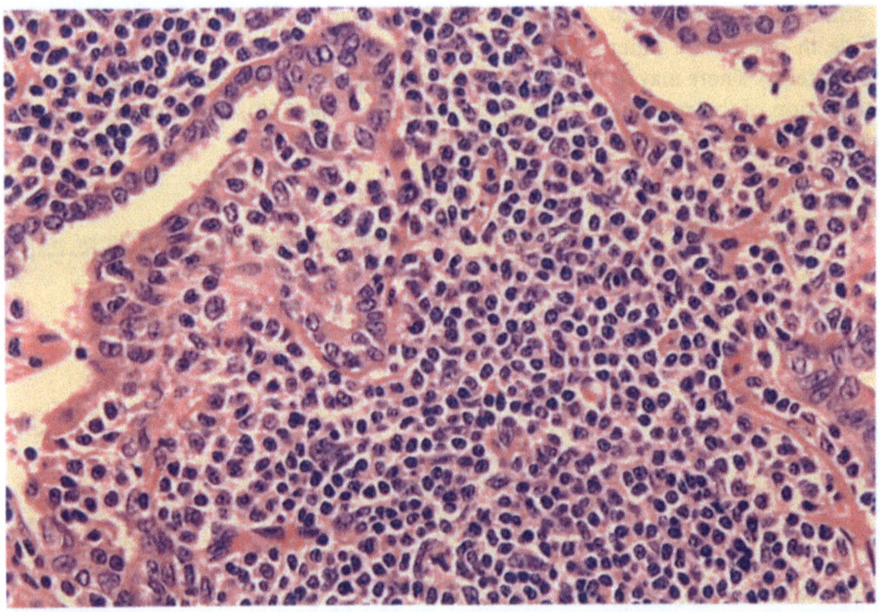

Fig. 6.52. Same patient as in Fig. 6.50. Note the diffuse infiltrate consisting of centrocyte-like cells and plasma cells (which were monotypic). A lymphoepithelial lesion is seen in the small bronchus (H and E stain)

Differential Diagnosis

In the past, many if not all of these BALT lymphomas were diagnosed as *pseudolymphoma*. This term is no longer used; instead, these tumors are now regarded as extranodal MALT lymphoma. The criteria of BALT lymphomas allows the rare secondary lung involvement of other small-B-cell lymphomas to be eliminated. Immunohistochemistry rules out T-cell lymphomas. Lung *inflammatory pseudotumor* can be difficult to distinguish. The absence of colonized germinal centers and lymphoepithelial lesions, the presence of sheets of collagenous fibrosis and nests of polyclonal plasma cells are good arguments in favor of the diagnosis of an inflammatory pseudotumor.

Finally, the differentiation from *lymphoid interstitial pneumonia* or *follicular bronchitis*, particularly in lung or bronchi biopsies, can be very difficult. Immunohistochemistry, and the etiologic conditions associated with lymphoid interstitial pneumonia can be useful, as well as the presence of heavy chain gene rearrangement. The possible association of MALT lymphoma of the lung and Sjögren's syndrome is another reason for the difficult differential diagnosis, as both lymphoid interstitial pneumonia and follicular bronchitis have been observed in Sjögren's syndrome.

Occurrence

Marginal zone lymphoma of MALT is the most frequent type of lymphoma occurring primarily in the lung, representing 69.4% of the cases in the series of Li et al. (1990) and 73% in the series of Fiche et al. (1995).

Clinical Presentation

The tumors have an indolent clinical course and are asymptomatic in half of the patients. Respiratory symptoms (cough, dyspnea, thoracic pain, hemoptysis) may be present. There are associated B symptoms in less than 25% of the patients (Le Tourneau et al. 1983; L'Hoste et al. 1984; Addis et al. 1988). Chest X-rays disclose one or sometimes multiple smaller or larger nodules in the parenchyma. The nodules can be unilateral or, less frequently, bilateral. In addition, such patients may show bronchovascular and/or pneumonic-alveolar features (Berkman et al. 1996). Pleural effusion may be present. Intrabronchial extension is responsible for dry cough, chest pain, dyspnea, hemoptysis, fever, and infection (pneumonia).

Prognosis is the same as for other MALT lymphomas. Relapse can occur even after 2 years in the lung or in other extranodal sites such as skin, stomach, and salivary glands (L'Hoste et al. 1984; Koss et al. 1985; Peterson et al. 1985; Addis et al. 1988). Transformation into DLBCL has been observed and represented approximately half of the large-B-cell lymphomas observed in two series of patients with primary lung lymphomas (Li et al. 1990; Fiche et al. 1995).

Overall survival at 5 years is more than 80% with a median survival of more than 10 years (L'Hoste et al. 1984; Kennedy et al. 1985; Koss et al. 1985; Addis et al. 1988; Li et al. 1990).

6.7.1.2 Primary Diffuse Large-B-Cell Lymphoma of the Lung

Diffuse large-B-cell lymphoma can occur as a primary tumor in the lung. In about half of the patients, the tumor arises secondarily or in association with a MZBCL of MALT (Li et al. 1990; Fiche et al. 1995).

In the majority of the patients, multiples nodules develop in one, or often in both, lungs. Morphologically these lymphomas are identical to the DLBCL types found in the lymph node.

Primary DLBCL of the lung represents about 10–20% of all lung primary lymphomas (Li et al. 1990; Fiche et al. 1995; Nicholson et al. 1995).Patients have a median age about 60 years, ranging from 30 to 80 years (L'Hoste et al. 1984; Kennedy et al. 1985; Koss et al. 1985; Li et al. 1990; Fiche et al. 1995). This type of lymphoma often occurs in patients with immunodeficiency, resulting either from HIV infection (Raphaël et al. 1991), or after organ transplantation, or during Sjögren's syndrome. Patients with immunodeficiency have EBV-positive tumors.

The patients complain of B symptoms, dyspnea, and thoracic pain. Conventional radiography shows a pulmonary mass and/or atelectasia. The prognosis and evolution are the same as for other sites of the tumor.

After surgery and polychemotherapy, 5-year overall survival is 40–60% (L'Hoste et al. 1984; Kennedy et al. 1985; Li et al. 1990; Fiche et al. 1995).

6.7.1.3 Primary Lung Intravascular Large-B-Cell Lymphoma

Rare cases of intravascular large-B-cell lymphomas have been reported in which the lymphoma is apparently confined to the lung (Remberger et al. 1987; Tan et al. 1988; Snyder et al. 1989; Yousem and Colby 1990).The large lymphoma cells are present in the lumen of capillaries and small arteries or venules. Sometimes they are trapped into a parietal fibrin clot thereby reducing the lumen of pulmonary arteries (see Chap. 6.18).

Patients present with dyspnea, fever and hypoxemia. Chest X-rays disclose diffuse infiltrates mimicking an interstitial pneumonia. Almost always, other typical localizations can be observed during evolution (skin, kidney, central nervous system).

The evolution is described in Chap. 6.18.

6.7.1.4 Large B-Cell Lymphoma[1] Secondary to Liebow's Lymphomatoid Granulomatosis[2] (ICD-O: 9680/3[1]; 9766/1[2])

Synonyms

- Kiel: Not listed
- REAL: Not listed
- WHO: Lymphomatoid granulomatosis
- Other: Liebow's disease (in part)
  Angiocentric immunoproliferative lesion (in part)

Definition

A large-B-cell lymphoma with angiocentric and angiodestructive features made up of a few tumor cells associated with numerous reactive cells comprising T-lymphocytes and histiocytes. This lymphoma is associated with EBV and represents the end stage (grade III) of an immunoproliferative disease occurring predominantly in the lung (Guinee et al. 1994; Jaffe and Wilson 1997). It was first described by Liebow et al. (1972) and Liebow (1973) as "lymphomatoid granulomatosis".

The normal cell counterpart is postulated to be a peripheral B-lymphocyte infected and transformed by EBV (Mittal et al. 1990; Guinee et al. 1994; Myers et al. 1995; Nicholson et al. 1996; Wilson et al. 1996; Jaffe and Wilson 1997; Haque et al. 1998).

Morphology

In the majority of patients, the lesions develop in the lung, forming nodules of variable size (Fig. 6.53). Distribution is often bilateral with a prevalence for the mid- and lower sections of the lungs. The largest nodules may cavitate due to central necrosis.

On biopsy material, the lung parenchyma is diffusely infiltrated by lymphocytes, plasma cells, and histiocytes. Granulocytes (neutrophils or eosinophils) are rare or absent. The small and medium-sized lymphocytes often show irregular and activated nuclei. Histiocytes and macrophages are dispersed or organized in small clusters, but typical granulomas are lacking.

The lymphocytes surround often the vessels which show a hypertrophic endothelium and infiltrate the wall imitating a lymphocytic vasculitis (Fig. 6.54a), sometimes with fibrinoid necrosis. Often the vessels wall is destroyed, leading to edema, hemorrhage, or ischemic necrosis of the pulmonary tissue.

Against this inflammatory background, numerous large cells are recognized, either dispersed or organized in clusters or sheets, sometimes surrounding or infiltrating the vessels (Fig. 6.54b). Their morphology is highly pleomorphic. Some resemble centroblasts or immunoblasts, others Hodgkin's cells. Multinucleated cells mimicking Reed-Sternberg cells can be observed.

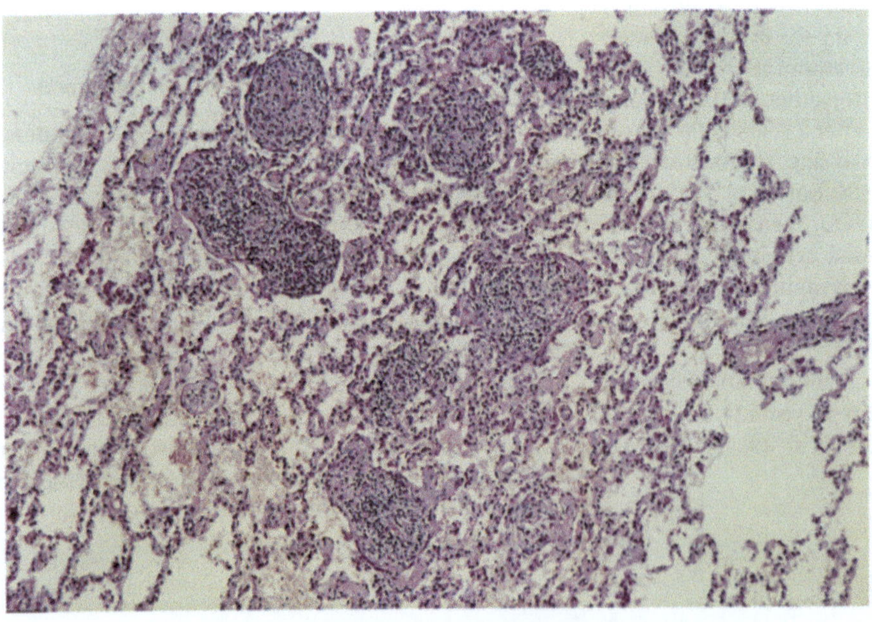

Fig. 6.53. Diffuse large-B-cell lymphoma secondary to Liebow's lymphomatoid granulomatosis. Nodular infiltrate of the lung (H and E stain)

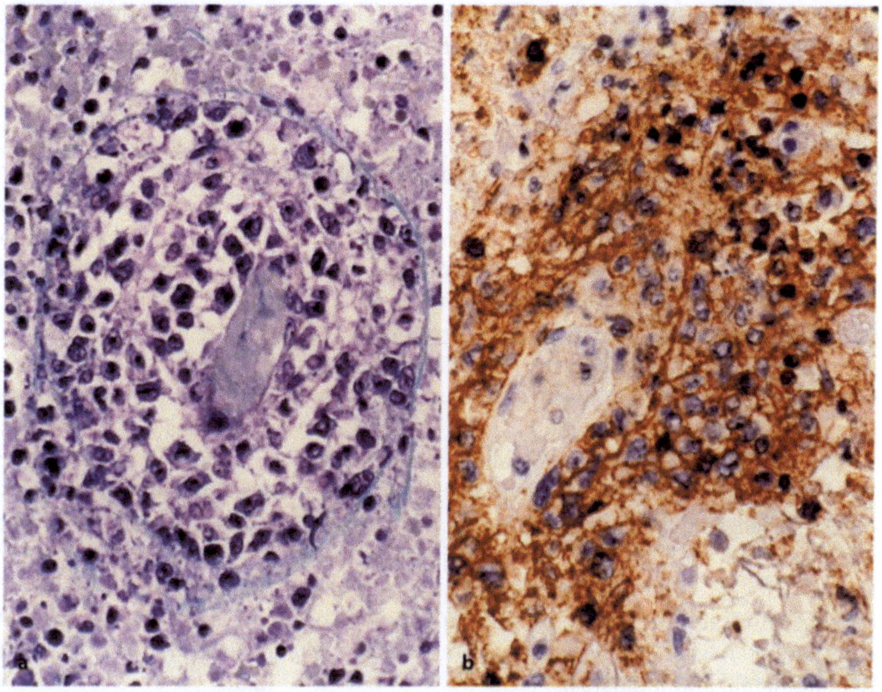

Fig. 6.54 a, b. Same patient as in Fig. 6.53. **a** Large tumor cells and reactive cells infiltrate the vessel wall (Giemsa stain). **b** These large cells express CD20 and are LMP-1- and EBER-1-positive (immunohistochemistry, peroxidase stain)

Necropsies discloses nodules also in the brain, kidney, and liver. Extension to the GI-tract, lymph nodes, and spleen are less frequent (Katzenstein et al. 1979; Koss et al. 1986; McNiff et al. 1996; Jaffe and Wilson 1997). Approximately half of the patients have skin or subcutaneous tissue involvement (Capron et al. 1985; McNiff et al. 1996).

The infiltration of sheets of B-cells and the dissemination justify the current classification of this tumor as large-B-cell lymphoma (Capron et al. 1985; Guinee et al. 1994; Nicholson et al. 1996; Taniere et al. 1998) and is interpreted as the last stage of the disease, *grade III*, which should be treated as an aggressive lymphoma.

The histopathological lesions show variations during their evolution. A grading system was therefore proposed by Lipford et al. (1987, 1988). *Grade I* is characterized by a polymorphic lymphoid cell infiltrate without extensive necrosis. Only a few B-immunoblasts can be recognized scattered throughout a background of T-lymphocytes. EBER-1-positive cells are also very scarce (less than 5 per high-power field).

In *grade II*, the lymphocytes in the background are often more activated and more atypical. The number of immunoblasts is much higher. Larger cells with a Hodgkin's cell morphology are often associated. Accordingly, the number of large-B-cells and EBER-1-positive cells is also higher (5–15 per high-power field).

Immunohistochemistry

The large cells express the B-markers CD20 (Fig. 6.54b) and CD79α (Capron et al. 1985; Guinee et al. 1994; Taniere et al. 1998; Wilson et al. 1996). They can be CD30-positive but are CD15-negative. Intracytoplasmic monoclonal immunoglobulin expression has been reported in some cases (Wilson et al. 1996). A prerequisite for the diagnosis is the detection of LMP-1 in the large-B-cell component.

The lymphocytes in the background have a mature T-cell phenotype with expression of CD3 and CD2. CD4-positive T cells predominate over CD8-positive ones. CD68-positive histiocytes are numerous.

Genetics

Many of the large-B-cells are EBER-1-positive by in situ hybridization. Clonality of EBV has been demonstrated (Medeiros et al. 1991). There is no rearrangement of the T-cell-receptor gene (Medeiros et al. 1991; McNiff et al. 1996).

Rearrangement of the immunoglobulin heavy-chain gene can be demonstrated (Guinee et al. 1994; McNiff et al. 1996). It is possible to show the presence of different clonal populations in different localizations (Mittal et al. 1990; Wilson et al. 1996).

Differential Diagnosis

The two most important diseases which should be distinguished are *Wegener's granulomatosis* and lung involvement by a nasal or *nasal-like NK/T-cell lymphoma.*

On biopsy material, Wegener's granulomatosis is characterized by the predominance of necrosis, the presence of giant cells, the absence of large-B-cells and the absence of EBV-positive cells. In addition, clinical information, such as the presence of renal manifestations, is important.

The differential diagnosis of nasal or *nasal-like NK/T-cell lymphoma* may be very difficult due to the angiocentric localization of the infiltrate and the frequent necrosis. The morphology of the NK/T-cells (see Chap. 6.3.3.2), their immunophenotype, and the absence of large-B-cells are the best arguments for eliminating a large-B-cell lymphoma secondary to lymphomatoid granulomatosis.

Occurrence

Large B-cell lymphoma secondary to Liebow's lymphomatoid granulomatosis is a rare disease that is observed mainly in adults, with a male preponderance (sex ratio = 2 : 1) (Katzenstein et al. 1979; Sordillo et al. 1982; Koss et al. 1986; Jaffe and Wilson 1997). This lymphoproliferative disorder appears in patients with an immunodeficiency and thus ineffective immune control of EBV. The etiology of this immunodeficiency can be allogenic organ transplantation, HIV infection, Wiskott-Aldrich syndrome, or X-linked lymphoproliferative syndrome (Mittal et al. 1990; Guinee et al. 1994; Haque et al. 1998). In other patients, only careful biologic analysis may disclosed some immune defect of unknown origin (Sordillo et al. 1982; Wilson et al. 1996).

The peculiar morphological picture as well as the clinical symptoms are mostly due to a high level of production of lymphokines and monokines.

Clinical Presentation

The patients present with fever, malaise, weight loss, rashes, arthralgias, myalgias, in addition cough, dyspnea or even chest pain. Chest X-rays disclose the presence of one or multiple nodules, sometimes cavitated dispersed to both lungs.

Some patients have also gastrointestinal symptoms. Neurological symptoms can be observed in patients with brain involvement. Subcutaneous nodules and superficial skin nodules or plaques may be seen (Katzenstein et al. 1979; McNiff et al. 1996; Jaffe and Wilson 1997).

The evolution is highly variable (Katzenstein et al. 1979; Fauci et al. 1982; Sordillo et al. 1982; Koss et al. 1986). Some patients may be more or less asymptomatic for a variable period. In many patients, the evolution is more aggressive, sometimes with one or numerous spontaneous remissions. Causes of death are mostly a progressive pulmonary extension or dissemination to other sites (e.g. cerebral).

Wilson et al. (1996) reported that grade I or II disease may present a regressive evolution of the lesions following α-interferon-2b treatment. This treatment will probably also prevent evolution to grade III (diffuse large-B-cell lymphoma). Aggressive chemotherapy is the only treatment for grade III lesions (Lipford et al. 1987, 1988). The course is often rapidly fatal.

6.7.1.5 Primary Lung Plasmacytoma

Primary lung plasmacytoma presents either as a hilar mass with involvement of major bronchi or as intraparenchymal nodules measuring 2.5 – 8 cm in diameter (Koss et al. 1998), mostly developing as a peribronchial lesion.

The infiltrate comprises large sheets of mature plasma cells associated with a variable number of more immature or atypical plasmacytoid cells resembling giant plasma cells, proplasmacytes, or plasmablasts. Crystal-like inclusions can be found in the tumor cells or in histiocytes. Immunoglobulin (Moriginaga et al. 1987) or amyloid deposits may be observed (Koss et al. 1998). Extension to peribronchial or mediastinal lymph nodes can occur.

Primary lung plasmacytoma is a very rare type of primary lung lymphoma and has to be distinguished from MALT lymphoma with a plasma cell component, from rare immunocytoma with or without serum macroglobulinemia, from plasma cell granuloma, a variant of inflammatory pseudotumor in which the plasma cells are polytypic, and, finally, from secondary pulmonary extension of multiple myeloma.

The median age of occurrence of primary lung plasmacytoma is between 40 and 50 years with exceptional cases in childhood and without gender predominance (Joseph et al. 1993).

The lymphoma is often disclosed by a chest X-ray as hilar or intralobar masses. A few patients present with clinical symptoms such as cough, dyspnea, and hemoptysis (Amin 1985; Joseph et al. 1993; Koss et al. 1998). Rarely, a peripheral blood monoclonal gammopathy is disclosed, which should disappear after surgical resection of the tumor.

This lymphoma is too rare to comment on the prognosis. Patients are mostly treated by surgery. In a series of 19 patients, local recurrences were rare, but three patients developed multiple myeloma (Joseph et al. 1993). In a group of five patients (Koss et al. 1998), two survived more than 20 years The overall 2- and 5-year survival are approximately 66% and 40% (Koss et al. 1998) (see Chap. 7.2).

6.7.1.6 Primary NK/T-Cell Lymphoma of the Lung

NK/T-cell lymphomas seem to present very rarely as primary tumors in the lung (Li et al. 1990).

Morphology
Three types presenting with predominant lung involvement have been occasionally observed:

- Peripheral T-cell lymphoma, unspecified (see Chap. 5.2.2.2)
- NK/T-cell lymphoma, nasal type (see Chap. 6.3.3.2)
- Anaplastic large-cell lymphoma (see Chap. 5.2.2.4) (Harrison et al. 1988; Close et al. 1993; Rush et al. 2000)

6.8 Lymphoma of the Pleura

6.8.1 Primary Lymphoma of the Pleura

Recently, two types of primary lymphoma of the pleura have been described.

6.8.1.1 Primary Effusion Lymphoma (ICD-O: 9678/3)

Synonyms
- Kiel: Not listed
- REAL: Not listed
- WHO: Primary effusion lymphoma
- Other: Primary body-cavity-based lymphoma

Definition
This lymphoma can develop in the pleura and in other body cavities without evolving tumor masses. It remains localized in the majority of patients, without extension to other organs or tissues. This lymphoma consists of large cells with a morphology between immunoblastic and anaplastic, with a peculiar B-cell immunophenotype. The cells show latent infection by EBV and human herpes virus 8/Kaposi's sarcoma herpes virus (HHV8/KSHV) (Cesarman et al. 1995, 1996; Jaffe 1996; Nador et al. 1996; Said et al. 1996a). It has been suggested that the two viruses may cooperate in the neoplastic transformation (Ohsawa et al. 1995; Cesarman et al. 1995, 1996; Ansari et al. 1996).

The postulated cell of origin is a post-germinal-center B-cell with plasmacytoid differentiation (Green et al. 1995; Ansari et al. 1996; Nador et al. 1996; Horenstein et al. 1997).

Morphology

Histology. The large neoplastic cells embedded in a fibrin network are present at the pleural surface (Fig. 6.55a). They may also diffusely infiltrate the pleural tissue without tumor formation. They have abundant, basophilic cytoplasm, roundish nuclei with occasional irregularities, and present with the morphology of immunoblasts, plasmablasts or anaplastic large cells (Fig. 6.55b). Herpes virus particles have been disclosed at the ultrastructural level in lymphoma cells (Said et al. 1996a).

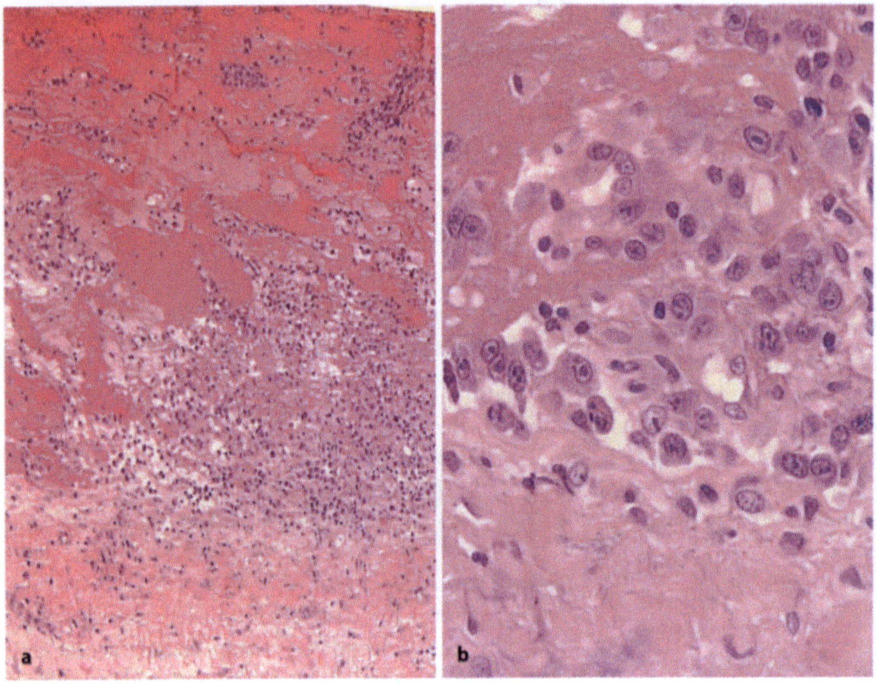

Fig. 6.55 a, b. Primary effusion lymphoma in an HIV-positive patient. **a** Large lymphoma cells in a fibrin network at the surface of the pleura without a tumor mass (H and E stain). **b** The tumor cells exhibit the morphology of immunoblasts or plasmablasts surrounded by fibrin (H and E stain)

Cytology. Smears obtained after cytocentrifugation of serous fluids and stained with May-Grünwald-Giemsa solution show large cells with abundant and basophilic cytoplasm, sometimes with vacuoles. The nuclei are also large, roundish, perhaps with some irregularities. Nucleoli are large, often single, and central. The morphology is that of an immunoblast, plasmablast with a perinuclear halo, or anaplastic large cell. Sometimes the neoplastic cells even have a Reed-Sternberg-like cytology

Immunophenotype

The tumor cells express CD45 and activation markers such as CD30 and/or EMA. They are often negative for CD19 and CD20 (Nador et al. 1996). Even CD79α is not always expressed. Often, markers of plasmacytoid differentiation, such as CD38 and CD138, are positive. Surface immunoglobulins are mostly not demonstrable. Rarely a monotypic immunoglobulin can be disclosed in the cytoplasm. Aberrant expression of CD3 in the cytoplasm has been observed. Exceptional cases with a T immunophenotype have also been reported (Green et al. 1995).

LMP-1 is negative. HHV8/KSHV-associated latent protein can be disclosed in the nuclei.

Genetic Features

In many cases studied (Cesarman et al. 1995, 1996; Ansari et al. 1996; Nador et al. 1996), the immunoglobulin heavy-chain gene was rearranged. Mutations are also observed. Aberrant rearrangement of the T-cell-receptor genes has been reported leading to the discussion of bigenotypic tumors (Ansari et al. 1996).

Cytogenetics failed to disclose chromosomal abnormalities. However, new technical developments such as comparative genomic analysis has demonstrated abnormalities similar to those observed in some HIV-associated lymphomas (Mullaney et al. 2000). These abnormalities include gains in chromosomes 12 and Y.

On paraffin section, EBER-1 can be demonstrated in the majority of the tumor cells (Horenstein et al. 1997) by in situ hybridization. In addition, the HHV8/KSHV genome is found in all cells (Ansari et al. 1996).

Tumor cells lack rearrangement of bcl-2, bcl-6, ras, p53 and c-myc genes. The presence of HHV8/KSHV and a c-myc rearrangement appears to be a mutually exclusive molecular event (Cesarman et al. 1995, 1996; Nador et al. 1996).

Differential Diagnosis
In the differential diagnosis *carcinomatous involvement* of the serous cavities should be considered first. The bizarre immunophenotype (CD20-negative) may be responsible for a misdiagnosis. Cytokeratins should be studied. They are always negative.

When the diagnosis of lymphoma is confirmed by the expression of CD45, secondary involvement of the serous cavity from other organ-based lymphomas or from *pyothorax-associated* lymphoma (see Chap. 6.8.1.2) should be excluded.

The best criteria for the diagnosis are the association of the bizarre cell morphology with an aberrant B-cell phenotype and HIV infection.

Occurrence
The age of the patients varies with the etiology: young or middle-aged HIV-positive patients (median age 42.5 years) (Nador et al. 1996) vs elderly HIV-negative patients (70–80 years), some with Kaposi's sarcoma (Said et al. 1996b; Strauchen et al. 1996).

This lymphoma represents about 2% of AIDS-associated lymphomas, occurring often in homosexual males (Knowles 1999; Nador et al. 1996; Said et al. 1996a).

However HIV is not the only condition associated with primary effusion lymphoma. The disease has also been described in HIV-negative patients (Said et al. 1996b), for example, in allograft recipients or elderly patients, mainly males, living in geographical areas in which a high incidence of HHV8 infection is known, i.e. Mediterranean countries. In some of these patients, Kaposi's sarcoma was present before primary effusion lymphoma(Strauchen et al. 1996).

Clinical Presentation
In addition to the pleural cavity, patients may present with effusion in the peritoneal or pericardial cavity, without any tumor or lymphadenopathies.

Localizations to other extranodal sites have also been described: GI-tract, soft tissue (Said et al. 1996b; Beaty et al. 1999).

Exceptional cases associated with multicentric Castleman's disease have been reported (Teruya-Feldstein et al. 1998).

The evolution is highly aggressive with a median survival of less than 6 months.

6.8.1.2 Pyothorax-Associated Primary Lymphoma

Definition
This is another type of large-B-cell lymphoma occurring primarily in the pleura in patients with long-standing pleural inflammation, which may result from therapeutic artificial pneumothorax or from tuberculos pleuritis associated with a latent EBV infection (Iuchi et al. 1989; Ibuka et al. 1994; Martin et al. 1994; Fukayama et al. 1995) without HHV8/KSHV infection.

Localized immunodepression secondary to chronic inflammation or treatment with immunosuppressive cytokines may be responsible for a clonal proliferation of EBV latently infected B-cells (Ohsawa et al. 1995).

Morphology
Histology. A tumor is present in the pleura (Fig. 6.56a) and extends to the lung parenchyma. This tumor comprises large cells with large, pale nuclei that are round, ovoid, or irregularly shaped and have large, often single and centrally situated nucleoli with abundant basophilic cytoplasm (Fig. 6.56b). A perinuclear halo is often present, demonstrating a plasmacytoid differentiation. Rare Reed-Sternberg-like cells can be observed.

Cytology. Examination of smears obtained after cytocentrifugation of pleural effusion fluid stained by May-Grünwald-Giemsa stain discloses large cells with the morphology of immunoblasts, plasmablasts, anaplastic large cells or even giant cells with a Reed-Sternberg-like morphology identical to those seen in pleural effusion lymphoma.

Immunohistochemistry
The immunoreactivity is almost identical to that of pleural effusion lymphoma, with a more frequent CD79α expression. Intracytoplasmic monotypic immunoglobulin, often α-heavy chain is observed (Martin et al. 1994).

LMP-1 is often positive, but the HHV8/KSHV-associated latent protein is missing (Cesarman et al. 1996; Nakatsuka et al. 2002). EBNA-2 is sometimes highly expressed (Sasajima et al. 1993). Rare biphenotypic tumors have been reported (Mori et al. 1996).

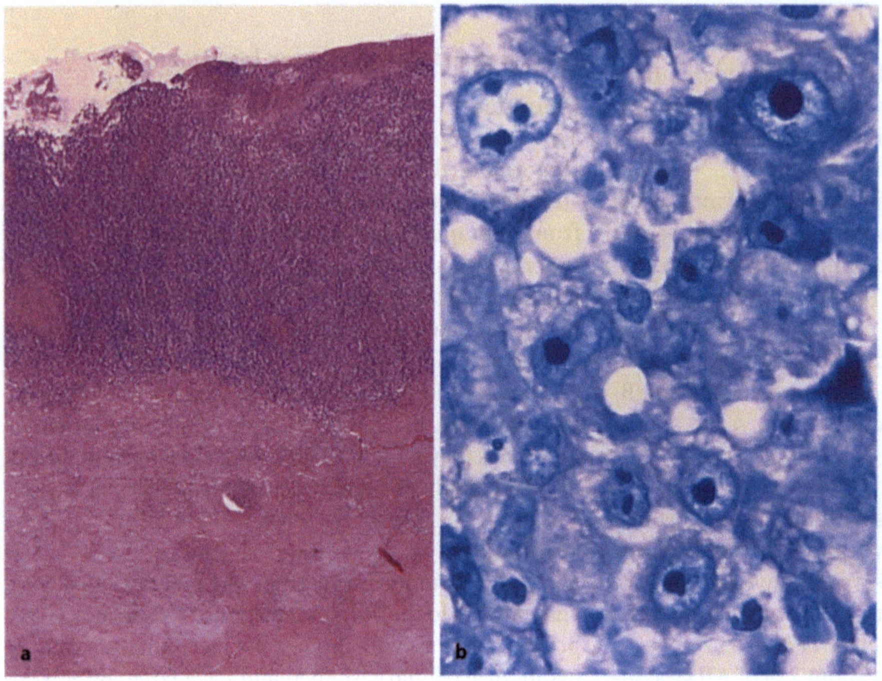

Fig. 6.56 a, b. Pyothorax-associated lymphoma. **a** The pleura is infiltrated by numerous neoplastic cells forming a large tumor (H and E stain). **b** The lymphoma cells have the morphology of immunoblasts, plasmablasts or anaplastic large cells. Many cells are necrotic (Giemsa stain)

Genetic Features

Ig heavy-chain genes are rearranged. Currently, no characteristic cytogenetic abnormality has been demonstrated.

In situ hybridization on paraffin section demonstrates in all cases in numerous tumor cells the presence of EBER-1 (Martin et al. 1994; Molinié et al. 1996). By contrast, the HHV8/KSHV genome is always absent (Cesarman et al. 1996).

Differential Diagnosis

Demonstration of CD45 positivity and cytokeratin negativity allows identification of a large-cell lymphoma and rules out the diagnoses *carcinoma and mesothelioma.*

The demonstration of intracytoplasmic immunoglobulins and/or of positivity for markers expressed by B-cells during plasmacytoid differentiation leads to a diagnosis of pyothorax-associated primary lymphoma.

The most important criteria to eliminate *primary effusion lymphoma* are:

- The absence of immunodeficiency and particularly serologic negativity for HIV
- The long history of pleural or pleuropulmonary chronic suppuration
- The presence of pleural tumor masses
- The absence of tumor cell infection by HHV8/KSHV

Occurrence

Patients have a median age of 63 years (Martin et al. 1994; Molinié et al. 1996) and are mostly male.

This type of primary pleural large-B-cell lymphoma develops in patients with a long history of pleural or pleuropulmonary chronic suppuration. Pyothorax-associated primary lymphoma resembles other large-B-cell lymphomas occurring in patients with long-standing suppurative diseases (Copie-Bergman et al. 1997; Nakatsuka et al. 2002). The production of cytokines with immunosuppressive activity may be responsible for a clonal proliferation of EBV latently infected B-cells (Ohsawa et al. 1995).

Most cases of pyothorax-associated primary lymphoma were reported in Japan (Iuchi et al. 1989; Ibuka et al. 1994; Fukayama et al. 1995; Ohsawa et al. 1995; Mori et al. 1996), but some cases have been observed in France (Martin et al. 1994; Molinié et al. 1996).

Clinical Presentation

Patients complain of chest or shoulder pain, dyspnea, and constitutional symptoms, such as fever or weight loss. Pleuritis is disclosed by clinical examination. Abnormal opacity is recognized by chest radiography. Computed tomography demonstrates the presence of a pleural mass with irregular pleural thickening.

These lymphomas often have a very rapid fatal outcome.

6.8.2 Secondary Pleural Lymphoma

Lymphomatous infiltration of pleura with effusion occurs mainly secondarily to primary or secondary lung lymphomas, to mediastinal lymphomas by contiguity or lymphatic spread, or by hematogenous dissemination from different lymphomas at nodal or extranodal sites.

Visceral and parietal serosa are thickened by a white tissue, revealing one or multiple pleural plaques or tumor masses with serous, hemorrhagic or, rarely, chylous effusion.

Cytological study of the effusion allows the presence of lymphoma cells of different types to be recognized in about 60–90% of the patients (Das et al. 1987).

Thirteen percent of malignant pleural effusions are due to lymphomas. Pleural effusions are disclosed at autopsy in about 76% of patients with NHL (Berkman and Breuer 1993). About 16% of patients with NHL have at presentation or will have during disease evolution a pleural involvement (Das et al. 1987).

About 20–70% of patients have mediastinal lymphoma (Das et al. 1987).

Large-B-cell lymphomas are more frequently associated with pleural effusion than are small-B-cell lymphomas. Any type of lymphoma may secondarily involve the pleura. Recently, in a series of patients with marginal zone lymphoma of nodal and splenic origin, pleural involvement was observed in 11% (Berger et al. 2000).

A secondary pleural effusion in a patient with a nodal or extranodal NHL is associated with a poor overall prognosis. Approximately 50% of these patients die within 2 years of this finding. Pleural effusion persists in about half of the 50% of surviving patients.

6.9 Lymphoma of the Heart

Cardiac lymphoma represents a rare example of extranodal malignant lymphoma that may involve all parts of the heart. These lymphomas are mostly secondary. In a series of 80 necropsies of patients with cardiac lymphoma, two patients presented with primary cardiac lymphoma and five with secondary (Petersen et al. 1976). In another survey of 12,485 consecutive autopsies in Hong Kong, no primary heart lymphoma was found, but secondary involvement by lymphoma was identified in 11.9% of males and 17% of females with secondary heart tumors (Lam et al. 1993). In the necropsy series of Ito et al. (1996), 14 patients out of 80 had secondary cardiac involvement by lymphoma (five B-cell and one T-cell lymphoma). A case of heart involvement during dissemination of a mycosis fungoides was reported (Servitje et al. 1999). Thus, the incidence of secondary heart involvement by lymphoma among heart tumors is between 8.7% and 17.8% (Petersen et al. 1976; McDonnell et al. 1982). Here, only primary lymphoma will be described.

6.9.1 Primary Cardiac Lymphoma

Definition

This condition has been defined as an extranodal lymphoma involving only the heart and the pericardium (McAllister and Fenoglio 1978). Today, massive cardiac involvement with only a minimal infiltration of other sites is also accepted as primary cardiac origin with early dissemination (Cairns et al. 1987; Wargotz et al. 1987; Ito et al. 1996).

Morphology

Macroscopy. Most patients are diagnosed at necropsy. Pericardial effusion is frequent, often with fibrinoid epicarditis. Nodules or polycyclic masses, gray-white and firm, are discovered in the myocardium, extending often to the epicardium but rarely to the endocardium. The topography of these nodules is variable, often occupying the left side of the heart.

Extension to the pleura with effusion or to mediastinal lymph nodes represents local spread of the lymphoma (Nagamine and Noda 1990).

Histology. The majority are large-B-cell lymphomas, immunoblastic type with plasmacytoid differentiation (Ito et al. 1996). Sometimes only the pericardium is infiltrated corresponding to a primary effusion lymphoma (see Chap. 6.8) occurring mostly in HIV-positive patients.

Rare cases belong to peripheral NK/T-cell lymphomas, unspecified, or anaplastic large-cell of T or null type.

Occurrence
Primary heart lymphoma is extremely rare. It occurs in adults, with a median age of 67 years, ranging from 38 to 90 years. A predominance of males has been reported (male : female, 4:1) (Ito et al. 1996). This lymphoma has also been observed in HIV-positive patients (Guarner et al. 1987) or in immunocompromised patients after organ transplantation.

Clinical Presentation
Patients complain of chest pain and dyspnea. Chest X-rays discloses an enlarged heart often with pleural effusion. Some patients present with pericardial effusion and perhaps cardiac tamponade (Nagamine and Noda 1990). Cytological study of pericardiac fluid obtained by puncture allows the diagnosis to be made, and immediate treatment by polychemotherapy to be initiated. This is the only chance for the patient to survive (Nand et al. 1991). Sternotomy for biopsy is required for the diagnosis (Chim et al. 1997). Some patients may die suddenly.

The prognosis of patients with primary cardiac lymphoma remains poor (Chim et al. 1997).

6.10 Splenic Lymphoma

Malignant lymphoma occurs in the spleen, either primarily or secondarily. The majority of these lymphomas develop in the white pulp; only a few occurs primarily in the red pulp. Secondary involvement is always due to hematogenous dissemination because of the absence of afferent lymphatic vessels. Splenic lymphoma disseminates mostly through the portal venous system, causing liver and then bone marrow involvement. Hilar lymph nodes are involved through the efferent lymphatic vessels of the spleen.

Lymphoma involvement of the spleen leads to an increase in the size and weight of the organ, from 300 g to 2,000–4,000 g or even more. Spontaneous rupture or rupture secondary to a minimal trauma may occur with subsequent intra-abdominal hemorrhage.

Macroscopic study of the spleen yields important diagnostic information in both primary and secondary splenic lymphomas, as most lymphomas of this type are associated with a distinct pattern of infiltration .

Dissection of the spleen should be done according to a precise protocol: the organ should be cut in parallel slices not thicker than 0.5 cm. Both sides of the slice should be carefully examined to be sure not to miss small nodules. Imprints should be always done, particularly any areas with nodules. Hilar lymph nodes should be dissected and included in the microscopic examination.

6.10.1 Primary Splenic Lymphoma or Lymphoma with a Splenic Predominance

- Small-B-cell lymphoma
  - Hairy cell leukemia
  - Marginal zone lymphoma
  - Lymphoplasmacytic lymphoma (immunocytoma)
  - Plasmacytoma
  - B-prolymphocytic leukemia
- Large-B-cell lymphoma
- Peripheral T-cell lymphoma
  - Hepatosplenic lymphoma
  - Chronic NK/T-cell leukemia with azurophilic granules
  - Peripheral T-cell lymphoma, unspecified
  - Aggressive NK-cell leukemia/lymphomas

Definition
Primary splenic lymphomas are less frequent than secondary ones (Burke 1981, 1985; Strauss et al. 1983; Narang et al. 1985; Spier et al. 1985; Diebold 1989). Ahmann et al. (1966), based on a series of 5,100 patients with malignant lymphoma, proposed an incidence of 1%, but Meuge et al. (1972) observed an incidence of 11.6% in a series of 274 patients with malignant lymphoma. In Japan, based on a series of 2,524 patients with malignant lymphoma studied between 1972 and 1977, the incidence of primary splenic malignant lymphoma was only 0.3% (Hara et al. 1985). Strauss et al. (1983) observed primary splenic lympho-

ma in 2.6 % of patients with malignant lymphoma clinical stage I or IE.

Such differences in the reported incidence can be partly explained by the fact that the definition of primary splenic lymphoma is still unclear. Initially, the definition was very strict. Only malignant lymphoma confined to the spleen without any other organ involvement was reported as primary splenic lymphoma. But, for many years now, the definition has been extended. It has now been accepted that primary splenic lymphoma is a lymphoma responsible for a huge spleen, without any other organ involvement that can be disclosed clinically. It is also accepted that these splenic lymphomas can be associated with an extension to the splenic hilar lymph nodes and with microscopic involvement of the liver and bone marrow that is only disclosed by systematic biopsies (Ahmann et al. 1966; Strauss et al. 1983; Hara et al. 1985; Narang et al. 1985; Spier et al. 1985; Diebold 1989).

The term *malignant lymphoma with predominant splenic involvement* was proposed as being equivalent to the term *primary splenic malignant lymphoma* (Spier et al. 1985; Narang et al. 1985; Diebold 1989).

Morphology

Macroscopy. Four main macroscopic patterns can be observed in both primary and secondary splenic lymphomas (Diebold 1989).

Multimicronodular Pattern

Primary splenic lymphoma comprises dispersed, numerous, small whitish nodules 0.5–1 cm in size (Fig. 6.57). The nodules represent lymphomatous involvement of enlarged follicles (Fig. 6.58). Often, the nodules are surrounded by a brown halo due to the accumulation of hemosiderin-laden macrophages. A diffuse dispersion of such multiple micronodules is observed in the majority of the small-B-cell lymphomas (*B-CLL*, *lymphoplasmacytic*, *follicular*, *mantle cell* and *marginal zone lymphomas*). Development on this background of larger nodules measuring more than 1 cm in diameter represents a localized transformation into *large-B-cell lymphoma* (Diebold 1989; Audouin et al. 1988; Duong et al. 2000). Often, tumorous lymphadenopathies are found in the hilum (Fig. 6.58). The most important diseases to consider in the differential diagnosis are *sarcoidosis*, *tuberculosis* due to hematogenous dissemination, or *reactive hyperplasia of follicles in some autoimmune disorders* mainly in children (Diebold 1989). Localized micronodules present only in one part of the spleen are observed only in *caseo-follicular tuberculosis* or in the early phase of classic Hodgkin's lymphoma, and in lymphocyte predominance Hodgkin's lymphoma, nodular type (nodular paragranuloma).

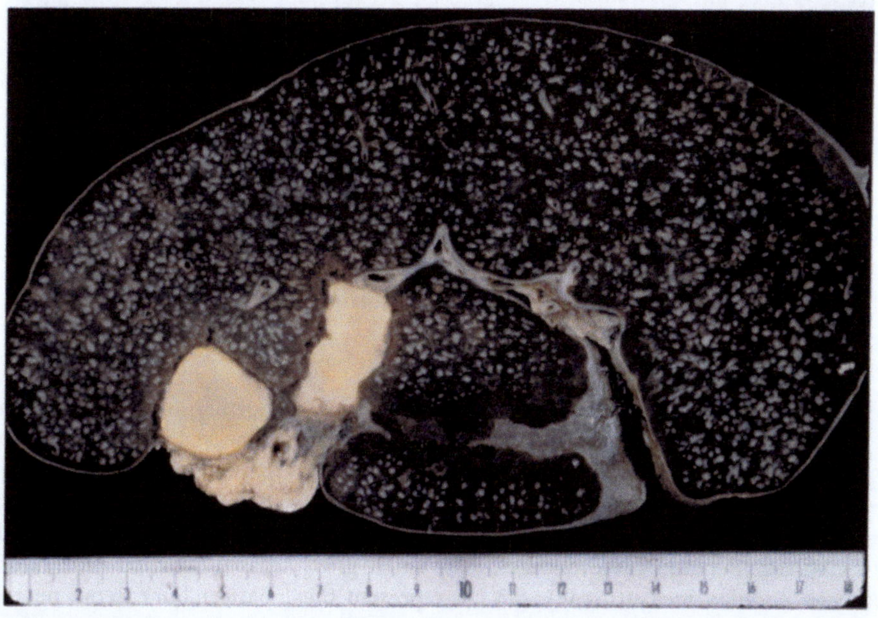

Fig. 6.57. Spleen with a micronodular pattern seen in many different types of small-B-cell lymphomas after formalin fixation. Here, a B-cell chronic lymphocytic leukemia (B-CLL) with two infarcts is shown

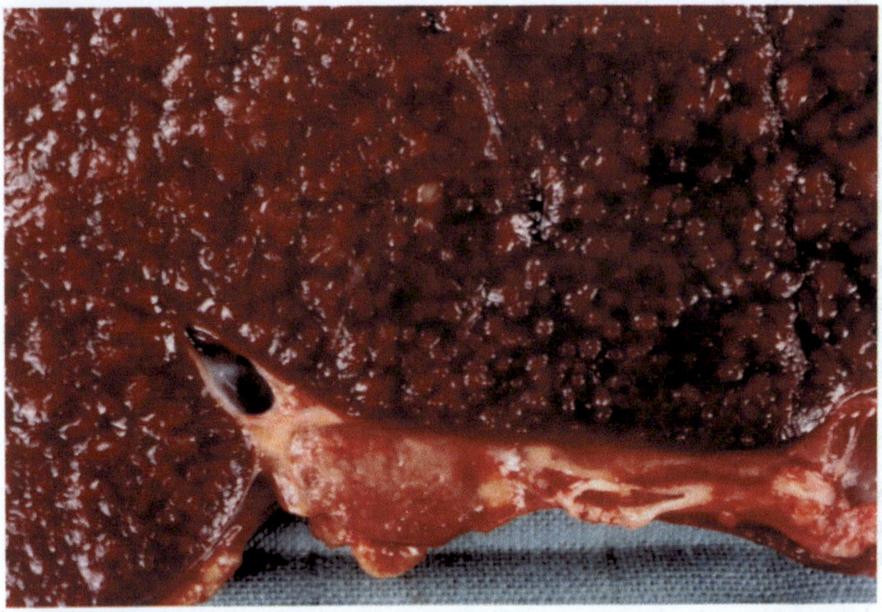

Fig. 6.58. Spleen with a micronodular pattern before fixation. This is a follicular lymphoma with hilar adenopathy and a nodular pattern

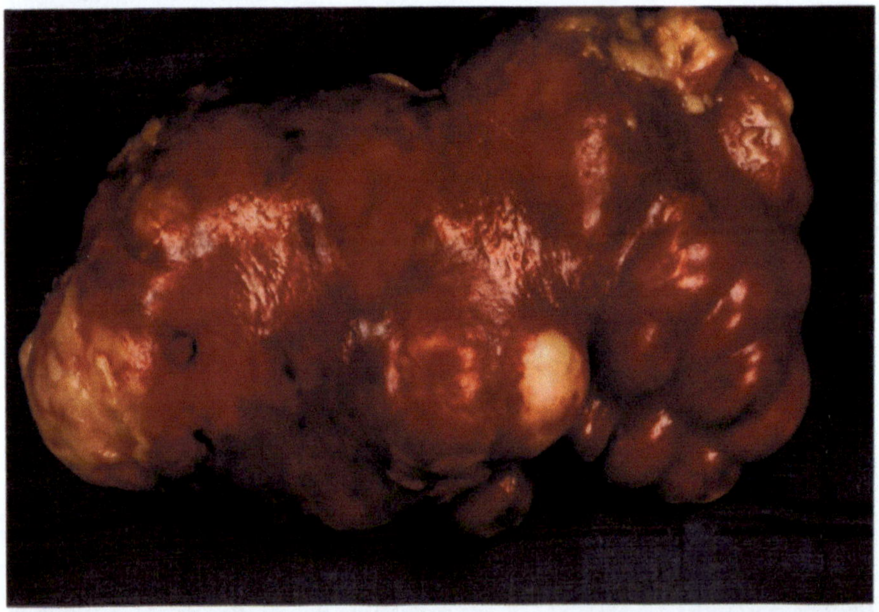

Fig. 6.59. Spleen with a large expansive mass that destroys the parenchyma is characteristic of large-B-cell lymphoma, for example, a polymorphic centroblastic type, shown here

Multimacronodular Pattern

The whitish nodules surrounded by a brown halo are somewhat larger, more than 1 cm and up to 5 cm in diameter. They are often localized in one or multiple areas of the spleen but are not dispersed throughout the spleen. Between these nodules, very small gray-brown nodules, measuring 0.1 – 0.3 cm represent the normal follicle (white pulp). This pattern can be observed in *Burkitt's lymphoma; peripheral T-cell lymphoma, unspecified; angioimmunoblastic T-cell lymphoma type* or *Lennert's lymphoma type*; as well as in *anaplastic large-cell* and *Hodgkin's lymphomas.* Some *caseo-follicular tuberculosis* may also present with this pattern but caseous necrosis is present.

Polycyclic Masses

Large whitish tumors with polycyclic outlines destroy a variable part of the organ, compressing the non-involved adjacent parenchyma. These masses often are confluent. They measure more than 5 cm in diameter, sometimes up to 10 or 20 cm (Fig. 6.59). In large nodules, yellow areas of central necrobiosis and/or dark red zones of hemorrhages may be seen. The shape of the spleen is often modified due to the protrusion of polycyclic masses. This pattern is observed in *large-B-cell lymphomas*, in *Hodgkin's lymphomas* but also in *non-hematopoietic tumors*.

Diffuse Pattern

The splenic parenchyma is firm and dense with a dark red color. No white nodules or masses can be seen (Fig. 6.60). This pattern is due to a diffuse infiltration of the red pulp often with atrophy of the white pulp and is seen in a few cases of *B-CLL*, in *hairy cell leuke*mia, in some *peripheral NK/T-cell lymphomas* (*hepatosplenic*, *peripheral T-cell, unspecified*, etc.), in *lymphoblastic lymphoma/acute leukemia* but also in different types of *chronic myeloproliferative disorders* (idiopathic myelofibrosis, CML, etc.).

6.10.1.1 Hairy Cell Leukemia (ICD-O: 9940/3)

Synonyms

- Kiel, REAL, and WHO: Hairy cell leukemia

Definition

This is a lymphoma characterized by a diffuse infiltration of the splenic red pulp and bone marrow by small-B lymphoid cells with an abundant pale cytoplasm surrounding an ovoid or sometimes kidney-shaped nucleus. On smears from peripheral blood and sternal puncture but not on imprints, the membrane of these cells exhibits long and thin projections, giving the cells a "hairy" appearance. The normal cell counterpart is not well defined. It is a peripheral B-cell of unknown post-germinal stage.

Morphology

Macroscopy. The spleen presents a homogeneous, dark red surface of the parenchyma after dissection without any visible nodules (Fig. 6.60). Hamartoma (splenoma) may be associated and appears as brown nodules of variable size (Diebold et al. 1977). The spleen weight in the majority of patients is more than 1,000 g and up to 4,500 g (Burke et al. 1974a, b; Diebold et al. 1977; Burke 1981; Burke and Rappaport 1984). The capsule can be

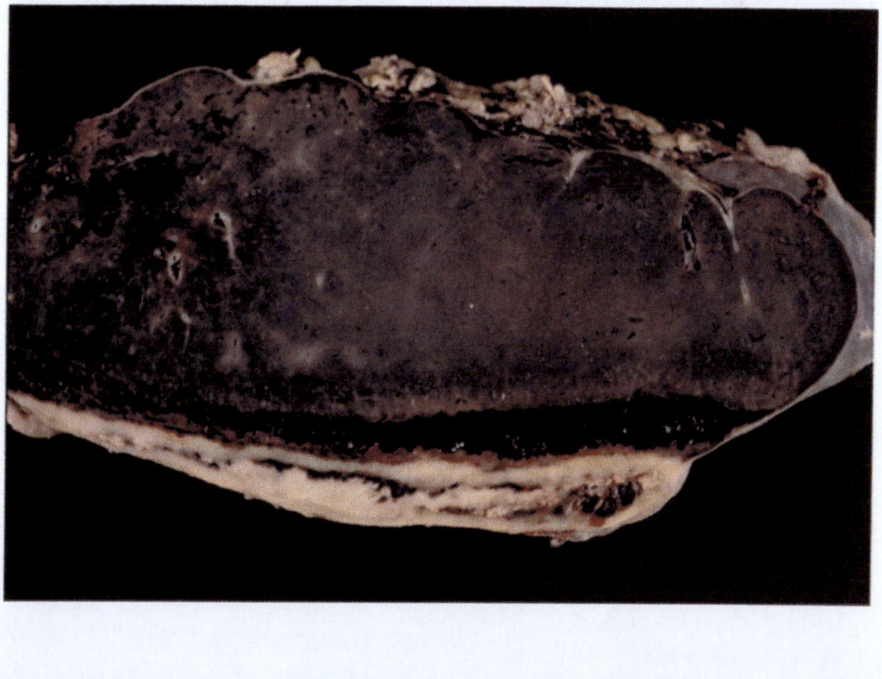

Fig. 6.60. Voluminous splenomegaly with a diffuse pattern such as most often observed in hairy cell leukemia (shown here) or NK/T-cell lymphomas. Note a subcapsular, organized, old hematoma and a recent one between the parenchyma and the old hematoma (after fixation)

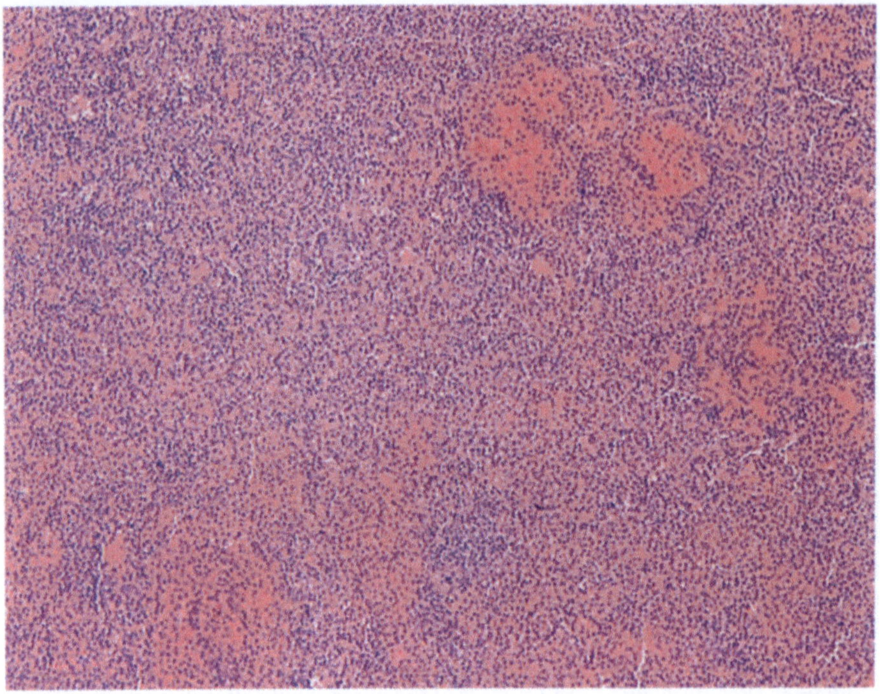

Fig. 6.61. Hairy cell leukemia. Diffuse infiltrate of the red pulp with atrophy of the white pulp. Notice the pseudo-angiomatous pattern due to distension of the sinuses (H and E stain)

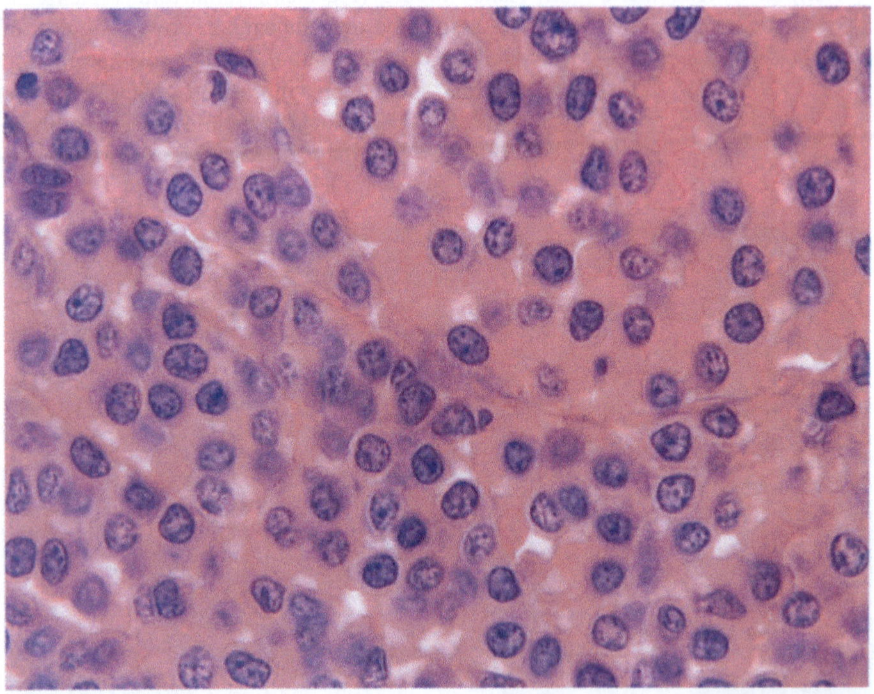

Fig. 6.62. Hairy cell leukemia. The hairy cells have a round or ovoid nucleus and a large cytoplasm. They infiltrate the cords and are present in the sinuses (H and E stain)

thickened. Sometimes hematomas, more or less organized, are observed beneath the capsule. A spontaneous rupture may occur.

Histology. The red pulp of the spleen is massively infiltrated by small to medium-sized cells (Fig. 6.61). Due to the abundant pale cytoplasm which is regularly disposed around each nucleus, at low magnification the pathologist has the impression of sheets of regularly dispersed nuclei, roundish, ovoid or kidney-shaped, with a wide pale space between them (Fig. 6.62). Cytoplasmic projections cannot be observed. The red pulp cords are filled and distended by the hairy cells. Sinuses contain also the leukemic cells. A pseudo-angiomatous pattern (Diebold et al. 1977; Nanba et al. 1977) resembling peliosis is observed in some areas (Fig. 6.61). These cavities are distended sinuses containing a large quantity of blood. Hairy cells can be recognized at the periphery of the vascular spaces, replacing the sinus endothelial cells (Diebold et al. 1977; Nanba et al. 1977; Burke et al. 1974a, b; Burke and Rappaport 1984; Burke 1985). The white pulp is atrophic.

For nodal involvement, see Chap. 4.2.1.3

Cytology. On smears, the cells are small to medium-sized. The cytoplasm is abundant and pale or faintly blue, with numerous long thin projections giving the cells their hairy appearance. In a few cells, rod-shaped inclusions can be recognized corresponding to the ribosome lamellar complex seen at the ultrastructural level (Burke et al. 1974b; Diebold et al. 1977). The nucleus is ovoid or kidney-shaped, with a homogeneous ground-glass chromatin not as clumped as in small lymphocytes. The nucleoli are absent or inconspicuous.

Numerous hairy cells show a strong, diffuse cytoplasmic positivity for tartrate-resistant acid phosphatase (TRAP) (Burke et al. 1974a; Burke 1981, 1985; Burke and Rappaport 1984).

Immunohistochemistry

The B-cell origin is demonstrated by the positivity of B-cell markers (CD20 and CD79α). Flow cytometry discloses surface monotypic immunoglobulin, mostly M, rarely G or A, but not D.

These cells strongly express CD11c, CD25, HLA-DR, FMC7, and CD103 (Visser et al. 1989; Moldenhauer et al. 1990; Möller et al. 1990). They also are strongly positive for DBA44, which is not specific, but often allows the villous cytoplasmic projections to be recognized on paraffin sections (Falini et al. 1990; Hounieu et al. 1992). Cyclin D1 is overexpressed in about half to two/thirds of the tumors (Ishida et al. 1999; Sole et al. 1999a). The hairy cells do not express CD5, CD10, or CD23. But CD5 and CD10 expression has been observed in Japan and, exceptionally, in Western patients (Robbins et al. 1993; Juliusson et al. 1994; Dunphy et al. 1999; Usha et al. 2000). The enzyme TRAP can now be detected by immunohistochemistry on paraffin section (Hoyer et al. 1997).

Genetic Features

Rearrangement of the heavy- and light-chain genes can be demonstrated by PCR (Korsmeyer et al. 1983; Wagner et al. 1994). Mutations of the Vκ gene have been shown in post-germinal-center cells (Wagner et al. 1994); bcl-6 mutations have been described (Capello et al. 2000).

There is no t(11;14) or bcl-1 rearrangement despite the overexpression of cyclin D1 (Ishida et al. 1999; Bosch et al. 1995; Sole et al. 1999a).

Characteristic cytogenetic abnormalities have yet to be described (Sole et al. 1999b). Trisomy 12 has been reported in a few patients (Vallianatou et al. 1999). Recent reports have shown some abnormalities involving mainly chromosome 5 (Haglund et al. 1994; Kluin-Nelemans et al. 1994). Some clonal chromosome abnormalities clustering to specific regions, i.e. RAS and RASA genes, have been reported (Haglund et al. 1994). An increased expression of the src proto-oncogene without any genetic abnormality has also been reported (Lynch et al. 1993).

A high incidence of p53 deletion has been reported in hairy cell leukemia (HCL) and in HCL-variant. The number of positive cells is higher in HCL-variant (mean 31%) than in HCL (mean 12%). This difference seems to correlate with the higher tendency for transformation and poor response to therapy in HCL-variant (Vallianatou et al. 1999).

Differential Diagnosis

The diagnosis of HCL is easy due to the very characteristic morphology of the cells in smears and sections. Regarding splenic localization, HCL is the only small-B-cell lymphoma with a predominant red pulp involvement. The infiltration is more homogeneous than in B-CLL with diffuse growth pattern. Although the infiltration pattern of the red pulp may be similar in *peripheral T-cell lymphomas* and in *chronic, subacute or acute myeloproliferative diseases*, the cytology is decisive.

Concerning the leukemic blood picture, HCL-variant as well as splenic MZBCL with villous lymphocytes should be considered in the differential diagnosis. The detailed phenotypes are described by Matutes et al (1994).

Occurrence

HCL represents no more than 2% of all lymphoid leukemias. Most of the patients are adults, with a median age of 55 years. There is a male predominance (sex ratio male:female = 5:1) (Bouroncle 1994).

Clinical Presentation

Splenomegaly is the major symptom; there is also a pancytopenia. At the beginning of the disease, the circulating hairy cells are absent or rare. A typical leukemia is only observed in more advanced cases and in HCL-variant (see below). Bone marrow biopsy in case of pancytopenia is mandatory for the diagnosis. Currently, the diagnosis is based on bone marrow histology. Hepatomegaly is very rare as are peripheral lymphadenopathies.

During the evolution, but rarely at presentation, voluminous abdominal lymph node tumor can occur, probably representing a kind of HCL transformation (Merciera et al. 1994; Pettit et al. 1999). Blastic transformation has also been reported (Nazeer et al. 1997).

Dysimmune disorders, opportunistic infections such as atypical mycobacteriosis, vasculitis, and some carcinomas have been described to occur in association with HCL.

The polychemotherapy regimens used to treat other types of B-cell lymphoma are not followed by a good response. Long-term remission (Spiers et al. 1987; Piro et al. 1990) can be obtained by the use of either interferon or dioxycoformycin or 2-chlorodioxyadenosine. This treatment currently replaces splenectomy, which in the past has been followed by long-term remission.

An unexpectedly high incidence of second neoplasms was reported in 10% of a cohort of HCL patients after treatment of with interferon-α 2B, compared to an age-matched population. These second neoplasms were hematopoietic tumors (malignant lymphomas, acute myelogenous leukemia, Langerhans' histiocytosis, polycythemia vera) or adenocarcinoma of various organs (Kampmeier et al. 1994).

Addendum: Hairy Cell Variant

Patients with this variant often have a large number of leukemic cells in the peripheral blood. The cells have a hairy cell cytology but with a prominent nucleolus thus mimicking a prolymphocyte. The histological pattern of both splenic and bone marrow infiltrates is similar to that of common HCL. These cells exhibit a B-cell phenotype, often expressing surface IgG. They lack CD25, sometimes CD103, and may be TRAP-negative. A high incidence of p53 deletion has been reported as well as the presence in some patients of a trisomy 12 (Vallianatou et al. 1999). The differential diagnosis to distinguish hairy cell variant from B-prolymphocytic leukemia and even from the villous lymphoid cells of splenic marginal zone lymphoma can be difficult. The survival is shorter than in common HCL due to poor response to treatment.

6.10.1.2 Splenic Marginal Zone Lymphoma (ICD-O: 9689/3)

- Kiel: Splenic immunocytoma (in part)
- REAL: Splenic marginal zone lymphoma (± villous lymphocyte)
- WHO: Splenic marginal zone lymphoma

Definition

This lymphoma develops in the follicles of the spleen and has a biphasic pattern. Medium-sized monocytoid B-cells are organized as a pale ring around the follicle with a marginal zone pattern. Small centrocyte-like lymphoid cells destroy the mantle zone and colonize the germinal centers. Diffuse, focally accentuated infiltration of the red pulp by lymphoid and monocytoid B-cells is also present (Isaacson et al. 1994; Isaacson 1996; Piris and Isaacson 1998; Mollejo et al. 1995; Duong et al. 2000; Franco et al. 2003).

In addition, in about half of the patients a monotypic plasma cell component is detected (Duong et al. 2000).

Some splenic marginal zone lymphomas (SMZLs) are associated with the presence of villous lymphocytes in the peripheral blood (Rousselet et al. 1992; Isaacson et al. 1994).

It has been postulated that the normal cell counterpart is the marginal zone cell (Jaffe et al. 2001). But in many cases these cells express IgD (Isaacson et al. 1994; Isaacson 1996; Duong et al. 2000) and are then impossible to be distinguish from mantle cells. Thus, the cell of origin of this lymphoma remains unclear, and the term "marginal zone" lymphoma is therefore perhaps inaccurate.

Morphology

Macroscopy. The enlarged spleen shows a typical multimicronodular pattern. The spleen weight in the majority of patients is more than 400 g and may even exceed 2,000 g.

Histology. The follicles are enlarged and are of variable size (Fig. 6.63). They present a marginal zone appearing as a pale corona surrounding the follicles (Figs. 6.63, 6.64). The marginal zone consists of medium-sized cells with an abundant pale cytoplasm and an ovoid nucleus with dispersed chromatin (Fig. 6.65). These cells exhibit a monocytoid B-cell morphology (Isaacson et al. 1994; Isaacson 1996; Mollejo et al. 1995; Melo et al. 1987a; Duong et al. 2000). The center of the follicles is either homogeneous, due to colonization by small centrocyte-like cells replacing mantle zone and the germinal center (Fig. 6.63, 6.64), or with a reactive germinal center surrounded by the same centrocyte-like neoplastic cells. Germinal centers with a regressive pattern can be seen.

In about 50 – 60 % of tumors, a third type of cell is present. These have a lymphoplasmacytic or plasmacytic morphology with monotypic intracytoplasmic Ig. They are observed in the marginal zone, in the follicle, in the infiltrated germinal centers, and sometimes in the cords. PAS-positive Dutcher-Fahey intranuclear vacuoles are present (Duong et al. 2000).

Large cells with an immunoblast morphology are very rare. Clusters of immunoblasts are not seen. An increase in the number of large cells around germinal centers (Fig. 6.66) or in the marginal zone may indicate transformation into a more aggressive lymphoma (Lloret et al. 1999; Cualing et al. 2000).

In the red pulp, a lymphoid cell infiltrate of variable intensity from minimal to extensive is observed. It mainly comprises centrocyte-like cells, sometimes associated with lymphoplasmacytoid cells and plasma cells. This infiltrate can be diffuse in the cords or nodular around terminal arteries. Often, these nodules are made up of monocytoid B-cells. Numerous lymphoid cells may also be present in the sinuses, particularly if there are villous lymphocytes in the peripheral blood (Melo et al. 1987a).

Hilar adenopathies are often disclosed. A clear zone of monocytoid B-cells or centrocyte-like cells with a

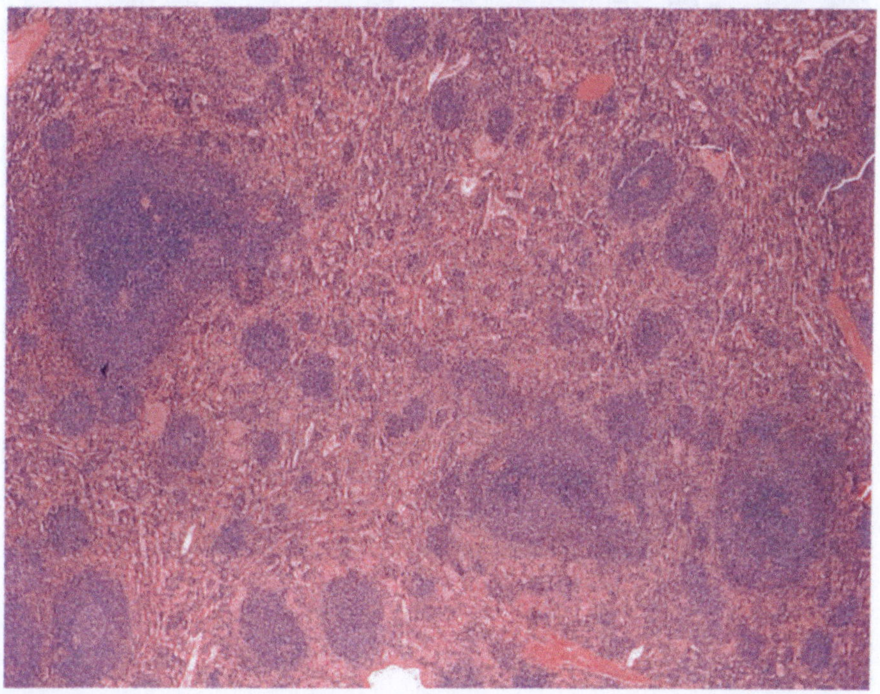

Fig. 6.63. Primary marginal zone lymphoma of the spleen. Follicles of variable size exhibit a marginal zone and a homogeneous germinal center. In the red pulp, there are diffuse and nodular infiltrates of the cords (H and E stain)

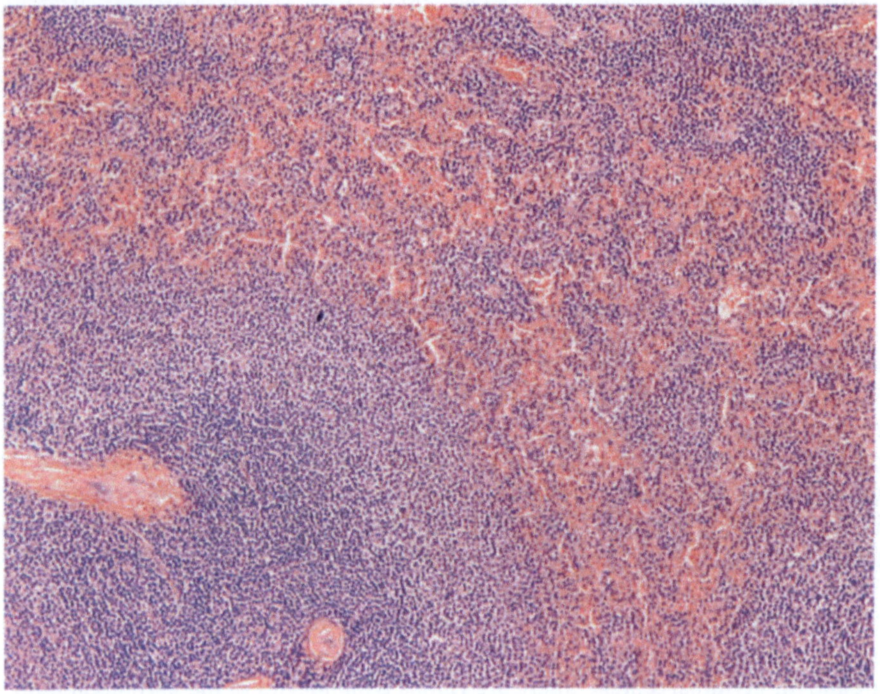

Fig. 6.64. Primary marginal zone lymphoma of the spleen. The pale marginal zone surrounds a colonized follicle. Note the infiltrate in the red pulp (H and E stain)

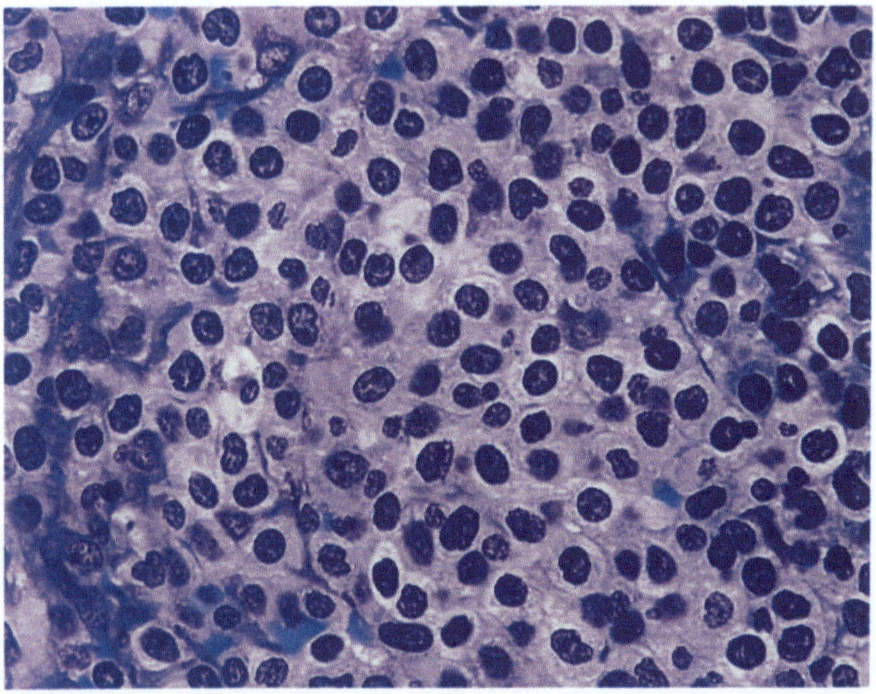

Fig. 6.65. Same patient as in Fig. 6.63. Monocytoid B-cells are seen in the marginal zone (Giemsa stain)

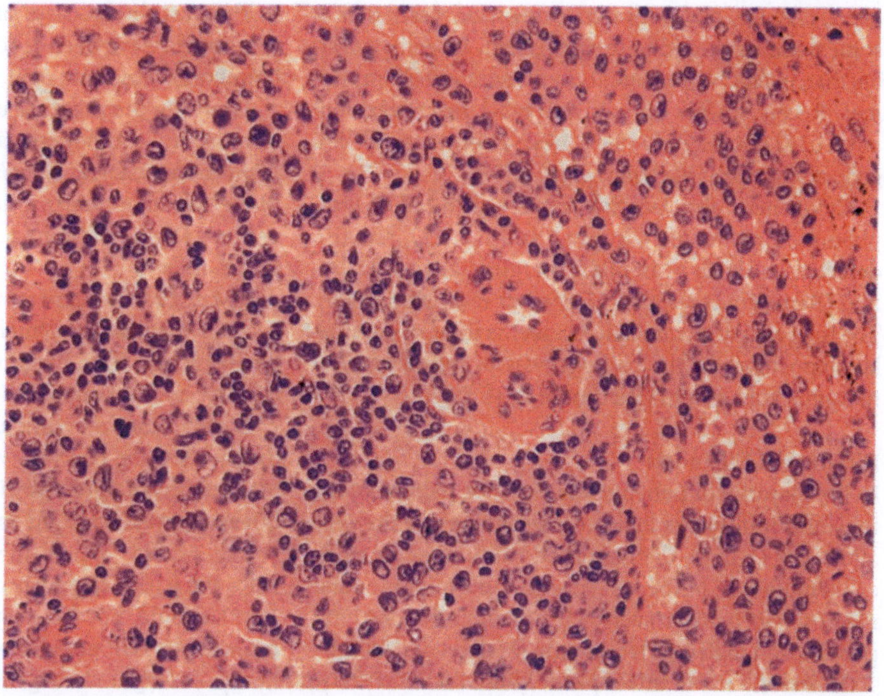

Fig. 6.66. Primary marginal zone lymphoma of the spleen transforming into a large-B-cell lymphoma. Near the centrofollicular artery; there are sheets of large cells with the morphology of centroblasts (H and E stain)

pale cytoplasm develops between the subcapsular and interfollicular sinuses and follicles. These follicles are homogeneous or present a reactive germinal center more or less infiltrated by centrocyte-like cells (Mollejo et al. 1995). The neoplastic involvement can be proven by immunohistochemistry.

Immunophenotype

The neoplastic cells, whatever the morphology is, express CD20, CD79α, CD45RA and are negative for CD5 (mostly), CD10, CD23, CD43 (Isaacson et al. 1994; Pawade et al. 1995; Wu et al. 1996; Duong et al. 2000; Thieblemont et al. 2003). There is also expression of monotypic surface IgM and sometimes IgD.

In some patients, IgD is expressed by all the neoplastic cells. In other patients, only some of the neoplastic cells are positive in the marginal zone, the follicle, and the red pulp. In two patients from our series (Duong et al. 2000), the neoplastic cells were negative, allowing recognition of the destruction of the mantle zone with persistence of only rare IgD-positive non-neoplastic mantle cells. In addition, CD21 and CD35 may be expressed by the tumor cells, as in the normal marginal zone.

The lymphoplasmacytic component has intracytoplasmic monotypic immunoglobulin, particularly IgM (Duong et al. 2000).

The neoplastic cells are bcl-2-positive, cyclin-D1-negative (Savilo et al. 1998) and express Ki-67 in less than 5% of the cells.

Immunophenotyping is very useful for the diagnosis of early spleen involvement in which the morphology is very difficult to distinguish from that of normal spleen with marginal zone hyperplasia.

Molecular Biology and Genetic Features

PCR discloses rearrangement of immunoglobulin heavy- and light-chain genes. Somatic mutations are usually present (Tierens et al. 1998). Ongoing mutations due to the presence of intraclonal variations have also been suggested (Zhu et al. 1995; Dunn-Walters et al. 1998).

In about 40% of SMZL patients there is an allelic loss of chromosome 7q31–32 (Mateo et al. 1999; Thieblemont et al. 2003). In patients with villous lymphocytosis, dysregulation of cyclin-dependent kinase 6(CDK6) gene expression has been shown to occur through chromosome 7q translocations (Corcoran et al. 1999).

There is no rearrangement of bcl-2 nor is there a t(14;18). Interpretation of reports of bcl-1 rearrangement, t(11;14), and cyclin D1 expression described in some patients should be very prudent. It seems possible that, in fact, these patients have mantle cell lymphomas. Recent studies did not find bcl-1 rearrangement or t(11;14) (Savilo et al. 1998). Rearrangements of bcl-6 gene also occur (Dierlamm et al. 1997).

Cytogenetic abnormalities observed in MALT lymphomas, for example trisomy 3 and t(11;18), are also detected in SMZL as in other marginal zone lymphomas (Remstein et al. 2000; Dierlamm et al. 1996, 2000). The long arm of chromosome 3 seems to be of particular importance in the pathogenesis of lymphomas of marginal zone origin (Dierlamm et al. 1996).

Differential Diagnosis

In the majority of patients, the biphasic pattern of the follicular infiltration and the morphology of the cells allows SMZL to be distinguished from other small-B-cell lymphomas of the spleen with multimicronodular macroscopic pattern, such as B-CLL, mantle zone lymphoma, and follicular lymphoma (Melo et al. 1987b).

However, a few of these splenic lymphomas may have or mimic a marginal zone pattern (Piris et al. 1998) which can be responsible for an incorrect diagnosis.

1. In some *mantle cell lymphomas*, the presence of remnants of reactive germinal centers surrounded by the neoplastic mantle cells form a biphasic pattern which can be misinterpreted as SMZL. Mantle cell lymphoma shows a more monotonous pattern without any blast cells. Immunophenotyping is necessary. Positivity for CD5 and cyclin D1 are decisive for mantle cell lymphoma.
2. Some *follicular lymphoma* also exhibit a biphasic pattern (inverse pattern) due to a marginal zone differentiation. The diagnosis is based on the absence of reactive germinal centers and on the morphology of centrocytes and centroblasts infiltrating the follicles. Here again, the typical immunophenotype of follicular lymphoma is useful.
3. *Splenic secondary localization of MALT lymphoma* presents a pattern that is similar to *primary splenic marginal zone lymphoma* (Du et al. 1997). But the spleen is not the initial site and/or the main organ involved. Precise clinical data are useful. The immunophenotype is more or less the same in SMZL as in MALT. The only difference is the expression in about half of the patients with SMZL of IgD, which is not expressed in MALT lymphoma.

In the past, many cases of SMZL with a plasmacytic component have been reported as lymphoplasmacytic lymphoma (Audouin et al. 1988; Duong et al. 2000).

However, the presence of a lymphoplasmacytic or a plasmacytic component can also be a source of error. *Lymphoplasmacytic lymphoma* developing primarily in the spleen homogeneously infiltrates the white pulp without a marginal zone pattern and without monocytoid B-cells.

In tumors that express CD5 and/or CD23, *lymphocytic lymphoma, lymphoplasmacytoid variant,* should be diagnosed. Such lymphomas are almost always secondary involvements of the spleen by *B-CLL.*

Finally, another difficult aspect of the differential diagnosis is the possibility of *reactive follicular hyperplasia with enlarged marginal zone.* This pattern is frequent or even constant in children, adolescents, and young adults. When the spleen weighs less than 300–400 g, the diagnosis of early PSZML (Rosso et al. 1995) should not be proposed in the absence of a monotypic cell population and of immunoglobulin heavy- and light-chain gene rearrangement (Dunphy et al. 1998).

Occurrence

Primary SMZL is a rare neoplasia, comprising about 1% of all lymphomas (Armitage and Weisenburger 2000). However the real incidence is perhaps still not well appreciated. Until the description of this entity in the late 1980s, confusion with many other small-B-cell lymphomas of the spleen was responsible for the lack of a precise definition.

Primary SMZL occurs mainly in patients older than 50 or 60 years, with a median age of 61–68 years (youngest patient: 22 years, oldest: 85 years) with an almost equal incidence in both sexes (Berger et al. 2000; Hammer et al. 1996; Duong et al. 2000).

Patients that are diagnosed with splenic lymphoma with villous lymphocytes, which seems to be the same disease, show a median age of 70 years (range 35–91).

Clinical Presentation

Patients present with a splenomegaly without hepatomegaly. Peripheral lymphadenopathies may be disclosed in about one-third of the patients. Peripheral blood cytopenia is often observed. The bone marrow is involved in the majority of patients (Duong et al. 2000). In some patients one or all of the following types of clinical and biological symptoms may be associated:

1. A peripheral blood monoclonal lymphocytosis sometimes with a villous lymphocyte morphology (Isaacson et al. 1994)
2. Autoimmune disorders, particularly autoimmune hemolytic anemia, immune thrombocytopenia (Murakami et al. 1997; Duong et al. 2000)
3. Coagulation abnormalities (Tefferi et al. 1997)
4. A serum monoclonal component (mainly IgM of variable quantity) up to 27% and sometimes more than 5 g/l, compatible with the diagnosis of Waldenström's macroglobulinemia (Duong et al. 2000; Parry-Jones et al. 2003)

The three last symptoms are always associated with the presence of a monotypic plasma cell population in the spleen (Duong et al. 2000).

In patients presenting with splenic lymphoma with villous lymphocytes, a monoclonal gammopathy (M band) was found in 28% of patients (Troussard et al. 1996).

Bone marrow involvement is not a sign of a poor prognosis (Berger et al. 2000). Splenectomy may be followed by a long indolent course (Audouin et al. 1988; Schmid et al. 1992; Duong et al. 2000).

Monochemotherapy can prolong patient survival but the response is mostly poor. Polychemotherapy seems to be a more effective treatment (Duong et al. 2000). Berger et al. (2000) showed that their series of 59 patients had a median time to progression longer than 5 years even in the absence of treatment or of complete response to therapy. A few patients died after transformation of their lymphomas into large-B-cell malignant lymphoma (Mulligan et al. 1991; Duong et al. 2000). Such transformation occurs in the spleen, in peripheral lymph nodes or in bone marrow. The median time to transformation was 4.5 years after the primary diagnosis (Berger et al. 2000).

6.10.1.3 Primary Splenic Lymphoplasmacytic Lymphoma

Synonyms

- Kiel: Immunocytoma, lymphoplasmacytic type/ splenic immunocytoma
- REAL: Lymphoplasmacytoid lymphoma
- WHO: Lymphoplasmacytic lymphoma

Definition

A lymphoma occurring primarily in the spleen and presenting a lymphoplasmacytic differentiation with secretion of a monotypic immunoglobulin, often associated with a serum monoclonal M component and/or cryoglobulinemia and sometimes with all the clinical and biological criteria of a Waldenström's macroglobulinemia.

The postulated normal cell counterpart is, as for nodal lymphoplasmacytic lymphoma, a splenic peripheral B-cell transforming to a plasma cell (see Chap. 4.2.1.2).

Morphology

Macroscopy. The spleen is huge, weighing more than 500 g and often up to 1000 or 2000 g. The cut surface of the parenchyma shows a multimicronodular pattern. In rare cases, the parenchyma is homogeneous and dark-red due to a diffuse infiltrate predominately in the red pulp (Audouin et al. 1988). Lymphadenopathies can be observed in the hilum.

Histopathology. The nodules represent remnants of the follicles of the white pulp which are diffusely infiltrated by a mixture of small lymphocytes, lymphoplasmacytoid cells, and mature plasma cells. A variable number of cells have PAS-positive intranuclear vacuoles (Dutcher-Fahey inclusions). Large B-cells with the morphology of immunoblasts may be recognized but these account for less than 20% of the cells. In tumors in which immunoblasts are more numerous, particularly when they begin to organize in small clusters, and in which there are associated plasmablasts or giant cells, transformation into a large-B-cell lymphoma of immunoblastic type has to be suspected. The follicles are homogeneous without active germinal centers or remnants, but sometimes with a regressive pattern without centrocytes or centroblasts and an onion-bulb-like structure. Infiltrated follicles do not compress the red pulp.

Cords of the red pulp are infiltrated diffusely by the same cell population. The sinuses are empty with only a small lumen. The architecture is preserved even in the presence of more massive infiltrates. Nests of epithelioid cells can be observed at the periphery of the infiltrated follicles. A variable number of mast cells and hemosiderin-laden histiocytes are dispersed throughout the infiltrates. There are no proliferation centers, no marginal zone, no centroblastic centrocytic population, and no monocytoid B-cells. The same macroscopic and histopathological presentation in the spleen has been described in Waldenström's macroglobulinemia.

In two cases of chronic cold agglutinin disease that we studied, the macronodules were follicles enlarged by the accumulation and proliferation of the same type of cell population as in other lymphoplasmacytic lymphoma, but with a large number of large-B-cells organized in sheets, reflecting a transformation into a large-B-cell lymphoma (Diebold et al. 1978).

Cytology. Imprints show a mixture of lymphocytes, lymphoplasmacytoid cells with the same type of nucleus as lymphocytes but with eccentric, more abundant basophilic cytoplasm and mature plasma cells. Large cells with the morphology of immunoblasts may be present but at less than 20%.

Immunohistochemistry

The cells exhibit the same immunophenotype as observed in nodal lymphoplasmacytic lymphoma (see Chap. 4.2.1.2).

MUM1/IRF4 (see Chap. 7.1) has been demonstrated by a new monoclonal antibody (MUM1p) in these lymphoplasmacytic lymphomas, which could be an argument in favor of their germinal center origin (Falini et al. 2000).

Differential Diagnosis

Lymphoplasmacytic lymphoma has to be distinguished essentially from a primary or secondary splenic localization of other small-B-cell lymphomas presenting with plasmacytoid differentiation and intracytoplasmic monotypic immunoglobulins.

Macroscopically, all of these lymphomas essentially demonstrate a multimicronodular pattern due to infiltration of the follicles of the splenic white pulp.

The differential diagnosis is based on the morphology of the cells, the infiltration pattern and the immunophenotype.

1. In *B-CLL, lymphoplasmacytoid variant*, the cells are small lymphocytes with some lymphoplasmacytoid cells including polytypic mature plasma cells. Proliferation centers can be recognized. A periarteriolar accumulation of lymphocytes in the red pulp is observed. The neoplastic cells express CD5, IgD, and CD23. These are all characteristics of a secondary splenic involvement of B-CLL.
2. *Splenic marginal zone lymphoma, either primary or secondary*, is defined by the presence of a marginal zone pattern, with monocytoid B-cells and colonization of follicles with some germinal centers remnants. The presence of a plasma cell population (Duong et al. 2000) has previously led to confusion with lymphoplasmacytic lymphoma (Audouin et al. 1988).
3. *Follicular lymphoma* may present with plasmacytic differentiation. However, the center of the nodules consists of a homogeneous population of centrocytes with a variable number of centroblasts. These cells are strongly CD10- and bcl-2-positive. Sometimes, the plasmacytic differentiation results in a signet-ring cell morphology (see Chap. 4.2.1.6), which has not been described in lymphoplasmacytic lymphoma. A rearrangement of the bcl-2 gene compatible with a t(14;18) can be disclosed by PCR.
4. *Mantle cell lymphoma* is characterized by cells with a different morphology and immunophenotype. Plasmacytoid differentiation with intracytoplasmic monotypic immunoglobulin is very rare; such cases may be difficult to distinguish from lymphoplasmacytic lymphoma. The expression of CD5, IgD and cyclin-D1, and the absence of typical plasmacytic differentiation allowed the two types of lymphomas to be distinguished from each other.

In rare cases featuring diffuse massive infiltration of all the splenic parenchyma, the diagnosis of *hairy cell leukemia* can be easily made based on the histology.

In *splenic plasmacytomas*, the monotypic plasma cells clearly predominate without a marked lymphocytic component.

Finally, if there are sheets of large-B-cells, a background of lymphoplasmacytoid and plasma cells should be present in order to propose the diagnosis of *large-B-cell lymphoma* (often immunoblastic type with plasma cell differentiation) secondary to lymphoplasmacytic lymphoma.

Occurrence

Primary splenic lymphoplasmacytic lymphoma occurs mostly in adults over 50 years of age, without any sex predominance. An association with hepatitis C virus infection has been stressed (Ascoli et al. 1998) (see Chap. 4.2.1.2).

Clinical Presentation

Splenomegaly with clinical symptoms due to the huge spleen is described. At presentation, peripheral lymphadenopathy is rarely present but may appear during relapses after splenectomy. Liver and bone marrow biopsies disclose microscopic involvement in almost all patients (Audouin et al. 1988).

The course is indolent but this lymphoma is not considered to be curable. Splenectomy has been followed by long-term remission even if in the majority of patients the liver and bone marrow are involved at presentation.

Monochemotherapy or polychemotherapy used in small-B-cell lymphomas may also induce long-term remission in patients with primary splenic lymphoplasmacytic lymphoma (Audouin et al. 1988).

In some patients, transformation of primary splenic lymphoplasmacytic lymphoma into a large-B-cell lymphoma in another site can be responsible for a rapid and fatal evolution.

6.10.1.4 Plasmacytoma

This is a lymphoma arising primarily in the spleen and characterized by the proliferation of mature plasma cells, sometimes associated with large-B-cells and proplasma cells, and representing less than 20 % of the neoplastic population.

Plasmacytomas seem to be extremely rare (Bjorn-Hansen 1973; Stavem et al. 1970) and are a still matter of discussion (van Krieken 1990; report of two cases). It has not been conclusively demonstrated that these tumors are neither *lymphoplasmacytic* nor *marginal zone lymphoma with predominance of the plasma cell component*. The diagnosis of primary plasmacytoma of the spleen can only be accepted when no multiple myeloma is disclosed.

Three macroscopic types of plasmacytoma have been described:

- A diffuse homogeneous type corresponding to a massive diffuse infiltrate
- A polycyclic solitary mass (van Krieken et al. 1989)
- A multimicronodular pattern (van Krieken et al. 1989)

Sheets of plasma cells infiltrate either the follicles, creating small nodules, or more or less replace the normal cells of the cords of the red pulp, resulting in a diffuse pattern without remnants of the white pulp.

On imprints, typical mature plasma cells, sometimes with two or three nuclei, are recognized. A few larger cells with the morphology of proplasma cells and plasmablasts or immunoblasts may be associated. Plasma cells are CD79α-, CD38- and CD138-positive but always CD20-negative. Immunoglobulin secretion with a light-chain restriction pattern is easily demonstrated. The most frequent heavy-chains are IgG and IgA.

The differential diagnosis includes more or less the same entities showing a plasma cell differentiation that have been discussed for lymphoplasmacytic lymphoma (see Chap. 4.2.1.2). Finally, two important points have to be mentioned:

1. A secondary manifestation of multiple myeloma or of primary plasmacytoma of the digestive tract has to be excluded.
2. Lymphoplasmacytic lymphoma and MZBCL with a predominant plasmacytic component also have to be excluded.

Patients complain of symptoms due to the splenomegaly. Various cytopenias can be observed (Bjorn-Hansen 1973). A monoclonal serum component is not always present.

6.10.1.5 B-Prolymphocytic Leukemia

Synonyms

- Kiel, REAL, WHO: B-prolymphocytic leukemia

The B-prolymphocytic leukemia is defined as a proliferation of medium-sized cells responsible for a leukemia with splenomegaly). The normal cell counterpart is a peripheral B-lymphocyte.

The size of the spleen is increased. The parenchyma shows either a multimicronodular or a homogeneous infiltration pattern. The medium-sized cells have round nuclei, open chromatin, and a prominent central nucleolus, with a weakly basophilic cytoplasm that is more abundant than in B-CLL.

These cells infiltrate the white pulp causing a multimicronodular pattern. In addition, they accumulate in the cords with a variable number of cells present in the sinus of the red pulp.

Sometimes, the infiltrate predominates in the red pulp, obscuring the normal architecture of the spleen, with a massive diffuse involvement.

B-prolymphocytes express B-cell markers mostly CD20, and strongly monotypic surface immunoglobulin. They are often negative for CD5, and usually for CD23.

B-prolymphocytic leukemia involving the spleen should not be confused with *B-CLL* featuring *large proliferation centers or transforming* into *so-called B-prolymphocytic variant.* In the latter variant, the distinction can only be made by clinical history. Another disease to be included in the differential diagnosis is *B-lymphoblastic lymphoma/acute B-cell leukemia.* The morphology of the lymphoblasts and their immunophenotype is completely different (see Chap. 4.1).

Demonstration of a B-cell phenotype eliminates the diagnosis of T-prolymphocytic leukemia.

Patients present with a splenomegaly but without adenopathies. Often the presence of a leukemia leads to discovery of the splenomegaly. In the majority of patients, the diagnosis is based on peripheral blood studies. The spleen is rarely removed, so pathologists only rarely have the opportunity to study it.

6.10.1.6
Large B-Cell Lymphoma of the Spleen

Any of the morphological variants of DLBCL (see Chap. 4.2.2) may develop primarily in the spleen (Diebold 1989; Harris et al. 1984).

These large-B-cell lymphomas always present as large, whitish polycyclic masses measuring more than 5 cm, and up to 10–20 cm, in diameter (Fig. 6.59). They compress the adjacent splenic parenchyma. The surface of the spleen is irregular due to protrusion of the tumors. The center of the more voluminous masses can be necrotic. Hemorrhages may present as black or dark red areas. The periphery of the tumor is often underlined by a brownish zone due to accumulation of hemosiderin-loaden macrophages. Adenopathies are often disclosed in the hilum.

The tumor masses consist of sheets of large cells replacing and destroying both the white and the red pulp (Fig. 6.67). Fibrosis is often associated.

The tumor cells exhibit the typical morphology of polymorphic, monomorphic, or multilobate centroblasts or of immunoblasts with or without plasmablastic differentiation (Fig. 6.68). Rarely, the appearance is that of a T-cell/histiocyte-rich B-cell lymphoma or of an intravascular large-B-cell lymphoma (see Chap. 4.2.2.2, 6.18).

There are individual description in which primary DLBCLs of the spleen are described in association with hepatitis C virus infection (Satoh et al. 1997).

The most important consideration in the differential diagnosis is massive spleen metastasis of different types of carcinomas and of malignant melanoma.

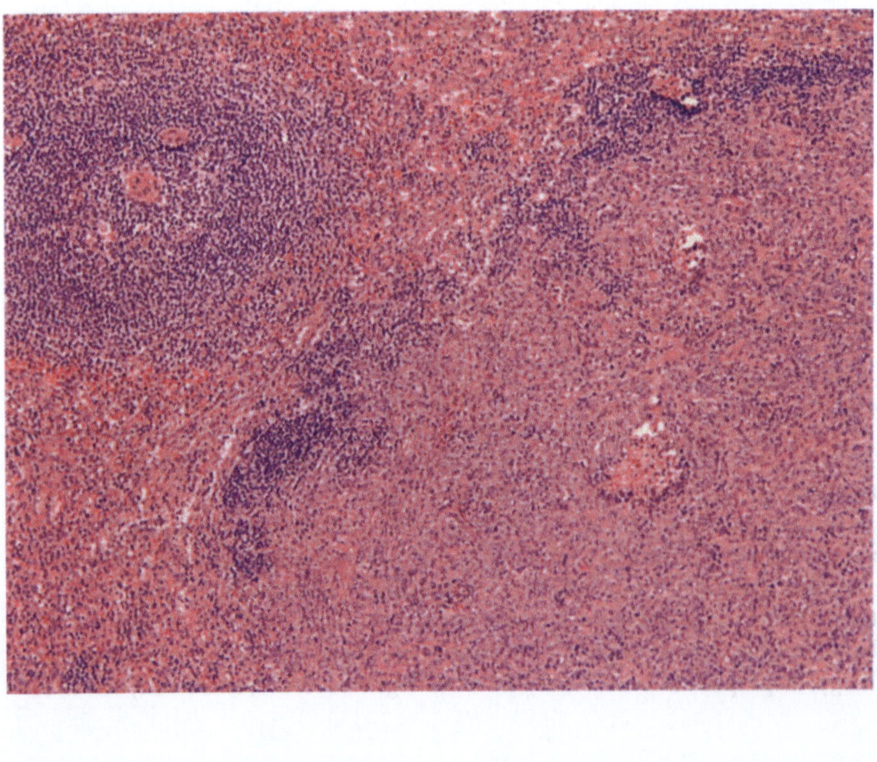

Fig. 6.67. Primary large-B-cell lymphoma (polymorphic centroblastic type). A voluminous mass has destroyed the splenic parenchyma (*right*). Note the persistence of white pulp at the periphery and a normal follicle (*upper left corner*) (H and E stain)

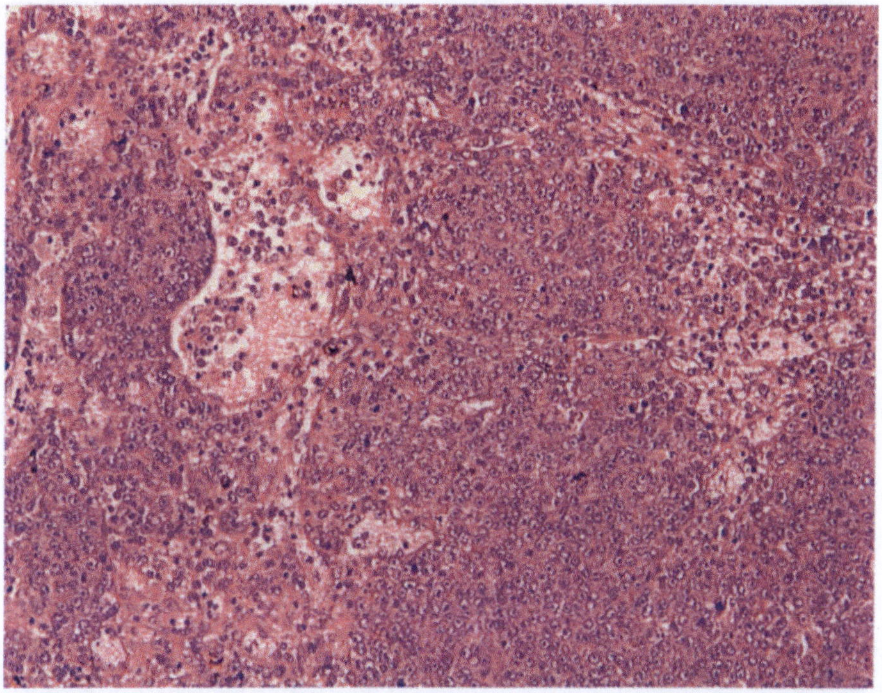

Fig. 6.68. Primary large-B-cell lymphoma of immunoblastic type. There is extension from the white pulp to the cords of the red pulp (H and E stain)

6.10.1.7 Hepatosplenic T-Cell Lymphoma* (ICD-O: 9716/3)

This rare lymphoma (HSTCL) entity has peculiar clinical, morphological, and phenotypic features (Farcet et al. 1990; Wong et al. 1995; Cooke et al. 1996). It occurs mainly in young adults, who present with splenomegaly and hepatomegaly, but without lymphadenopathy. Today, this clinical picture represents a well defined clinicopathological entity. Primarily such lymphomas have been described to be of γδ-T-cell origin. However, very recently, rare similar tumors with an αβ-phenotype have been described. Another characteristic feature is the non-activated cytotoxic profile (TIA-1+, perforin–, granzyme B–) of the γδ-neoplastic cells (Cooke et al. 1996; Boulland et al. 1997). Cytogenetic analysis of several HSTCLs reported a frequent association with isochromosome 7q (Colwill et al. 1990; Wang et al. 1995; Alonsozana et al. 1997). Some of these lymphomas are found in patients with immune defects, especially following organ transplantation (Ross et al. 1994; Khan et al. 2001). The disease has a highly aggressive course despite the use of an intensive chemotherapy regimen.

* This chapter has been written by Prof. Philippe Gaulard, Paris

Synonyms

- Kiel: Not listed
- Real: Hepatosplenic γδ-T-cell lymphoma (provisional entity)
- WHO: Hepatosplenic T-cell lymphoma

Definition

A neoplastic proliferation usually consisting of monomorphic medium-sized T-cells expressing in most instances the γδ-T-cell receptor and disclosing a peculiar pattern of infiltration within the splenic red pulp, the sinusoids of the liver- and the sinuses of the bone marrow. This is a rare lymphoma with an hepatosplenic clinical presentation without adenopathy and an aggressive clinical course. It is associated with a recurrent cytogenetic abnormality, the isochromosome 7q.

Morphology

Macroscopy. The *spleen* is enlarged (commonly weighting 1,000–3,500 g) with a homogeneous pattern without nodules. The cut surface is homogeneous red-purple. Hilar lymph nodes are not enlarged.

Histology. There is marked reduction or complete loss of the white pulp whereas the red pulp is hyperplastic

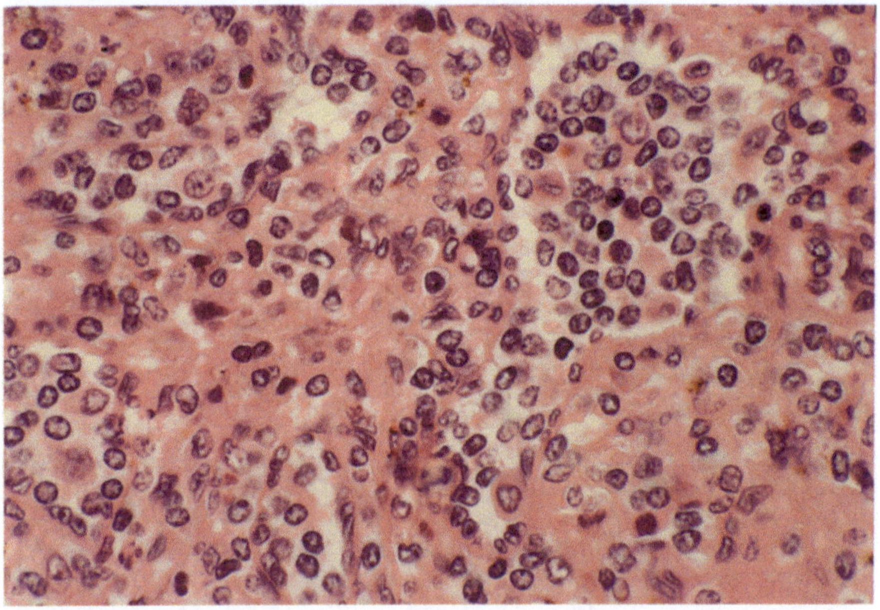

Fig. 6.69. Hepatosplenic T-cell lymphoma infiltrating the spleen. The neoplastic monomorphic medium-sized cells infiltrate the sinuses and the cords of the red pulp (H and E stain)

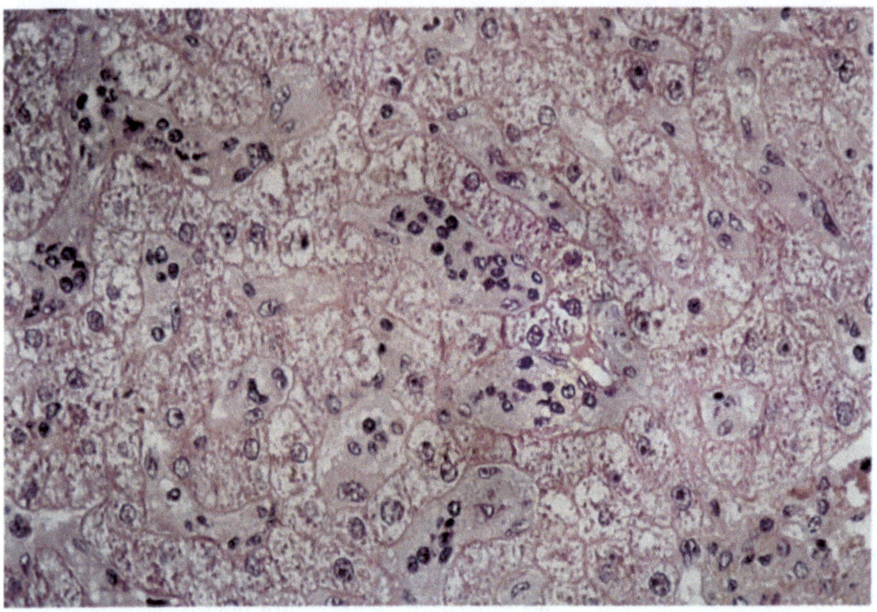

Fig. 6.70. Hepatosplenic T-cell lymphoma. A liver section shows infiltration of the sinusoids by atypical lymphoid cells (H and E stain)

(Fig. 6.69) . The latter contains a more or less sparse or dense infiltration frequently consisting of monomorphic medium-sized lymphoid cells, with round/oval or slightly irregular nuclei showing slightly dispersed chromatin and inconspicuous nucleoli. The cytoplasm is pale and azurophilic granules are not often seen on smears or imprints. These atypical cells are present within the cords and, to a variable extent, the sinuses of the red pulp (Fig. 6.69). In some/many instances, dilated sinuses filled by sheets of neoplastic cells can be observed. A few small lymphocytes are scattered throughout the tumor and plasma cells are rare. Histiocytes with hemophagocytic features may be admixed.

Hilar lymph nodes, although usually not significantly enlarged, commonly show some involvement which is confined to sinuses or perisinusal areas (Charton-Bain et al. 2000a).

Hepatomegaly without nodules is very common. Histologically, involvement of the *liver* is quite constant. It always consists of a sinusoidal pattern that may resemble "pseudopeliotic lesions" (Gaulard et al. 1986) (Fig. 6.70). In addition, a portal and periportal lymphomatous infiltrate may be observed.

Bone marrow involvement is a consistent finding and a very useful diagnostic feature, although it may be difficult to recognize and often requires immunohistochemistry for its demonstration. Indeed, the initial diagnostic bone marrow biopsy specimens are usually hypercellular, and may be first misdiagnosed as myelodysplastic or myeloproliferative syndrome – with a subtle, or *predominately sinusal infiltrate* of atypical small to medium-sized lymphoid cells (Gaulard et al. 1991; Vega et al. 2001) (Fig. 6.71). Aspirate smears may be helpful to recognize this slight marrow infiltration, which is composed of cells that may resemble blasts on smears, some with fine cytoplasmic granules.

Cytological variants, i.e. a large-cell or blastic appearance, have been described either during the course of the disease or observed at diagnosis (Farcet et al. 1990; Mastovich et al. 1994; François et al. 1997). The variants have the same tissue distribution as classical HSTCL. With progression, at a late disease stage, the pattern of bone marrow involvement has a tendency to become more intense, diffuse, and interstitial, and not only sinusal, whereas the neoplastic cells become larger.

Immunohistochemistry

On paraffin sections, all HSTCLs feature a CD3+ T-cell phenotype (Fig. 6.72). The general pattern of expression of T-cell antigens is CD3+, CD2+, CD5–, CD7+/– and CD4–/CD8– or more rarely CD4–/CD8+. Most tumors are CD56+. Virtually all HSTCLs have a non-activated cytotoxic phenotype (TIA-1+, granzyme B–/perforin–). On frozen sections, most tumor cells express the γδ-T-cell receptor and the γδ-(βF1–/TCRδ-1+)-T-cell phenotype has been part of the definition of the entity, initially named *hepatosplenic γδ-T-cell lymphoma*. Most tumors, but not all, seem to derive from the subset of γδ-T cells with the Vδ1 phenotype (Gaulard et al. 1990; Przybylski et al. 2000). Recently, HSTCLs with an αβ-T-cell receptor phenotype (βF1+/TCRδ-1–) but with the same clinicopathological and cytogenetic features have been reported (Lai et al. 2000; Suarez et al. 2000; Macon et al. 2001).

Genetics

Molecular Studies. Whatever their γδ- or αβ-phenotype, HSTCLs show a clonal rearrangement of the TCRγ gene. Most tumors have the genotype of γδ-T cells and disclose a biallelic rearrangement of the δ-

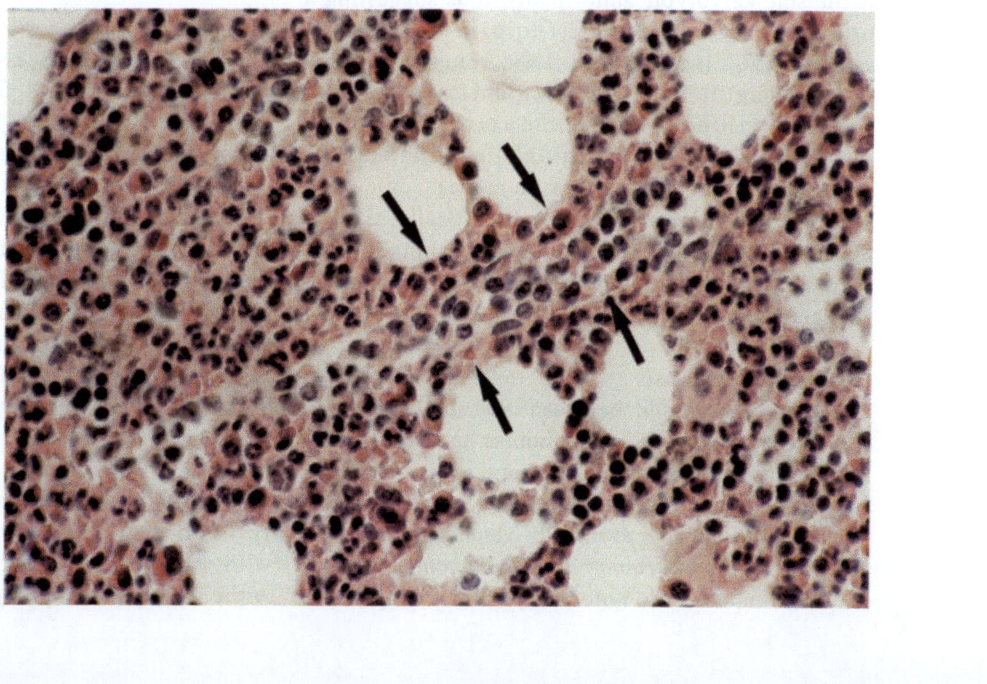

Fig. 6.71. Hepatosplenic T-cell lymphoma. H and E staining of a section from a bone marrow biopsy demonstrates the presence of a moderate infiltration consisting of small to medium-sized cells located within the sinuses

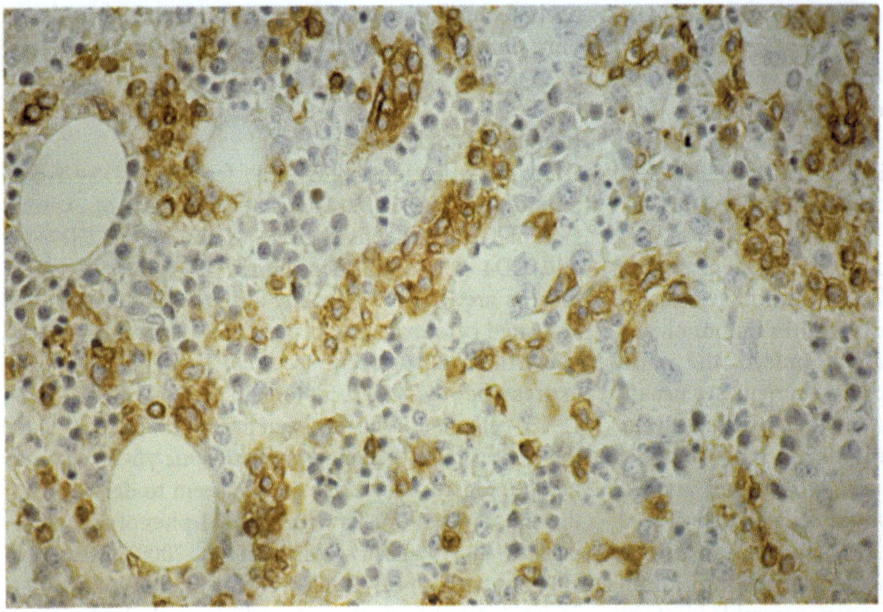

Fig. 6.72. Hepatosplenic T-cell lymphoma. CD3 staining of a bone marrow section highlights the sinusal infiltration of the bone marrow by neoplastic T-cells (immunohistochemistry, peroxidase)

chain (Kanavaros et al. 1991). Unproductive rearrangements of the β-chain have been reported in some cases of HSTCL. Most tumors with an αβ-phenotype disclose clonal rearrangements of the γ- and β-chains.

Cytogenetics. As revealed by conventional cytogenetics and by FISH, most tumors are characterized by the presence of an isochromosome 7q, which occasionally is the sole karyotypic abnormality, thus suggesting a primary and possible role of i(7)(q10) in the pathogenesis of HSTCL (Colwill et al. 1990; Wang et al. 1995; Alonsozana et al. 1997). Trisomy 8 and loss of chromosome Y seem to be associated with a progression of this disorder. Interestingly, i(7)(q10) is found in HSTCLs with a γδ-phenotype as well as in at least some cases with an αβ-phenotype (Suarez et al. 2000; Lai et al. 2000; Macon et al. 2001), thus providing another argument that both HSγδ- and HSαβ-TCL are variants of the same entity.

Differential Diagnosis

The diagnosis should be essentially discussed with respect to other T-cell lymphomas that commonly manifest as hepatosplenic disease and show an infiltration of the splenic red pulp: *T-cell large granular lymphocytic leukemia, aggressive NK-lymphoma/leukemia,* and some types of *primary T-cell lymphoma, unspecified.* It is important to note that γδ-T-cell lymphomas may arise initially in other organs, such as the skin, nasopharyngeal region, and intestine – thus belonging to other disease entities – and secondarily involve the spleen and/or liver (Arnulf et al. 1998).

Due to the distribution pattern in the splenic red pulp, only *hairy cell leukemia*, among the B-NHLs, and acute lymphoid or myeloid leukemias have to be discussed .

Occurrence

The disease represents less than 5% of all peripheral T-cell lymphomas and is characterized by a male predominance (sex ratio, 2:1) and its occurrence in young adults (median age 34 years). HSTCL occurring in adolescents has been reported (Lai et al. 2000).

A number of cases have been reported in patients with immune defect manifestations or with a previous history of an immune defect, especially in patients receiving long-term immunosuppressive therapy for solid organ transplantation (Ross et al. 1994; François et al. 1997; Reyes et al. 1997; Khan et al. 2001).

As of yet, no consistent viral association has been reported.

Clinical Presentation, Evolution, and Prognosis

HSTCL occurs mainly in young adults. Patients present with splenomegaly and most often hepatomegaly, but without lymphadenopathy. Most patients have B symptoms. Thrombocytopenia is a consistent feature and is associated with anemia and/or leukopenia in more than half of the patients. A leukemic picture is rare at presentation, but more common during the course of the disease. An association with hemophagocytic syndrome is possible. The disease has a highly aggressive course. Following treatment with an intensive chemotherapy regimen, about 70% of the patients achieved complete remission, but most of them relapsed during the first 2 years. Relapses occur in initially involved sites, i.e. spleen (when splenectomy not performed at diagnosis), bone marrow, liver. and sometimes blood. Relapses in skin or mucosae may be rarely observed. Overall, the prognosis is poor, with a median survival time of 13 months according to a recent series of 20 patients (Reyes et al. 1997). Features of cytological progression to large-cell lymphoma with slight pleomorphism or with a blastic appearance is common during relapses. It can be associated with a "loss" of T-cell antigens including the TCR, thus leading to a "TCR-silent" phenotype.

6.10.1.8 T-Cell Large Granular Lymphocytic Leukemia (ICD-O: 9831/3)

Synonyms

- Kiel: Chronic T-CLL
- Real: T-cell large granular lymphocyte leukemia
- WHO: T-cell large granular lymphocytic leukemia

Definition

This disease is characterized by a slight increase in the peripheral blood of medium-sized lymphocytes showing a large pale cytoplasm containing a variable number of azurophilic (red) granules. The lymphocytosis increases over the course of months to years. Cytopenia may occur. Often, a splenomegaly develops also very slowly. This progressive evolution lasts for 10–25 years. The normal cell counterparts are αβ-CD8-positive large granular lymphocytes (LGLs) representing 10–15% of peripheral blood mononuclear cells (Loughran 1993). LGLs are now divided into two major groups according to the expression or absence of expression of CD3.

CD3-negative LGLs are NK-cells that do not express the CD3 TCR complex or rearranged TCR genes. These cells mediate *non-major histocompatibility complex (MHC)-restricted cytotoxicity. CD3-positive LGLs* are T-cells that do express the CD3/TCR complex and rearranged TCR genes. These cells mediate *non-MHC-restricted cytotoxicity in vitro and may represent in-vivo-activated cytotoxic T-lymphocytes* (Loughran 1993). *CD3- and CD8-positive αβ-T-cells* from the peripheral blood seem to represent the normal counterparts of the common types of LGL leukemia cells (Loughran 1993). The postulated normal cell for the rare leukemia cell with a γδ-TCR is represented by a subset of Tγδ-lymphocytes (Chan et al. 2001).

Morphology

Histology. In the majority of cases, the pathologist must study either the removed spleen, an iliac crest bone marrow trephine biopsy, or a liver biopsy (Agnarsson et al. 1989).

The spleen, which weighs 300–500 g, has a normal architecture. The white pulp is quite normal. The organization of the red pulp in cords and sinuses is preserved. A variable number of medium-sized lymphocytes with a clear cytoplasm infiltrate the cords and some are present in the sinuses (Fig. 6.73). A reactive plasmacytosis is frequently seen around the terminal arterioles in the cords. Azurophilic granules cannot be recognized on paraffin sections. Only immunohistochemistry allows identification of the disease.

The bone marrow shows a normal cellularity made up of cells of all three main hematopoietic cell lines and at different stages of maturation. There is an interstitial infiltrate of variable degree, sometimes with focal aggregates, and comprising medium-sized lymphocytes with a pale cytoplasm.

The architecture of the liver is preserved. Numerous lymphocytes with round nucleus and large pale cytoplasm are present in the sinusoids. A small number of the same type of lymphoid cells accumulates in the portal spaces.

Cytology. Evaluating peripheral blood or bone marrow smears as well as imprints of the spleen is the easiest way to reach a diagnosis. The typical lymphocytes have a large pale cytoplasm surrounding a round or oval nucleus with condensed chromatin present in small blocks as well as a small nucleolus. Coarse or fine intracytoplasmic granules (Fig. 6.74) are observed and appear as azurophilic (Brouet et al. 1975; McKenna et al. 1977; Semenzato et al. 1997).

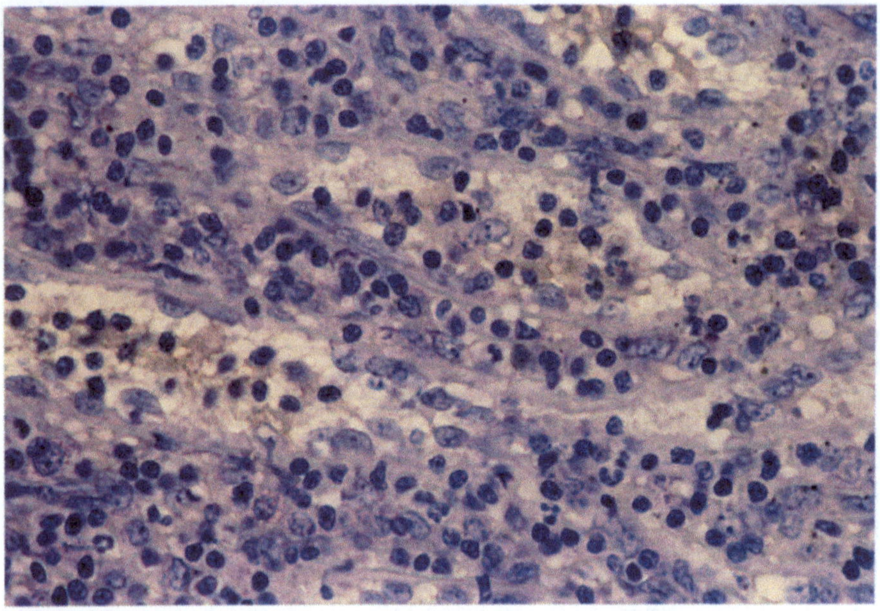

Fig. 6.73. T-LGL with large granular cells. Lymphoid cells with dark nuclei infiltrate the cords of the red pulp (Giemsa stain)

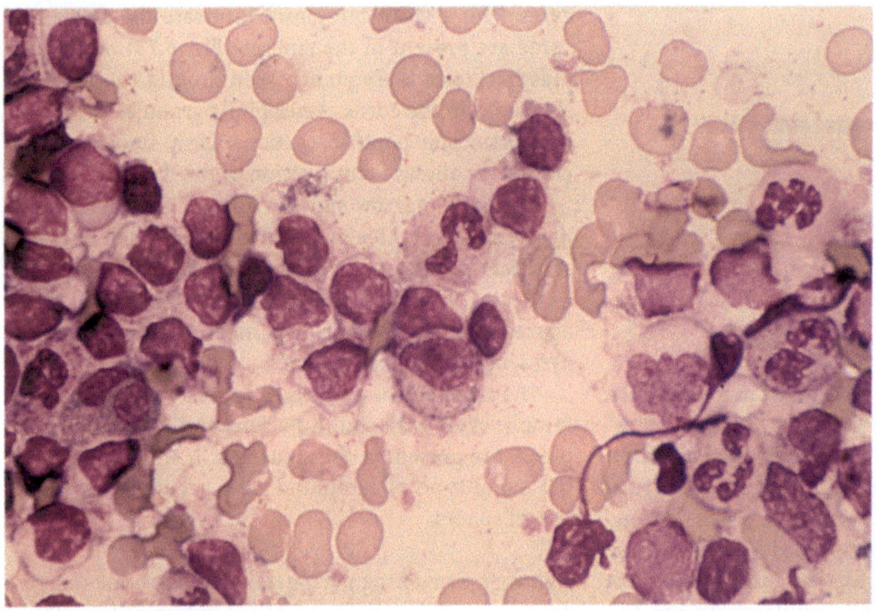

Fig. 6.74. T-LGL with large granular cells. In this imprint of the spleen, numerous lymphocytes with pale cytoplasm containing azurophilic granules are easily recognized (May-Grünwald-Giemsa stain)

Immunohistochemistry

Many tumor cells express CD3 on paraffin section (Chan et al. 1986; Pandolfi et al. 1990; Oshimi et al. 1993; Semenzato et al. 1997). The *common variant* (80% of the cases) is CD3-, CD8- and TCRαβ-positive but CD4-negative. Rare variants have been reported: CD4-positive and CD8-negative, positive for both CD4 and CD8, and CD3-positive with a γδ-TCR (Vie et al. 1989).

In addition, most T-cell large granular lymphocytic leukemias, particularly the common type, are CD57- (Lamy and Loughran 1999) and TiA-1-positive. Expression of CD11b, CD16 and CD56 is highly variable.

In other cases, the tumors are CD3- and TCRαβ-negative. These correspond to NK-cell lymphoproliferations often with CD56 positivity.

The leukemic cells also express CD95(Fas) and Fas-ligand (Chan et al. 2001).

Genetics

The TCRβ gene is rearranged in the majority of these tumors (Rambaldi et al. 1985; Loughran et al. 1988). A few have only a TCR-γ rearrangement. Chromosomal translocations have occasionally been demonstrated (Loughran et al. 1985).

Differential Diagnosis

The discussion includes the possibility of a slight reactive peripheral *blood lymphocytosis*. The discovery on smears of large azurophilic granules and the immunophenotype allow the disease to be recognized. The major differential diagnosis is that of a *reactive hyperplasia of large granular lymphocytes*, which is found in patients with rheumatoid arthritis and which is present in some viral diseases. In such cases monoclonality should be tested.

Occurrence

This type of chronic T-cell leukemia represents no more than 2–3% of all leukemias made up of small lymphocytes (Chan et al. 2001). There is no sex predominance and the median age is 55 years with a range of 4–88 years (Loughran 1993). Exceptional cases have been described in children.

Clinical Presentation

Patients present with severe neutropenia, associated or not with anemia. A peripheral blood lymphocytosis of variable intensity ($2-20\times10^9$/l) is consistently found (Chan et al. 2001). Recurrent bacterial infections may occur as a consequence of neutropenia, involving the skin, nasal sinuses and perirectal areas; more rarely pneumonia or sepsis may result (Loughran 1993). A splenomegaly is disclosed in the majority of patients. The size of the spleen remains mostly moderate. In the past, splenectomy was performed when the anemia or the cytopenia was clinically relevant. Hepatomegaly and lymphadenopathy are exceptionally observed.

Often patients have rheumatoid arthritis. They also present with biologic disorders including polyclonal hypergammaglobulinemia and circulating immune complexes (Loughran et al. 1985, 1988; Chan et al. 1986; Oshimi et al. 1993; Lamy and Loughran 1999). Recently, high levels of circulating Fas ligand have additionally been demonstrated. This is associated with a defective CD95 apoptotic pathway leading to the resistance of LGLs to Fas-induced apoptosis (Lamy and Loughran 1999). The possibility of a immun disorder with reactive but clonal lymphocytosis has been hypothesized.

In many patients, the disease has a long indolent course, whereas in others it is more aggressive (Gentile et al. 1994). One of our patients was a female who presented after 20 years of indolent disease evolution with a tumor of the small intestine that caused bleeding. The tumor consisted of medium-sized lymphocytes with azurophilic granules.

Transformation into a peripheral NK/T-cell lymphoma with large-cell predominance has been discussed. Splenectomy has been performed in patients with large spleens but had no effect on either the anemia or the cytopenia.

6.10.1.9
Other Types of Lymphoma

All other lymphomas may also present as primary splenic lymphoma but only very rarely, for example: follicular lymphoma, mantle cell lymphoma, peripheral T-cell lymphoma, unspecified (Falk et al. 1990). More frequently, they involve the spleen secondarily. These other types of lymphoma are discussed below.

6.10.2
Secondary Splenic Lymphoma

Systematic laparotomy in patients with malignant lymphoma in a nodal or extranodal site shows lymphoma involvement in 40–50% of the patients (Rosenberg et al. 1978; Strauss et al. 1983). Spleen involvement is even more frequently revealed at autopsy, which disclosed lymphoma infiltration in about 50–80% of the patients (Risdall et al. 1979; Strauss et al. 1983).

Secondary spleen involvement is often associated with a liver and/or bone marrow localization (stage IV), and worsens the prognosis

6.10.2.1
Small-B-Cell Lymphoma

B-CLL/Small Lymphocytic Lymphoma (see Chap. 4.2.1.1)

The majority of these patients present with tumors having a multimicronodular pattern. A few such tumors, often at the end of disease evolution, have a

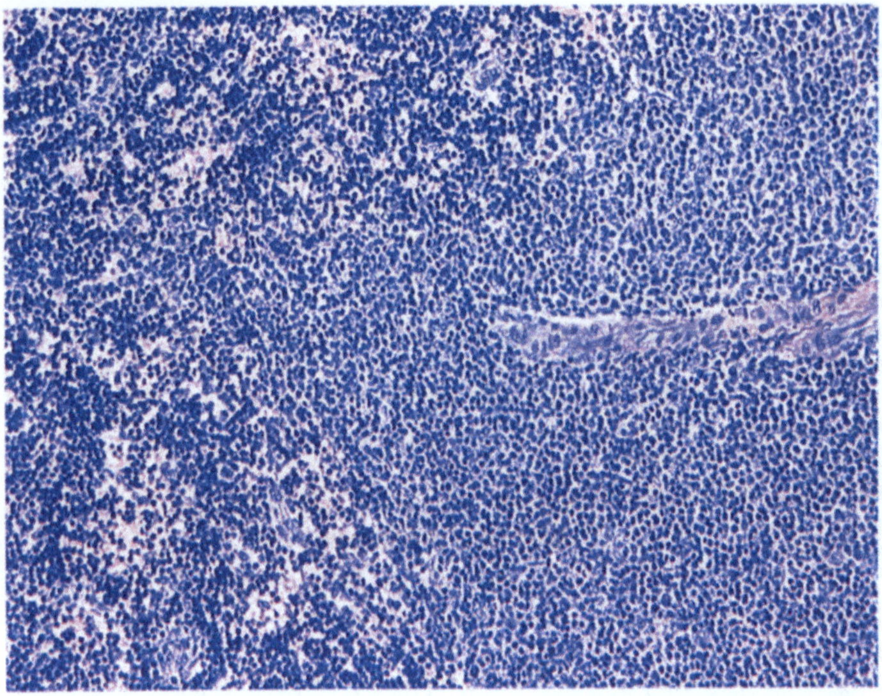

Fig. 6.75. B-CLL. Homogeneous follicle with a severe infiltrate of the red pulp, predominately in the cords (Giemsa stain)

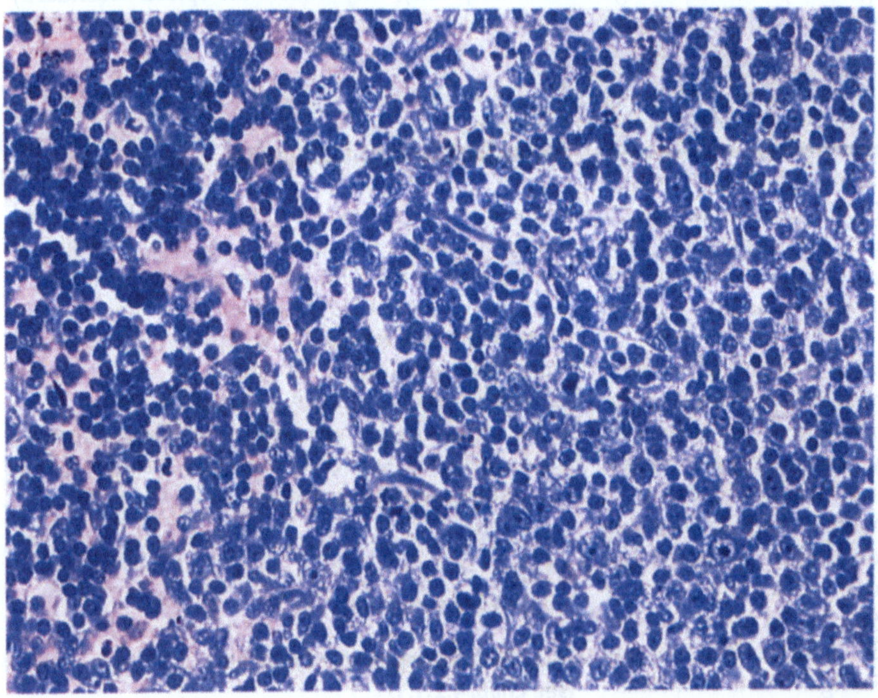

Fig. 6.76. In this B-CLL, a proliferation center, containing prolymphocytes and paraimmunoblasts (*right*), in a homogeneous infiltrated follicle are present (Giemsa stain)

diffuse splenic infiltration (Diebold 1989; Wolf and Neiman 1989).

The follicles appear homogeneous due to a diffuse accumulation of typical small-B-cells (Fig. 6.75), obscuring germinal center and mantle zone (Wolf and Neiman 1989; Diebold 1989). Some proliferative centers can be recognized but less easily than in lymph nodes. The cords of the red pulp are infiltrated either diffusely or by nodules surrounding terminal arteries (Fig. 6.76). The lumens of the sinuses contain a variable number of small lymphocytes with a round nucleus and dense chromatin. In a few cases, the red pulp is so massively and diffusely infiltrated that it is difficult to recognize remnants of red and white pulp. In such cases, proliferative centers are more easily seen, appearing as round pale areas.

A splenomegaly may be disclosed during the evolution of a B-CLL, corresponding to a progressive extension of the disease with a more (Rai et al. 1975) aggressive stage (Binet et al. 1977, 1981; Wolf and Neiman 1989).

A splenomegalic variant of B-CLL, often with a mild or absent peripheral blood lymphocytosis, and presenting a more favorable prognosis (Binet et al. 1977; Dighiero et al. 1979) has been described. This variant with massive splenomegaly probably represents less than 10–15% of the cases (Wolf and Neiman 1989).

Marked splenomegaly associated with severe anemia or thrombocytopenia is a poor prognostic sign (Binet et al. 1977; Rai et al. 1975).

Variants

Richter's syndrome (Diebold 1989) can be recognized by the presence of a variable number of nodules measuring more than 1 cm in diameter and consisting of large-B-cells, often paraimmunoblasts and plasmablasts. *"Prolymphocytoid" transformation* (Enno et al. 1979; Arber et al. 1997) may occur in the spleen and is morphologically identical to the entity described as nodal lymphoma.

Follicular Lymphoma

A multimicronodular pattern is the most frequent presentation. In addition, confluence of the nodules results in the formation of larger nodules, sometimes causing polycyclic masses. This reflects transformation into large-B-cell lymphoma (Diebold et al. 1987).

The follicles are increased in size and homogeneous

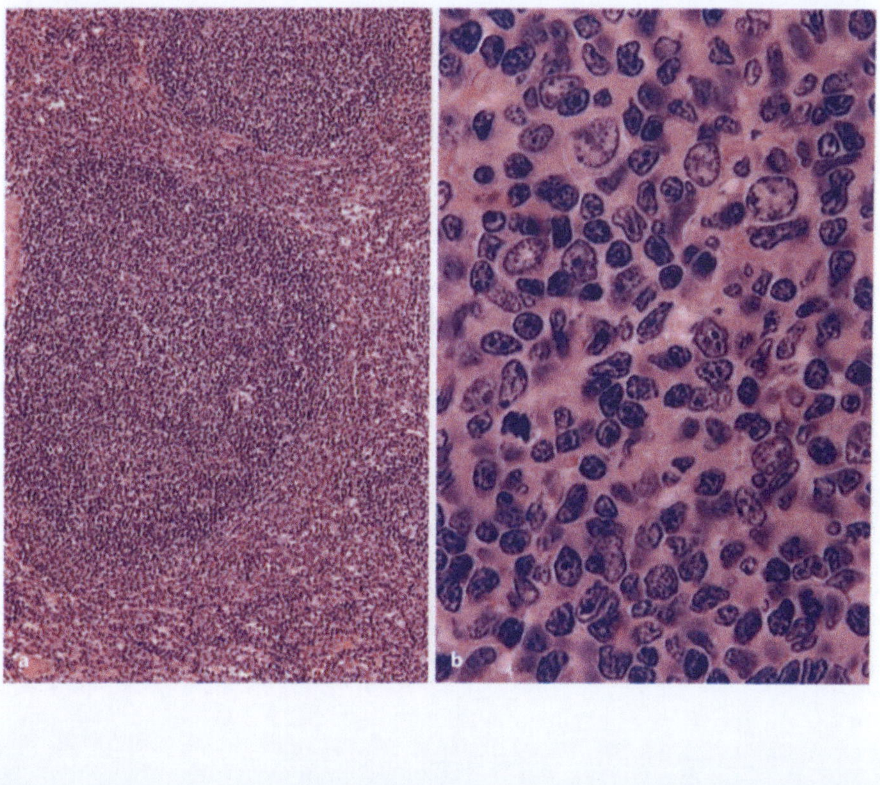

Fig. 6.77 a, b. Follicular lymphoma. **a** The neoplastic follicle are homogeneous and increased in size (H and E stain). **b** The cell population consists of centrocytes and a few centroblasts (H and E stain)

(Fig. 6.77a) due to infiltration by a mixture of typical centrocytes (small/medium-sized cells with cleaved nuclei) (Fig. 6.77b) and a variable number of centroblasts. Reactive germinal centers are absent. The tumors should be graded according to the score proposed by the WHO classification (see Chap. 4.2.1.6). Sometimes a marginal zone differentiation may be seen making the differentiation from a primary SMZL difficult (Alkan et al. 1996) (see Chap. 4.2.1.6). The red pulp is compressed by the expanding neoplastic follicles. Small tumorous nodules develop around arteries in the cords.

Splenomegaly may be disclosed either at presentation, associated with peripheral adenopathies corresponding to clinical stage II or III, or during relapse, reflecting dissemination of the disease. Transformation into large-B-cell lymphoma is mostly observed in this condition.

Rarely, patients present with a predominant splenic involvement (primary splenic follicular lymphoma).

Mantle Cell Lymphoma

The spleen is huge, weighing 700 – 2.000 g with a mean weight of 1,491 g (Arber et al. 1997). The parenchyma has a multimicronodular pattern with numerous small whitish nodules dispersed throughout the spleen. The presence of one or more nodules larger than 1 cm in diameter represents transformation into a more aggressive type of lymphoma. This was observed in three patients out of a personal series of eight (Molina et al. 2000). Spontaneous rupture of the spleen has been reported in patients with blastoid variant (Oinonen et al. 1997). Hilar adenopathies are frequently observed.

The nodules correspond to homogeneous follicles (Fig. 6.78a) due to the proliferation of small to medium-sized cells with either irregular cleaved nuclei or roundish nuclei resembling B-CLL (Fig. 6.78b). The chromatin is clumped and the nucleoli inconspicuous.

Three patterns can be recognized:

1. A huge mantle zone surrounding a reactive germinal center
2. A huge mantle zone with small remnants of germinal center obscured and colonized by mantle cells
3. Homogeneous follicles completely infiltrated by neoplastic lymphoid cells

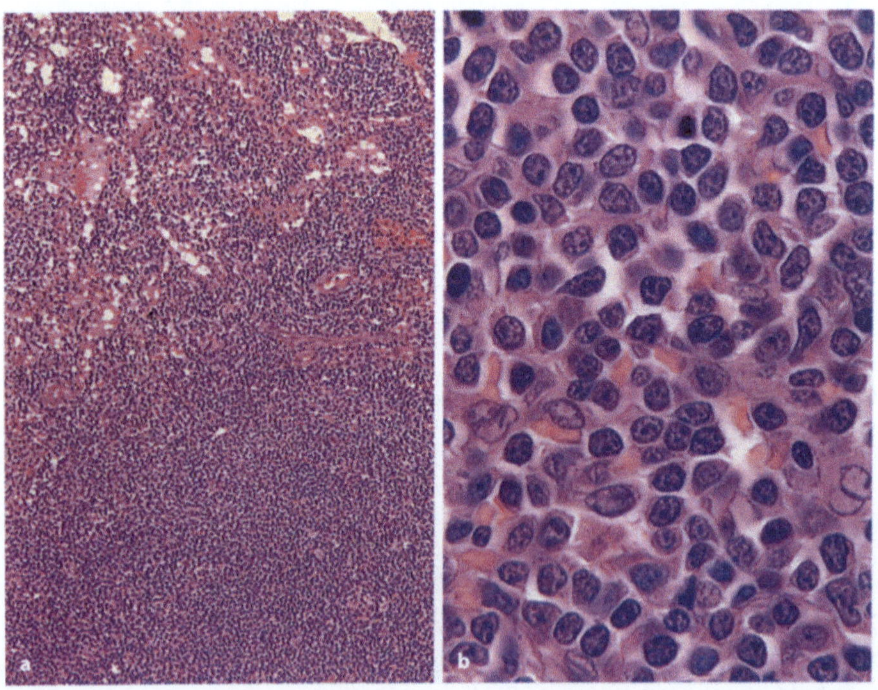

Fig. 6.78 a, b. Mantle cell lymphoma. **a** Homogeneous follicles with infiltration of the cords (H and E stain). **b** Mixture of small lymphoid cells with round or irregular nuclei. Note the presence of two activated histiocytes without tingible bodies (H and E stain)

The red pulp, mostly the cords, is always infiltrated by the same neoplastic lymphoid population. In the diffuse areas, there are no proliferative centers, which is a good argument against B-CLL. Dispersed large activated histiocytes with abundant pale cytoplasm without tingible bodies and large clear ovoid nuclei are seen.

In tumors with larger nodules, cells with a blastic morphology, or even large-B-cells with a centroblastic morphology, infiltrate the follicles and the red pulp reflecting transformation into a more aggressive lymphoma (Molina et al. 2000).

Mantle cell lymphoma can mimic *B-CLL* when the majority of the neoplastic cells have a round nucleus and when the follicles are diffusely infiltrated. The absence of proliferative centers, and the immunophenotype () help in making the distinction. The diagnosis of *B-CLL* is particularly difficult in lymphomas with a leukemic phase. Expression of cyclin D1 is of great importance (Molina et al. 2000).

Follicular lymphoma may be difficult to distinguish when the neoplastic mantle cells exhibit a centrocyte-like morphology. The absence of centroblasts, and the immunophenotype are mandatory for the diagnosis.

The distinction from *primary splenic marginal zone lymphoma* may be difficult in some cases due to a possible marginal zone pattern occurring in mantle cell lymphoma. Again, an immunophenotype showing negativity for CD5, CD43, and cyclin D1 plays a decisive role.

Finally, the blastic variant of mantle cell lymphoma may be difficult to differentiate from *lymphoblastic lymphoma* or *acute leukemia* or from *large-B-cell lymphomas* (centroblastic type). But in the spleen, transformation of mantle cell lymphoma develops mostly in small areas associated with a typical multimicronodular pattern. The macroscopic pattern is very important: lymphoblastic lymphoma and acute leukemia infiltrate the red pulp diffusely whereas large-B-cell lymphoma is characterized by voluminous polycyclic masses.

Patients present with splenomegaly and peripheral blood lymphocytosis mimicking B-CLL with a median peripheral blood lymphocytosis of 38×10^9/l (Molina et al. 2000). Often, patients have anemia, granulocytopenia, and thrombopenia. Peripheral adenopathies are absent (Molina et al. 2000). Thus, the presentation is not really that of a primary splenic lymphoma. The presence of leukemia and splenomegaly indicates an aggressive course.

The prognosis is poor, particularly with hyperleukemic disease (Weisenburger et al. 1981; Pombo de Oliveira et al. 1989; Duggan et al. 1990; Swerdlow and Williams 1993; Daniel et al. 1995; Vadlamudi et al. 1996; Molina et al. 2000).

In a recent series (Molina et al. 2000), disease in all of the eight patients progressed rapidly; the median overall survival was 8 months.

6.10.2.2 Other Types of B-Cell Lymphoma

The following lymphomas present with the same pattern as observed in the primary disease and thus are not described in detail: *lymphoplasmacytic lymphoma, marginal zone lymphoma of MALT, large-B-cell lymphoma and Burkitt's lymphoma.*

6.10.2.3 Peripheral NK/T-Cell Lymphoma

Any type of peripheral NK/T-cell lymphoma and leukemia can secondarily spread to the spleen. Below, only examples of the major categories of disease that can involve the spleen are discussed.

NK/T-cell lymphoma, leukemic or disseminated
In the group comprising T-prolymphocytic leukemia, aggressive NK/T-cell leukemia, and adult lymphoma/leukemia HTLV-1-associated, the spleen may be infiltrated but not primarily. The splenomegaly is mostly moderate. The other symptoms and particularly the leukemia are of greater clinical importance. Splenectomy is rarely performed. Only during necropsies do pathologists have the possibility to study such spleens. As in the majority of leukemias, the spleen is diffusely infiltrated. The architecture of the red pulp can be recognized if the infiltration is not too dense. The white pulp is often atrophic. The morphology of the cells, the immunophenotype, and the clinical presentation permit the proper diagnosis.

Nodal NK/T-cell lymphoma
In nodal NK/T-cell lymphomas, the spleen may be involved, although in the majority of patients not at first presentation but during disease evolution. *Peripheral NK/T-cell lymphoma, unspecified, or of the* "angioimmunoblastic lymphadenopathy with dysproteinemia" (*AILD*) *type* infiltrate primarily into the white pulp with all the characteristics of the nodal manifestations. *Anaplastic large-cell lymphoma* (Audouin et al. 1989) infiltrates the white pulp (follicles and periarteri-

olar sheets) in sheets or clusters. Giant cells with a typical Reed-Sternberg morphology are often associated.

Extranodal NK/T-cell lymphomas

The spleen is only involved secondarily, with the exception of in *hepatosplenic lymphoma* (see Chap. 6.10.1.7). Such involvement has been described in mycosis fungoides/Sézary's syndrome (Epstein et al. 1972; Long and Mihm 1974; Rappaport and Thomas 1974) and is sometimes revealed by a spontaneous rupture (Bennett et al. 1984), or in primary intestinal NK/T-cell lymphoma and primary NK/T-cell nasal lymphoma.

6.10.2.4 Precursor Cell Neoplasias: B- and T-Lymphoblastic Lymphoma/Acute Leukemia

The spleen is moderately increased in weight, the parenchyma is homogeneous and firm with a reddish color, and without any tumor. Medium-sized cells with the typical morphology of lymphoblasts massively infiltrate the cords and the sinuses of the red pulp, effacing the architecture and the white pulp. Immunohistochemistry demonstrates the B- or T-cell origin. Rarely, a splenomegaly is detected at the beginning of the disease. Sometimes a large spleen is found during relapse. Spontaneous rupture has occurred in some patients.

6.11 Lymphoma of the Liver

The liver can be involved primarily by a lymphoma, presenting either as a primary liver tumor or as hepatic failure that is usually severe. Most lymphomas infiltrating the liver are in fact secondary in nature.

The most common lymphomas involving the liver either primarily or secondarily are large-B-cell lymphomas, representing 64.5% of the cases, while peripheral NK/T-cell lymphomas represent only 9.7%, follicular lymphomas 4.8%, and primary hepatic marginal zone lymphomas of MALT about 1.6% (Dargent et al. 1998).

6.11.1 Primary Lymphoma of the Liver

Definition

A lymphoma of the liver is regarded as primary when only the liver is involved without lymphadenopathy or splenomegaly, with normal abdominal and thoracic CT scans, and normal bone marrow and blood counts, for at least 6 months after the diagnostic biopsy (Caccamo et al. 1986).

Primary liver lymphoma can present in two different ways (Scoazec et al. 1991; Zafrani and Gaulard 1993).

6.11.1.1 Primary Lymphoma Presenting as a Tumorous Infiltrate of the Liver

Macroscopy

The liver is occupied either by a solitary mass or, less frequently, by multiples nodules 4–18 cm in diameter, or, exceptionally, by diffuse lesions without nodule formation (Anthony et al. 1990; Scoazec et al. 1991; Ohsawa et al. 1998).

Histology

1. A variable topography of the liver involvement can be recognized (Walz-Mattmüller et al. 1998).
   The nodules consist of sheets of tumor cells that destroy the liver and compress the surrounding parenchyma (Fig. 6.79). Areas of necrosis are frequent.
   The infiltration can be diffuse initially in the portal tract, then penetrating the parenchyma but without hepatocellular destruction. This pattern is sometimes difficult to distinguish from that observed in chronic hepatitis, particularly on small liver biopsies.
   Intrasinusoidal infiltration can also be observed as in secondary liver lymphoma.
2. Different histological types of lymphomas have been reported.
   Diffuse large-B-cell lymphomas are the most frequent in normal (Collins et al. 1993; Anthony et al. 1990; Reman et al. 1990; Scoazec et al. 1991; Ohsawa et al. 1992; Aozasa et al. 1993a; Lei et al. 1995; Rubbia-Brandt et al. 1999) or immunodeficient patients (Nalesnik et al. 1988; Raphaël et al. 1991; Swerdlow 1992; Scerpella et al. 1996; Diebold et al. 1997; Mossad et al. 2000).
   Burkitt's lymphoma has on rare occasion also been observed in patients, some with immunodeficiency,

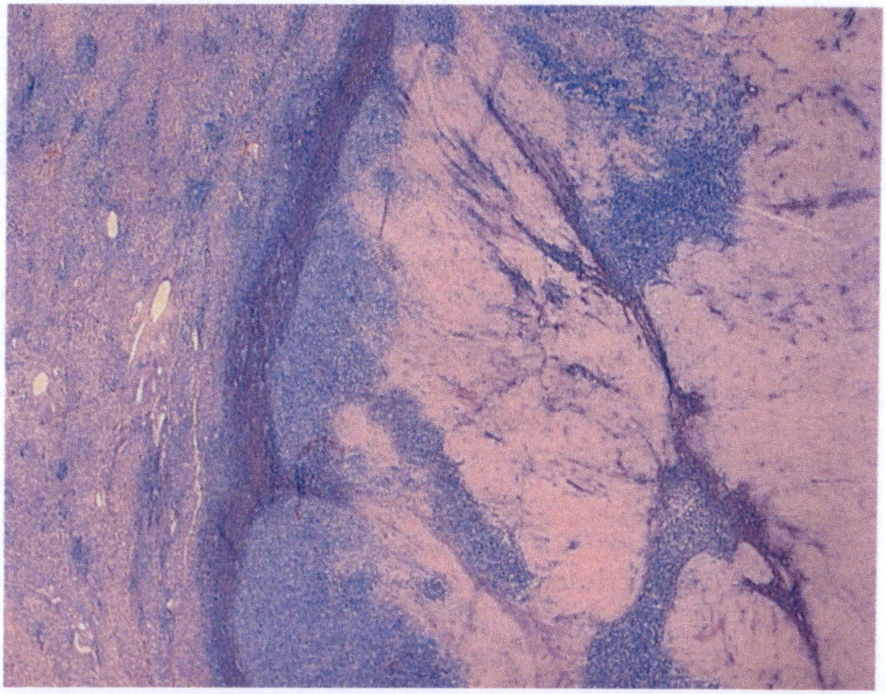

Fig. 6.79. Diffuse large-B-cell lymphoma developing as a primary tumor in the liver. The voluminous expansive tumor has destroyed the parenchyma; large areas of necrosis (pink areas) are seen (Giemsa stain)

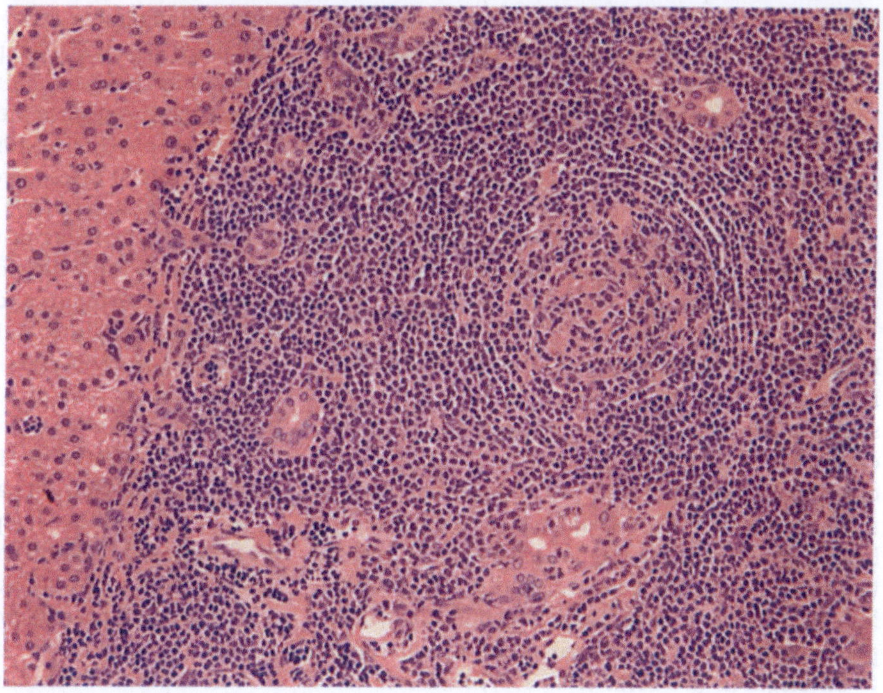

Fig. 6.80. Primary hepatic marginal zone B-cell lymphoma of MALT. There is a diffuse infiltrate of the portal spaces with a follicle showing a reactive germinal center that is partially colonized (H and E stain)

without any other localization besides the liver (Huang et al. 1997).

Marginal zone lymphoma of MALT developing primarily in the liver was initially reported by Isaacson et al. (1995). The tumor presents as solitary or multiple nodules destroying the liver parenchyma. Portal spaces are diffusely infiltrated by centrocyte-like lymphocytes and sometimes monocytoid B-cells and plasma cells. Reactive germinal centers that are more or less colonized can also be recognized (Fig. 6.80). There may be lymphoepithelial lesions in bile duct epithelium (Ohsawa et al. 1992; Ueda et al. 1996; Maes et al. 1997; Prabhu et al. 1998; Kirk et al. 1999; Chen et al. 2000; Ye et al. 2000). Two cases were associated with primary biliary cirrhosis (Prabhu et al. 1998; Ye et al. 2000).

Individual cases of small-B-cell lymphoma, such as *follicular, mantle cell* (Ohsawa et al. 1992; Lei et al. 1995), *lymphoplasmacytic lymphoma* (Borgonovo et al. 1995), and *plasmacytoma* (Weichhold et al. 1995; Demirhan et al. 1997; Solves et al. 1999), have been reported.

NK/T-cell lymphoma represents only a few cases and includes *peripheral T-cell lymphoma, unspecified* (Gaulard et al. 1986; Anthony et al. 1990; Scoazec et al. 1991; Bowman et al. 1994; Taketomi et al. 1996; Kim et al. 2000a; Schweiger et al. 2000), *anaplastic large-cell lymphoma* also in AIDS patients (Lei et al. 1995; Baschinsky et al. 2001), and *hepatosplenic lymphoma*, which represents the most frequent NK/T-cell lymphoma occurring primary in the liver – about 45 cases have been reported (Zafrani and Gaulard 1993; Weidmann 2000) (see Chap. 6.10.1.7).

Differential Diagnosis

Lymphoma presenting as a primary hepatic tumor should be distinguished from primary and metastatic carcinoma. While clinical data and radiological findings often allow this distinction (De Ment et al. 1987), in many cases only the histopathological study of a good liver biopsy permits the diagnosis. It should be stressed that sometimes the differential diagnosis at the histological level between large-B-cell lymphoma and some poorly differentiated carcinomas can be difficult leading to misdiagnosis (De Ment et al. 1987; Andreola et al. 1988). Immunohistochemistry is therefore mandatory.

The differential diagnosis between MALT lymphoma and mantle cell lymphoma is very difficult (Ueda et al. 1996; Kirk et al. 1999).

On liver biopsy, some small-B-cell lymphomas and, more often, peripheral T-cell lymphomas can be difficult to distinguish from inflammatory processes such as chronic active hepatitis and primary biliary cirrhosis. Again, immunohistochemistry and molecular genetics are very useful. The difficulty in this differential diagnosis is even more pronounced since the two diseases may be associated (see Chap. 4.2.1).

Finally, a very rare and unusual lymphoid infiltrate forming nodular macroscopic masses in the liver and made up of reactive T- and B-lymphoid cells has been reported (Sharifi et al. 1999). This "nodular lymphoid lesion of the liver" is very difficult to distinguish clinically and radiologically from primary liver lymphoma. At the histopathological level, the nodules consist of a very polymorphic cell population comprising small lymphocytes, plasma cells, and immunoblasts with scattered lymphoid follicles and acute inflammatory cells. The evolution is benign. Immunohistochemistry and molecular studies are required to rule out some lymphomas, particularly MALT lymphomas.

Occurrence

Primary lymphoma of the liver is extremely rare. As with many extranodal lymphomas, it is more common among immunocompromised patients and their number has increased since the onset of AIDS (Reichert et al. 1983; Raphaël et al. 1991; Diebold et al. 1997). In 1993, about 100 cases were reported in the literature (Zafrani and Gaulard 1993).

Primary lymphoma of the liver occurs during the fifth decade of life, with a male preponderance (Anthony et al. 1990; Avlonitis and Linos 1999). In a review of the literature published in 1992, Ohsawa et al. reported a median age of 55 years (range 7–87 years) with a male:female sex ratio of 3.1 : 1. The authors also noted that chronic hepatitis or cirrhosis preceding the lymphoma was observed in 44 % of Japanese patients but only in 9.6 % of Western patients.

Some primary liver lymphomas of the diffuse large-B-cell type, particularly those occurring in immunodeficient patients, may be associated with EBV.

In a few patients with primary liver lymphomas, an association with either a chronic hepatitis B or a chronic hepatitis C infection has been reported (Matano et al. 1998; Charton-Bain et al. 2000b; Mohler et al. 1997; Rubbia-Brandt et al. 1999; Chowla et al. 1999; Mizorogi et al. 2000; Kim et al. 2000b; Suriawinata et al. 2000).

Clinical Presentation

Patients complain of abdominal pain, night sweat, weight loss, and fever and present with hepatomegaly. Liver function tests are usually abnormal. The LDH level is high (Osborne et al. 1985; Anthony et al. 1990). Sometimes, primary lymphoma of the liver is an incidental finding during evaluation of a patient with cirrhosis or AIDS (Scoazec et al. 1991). Some patients present with jaundice as seen in chronic active hepatitis or granulomatous cholangitis (Anthony et al. 1990). Pleural effusion and immune thrombocytopenic purpura have been also observed.

Ultrasonography, CT and MRI can aid in the diagnosis (Scoazec et al. 1991); but only the histological examination of a biopsy specimen confirms the diagnosis (Scoazec et al. 1991).

Due to the small number of cases, the therapeutic strategy and the prognosis are not well known. Patients with hepatic lymphoma have a relatively favorable prognosis when the disease is recognized early (Ohsawa et al. 1992; Aozasa et al. 1993a) even if it is of the aggressive histological type. Resection, in association with radiotherapy and polychemotherapy, is usually recommended (Osborne et al. 1985; De Ment et al. 1987; Redondo et al. 1987; Pescovitz et al. 1990; Scoazec et al. 1991).

6.11.1.2 Primary Hepatic Lymphoma Presenting as Severe Hepatic Disease

Severe hepatocellular insufficiency can reveal a primary hepatic tumor (Zafrani and Gaulard 1993).

The liver parenchyma is massively infiltrated and destroyed by sheets of lymphoma cells, with sinusoidal infiltration and necrosis.

This pattern is mostly associated with Burkitt's lymphoma, DLBCL, or some anaplastic large-cell lymphoma, often reported in the past as "malignant histiocytosis".

Patients present with a rapidly worsening hepatomegaly associated with severe hepatocellular insufficiency and hyperlactatemia (Zafrani et al. 1983). The evolution is rapid and fatal. Only prompt polychemotherapy based on an early precise diagnosis can avoid a fatal outcome (Zafrani et al. 1983).

6.11.2 Secondary Lymphoma of the Liver

The liver is one of the most frequently involved organs in patients with NHL (Kim et al. 1976; Wright 1979).

DLBCLs are often responsible for large tumoral masses, either nodular or polycyclic. The T-cell-rich variant has been reported to infiltrate the portal tracts (Castroagudin et al. 1999). In small-B-cell lymphoma, the infiltrate predominates in the portal spaces penetrating the hepatic parenchyma which is progressively destroyed. Nodular infiltration is present mainly in follicular lymphomas. Diffuse infiltration is observed in B-CLL, mantle zone lymphoma, MALT lymphoma, and in peripheral NK/T-cell lymphoma. In small-B-cell lymphoma, particularly of the spleen, histological involvement of the liver is often disclosed at biopsy without any negative influence on the prognosis. The finding of a peculiar, preferentially intrasinusoidal infiltrate should be stressed.

1. In early phases of *hairy cell leukemia*, the cells are only present in the sinusoids and are in close contact with the endothelial cells (Diebold et al. 1977; Zafrani and Gaulard 1993). Diffuse infiltration of the portal tract is observed in more advanced cases (Diebold et al. 1977).
2. In *primary splenic marginal zone lymphoma* (Fig. 6.81), *T-cell large granular lymphocytic leukemia*, and *hepatosplenic lymphoma*, the pattern is the same, only the morphology of the cells is different (see corresponding chapter).
3. In *intravascular large-B-cell lymphoma*, the sinusoids are often full of large tumor cells and distended. One case after a nodal follicular lymphoma has been observed (Carter et al. 1996). Another was associated with hemophagocytic histiocytosis (Okada et al. 1994).

Secondary liver lymphoma is observed at staging in 15–40% of NHLs (Scoazec and Brousse 1991), often associated with splenic involvement.

Hepatomegaly with or without modification of hepatic function tests is the most frequent symptom. Ultrasonography or CT scan discloses nodular masses.

In some cases, only systematic liver biopsy demonstrates liver involvement.

In large-B-cell lymphomas and most T-cell lymphomas, such secondary involvement represents an advanced stage of the disease and is indicative of a poor

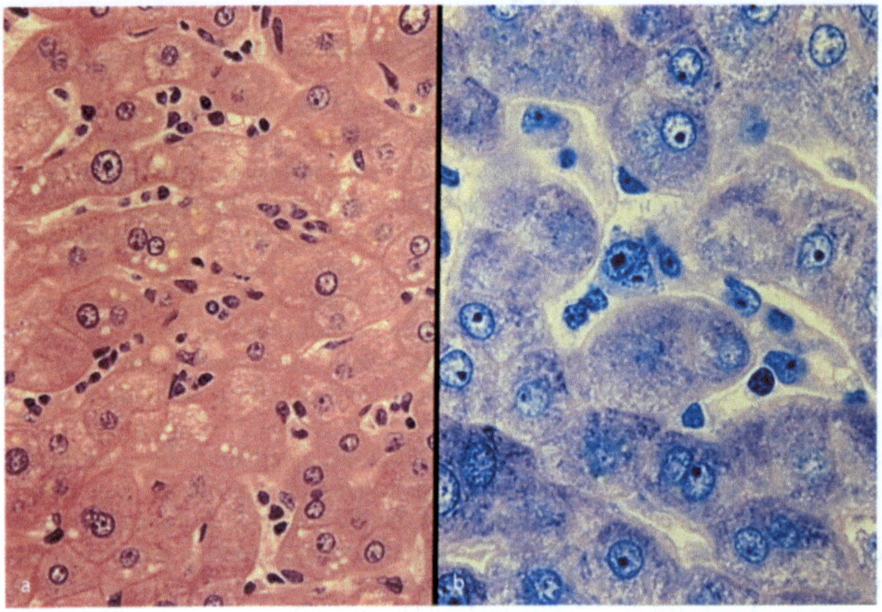

Fig. 6.81 a, b. Secondary liver extension by a primary splenic marginal zone lymphoma transforming into a large-B-cell lymphoma. Small and large cells are dispersed throughout the hepatic sinusoids. (**a** H and E stain, **b** Giemsa stain)

prognosis. Finally, fulminant hepatic failure can also occur, sometimes revealing a lymphoma involving the liver. This pattern is found mostly in patients with Burkitt's lymphoma and DLBCL including anaplastic large-B-cell lymphoma (Myszor and Record 1990). In small-B-cell lymphoma, this type of presentation may reflect transformation into a large B-cell lymphoma, for example, in lymphoplasmacytic lymphoma.

Large-cell lymphoma of B- or T-type can be difficult to distinguish from hepatocarcinoma or from metastatic carcinoma. The rare T-cell-rich variant of large-B-cell lymphoma predominates in the portal tract and can be difficult to differentiate not only from Hodgkin's lymphoma but also from inflammatory diseases (Dargent and De Wolf-Peeters 1998). Without immunohistochemistry and molecular studies, small B- and NK/T-cell lymphomas are also often difficult to distinguish from chronic inflammation.

- Primary lymphoma
  - Small-B-cell lymphoma
    Follicular lymphoma
    Marginal zone lymphoma, MALT
  - Diffuse large-B-cell lymphoma (the most frequently occurring type)
  - Burkitt's lymphoma
  - Peripheral NK/T-cell lymphoma
- Secondary lymphoma
  In principal, all lymphoma types may occur as secondary lymphomas. The most frequent ones are the same as listed under primary lymphoma.

6.12 Lymphoma of the Breast, Reproductive, and Urinary Systems

The various lymphomas discussed in this section occur in the following organs: breast, uterus, ovary, testis, prostate, kidney, and urinary bladder.

6.12.1 Malignant Lymphoma of the Breast

6.12.1.1 Primary Lymphoma of the Breast

Morphology

Macroscopy. One or multiples nodules, roundish or polycyclic, apparently well demarcated with a whitish, firm, homogeneous aspect. The nodules measure 1–10 cm in diameter (Mattia et al. 1993; Arber et al. 1994) and can develop at any site in the mammary gland, including near the nipple. Large tumors may invade the skin with possible ulceration. Some lymphomas massively infiltrate the entire gland, sometimes bilaterally. Inflammatory skin changes can be noted. Local adenopathies are often associated in the axilla.

Histology. The neoplastic cells infiltrate the soft tissue between the glandular lobules but also extend intralobularly. Sometimes, the glandular tissue is completely destroyed.

The majority of the lymphomas have a B-cell immunophenotype (Lamovec and Jancar 1987; Hugh et al. 1990; Cohen and Brooks 1991; Giardini et al. 1992; Mattia et al. 1993). Some are small-B-cell lymphomas, mainly *follicular* (Prévot et al. 1990; Hugh et al. 1990; Aozasa et al. 1992; Hansen et al. 1992; Mattia et al. 1993) or of *MALT* (Fig. 6.82) (Lamovec and Jancar 1987; Hugh et al. 1990; Cohen and Brooks 1991; Giardini et al. 1992; Aozasa et al. 1992; Bobrow et al. 1993; Mattia et al. 1993). It should be stressed that lymphoepithelial lesions are rarely seen in these MALT lymphomas. Lymphocytic lobulitis, mostly associated with MALT lymphoma, has been observed in some patients (Aozasa et al. 1992; Rooney et al. 1994; Le Pessot et al. 2001).

Diffuse large-B-cell lymphoma (centroblastic, immunoblastic) and *Burkitt's lymphoma* are probably the most frequent types of lymphoma observed (Prévot et al. 1990; Trojani et al. 1990; Hugh et al. 1990; Jeon et al. 1992; Hansen et al. 1992; Bobrow et al. 1993; Mattia et al. 1993; Arber et al. 1994; Abbondanzo et al. 1996). Some are secondary to MALT lymphomas (Fig. 6.83).

Primary breast lymphomas are rarely of NK/T-cell type: one case of peripheral T-cell lymphoma, unspecified, out of 14 cases of primary breast lymphomas (Prévot et al. 1990), one case of adult T-cell leukemia lymphoma, HTLV-1-associated (Kosaka et al. 1992), and one case of lymphoma featuring cells with multilobate nuclei (Pettinato et al. 1991) have been reported.

Differential Diagnosis

Large-B-cell lymphoma has to be distinguished from carcinomas. In the majority of the cases, morphology alone is sufficient. In a few cases, demonstration of cytokeratin expression and CD45 negativity are necessary to diagnose carcinoma.

Lymphocytic lobulitis, sometimes even associated with follicular hyperplasia, should not be misinterpreted as early small-B-cell lymphoma of MALT. The topography of the infiltrate in the lobules, the absence of a diffuse infiltrate destroying the lobules, the absence of lymphoepithelial lesions, and the presence

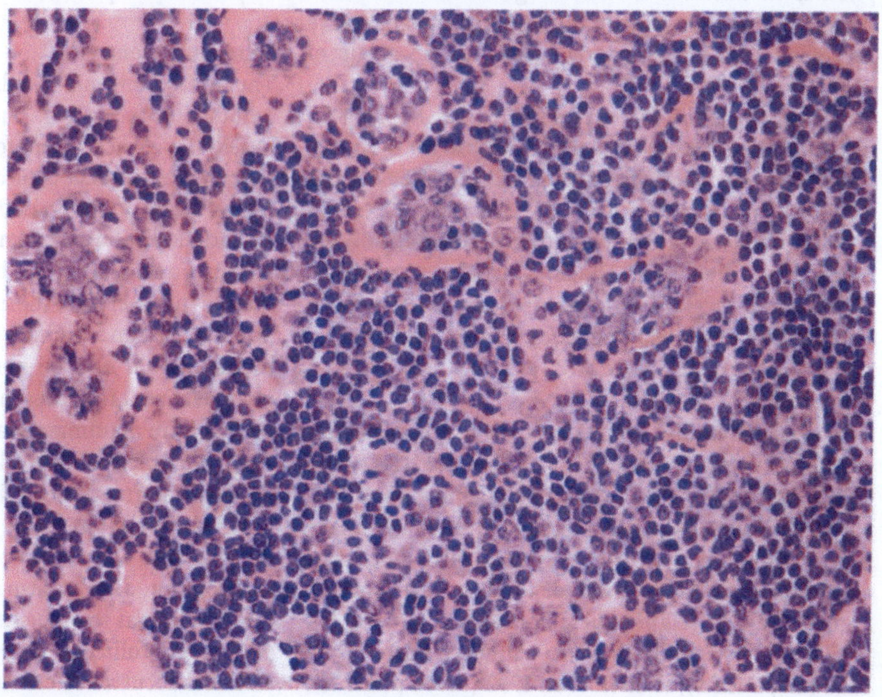

Fig. 6.82. Primary marginal zone lymphoma, MALT, developing in a female breast. There is a diffuse infiltrate of small-B-cells with a centrocyte-like morphology between the glands, and colonization of a reactive germinal center near the right border (H and E stain)

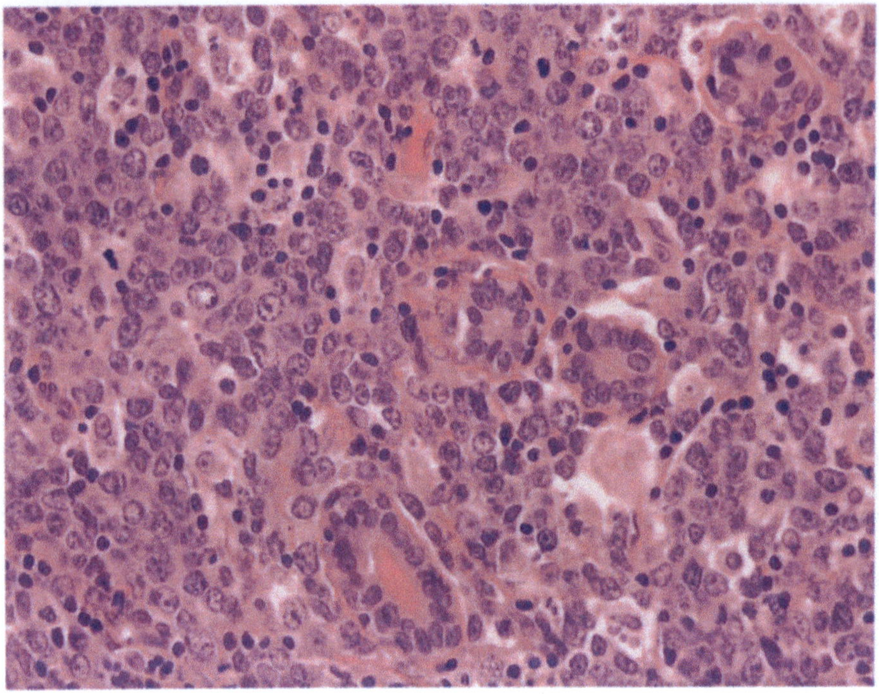

Fig. 6.83. Large-B-cell lymphoma of the breast. A diffuse infiltrate of a glandular lobule by large-B-cells characteristic of a polymorphic centroblastic lymphoma. This lymphoma was secondary to a marginal zone lymphoma of MALT (H and E stain)

of a majority of T-cells are helpful in ruling out MALT lymphoma. In the past, most of the small B-cell lymphomas in different extranodal glandular sites were designated as immunocytomas. Today, we are aware that almost all of these cases belong to the group of MALT lymphomas.

Finally, *myeloid sarcoma* should also be kept in mind; immunohistochemistry is useful to show the expression of myeloperoxidase, CD15, CD68, and CD34.

Also, when using intraoperative frozen sections, the differential diagnosis should include carcinoma, DLBCL, and myeloid sarcoma. In such cases a touch imprint is of great help in making a final diagnosis.

Occurrence

Primary lymphomas constitute 0.04–0.5% of malignant breast neoplasms, 1.7% of extranodal NHLs, and 0.7% of all NHLs (Dixon et al. 1987; Lamovec and Jancar 1987; Hugh et al. 1990; Mattia et al. 1993). Primary breast lymphoma occurs mostly in older women and exceptionally in men. Based on seven series: Lamovec and Jancar 1987 (eight patients), Prévot et al. 1990 (14 patients), Jeon et al. 1992 (seven patients), Aozasa et al. 1992 (19 patients), Hansen et al. 1992 (seven patients), Mattia et al. 1993 (nine patients), and Abbondanzo et al. 1996 (31 patients), the mean age is between 42 and 69 years with a peak around 60 years.

Clinical Presentation

The first symptom is usually the fortuitous discovery of a nodule in the breast. The diagnosis cannot be made based on clinical symptoms or on mammographic aspects. Only needle aspiration of the nodule and cytological study or biopsy of the nodule with histopathology and immunohistochemistry can recognize the lymphomatous origin of the breast nodule. Adenopathies may be discovered in the axilla or in any other regional nodal areas and should be biopsied. Bone marrow biopsy should also be performed even if there is no involvement at first presentation. Bilateral involvement of the entire mammary gland with inflammatory signs and sometimes pain, developing in pregnant women or during puberty, are mostly observed in patients with Burkitt's lymphoma. The evolution of the disease is rapidly fatal.

Evolution after treatment is the same as discussed for lymphomas in other sites. Patients with MALT lymphoma and follicular lymphoma have a longer survival. Local recurrence can occur, as well as transformation into a large-B-cell lymphoma, which is more aggressive. In a series of 31 patients (Abbondanzo et al. 1996) treated by surgery, chemotherapy, and/or radiation therapy, the median survival was 36 months, demonstrating the poor prognosis.

6.12.1.2
Secondary Lymphoma of the Breast

Diffuse large-B-cell lymphoma is the most frequent type (Cohen and Brooks 1991). *Burkitt's lymphoma* can also be observed, particularly in pregnant female. In the series of Mattia et al. (1993), there were 13 patients with *small-B-cell lymphoma,* nine with *follicular* lymphoma, four with *MALT lymphoma*, and eight with large-B-cell lymphoma. Thus, the majority of the tumors had a B-cell phenotype. The occurrence of *NK/T-cell lymphoma* is rare (one out of 21 in the preceding series).

Secondary breast involvement by lymphoma remains seldom. In a 24-year series of 5,111 patients with breast neoplasias, only four such patients (0.07%) were observed (Lamovec and Jancar 1987). In 31 patients with malignant lymphomas involving the breast, 22 had secondary involvement (Mattia et al. 1993). Only one patient was a male. The median age in this series was 60 years (range 39–83 years).

Lymphoma with secondary breast involvement occurs mostly in the context of widespread, preexisting nodal or, less frequently, extranodal primary lymphoma. Rarely, it occurs at presentation in more or less generalized lymphoma. More often, breast involvement develops during the course of the disease and is detected during relapse. Secondary breast MALT lymphomas can occur as isolated relapses from other extranodal sites, with a possibility for disease-free survival after local therapy.

The evolution is identical to that of disseminated large-B-cell lymphoma or follicular lymphoma; thus, patients have a poor prognosis. Only MALT lymphoma may have a longer, less aggressive course (Mattia et al. 1993).

6.12.2
Malignant Lymphoma of the Uterus

Definition

Lymphoma involving the endometrium or the cervix, either primarily or sometimes secondarily.

6.12.2.1
Primary Uterine Lymphoma

Morphology

Macroscopy. A polycyclic mass develops in the uterine cervix or in the corpus with involvement of the endometrium extending to the myometrium. Hemorrhagic and necrotic areas may be present.

Histology. All published cases have been either DLBCLs, immunoblastic or centroblastic (Aozasa et al. 1993b; Latteri et al. 1995; Alvarez et al. 1997; Matsuyama et al. 1989; Harris and Scully 1984) or Burkitt's lymphoma (Harris and Scully 1984; Renno et al. 2002). However, rare cases of follicular lymphoma have also been reported (Muntz et al. 1991; Harris and Scully 1984).

Differential Diagnosis

Lymphoma of the uterine corpus and cervix should be distinguished from anaplastic carcinoma and myeloid sarcoma. In addition, stromal endometriosis and poorly differentiated leiomyosarcoma have to be taken into account in the presence of a corpus localization.

Occurrence

In a National Cancer Institute (USA) review of 1,467 patients with extranodal lymphomas, primary NHL of the uterine corpus accounted for about 0.002% of all cases (Latteri et al. 1995). In a recent review of the literature done to complete the report of a case of primary NHL of the uterine corpus, eleven other cases were discovered (Rennoet al. 2002). Cervical involvement represented 0.008% of primary cervical tumors (Aozasa et al. 1993b). This type of lymphoma is clinically confined to the corpus or the cervix for a longer period without dissemination (Alvarez et al. 1997).

Primary uterine lymphoma develops mostly in patients over 50 years old. Cases appearing in children are exceptional (Renno et al. 2002).

An association with endometrial carcinoma has been observed (Vang et al. 2000).

Clinical Presentation

Symptoms revealing primary uterine corpus lymphoma are vaginal bleeding, and abdominal or pelvic pain (Alvarez et al. 1997; Renno et al. 2002). A pelvic mass is disclosed (Alvarez et al. 1997). Clinical staging shows that some tumors are limited to the cervix with a stage

IC (Muntz et al. 1991; Rennoet al. 2002) During disease evolution, extension to other sites, nodal or extranodal, can occur (Renno et al. 2002).

Treatment comprises surgery, radiation therapy, and chemotherapy. The number of cases is too small to be able to evaluate disease evolution and the effects of treatment. Localized tumors seems to have a favorable evolution.

6.12.2.2
Addendum: Primary Lymphoma of the Vagina

Primary lymphoma of the vagina is extremely rare. Less than 25 cases have been reported (Prévot et al. 1992; Höffkes et al. 1995).

It presents as a circumferential tumor around the superior part of the vagina with extension to the pouch of Douglas, the parametrium, and the bladder.

Höffkes et al. (1995) reported a case of DLBCL (centroblastic type) and reviewed 18 cases. It is not possible to interpret the diagnoses in old cases but the two most frequent types seem to be DLBCL and follicular lymphoma, and less frequently lymphoblastic lymphoma.

In an additional personal series (Prévot et al. 1992), we reported two cases of DLBCL (polymorphic centroblastic type) and one case of peripheral NK/T-cell, unspecified, with angiocentrism.

Such vaginal lymphoma occurs mostly in premenopausal patients with a median age of 50 years, ranging from 20 to 79 years (Prévot et al. 1992; Höffkes et al. 1995). Some patients seem to be asymptomatic. Other patients present with vaginal bleeding. Rarely, an ulcerated mass is discovered.

It is our experience that cervicovaginal smears are not useful for the diagnosis; instead vaginal biopsies are required (Prévot et al. 1992).

Disease evolution is not easy to evaluate due to the very small number of reported cases. Pelvic irradiation with or without radical surgery is followed by remission. Chemotherapy is recommended in young patients, sometimes with salvage radiotherapy (Perren et al. 1992).

6.12.2.3
Secondary Uterine and Vaginal Lymphoma

This type of involvement is observed in at least 40 % of patients with disseminated lymphoma of any histological type (Höffkes et al. 1995).

Treatment is based on limited surgery followed by local radiotherapy associated with polychemotherapy. Nonetheless, one-third of the patients died within 17 months of diagnosis (Höffkes et al. 1995). Patients who survived free of disease had a mean follow-up period of 75 months (Prévot et al. 1992).

6.12.3
Malignant Lymphoma of the Ovary

6.12.3.1
Primary Lymphoma of the Ovary

Definition

Primary lymphoma of the ovary is still controversial (Woodruff et al. 1963; Freeman et al. 1972; Chorlton et al. 1974; Paladugu et al. 1980; Rotmensch and Woodruff 1982; Osborne and Robboy 1983; Yamane et al. 1989; Monterroso et al. 1993; Ferry and Young 1991; Skodras et al. 1994).

A primary lymphoma of the ovary can be defined as a lymphoma involving one ovary without regional extension to the peritoneum, or to regional lymph nodes (lateroaortic), or to any organ at distance. These criteria suggest that the lymphoma develops first in the ovary (Monterroso et al. 1993) but reports of bilateral involvement that is apparently primary have been published (Piura et al. 1986).

This definition is perhaps too strict; but due to the rarity of the cases, it is not possible to collect enough information for a more precise definition.

Morphology

Macroscopy. One ovary is transformed into a huge mass, homogeneous, whitish and firm, with areas of necrosis or hemorrhage, or is distorted by multiple whitish nodules of different sizes. These lymphomas can measure 3–8 cm or more in diameter (Monterroso et al. 1993). The fallopian tubes and uterus should not be involved primarily, neither should regional lymph nodes or omentum.

Histology. Only a few of these lymphomas have been reported as primary lymphoma of the ovary. All were B-cell lymphomas (Monterroso et al. 1993; Skodras et al. 1994).The majority are DLBCL (centroblastic and immunoblastic type) and Burkitt's lymphomas (Osborne and Robboy 1983; Monterroso et al. 1993; Skodras et al. 1994). One case that was perhaps a pri-

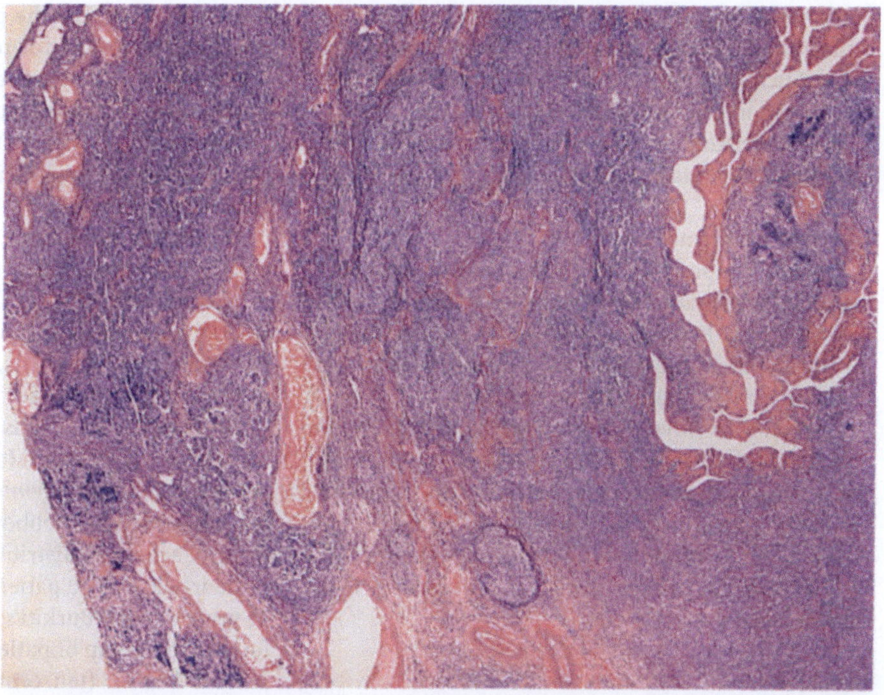

Fig. 6.84. Primary ovarian follicular lymphoma. Multiple lymphomatous follicles infiltrate the ovarian stroma and extend to the mesosalpinx. On the *right*, the lumen of the infiltrated salpinx can be seen (H and E stain)

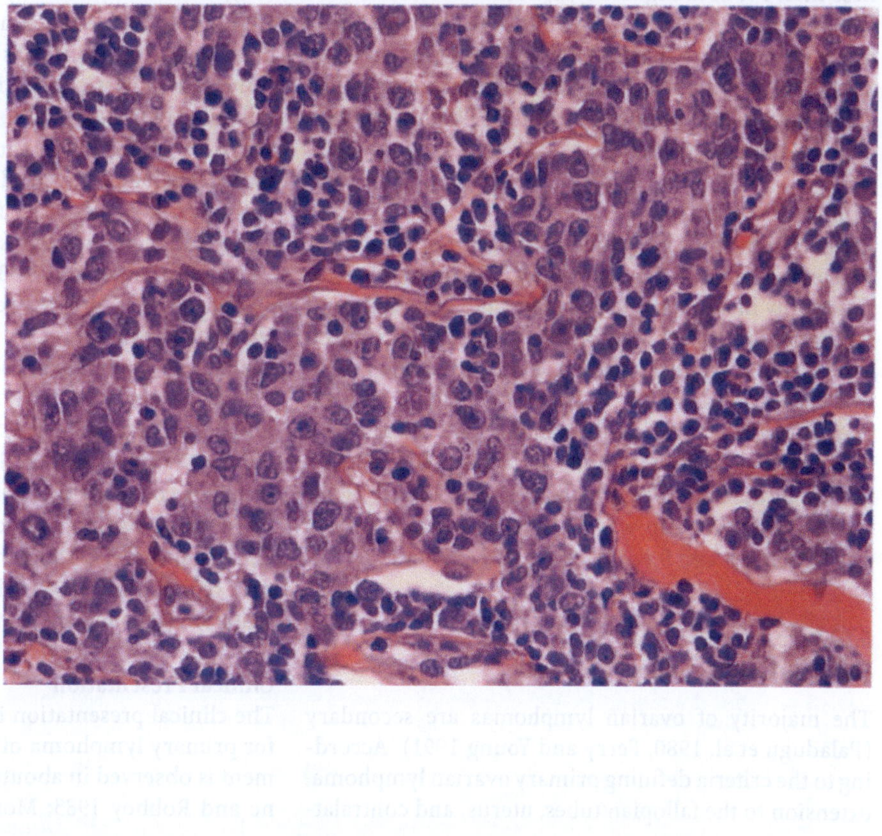

Fig. 6.85. Primary ovarian follicular lymphoma. Same patient as in Fig. 6.84. In the diffuse areas, there are sheets of large B-cells corresponding to a diffuse large-B-cell lymphoma, monomorphic centroblastic type, and secondary to the follicular lymphoma (H and E stain)

mary lymphoma of the ovary was instead a DLBCL secondary to follicular lymphoma (Monterroso et al. 1993). Such follicular lymphomas are infrequent. They can extend into the salpinx (Figs. 6.84, 6.85).

An association with serous carcinoma has been described (Skodras et al. 1994).

Differential Diagnosis

Malignant lymphomas are in some cases difficult to distinguish from *ovarian tumor of granulosa* or *germinal cell origin*. Precise study of the architectural organization of the tumor and immunohistochemistry are useful in establishing a precise diagnosis.

Granulocytic (myeloid) sarcoma can also involve the ovaries and should be distinguished from lymphoma. Again, the morphology of the cells, the use of imprints, the demonstration of a naphthol-ASD-chloracetate-esterase, and immunohistochemistry (particularly myeloperoxidase) allow the proper diagnosis to be established.

Occurrence

Less than 1 % of malignant lymphoma involve the ovaries; among these, only a few fulfill the criteria of primary lymphoma (Chorlton et al. 1974; Freeman et al. 1972). These lymphomas occur mostly in young women. In the series of Monterroso et al. (1993), the median age was about 38 years.

Clinical Presentation

Patients complain of a pelvic or abdominopelvic mass with pain in about 65 % of the cases. This mass is sometimes only incidentally discovered. Only about 10 % of the patients present with B symptoms. By definition, these cases comprise stage I according to the Fédération Internationale de Gynéco-Obstétrique (FIGO) classification of ovarian tumors. Precise information on survival rates after treatment is lacking. In the series of four patients reported by Monterroso et al. (1993), the clinical follow-up was 15 months for one patient and between 4 and 8 years for the three others.

6.12.3.2 Secondary Lymphoma of the Ovary

The majority of ovarian lymphomas are secondary (Paladugu et al. 1980; Ferry and Young 1991). According to the criteria defining primary ovarian lymphoma, extension to the fallopian tubes, uterus, and contralateral ovary as well as the presence of a retroperitoneal mass, with omentum or regional lymph node involvement, is regarded as secondary lymphoma. Secondary involvement is evident due to the existence of a lymphoma in another site at the time of patient presentation or subsequent to an either previously diagnosed or treated lymphoma.

Secondary lymphoma differs from primary lymphomas according to the following: larger size (5 – 21 cm in diameter in the series of Monterroso et al. 1993), bilateral localization, and extension to the fallopian tubes, uterus, pelvis, omentum, or lymph nodes, particularly lateroaortic.

All cases reported thus far have been B-cell lymphomas: *diffuse large-B*-cell (either centroblastic or immunoblastic), *Burkitt's lymphoma*, or *follicular lymphoma*. Osborne and Robboy (1983) showed the importance of age in the distribution of the histological type. In their series of 40 patients, 14 females were less than 20 years old and Burkitt's lymphoma was diagnosed in four. In the group of patients between 29 and 74 years, 19 had DLBCL (ten centroblastic, nine immunoblastic), and six follicular lymphoma. Monterroso et al. 1993 showed almost a similar distribution of lymphomas: 14 cases of Burkitt's lymphomas, ten of DLBCL (nine centroblastic including three cases secondary to follicular lymphoma, and one immunoblastic secondary to a B-CLL), one follicular and diffuse, two "diffuse mixed small and large cells" of probable follicular origin, and only one case of T-cell lymphoma with the morphology of an anaplastic large-cell lymphoma.

Monterroso et al. (1993) accepted in their series of 39 cases, only four as being primary and eight for which the primary origin was uncertain. Thus, 27, or perhaps 35, patients had secondary involvement.

Such secondary lymphoma of the ovary may be the initial manifestation of occult nodal or extranodal lymphoma (Monterroso et al. 1993). Sometimes, the ovaries are involved during the disseminated phase of a lymphoma. Ovaries are not infrequently involved at necropsy (Chorlton et al. 1974). However, less than 1 % of patients with lymphoma have ovarian localization at initial presentation (Freeman et al. 1972; Chorlton et al. 1974).

Clinical Presentation

The clinical presentation is identical to that described for primary lymphoma of the ovary. Bilateral involvement is observed in about 55 % of the patients (Osborne and Robboy 1983; Monterroso et al. 1993). In the series of Osborne and Robboy (1983), 36% of the patients had a FIGO stage I, 12% a stage II (extension to fallopian tubes and uterus), 45% a stage III (with extension to the peritoneum and/or lumboaortic lymph nodes). Concerning the histological type, follicular lymphoma had a better prognosis than the other B-cell lymphomas (Osborne and Robboy 1983). In the same report, after treatment (surgery completed by radiotherapy with or without chemotherapy), the 5-year overall survival was 35%. Disseminated lymphoma localized only secondarily to the genital tract (FIGO I) seemed to have a better outcome. Therefore, in secondary lymphoma of the ovaries, two factors are associated with a more favorable prognosis: localized stage and a follicular lymphoma.

6.12.4 Lymphoma of Testis

Definition

Lymphomas arising primarily in the testis remain rare. They are studied together with lymphomas involving the epididymis (McDermott et al. 1995) and spermatic cord, which are even rarer (Ferry et al. 1994).

A few cases represent extension or often relapse of lymphomas of other initial sites (Ferry et al. 1994).

Morphology

Macroscopy. The size of the affected testis ranges from 3 to 9 cm. The cut surface appears homogeneous, granular, or slightly lobulated. The tumor tissue is firm, gray or brown-white with small foci of hemorrhage and/or necrosis. Most often, the tunica albuginea is distended but not invaded; however sometimes macroscopic extension can be seen (Moller et al. 1994).

Histology. The testis is diffusely infiltrated and more or less destroyed. Seminiferous tubuli are atrophic, sometimes invaded (Ferry et al. 1994; Moller et al. 1994). Focal or extensive bands of fibrosis may be present (Ferry et al. 1994). Vascular invasion is disclosed in 30% of patients.

Diffuse large-B-cell lymphoma is the most frequent type (50–80%)- occurring primarily in the testis. Most of these DLBCLs are *centroblastic lymphoma* and less frequently of *immunoblastic type with or without plasmacytoid differentiation* (Paladugu et al. 1980; Ganem et al. 1985; Nonomura et al. 1989; Ferry et al. 1994).

A few cases of *Burkitt's lymphoma* have been reported in elderly patients (Root et al. 1990; Ferry et al. 1994).

Follicular lymphomas are extremely rare (Ferry et al. 1994; Moertel et al. 1995).

Rarely, *peripheral NK/T-cell lymphoma* has been recognized. In the series of Ferry et al. (1994), one large-cell lymphoma was of T-cell immunophenotype.

In another series, based on 39 patients, 89% of the large-cell lymphomas were of B-immunophenotype and 11% of T-immunophenotype (Moller et al. 1994).

In children, *T- or B-cell lymphoblastic leukemia or lymphoma* and *Burkitt's lymphoma* are the most frequent types of primary lymphomas of the testis, often in association with a multifocal disseminated disease.

The same histological type of lymphoma is recognized in secondary testis involvement.

Occurrence

Lymphomas with a primary testicular localization are rare, representing approximately 0.5–2% of all NHLs (Turner et al. 1981; Ganem et al. 1985; Ferry et al. 1994), 1.5% of all extranodal lymphomas (Freeman et al. 1972), and 26–44% of all testicular tumors. In a Danish population-based lymphoma registry, the recorded incidence was 0.26 per 10,000 per year (Moller et al. 1994). It is the most frequent tumor in men older than 60 years of age (Turner et al. 1981; Root et al. 1990).

In the large series published by Ferry et al. (1994), the age range was from 16 to 91 years (mean: 56), but children can also be affected (Kellie et al. 1989).

At autopsy of patients treated for lymphomas of different localization, the testes were involved in about 10–20% of the cases (Givler 1969).

Clinical Features

Patients complain mostly of a scrotal mass which may be present from 1 week to 5 years (Ferry et al. 1994). The mass is hard and painless but sometimes associated with a feeling of heaviness (Moller et al. 1994). A few patients complain of pain and tenderness. Hydrocele can be observed (Moller et al. 1994).

Bilateral involvement is rare at initial presentation – less than 10% of patients (Ostronoff et al. 1995). By contrast, bilateral involvement is more frequent in secondary testicular lymphomas. Most patients present with stage I or stage II disease (Zucca et al. 2003).

In primary testis lymphomas, dissemination varied among several series, ranging from 13% to 66%

(Ganem et al. 1985; Martenson et al. 1988). An aggressive evolution is mostly seen in patients with DLBCL.

The most striking feature in primary testis lymphoma is the propensity for extranodal dissemination, particularly to the nasopharynx and the central nervous system. The risk of neuromeningeal extension is five times greater than in DLBCL of other sites (Paladugu et al. 1980; MacIntosh et al. 1982; Ganem et al. 1985; Zucca et al. 2003).

The frequency of cerebral extension has increased due to the prolonged survival obtained by treatment (Ganem et al. 1985). Systemic treatment for preventing such dissemination should always be done (MacIntosh et al. 1982; Moller et al. 1994). Today, intensive polychemotherapy, including anthracyclin, and intrathecal chemotherapy has made treatment as efficient as for other DLBCLs (Ganem et al. 1985; Connors et al. 1988; Ferry et al. 1994; Ostronoff et al. 1995).

Due to a rather bad penetration of the testis by chemotherapeutic agents, radiotherapy is still used to treat localized disease. One study (Connors et al. 1988) reported good results in localized lymphoma after CHOP followed by locoregional radiotherapy.

The following factors are associated with a poor prognosis: high International Prognostic Index (IPI), particularly together with involvement of the epididymis and spermatic cords (Ferry et al. 1994; Moller et al. 1994).

Ferry et al. (1994) stressed the prognostic value of fibrosis. In their series, extensive fibrosis was strongly associated with stage I disease and may be a predictor of long disease-free survival.

During a median follow up of 7.6 years, 52% of the patients relapsed (Zucca et al. 2003).

6.12.5 Malignant Lymphoma of the Prostate

Definition

The prostate gland is very rarely involved by lymphomas either primarily but more often secondarily (Bell et al. 1995). Exceptional cases of lymphomas of the epididymis have also been reported. For example, there was one case of follicular lymphoma with large-cell predominance (McDermott et al. 1995).

Morphology

Macroscopy. The prostate gland is partially or totally destroyed by polycyclic or diffuse whitish masses compressing the urethra. Small foci of necrosis (yellow) or hemorrhages (dark red) can be seen.

Histology. Primary lymphomas comprise small lymphocytic lymphomas, as well as mantle cell lymphoma, follicular lymphoma, Burkitt's lymphoma (Bostwick and Mann 1985; Bostwick et al. 1998), and, most often, DLBCL (Bostwick and Mann 1985; Bostwick et al. 1998; Mounedji-Boudiaf et al. 1994) of centroblastic or immunoblastic type (Sarlis et al. 1993).

The same types have been reported as secondary lymphomas. Thus far, NK/T-cell lymphomas have been reported only as occurring secondarily (Bostwick and Mann 1985; Bostwick et al. 1998).

Occurrence

Malignant lymphomas of the prostate occur mostly in elderly men. The mean age is 62 years, age ranging from 5 to 89 years (Bostwick and Mann 1985; Bostwick et al. 1998). In a series of 62 patients (Bostwick et al. 1998), 35% had primary prostatic lymphomas and 48% had a prior nodal or extranodal lymphoma. In ten patients, the disease could not be classified as either primary or secondary.

Clinical Presentation

The majority of the patients complain of urinary disorders, similar to lower urinary tract obstruction. Physical examination discloses a prostatic mass. The serum acid phosphatase level is not elevated. Only prostate biopsy allows the diagnosis.

Secondary prostate gland involvement is mainly observed during disease evolution, as a relapse, between 2 and 60 months (mean 14 months) (Bostwick and Mann 1985).

The number of cases is so small that little information is available concerning disease evolution and prognosis. In the series of 62 patients reported by Bostwick et al. (1998), 25 died of malignant lymphoma, 14 died of unknown or other causes, 18 were alive 12–20 months after diagnosis (eight primary, ten secondary), and five were lost to follow-up. Survival was 64% at 1 year, 50% at 2 years, 33% at 5 and at 10 years. The evolution is the same for both primary and secondary prostatic lymphoma (23 months vs 28 months, respectively).

6.12.6 Lymphoma of the Kidney

6.12.6.1 Primary Lymphoma of the Kidney

Definition

Malignant lymphomas first seen as a renal mass have been reported, but remain very rare (Rosenberg et al. 1961; Kandel et al. 1987; Okuno et al. 1995; Ferry et al. 1995).

Exceptional cases of lymphoma of the ureter have also been reported (Buck et al. 1992), sometimes secondary to extension from retroperitoneal nodal lymphoma or from kidney lymphoma.

Morphology

Macroscopy. Mostly, there is a single mass, which is tan, gray-pink, or yellow-white , either soft and fleshy or firm or even stony hard. Such masses measure from 5 to 25 cm in diameter. Sometimes areas of necrosis or hemorrhage are present. In rare cases, multiple nodules are found. In a few cases, the disease is bilateral (Brouland et al. 1994).

Extension of the lymphoma to the perinephric fat is frequent. Adrenal glands, renal vessels, ureters, psoas muscle, diaphragm, and liver may also be involved (Ferry et al. 1995).

Histology. Most primary lymphoma of the kidney are B-cell lymphomas (Osborne et al. 1987; Richards et al. 1990; Morel et al. 1994; Ferry et al. 1995; Okuno et al. 1995). The majority of the patients have either DLBCLs, mostly of centroblastic type (Richards et al. 1990; Brouland et al. 1994; Ferry et al. 1995), Burkitt's lymphoma, or "small non-cleaved non Burkitt's lymphoma", the latter being difficult to translate into the WHO classification (Okuno et al. 1995; Osborne et al. 1987; Ferry et al. 1995; Richards et al. 1990). Small-B-cell lymphomas can also occur. For example, in a series classified according to the up-dated Kiel classification (Ferry et al. 1995), two patients had immunocytomas (one with a serum monoclonal component as in Waldenström's macroglobulinemia) and three with centroblastic-centrocytic follicular lymphomas were observed out of a total of 11 patients. One of the immunocytomas showed features suggestive of MALT lymphoma (Ferry et al. 1995). Another case of MALT lymphoma was also reported (Parveen et al. 1993). Intravascular large-B-cells have also been observed (Axelsen et al. 1991).

T-cell lymphomas are extremely rare. There is one report of T-lymphoblastic lymphoma with bilateral renal involvement (Camitta et al. 1986) and one of a peripheral NK/T-cell lymphoma with large cells (Miyake et al. 1990).

The lymphomas largely destroy the normal parenchyma, forming expansive masses obliterating the neighboring normal parenchyma. Often, extension of the lymphoma is observed between glomerules and tubules; there may also be intravascular invasion.

Occurrence

In a series from the Mayo Clinic, only five out of 176 cases met the criteria for primary renal lymphoma (Okuno et al. 1995). Brouland et al. (1994) reported one case and found only 36 other cases of primary renal lymphoma in the literature. The tumor develops mainly in adults, between 40 and 80 years of age with a median age of 67 years (Ferry et al. 1995) or 60 years (Okuno et al. 1995) without sex predominance. A few cases have been reported in children (Donnadieu et al. 1992). It is interesting to stress that, in the series of Ferry et al. (1995), some patients had preceding other malignancies: colonic or prostatic carcinoma, various cutaneous neoplasias, or Hodgkin's lymphomas. One case appearing in a renal transplant recipient has been reported (Gassel et al. 1991).

Finally, primary renal lymphoma, usually aggressive B-cell lymphoma, is one of the extranodal localizations occurring in HIV-infected patients (Tsang et al. 1993; Meulders et al. 1993).

Differential Diagnosis

Most of the patients have been diagnosed clinically as having *renal carcinoma*, often with vascular involvement. Hydronephrosis due to ureteral obstruction by lymphomatous adenopathies or pyelonephritis have also been discussed.

Clinical Presentation

Some patients are completely asymptomatic and the renal tumor is disclosed by chance. Other patients complain of B symptoms and sometimes of pain (in the back, flank, or abdomen). Patients may also present with hematuria or renal insufficiency (Bertoncelli et al. 1993; Meulders et al. 1993), particularly in cases of bilateral renal lymphoma (Van Gelder et al. 1992; Brouland et al. 1994).

Intravenous urography, angiography, sonography,

CT, and MRI disclose focal or diffuse renal involvement by a tumor. The final diagnosis is only made by biopsies (Brouland et al. 1994) or after nephrectomy (Ferry et al. 1995).

In two patients, a monoclonal serum IgM component was found, indicating a Waldenström's macroglobulinemia (Ferry et al. 1995).

Follow-up is not easy to summarize due to the rarity of the disease, the absence of precise information, and the variety of treatments. In the series of Ferry et al. (1995), the follow-up of the 11 patients ranged from 1 week to 169 months (median 15 months). Five of the eight treated patients achieved complete remission; three patients had relapses in lymph nodes, bone marrow, or kidney. In the series of Okuno et al. (1995), the median survival was 8 months (range 3–93 months) but two patients out of five achieved complete remission longer than 80 months following therapy. Treatment consisting of complete resection followed by chemotherapy and consolidation radiotherapy may be followed by long disease-free survival, while bilateral involvement and no debulking of the renal lymphoma are associated with poor survival (Okuno et al. 1995).

6.12.6.2 Secondary Kidney Lymphoma

All types of lymphomas may be observed, with a predominance of DLBCL (centroblastic mostly) and Burkitt's lymphoma. One case of adult NK/T-cell lymphoma extending to the kidney was reported (Srinisava et al. 1990). During the clinical follow-up of 1,269 patients with lymphoma, Rosenberg et al. (1961) reported on 11 cases of renal involvement, none of which were observed at initial presentation. Since the introduction of CT, early renal localization in patients with lymphomas that developed in other areas can be disclosed in about 2.7–6% of the cases (Richards et al. 1990). At necropsy, renal involvement is observed in about 50% of the cases (Strauss et al. 1983; Kandel et al. 1987; Morel et al. 1994; Wentzell and Berkheise 1995).

Renal involvement in the course of a lymphoma developing in another site is often asymptomatic (Rosenberg et al. 1961; Richards et al. 1990). The kidneys are involved mostly during progression of the disease or at relapse. Rarely, renal involvement is responsible for renal insufficiency, associated with a fatal disease evolution. Evolution is mostly rapidly unfavorable.

6.12.7 Malignant Lymphoma of the Urinary Bladder

Morphology

Macroscopy. The lymphoma infiltrates the urinary bladder wall at various sites but often in the trigone and base. The wall is thickened by a whitish firm tissue that destroys the normal components. Polypoid masses can be seen protruding into the lumen (Siegel and Napoli 1991). Often, the overlying mucosa is intact. In some patients, geographic ulceration is present. More advanced lymphoma may extend to the abdominal wall, the uterus, or to the entire pelvis. Ileo vesical fistula has also been reported.

Histology. Due to the rarity of this disease, it remains difficult to know precisely which kind of lymphoma involves the urinary bladder.

Small-B-cell lymphomas do occur, for example, follicular lymphoma, immunocytoma (De Bruyne et al. 1987), and MALT lymphoma (Pawade et al. 1993) have been mentioned. DLBCLs are also found. One case of large-B-cell lymphoma that expressed CD20 with eosinophilic, PAS-positive cytoplasmic inclusions forming a signet-ring pattern has been reported (Siegel and Napoli 1991).

Occurrence

Lymphoma of the urinary bladder represents 2% of all bladder neoplasms (Bates et al. 2000). Primary involvement of the urinary bladder by lymphoma is very rare (Ohsawa et al. 1993). It occurs mostly in elderly women. A review of the literature through 1989 revealed a total of 73 published cases (Siegel and Napoli 1991).

In a recent series of 11 patients, there were only ten cases of NHL (Bates et al. 2000). Six were primary lymphomas (three marginal zone lymphomas of MALT with lymphoepithelial lesions, three DLBCLs) and four were secondary DLBCLs, one occurring subsequent to a follicular lymphoma.

Clinical Presentation

Dysuria, polyuria, and hematuria are the first clinical symptoms in many patients. In other patients, a pelvic mass is disclosed by physical examination. A CT scan of the abdomen and pelvis shows a mass in the urinary bladder with possible extension to the anterior abdominal wall or to the uterus. Cystoscopy also discloses the tumor and allows for a biopsy.

In patients having a lymphoma of another organ,

urinary bladder involvement has been demonstrated often only during relapses.

The evolution seems to be unfavorable in both primary and secondary involvement, but information concerning the type of lymphoma, the type of treatment, and follow-up are missing in many reported cases. Recently, Bates et al. (2000) report on ten cases. Patients with secondary lymphomas died of disease within 13 months after diagnosis. Primary lymphomas followed a more indolent course.

6.13 Endocrine Gland Lymphoma

Initial manifestation of malignant lymphoma in endocrine glands is a rare event. We will focus on two endocrine glands, the adrenal glands and the thyroid, as they are the most frequently involved.

Secondary involvement of the adrenal glands and the thyroid has been found at autopsy of patients with different types of lymphomas.

6.13.1 Malignant Lymphoma of the Thyroid Gland

Definition

A malignant tumor composed of lymphoid cells and which involves primarily the thyroid gland, or which is due to secondary involvement by lymphomas arising in another site.

Primary lymphomas of thyroid gland are associated in more than 80% of patients with Hashimoto's thyroiditis or lymphocytic thyroiditis. This autoimmune disease, resulting from chronic antigenic stimulation, is responsible for a clonal selection of B-cells and development of a marginal zone cell lymphoma of the MALT that can transform into DLBCL (Aozasa et al. 1986a, 1987; Hyjec and Isaacson 1988; Matsuzuka et al. 1993; Pedersen and Pedersen 1996).

List of Entities

- Diffuse large-B-cell lymphoma
- Marginal zone lymphoma of MALT
- Follicular lymphoma
- Plasmacytoma
- Peripheral NK/T-cell lymphoma

Morphology

Macroscopy. The thyroid gland is totally or partially replaced by a solid homogeneous mass with a typical fish-flesh appearance. There is no capsule between the neoplastic tissue and the remnants of the thyroid gland. Nodular extension outside the gland capsule into the adjacent soft tissue is often seen.

Histology

1. The most frequent type of lymphoma is *diffuse large-B-cell lymphoma*. The thyroid parenchyma is diffusely infiltrated by large cells destroying the follicles, infiltrating between the follicles, penetrating between the cells of the follicles, and accumulating in the follicle lamina. Fibrotic bands are responsible for compartmentalization of the tumorous tissue, similar to what occurs in nodal or mediastinal lymphomas. The lymphoma cells surround and spread along the vessels and sometimes infiltrate and accumulate beneath the intima, occasionally bulging into the lumen. The large-cells have the morphology of centroblasts or immunoblasts. The most frequent DLBCL subtype is monomorphic or polymorphic *centroblastic lymphoma. Immunoblastic lymphoma with or without plasmablastic differentiation* is less frequent.
2. The second type of lymphoma of the thyroid gland is *marginal zone cell lymphoma of MALT* appearing as diffuse areas with reactive germinal centers (Fig. 6.86) that consist of small centrocyte-like cells surrounding and colonizing the follicles (Fig. 6.87). Often, a lymphoplasmacytic component is present. Sheets of monocytoid B-cells may be seen between the lymphoplasmacytic and the centrocyte-like components. Lymphoepithelial lesions are often found (Fig. 6.88) (Anscombe and Wright 1985; Hyjek and Isaacson 1988). DLBCL may be associated and is interpreted as transformation from MALT lymphoma into a large-B-cell lymphoma. In such DLBCLs, remnants of marginal zone cell lymphoma of MALT are often found, as well as lymphoepithelial lesions with large cells. These secondary lymphomas are reported to have a more aggressive behavior (Higgins and Warnke 2000; Skacel et al. 2000).
3. Rare cases of apparently *primary follicular lymphoma* have been described, as well as a few cases of *plasmacytic lymphoma (primary plasmacytoma)* (Aozasa et al. 1986b; Rubin et al. 1990; Rosaï et al. 1992) (see Chap. 7.2).

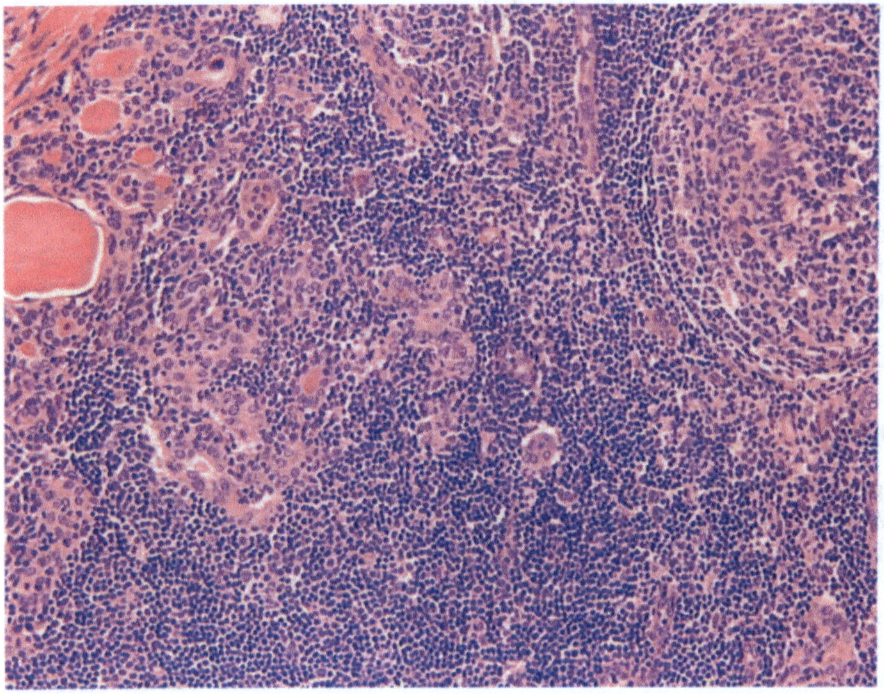

Fig. 6.86. Primary thyroid marginal zone lymphoma of MALT. A diffuse infiltrate of the glandular parenchyma and a reactive germinal center (*upper right corner*) are shown (H and E stain)

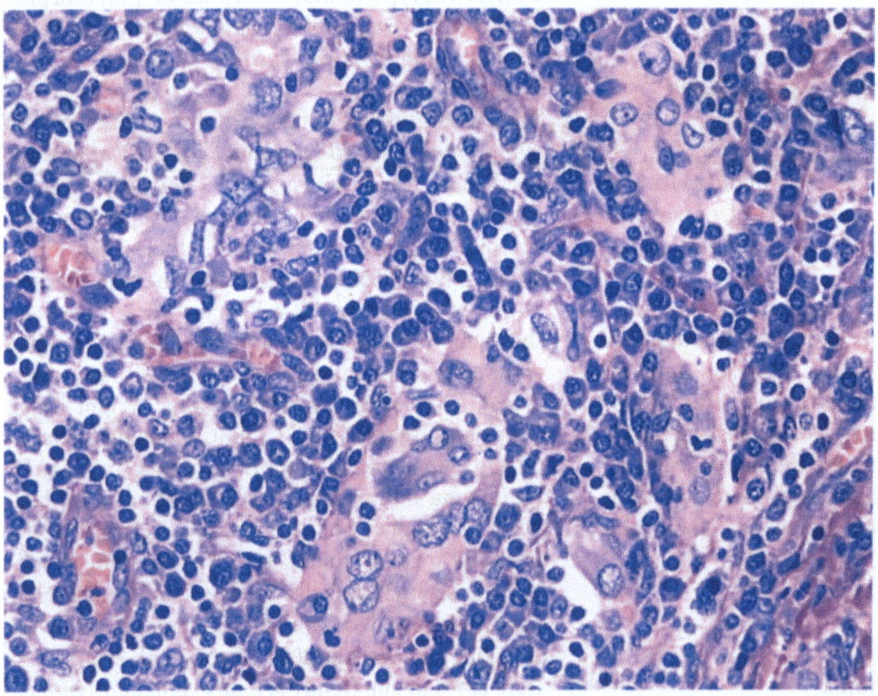

Fig. 6.87. Primary thyroid marginal zone lymphoma of MALT. Same patient as in Fig. 6.86. There is a diffuse infiltrate consisting of monocytoid B-cells and plasma cells, with destruction of the thyroid follicles (Giemsa stain)

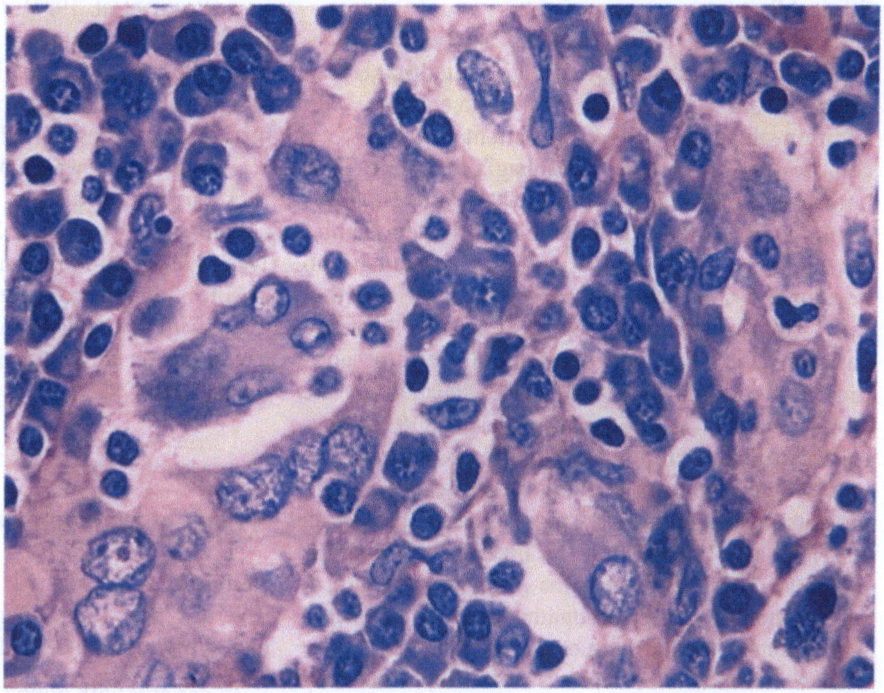

Fig. 6.88. Primary thyroid marginal zone lymphoma of MALT. Same patient as in Figs. 6.86, 6.87. Lymphoepithelial lesions in thyroid follicles and a diffuse infiltrate comprising mostly plasma cells are seen (Giemsa stain)

4. A few cases of *peripheral T-cell lymphoma, unspecified,* have also been reported (Mizukami et al. 1987), as well as a case of anaplastic large-cell lymphoma of T/null-phenotype (Skacel et al. 2000).

Immunohistochemistry

The majority of the primary lymphomas of the thyroid gland express a B-cell immunophenotype (Rosaï et al. 1992), particularly CD20. In addition, immunoglobulins with a light-chain restriction can be demonstrated in the cytoplasm (Aozasa et al. 1987). Anti-cytokeratin as well as anti-thyroglobulin are useful to confirm the diagnosis. Cytokeratin staining allows observation of lymphoepithelial lesions in the follicles.

Differential Diagnosis

Large-B-cell lymphomas have to be distinguished from *undifferentiated carcinoma.* The size of the cells, the architecture, and immunohistochemistry are very useful in differentiating between the two. In addition, *MALT lymphoma* has to be distinguished from *Hashimoto's chronic thyroiditis,* which consists of a diffuse lymphoid infiltrate comprising follicles with hyperplastic germinal centers and associated with an oncocytic metaplasia of the thyroid . The differential diagnosis can be very difficult and immunohistochemistry is often useful to demonstrate a monoclonal population (Hyjek and Isaacson 1988). In addition, a progressive evolution from Hashimoto's thyroiditis to marginal zone cell lymphoma of MALT is possible with intermediate phases. Follicular hyperplasia in MZBCL has to be differentiated from primary follicular lymphoma (see Chap. 4.2.1.6).

Occurrence

Secondary involvement of the thyroid gland by different types of lymphoma is observed at autopsy in about 10% of the cases (Shimaoka et al. 1962).

Primary thyroid lymphoma constitutes approximately 8% of all neoplasias of the thyroid gland (Heimann et al. 1978). They occur in middle-aged or elderly patients, around 60 years of age. The predominance in women is shown by the sex ratio, which ranges from 2:1 to 8:1 according to different series of patients (Anscombe and Wright 1985). A recent series of 53 patients with primary lymphoma of the thyroid, reported by Skacel et al. (2000), confirmed the female predominance (38 females vs 15 males) and the older age (mean: 66.3 years, range 38–90).

Clinical Features

Patients present in 33–60% of the cases with enlargement of the thyroid gland, forming a goiter that is firm or hard (Aozasa et al. 1986a; Matsuzuka et al. 1993). In addition, about 25–30% of the patients complain of a compressive syndrome: dysphagia, dyspnea, or hoarseness (Matsuzuka et al. 1993). Cord paresis occurs in 17% of the patients. Cervical adenopathies may be present. The majority of the patients have no hormonal dysfunction. Only 25–40% show hypothyroidy (Matsuzuka et al. 1993). In 65–80% of the patients, circulating anti-thyroglobulin and/or anti-thyroid microsome antibodies are detected in the blood (Aozasa et al. 1986a; Matsuzuka et al. 1993). Thyroid scan discloses in some patients the presence of one or more cold nodules in the goiter. The majority of patients present with early-stage disease (Rosaï et al. 1992). An associated GI-tract localization is frequent in patients with MALT lymphoma (Stone et al. 1986). A serum monoclonal gammopathy can be associated with plasmacytoma (Rubin et al. 1990).

Treatment often comprises total thyroidectomy (Rosaï et al. 1992), followed by high-dose irradiation. In patients with extrathyroid involvement, surgical resection should be avoided and replaced by irradiation (Rosaï et al. 1992). Chemotherapy is mandatory particularly in patients with stage III–IV disease. The most important prognostic factors are the presence or absence of extrathyroid extension and the stage of the disease. In a series from the Mayo Clinic, the overall 5-year survival rate was 50% (Devine et al. 1981).

A survey of disease evolution showed that all patients with “low grade MALT” were alive at 5 years. There are some indications that secondary “high grade MALT” lymphomas have a more aggressive course than primary DLBCL and patients with the former have a shorter survival (Higgins and Warnke 2000; Skacel et al. 2000).

6.13.2 Malignant Lymphoma of the Adrenal Gland

Definition

Several types of adrenal gland involvement by malignant lymphomas can be distinguished:

1. In patients with lymphomas of other sites, the adrenal glands may be involved at a microscopic level, disclosed only at autopsy, and with a silent clinical presentation.

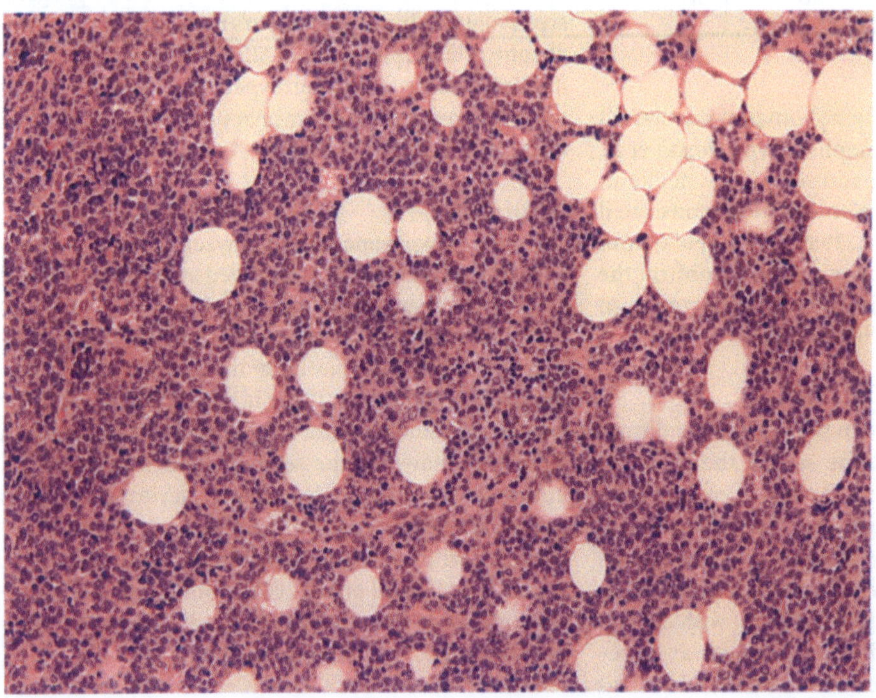

Fig. 6.89. Primary adrenal gland large-B-cell lymphoma extending into the surrounding adipose tissue (H and E stain)

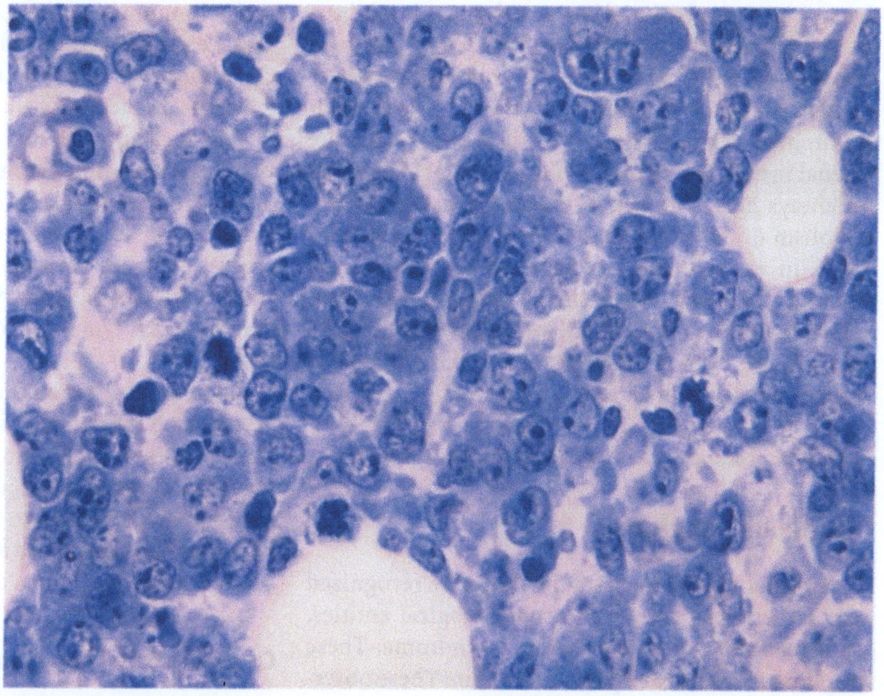

Fig. 6.90. Primary adrenal gland large-B-cell lymphoma. Same patient as in Fig. 6.89. Diffuse polymorphic centroblastic lymphoma (Giemsa stain)

2. In other patients, masses may develop, destroying one or both adrenal glands, sometimes leading to hypoadrenalism (Gamelin et al. 1992). This type of involvement is mostly observed in DLBCL (Figs. 6.89, 6.90). A few patients present with primary lymphoma, without any other tumor site (Ohsawa et al. 1996, review of the literature).

List of Entities

- Diffuse large-B-cell lymphoma (the most frequently occurring)
- Follicular lymphoma
- Small B-cell and NK/T-cell lymphomas (rare)

It can be difficult to distinguish malignant lymphoma of the adrenal gland from primary carcinoma of the cortex or the medulla or metastasis of carcinomas of various organs. Immunohistochemistry is mandatory for the diagnosis.

Secondary involvement of adrenal glands occur in about 4% of patients with a lymphoma (Paling and Williamson 1983). In a large study, 24.9% of adrenal gland involvements were disclosed at autopsy (Rosenberg et al. 1961). The adrenal glands are mostly involved by lymphoma with initial localization in the kidney or urogenital tract, the gonads (ovary, testis), and the mediastinum. Bilateral destruction of adrenal glands and hypoadrenalism are rare (Carey et al. 1987; Huminer et al. 1988; Gamelin et al. 1992).

Only a very few adrenal gland lymphomas are really primary and not all patients present with hypoadrenalism. Ohsawa et al. (1996) reported on 20 patients from a nation-wide study conducted in Japan. They also found 27 cases published in Western countries and five from Japan in the English literature. In addition to these cases, at least four others have been published (Delafaye et al. 1990; Utsunomiya et al. 1992; Miyamura et al. 1993; Levaltier et al. 1994; Perrier et al. 1994).

Apparently, primary adrenal gland lymphoma with adrenal gland insufficiency occurs mostly in adults (Gamelin et al. 1992; Ohsawa et al. 1996) 40–87 years of age (median: 65 years). There is a slight female predominance.

Clinical Features

Patients complain of anorexia, weight loss, and abdominal pain. Weakness and hypotension suggest adrenal insufficiency. Radiography and CT scan disclose bilateral adrenal gland tumor masses. When adrenal insufficiency is suspected, basal hormonal serum levels have to be evaluated. Often they are borderline and only stimulation tests can prove the hormonal failure (Gamelin et al. 1992). Such tests should be done prior to initiation of chemotherapy because of risk of acute adrenal insufficiency (Gamelin et al. 1992). LDH levels are always high. The risk of death due to pulmonary embolism or infectious shock syndrome is significant (Gamelin et al. 1992). Recovery of normal adrenal function following successful treatment has been reported (Carey et al. 1987). Dissemination of the lymphoma to the liver and the central nervous system has been found (Carey et al. 1987).

6.14 Cutaneous Lymphoma

Some primary lymphomas of the skin were recognized early on as being unique clinicopathological entities, e.g. mycosis fungoides and Sézary's syndrome. These lymphomas are observed only in the skin. These observations started a long lasting discussion on the classification of cutaneous lymphomas. In 1980, Edelson introduced the term cutaneous T-cell lymphoma. Around 1987, it became obvious that cutaneous lymphomas of B-cell type without extracutaneous manifestation behave quite differently than their nodal counterparts. This led to the basic concept of cutaneous T- and B-cell lymphomas (CTCL and CBCL). A major breakthrough was achieved with a proposal by a Dutch group in 1994, and the publication of the EORTC classification in 1997 (Willemze et al. 1994, 1997). These investigators clearly distinguished B- and T-cell types and divided them, according to their clinical aggressiveness, into indolent, intermediate, and aggressive lymphomas. Overall, there is still a morphological basis to the classification, which to some extent correlates with the Kiel classification. However, the clinical aspect, especially in terms of prognosis, dominates. Thus in some entities the clinical aspect has priority, in others immunophenotypic antigen expression. For example, in lymphomas of the B-cell lineage, large-cell lymphoma of the leg is described as a distinct clinicopathological entity due to the primary occurrence of this lymphoma on the leg. In the group of CTCLs, the morphology has secondary priority, especially regarding the small, medium, and large pleomorphic subtypes. The EORTC classification gave priority to the immunohistochemical expression of CD30 and thus classified these lymphomas as CD30-positive and CD30-negative, which to some extent correlates with the clinical outcome.

This strategy was not completely in line with the WHO classification (Willemze and Meijer 2000). The major discrepancies and remaining questions are the following: Does CD30 expression take precedence over other criteria? Do we need a separate NK/T-cell category for the skin? Is primary CBCL a better description than follicular lymphoma? Do we need a separate entity for CLBCL of the leg?

All of these questions are of clinical relevance. Here, we describe the cutaneous lymphomas primarily with respect to their morphology. Mostly we have followed the EORTC classification, indicating the relationship of the individual entities to the WHO classification. We have also indicated those aspects that might be of clinical relevance.

Cutaneous B-Cell Lymphoma

- Extranodal marginal zone B-cell lymphoma of MALT
  - Skin-associated lymphomoid tissue (SALT) lymphoma, including immunocytoma
- Follicular lymphoma
- Diffuse large-B-cell lymphoma
  - Centroblastic/immunoblastic, including large-B-cell lymphoma of the leg
  - Intravascular large-B-cell lymphoma
  - T-cell-rich B-cell lymphoma
- Plasmacytoma
- Addendum: Infectious diseases and primary cutaneous B-cell lymphomas

Cutaneous T-Cell Lymphomas

- Mycosis fungoides
  - Classical type
  - Follicular mucinosis variant
  - Pagetoid reticulosis variant
  - Granulomatous slack skin disease
- Sézary's syndrome
- Primary cutaneous CD30-positive lymphoproliferations
  - Anaplastic large-cell lymphoma
  - Lymphomatoid papulosis
  - Borderline lesions

- Peripheral T-cell lymphoma, unspecified
  - Pleomorphic small-cell, pleomorphic medium- and large-cell
  - Adult T-cell lymphoma/leukemia (ATL) with skin involvement
- Primary cutaneous NK/T-cell lymphomas
  - Cutaneous NK/T-cell lymphoma, nasal type
  - CD8 epidermotropic T-cell lymphoma
  - Blastic NK/T-cell lymphoma
  - Subcutaneous panniculitis-like T-cell lymphoma

6.14.1 Primary Cutaneous B-Cell Lymphoma

6.14.1.1 Cutaneous Marginal Zone B-Cell Lymphoma/SALT Lymphoma, Including Immunocytoma (ICD-O: 9699/3)

Until 1994, primary lymphocytic infiltrates of the skin were designated as immunocytoma according to the Kiel classification. After the MALT concept was developed, it became increasingly clear that at least a number of these primary skin lymphomas belong to the MALT system due to the dissemination to other typical MALT localizations and to the immunophenotype. Moreover, the same cellular constituents could be found in the different sites, including the skin. Although the MALT concept, including the skin as SALT lymphomas, was not included into the EORTC classification, and although there is an ongoing discussion whether primary immunocytomas of the skin do exist, the concept of including such skin lymphomas into the group of extranodal marginal zone lymphomas is now mostly accepted. Whatever the truth in this controversy is, both groups of lymphomas show strong overlap, which makes it difficult or even impossible to distinguish between them with certainty. Therefore, we will use the term immunocytoma, equivalent to SALT lymphoma, to include primary skin immunocytoma (Duncan and LeBoit 1997).

Synonyms

- Kiel: Immunocytoma
- REAL: Extranodal marginal zone B-cell lymphoma
- WHO: Extranodal marginal zone B-cell lymphoma of MALT

Definition

Primary SALT lymphoma is a predominately nodular infiltrate present throughout the dermis and infiltrating into the subcutaneous fat. The neoplastic cells consist of small lymphocytes, plasmacytoid cells, and plasma cells, as well as monocytoid and centrocyte-like cells. Sometimes this infiltrate surrounds reactive follicles and may even colonize them.

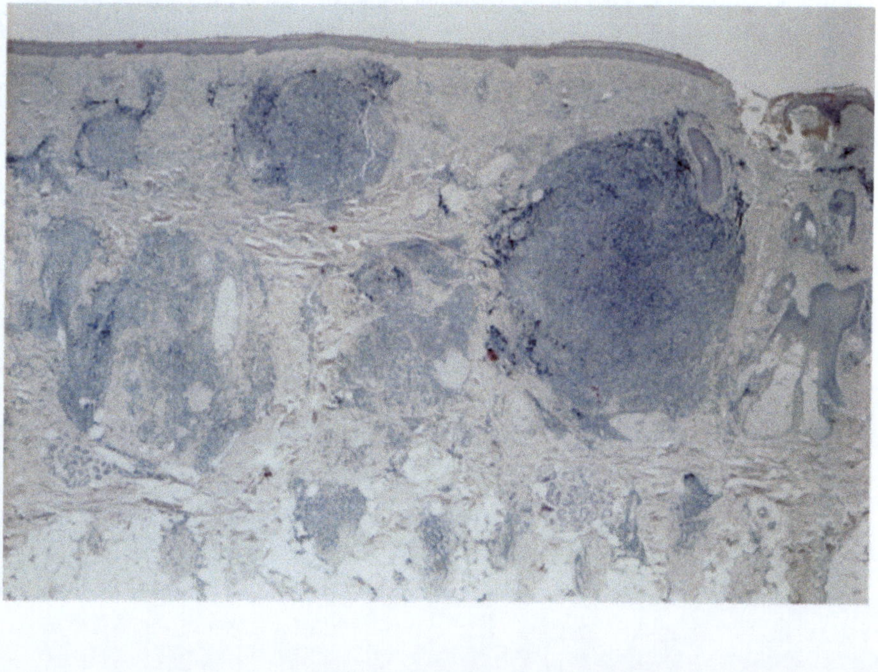

Fig. 6.91. Skin-associated lymphoid tissue (SALT) lymphoma with a lymphocytic infiltrate in the dermis sparing the dermo-epidermal junction (Giemsa stain)

Morphology

Under low-power magnification, the infiltrate is mostly nodular, less frequently diffuse (Figs. 6.91, 6.92), and dominates the deep dermis, sometimes infiltrating the subcutaneous fat. An epidermotropism is absent; moreover, the upper dermis is mostly spared by the infiltrate. Sometimes the nodular pattern is dominated by follicular structures with reactive germinal centers (Fig. 6.93). These show a starry-sky pattern and are rich in blasts. The arrangement of the cellular infiltrate is highly variable (Fig. 6.94). Small lymphocytes may predominate with plasmacytoid and plasma cells. These tumors were described as immunocytomas in the earlier literature and show a more diffuse growth pattern. Intranuclear PAS-positive inclusions can be observed. Sometimes, monocytoid cells with a clear

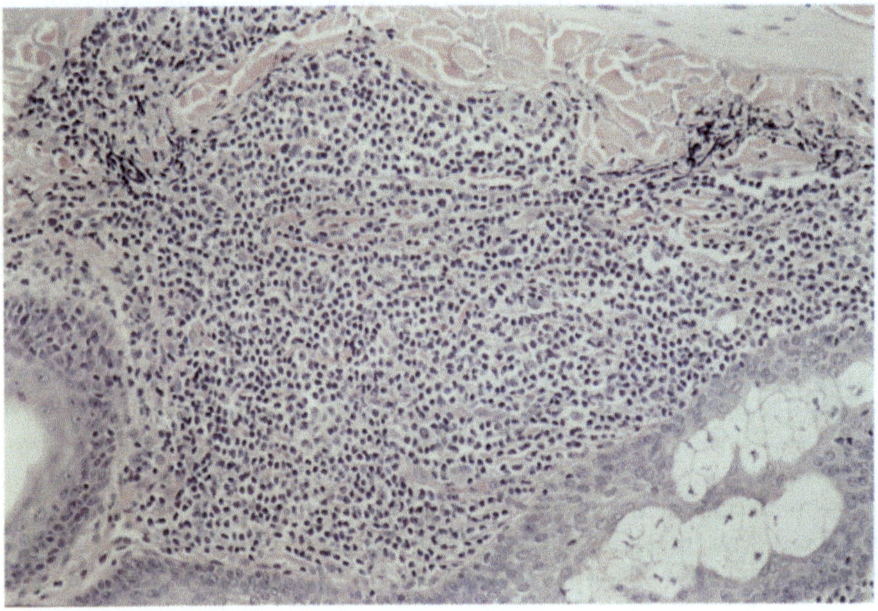

Fig. 6.92. SALT-lymphoma with a quite monotonous infiltrate of small, partly centrocyte-like cells (H and E stain)

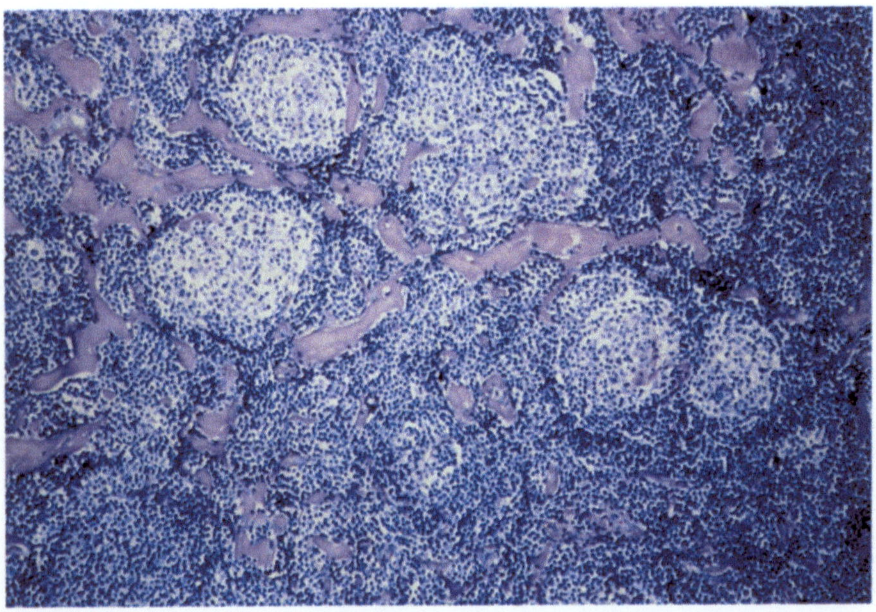

Fig. 6.93. SALT-lymphoma with a neoplastic infiltrate between reactive follicles (Giemsa stain)

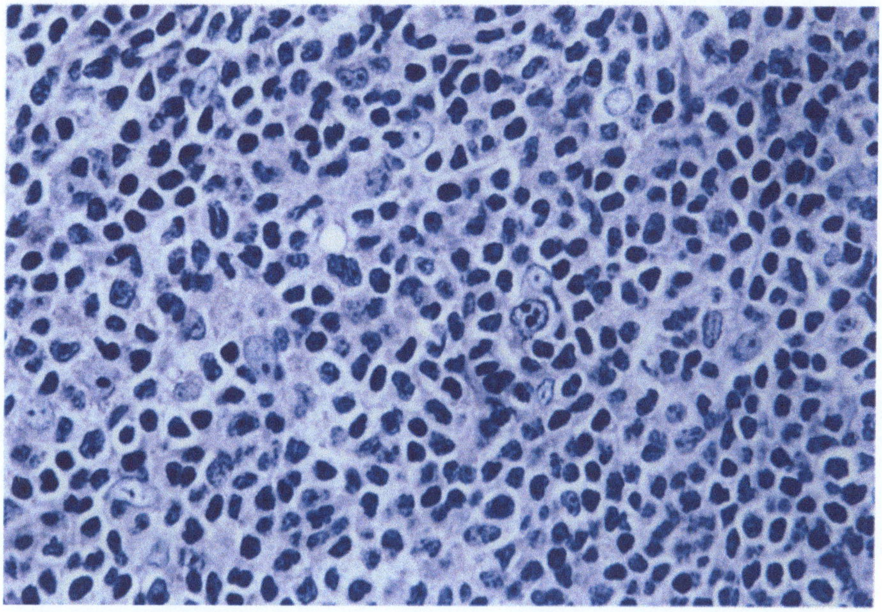

Fig. 6.94. SALT-lymphoma with a monotonous cellular infiltrate with centrocyte-like cells and a few blasts (Giemsa stain)

cytoplasm and centrocyte-like cells are found in large sheets. Finally, some tumors have an overwhelming number of plasma cells, especially in the interfollicular areas, with prominent germinal centers, or at the outer zone of the infiltrate. Some blasts are always intermingled.

Immunohistochemistry

All tumors stain positive for CD20 and CD79α and are consistently negative for CD5 and CD23, in contrast to nodal small lymphocytic lymphoma (B-CLL) and its variant lymphoplasmacytoid immunocytoma. The neoplastic cells are also negative for CD43 and CD10, whereas the reactive germinal centers may show weak reactivity for the latter antibody. A light-chain restriction can be found in about 60–90% of the tumors depending on the sensitivity of the staining method. About 50–60% have detectable *surface Ig* staining with light-chain restriction. In the majority of tumors, a more or less dominating plasma cell clone shows monoclonal *cytoplasmic Ig* light-chain expression (Fig. 6.95a, 6.95b) (Servitje et al. 2002). The heavy-chain can be IgG or IgM. Almost all tumors have detectable remnants of follicular dendritic cells, as shown by staining for either CD21 or CD23. In lymphomas with reactive germinal centers, this network is pronounced and well-preserved. The proliferation rate (Ki-67) is low, between 15 and 25%. If this proliferation rate increases focally, it may indicate focal transformation into a DLBCL.

Genetics

Typical chromosomal abnormalities have not been described in a larger series.

Almost all tumors have detectable monoclonal Ig heavy-chain gene rearrangement.

Differential Diagnosis

Reactive Cutaneous Lymphoid Infiltrates (Pseudolymphoma). In tumors that are predominantly nodular with many follicles, lymphoid hyperplasia (so-called pseudolymphoma) together with *follicular lymphoma* is the major differential diagnosis (but also see chapter on follicular lymphoma). Both occur at more or less the same sites. In lymphoid hyperplasia as well as in SALT lymphoma, the germinal centers are reactive (see Chap. 4.2.1.5., Differential Diagnosis). Thus, immunohistochemistry is required for a correct diagnosis. It is of major importance to note that plasma cells can be monoclonal in follicular lymphoma with plasmacellular differentiation as well as in SALT lymphoma. In such cases, the structure and the cellular components of the follicles are decisive. The germinal centers are reactive in SALT lymphoma, mostly with a high content of blasts and a high proliferation rate (Ki-67).

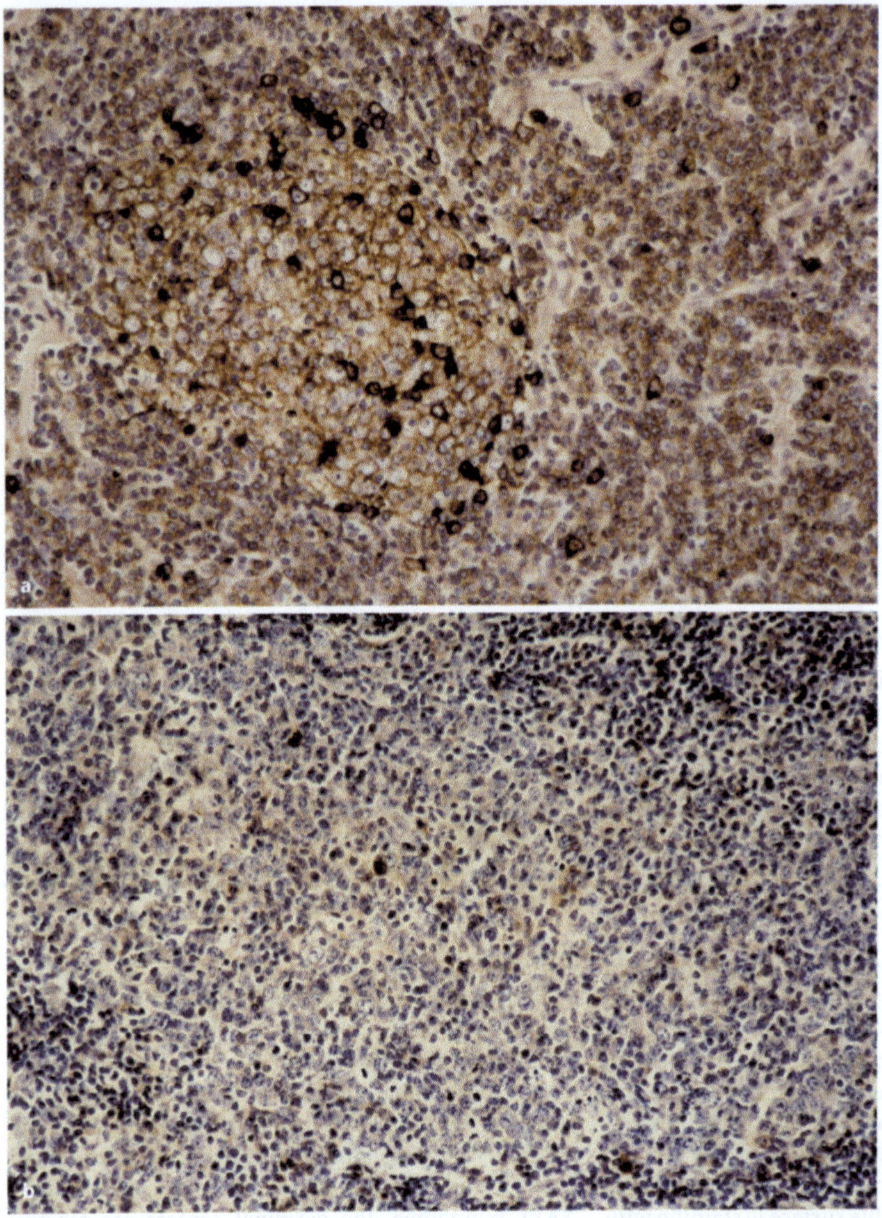

Fig. 6.95 a, b. Immunohistochemical staining for Ig-light chain. **a** The reactive follicle is colonized by monoclonal plasma cells. The surrounding infiltrate shows surface κ-light-chain. **b** Some reactive Ig-λ-positive plasma cells within the reactive follicle (immunohistochemistry, peroxidase stain)

Sheets of marginal zone cells should be carefully searched for, as these do not occur in lymphoid hyperplasia. The same is true for intranuclear inclusions. In lymphoid hyperplasia, T-cells usually clearly dominate the infiltrate, in contrast to MZBCL (Baldassano et al. 1999).

Secondary MALT or Extracutaneous (Nodal) Immunocytoma. The infiltration pattern and the cellular constituents are identical to those of primary disease. Also, the immunophenotype is the same except in cases of primary nodal lymphocytic lymphoma (lymphoplasmacytoid immunocytoma) which spread secondarily to the skin. Such tumors may be CD5- and/or CD23-positive. In all other cases, clinical data are essential.

Similar to other CBCLs, also SALT can be associated with a *Borrelia burgdorferi infection*. The detection of a serum titer characteristic for a florid infection does not by itself exclude the diagnosis of lymphoma (see Chap. 6.14.1.4).

Occurrence

SALT lymphomas make up about one-third of all CBCLs. The medium age is between 50 and 55 years, thus the patients are younger than those with DLBCLs. There is a slight male preponderance (Bailey et al. 1996; Cerroni et al. 1997a).

Clinical Presentation and Prognosis

The patients mostly present with solitary nodules, larger papules, or plaques occurring mostly on the extremities and less frequently on the trunk (Servitje et al. 2002). About 20% of the patients have multiple infiltrates from the onset. A few patients present with a monoclonal gammopathy. A minority has bone marrow involvement and/or other sites of involvement, especially typical sites of MALT lymphoma (lung, breast, orbit). The opposite may also occur; that is, skin involvement can be secondary to a primary MALT lymphoma at another site. In general, an additional extracutaneous manifestation slightly worsens the prognosis in that such patients have persistent disease (Bailey et al. 1996; Cerroni et al. 1997a; de la Fouchardiere et al. 1999).

The 5-year survival is between 90 and 100% mostly following radiotherapy.

6.14.1.2 Follicular Lymphoma

Synonyms

- Kiel: Centroblastic-centrocytic
- REAL: Follicular lymphoma
- WHO: Follicular lymphoma

Definition

Follicular lymphoma consists of a non-epidermotropic infiltrate with a more or less pronounced follicular or nodular growth pattern. The cellular constituents are centrocytes and centroblasts with a large number of intermingled T-cells. A pattern of tingible body macrophages is absent. Mostly, the infiltrate is evenly distributed throughout the dermis, frequently with extension into the subcutaneous fat.

Morphology

The patients present with solitary or multiple small plaques, papules, or reddish nodular lesions that predominate in the head and neck areas (Fig. 6.96).

Histology mostly shows an extended infiltrate throughout the dermis, sometimes bottom-heavy with infiltration of the subcutaneous fat. There is no epidermotropism; hair follicles may be infiltrated. A follicular or nodular growth pattern, and sometimes a predominately diffuse pattern is detectable under low-power

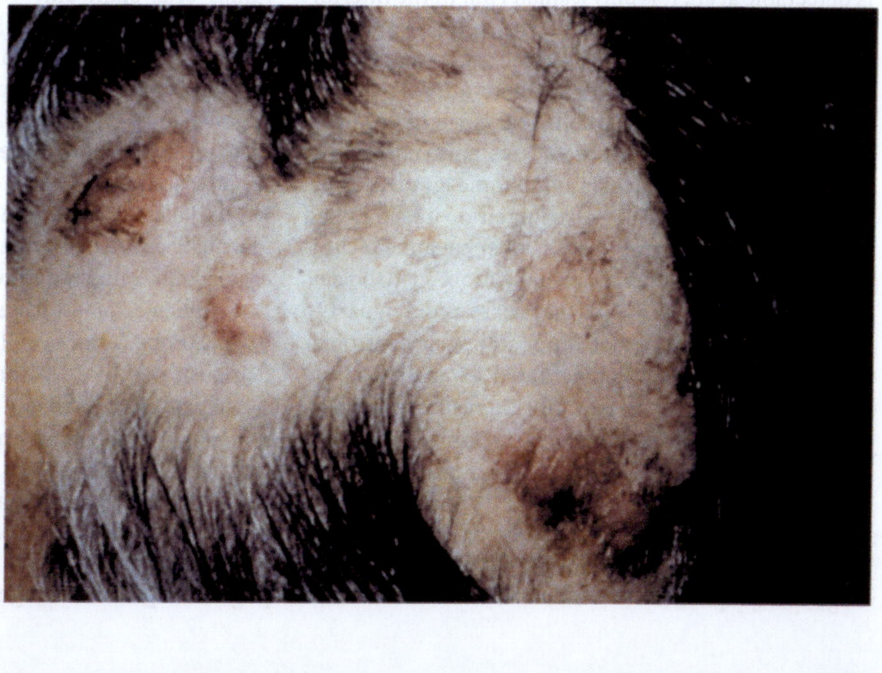

Fig. 6.96. Follicular lymphoma with multiple nodular lesions on the head

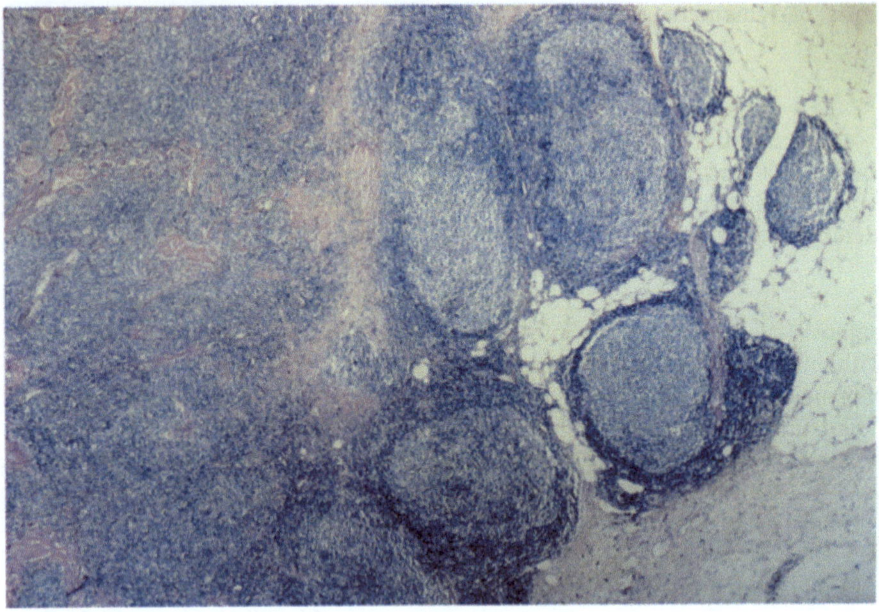

Fig. 6.97. Follicular and diffuse infiltrate of a follicular lymphoma in the dermis infiltrating the subcutaneous fat (Giemsa stain)

magnification (Fig. 6.97). Sometimes, both patterns are observed. Silver impregnation or CD20 staining makes the follicular pattern more easily visible. The follicular structures are usually close to each other. A few reactive follicles may be found. These show a typical starry-sky pattern and possibly zonal compartments. The neoplastic follicles are not well-demarcated from the interfollicular areas. If a follicular mantle zone is detectable at all, it is only a small rim. In the interfollicular areas, a diffuse infiltrate with a high content of small-T-cells intermingled with centrocytes and centroblasts is found. Beyond that, there are also plasma cells and histiocytes. The follicular structures themselves mostly consist of centrocytes and centroblasts corresponding to follicular lymphoma grades 1–3a. The blasts are irregularly distributed or intermingled with the smaller centrocytes. Lesions that appear clinically more tumorous may contain more centroblasts (Pimpinelli et al. 1990). This may correspond in part to follicular lymphoma grade 3b or follicular centroblastic lymphoma according to the Kiel classification. However, the prognosis and thus the value of grading in primary cutaneous follicular lymphoma do not have the same value as in primary nodal lymphomas. Some tumors may show transformation into a higher grade with a large number of blasts, which may occur in sheets. Such tumors may then transform into diffuse large-cell lymphoma.

Immunohistochemistry

The neoplastic cells stain uniformly for CD20 and CD79α. This staining as well as the staining for CD10 clearly demonstrates a follicular growth pattern. The neoplastic follicles or nodules are stained by CD10 in about 30–50% of tumors (Cerroni et al. 2000; Bergmann et al. 2001). The number of positive cases is variable in the literature, perhaps due to the fact that some tumor cells stain only very weakly and thus can be missed by conventional immunostaining without enhancing techniques. Some of the positive cells may have an enhanced strong positivity. The tumor cells are negative for CD5 and CD43 (Berti et al. 1990). In most cases, although the follicles are neoplastic they are also negative for bcl-2 (Kerl and Cerroni 1997; Cerroni et al. 1994, 2000; Child et al. 2001; Bergmann et al. 2001). Lawnicki (2002) described up to 40% bcl-2 positive cases. Expression was inversely related to the grade. Both follicular mantle cells and T-cells stain positive for bcl-2. Almost always, follicular dendritic cells can be demonstrated by CD21 or CD23 expression. However, the network is usually not as dense as in primary nodal follicular lymphomas. The number of Ki-67-positive cells is clearly lower than in reactive germinal centers. The positive cells are irregularly distributed throughout the neoplastic follicles, compared to a zonal pattern in reactive germinal centers. Plasma cells normally show a polyclonal pattern for light-chain staining.

Genetic Features

Monoclonal Ig gene rearrangement patterns were observed in up to 94% of the primary cutaneous follicular lymphomas using Southern blot techniques (Bergman et al. 2001). Other studies detected B-cell clonality with the same technique in only 40% of the tumors (Neri et al. 1995). PCR amplification revealed a large number of clonally derived tumors; this frequency is enhanced by microdissection, which increases the detection of a B-cell clone to more than 90% of primary cutaneous follicular lymphomas (Signoretti et al. 1999).

During testing for bcl-2 rearrangement, a t(14;18) was found only occasionally. The vast majority of primary cutaneous follicular lymphomas do not have this translocation, in contrast to primary nodal follicular lymphomas (Gronbaek et al. 2000; Cerroni et al. 2000; Bergman et al. 2001; Child et al. 2001).

The number of cases studied by classical cytogenetics is very limited, and systematic conclusions cannot be drawn .

Differential Diagnosis

Three major possibilities have to be taken into account:

1. *Reactive cutaneous lymphoid infiltrate (pseudolymphoma).* The number and the significance of morphological criteria for differentiating these two entities are very limited. Most of the criteria given below describe a tendency but are not absolute for distinguishing benign from malignant. Follicular lymphoma more frequently shows an infiltration of the trunk with a bottom-heavy infiltrate and extension into the subcutaneous fat. The follicles are not well-demarcated and do not show a starry-sky pattern or a zonal arrangement. The blasts are irregularly distributed, the CD20 B cells extend throughout the follicles, and a well developed follicular mantle is absent.
   Immunohistochemistry is mandatory but it is hard to demonstrate light-chain restriction within the follicles. The latter always requires several-step titration of antibody dilution for κ and λ; additionally, an enhancing technique has to be used. This procedure will give diagnostic results in about 30–50% of the cases.
   PCR to detect a rearrangement of Ig heavy-chain genes has to follow. This can be decisive in about 70% of the cases, demonstrating either a dominating band for a clonal B-cell proliferation or a smear (Brady et al. 1999). However, even the demonstration of a clonal rearrangement cannot be used as an absolute criterion for diagnosing follicular lymphoma (Wood et al. 1989; Rijlaarsdam et al. 1992).
   Therefore, clinical data should be included in these doubtful cases; in particular, an infection with *B. burgdorferi* has to be ruled out. Nonetheless, even demonstration of a positive serum titer does not completely exclude a follicular lymphoma as the two may be associated with each other. Moreover cases have been reported in which CBCL developed from a lymphoid hyperplasia associated with *B. burgdorferi* infection (Jelic and Filipovic-Ljeskovic 1999; Goodlad et al. 2000a,b; Slater 2001). The prognosis of both diseases is very favorable so that even a 5-year disease-free follow-up is not completely decisive (see Addendum).
   The conclusion from these observations is that the clinical behavior of individual doubtful cases that have been investigated with all of the above-described techniques have to be followed carefully, and new efflorescences have to be rebiopsied (Willemze and Meijer 1998).
2. *Marginal zone B-cell lymphoma/SALT lymphoma*: Small lymphocytes and plasma cells as well as centrocyte-like and monocytoid cells in a diffuse growth pattern or associated with reactive germinal centers characterize SALT lymphoma. Frequently, a monotypic plasma cell component is detected that is mostly interfollicular or at the margin of the lymphoid infiltrate.
3. *Secondary follicular lymphoma of the skin/systemic follicular lymphoma:* Rare cases occur in which a *follicular lymphoma* secondarily infiltrates the skin. These are morphologically almost indistinguishable from primary nodal *follicular lymphomas.* In secondary disease, the follicular structures are slightly more pronounced. If there is no doubt about the neoplastic nature of the infiltrate, immunohistochemistry is extremely helpful in classifying the disease. Systemic *follicular lymphoma* usually features up-regulated CD10 staining and, even more significant, bcl-2 positivity of the neoplastic germinal centers. This means that a bcl-2-positive germinal centers in the skin should raise suspicion of a systemic follicular lymphoma.

Occurrence
In most reports, follicular lymphoma is the most frequent primary CBCL. However, in the past a number of marginal zone lymphomas may have been misinterpreted as follicular lymphoma. The frequency is thus 30–70% of all CBCLs. There seems to be a slight male preponderance. The median age is around 50–60 years (Bergman et al. 2001; Cerroni et al. 2000; Yang et al. 2000).

Clinical Presentation and Prognosis
Patients mostly present with solitary lesions, especially on the head and neck; about one-third have multiple nodules or efflorescences on their arms or back. If the lesions are untreated, they increase slowly in size over months and years. About 50% of patients will have recurrences. Nevertheless, the overall prognosis is excellent, with a survival rate over 90% (Yang et al. 2000; Bergman et al. 2001).

6.14.1.3 Plasmacytoma

Synonyms
- Kiel: Plasmacytic lymphoma/plasmacytoma
- REAL: Plasmacytoma/plasma cell myeloma
- WHO: Extraosseous plasmacytoma

Primary plasmacytomas of the skin is an extremely rare disease within the heterogeneous spectrum of plasma cell neoplasms (Muscardin et al. 2000). They present either as solitary lesions, or as multiple lesions in the same area. There is a predilection for the head and trunk. The infiltrate spares the epidermis. It shows a circumscribed, non-capsulated nodular or diffuse growth pattern sometimes penetrating the subcutaneous fat. The neoplastic cells are mostly mature-appearing plasma cells, although sometimes anaplastic infiltrates are observed. Other non-neoplastic cells are rare. If a monotonous infiltrate of plasma cells is found, the clonality of this infiltrate always has to be checked, as even reactive infiltrates – sometimes described as plasma cell granulomas – may appear monotonous and tumor-like. Plasmacytoma of the skin also has to be differentiated from lymphoplasmacytic immunocytoma and marginal zone lymphoma with marked or even predominant plasmacytic differentiation. The median age is around 60 years. The survival after 5 years is around 40–50% (Wong et al. 1994; Muscardin et al. 2000).

Details are given in Chap. 7.2.

6.14.1.4 Diffuse Large-B-Cell Lymphoma

Morphological and Clinical Variants
- Centroblastic/immunoblastic
- T-cell-rich B-cell
- Intravascular large-B-cell lymphoma

These lymphomas may occur primarily in the skin. Their morphology is described in detail in the chapter on nodal lymphomas. Intravascular large-B-cell lymphoma mostly shows additional manifestations, such as CNS, bone or soft tissue. If the large-cell lymphomas are localized, the prognosis is favorable. Large-B-cell lymphoma of the leg is described separately as it has some distinct features in terms of the antigen profile and the prognosis. In contrast to nodal DLBCLs, they do not exhibit a t(14;18) translocation (Kim et al. 2003).

Beyond that DLBCL is described in Chap. 4.2.2.

Large-B-Cell Lymphoma of the Leg

Synonyms
- Kiel: Centroblastic/immunoblastic
- REAL: Diffuse large-B-cell
- WHO: Diffuse large-B-cell lymphoma

Definition
The cutaneous infiltrate is made up of non-epidermotropic large-B-cells, mostly centroblasts and immunoblasts. Due to the different clinical behavior of this lymphoma, localized and multifocal occurrences have to be distinguished as well as specific localization on the leg. Large-B-cell lymphoma of the leg is described as a distinct entity in the EORTC classification (Willemze and Meijer 1999). However, recent descriptions of Paulli et al. (2002) dispute that this entity differs from other DLBCLs in terms of immunohistochemistry and molecular genetics.

Morphology
The reader should refer to the chapter on nodal lymphomas (Chap. 4.2.2), as the cytology of lymphoma types that may occur primarily in the skin is almost the same as that in the lymph node. In principle, the infiltrate is clearly dominated by blasts, except in T-cell-rich B-cell lymphoma (TCRBCL), and forms sheets of neoplastic cells present mostly throughout the dermis and frequently extending into the subcutaneous fat (Fig. 6.98).

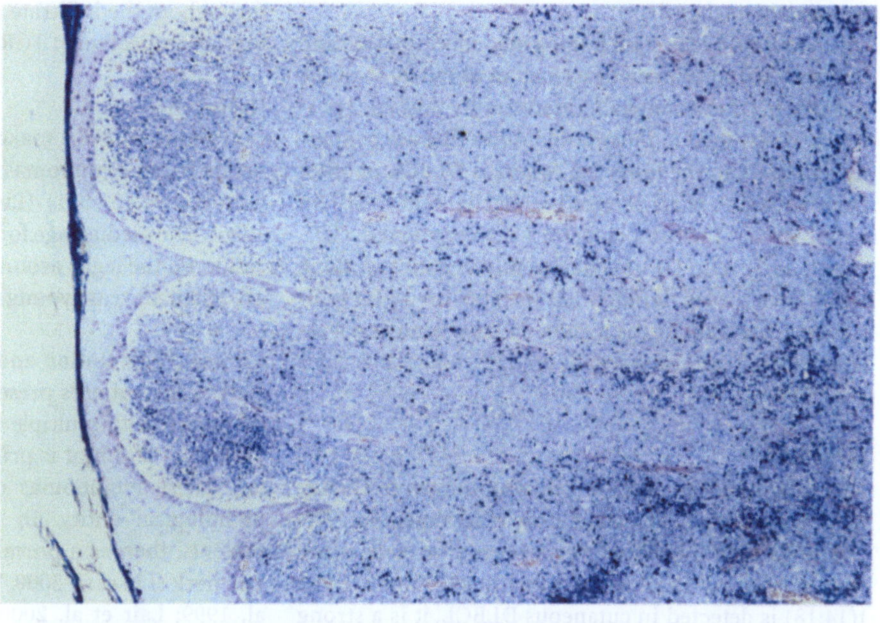

Fig. 6.98. Primary diffuse large-B-cell lymphoma of the skin infiltrating the upper and lower dermis without epidermotropism

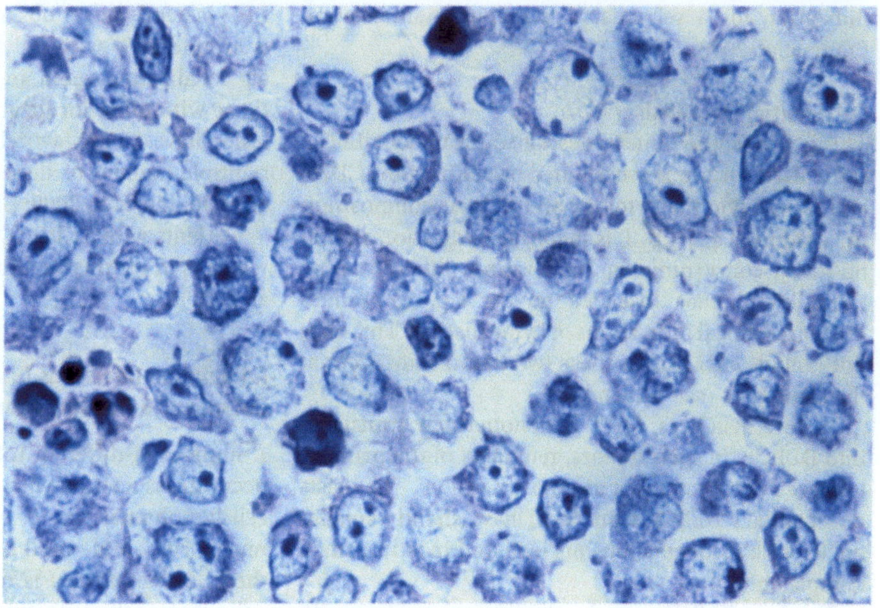

Fig. 6.99. Primary diffuse large-B-cell lymphoma of the skin, variant centroblastic lymphoma (Giemsa stain)

Overall, the arrangement is identical to that seen in nodal DLBCL with a variable amount of centroblasts, immunoblasts and large centrocyte-like cells (Fig. 6.99). Also, some multilobulated cells are present. The infiltration pattern is almost always diffuse; follicular structures are rarely found. Some small lymphocytes are intermingled. Mitotic figures are frequent.

TCRBCL has the same infiltration pattern, frequently extending into the subcutaneous fat. The majority of cells are mature non-neoplastic T-cells intermingled with some large atypical cells (B-blasts).This variant has to be kept in mind as it is of importance for the differential diagnosis of lymphoid hyperplasia (pseudolymphoma) and pleomorphic CD30-negative T-cell lymphoma (peripheral T-cell lymphoma, unspecified).

Immunohistochemistry
The neoplastic cells stain homogeneously for CD20 and CD79α. CD10 has been described in about 30% of the tumors, bcl-2 in about half. Interestingly this bcl-2 positivity is confined to those lymphomas that are primarily localized on the lower leg, whereas DLBCL in other cutaneous sites is bcl-2-negative (Geelen et al. 1998). In about 50% of the tumors, bcl-6 is also expressed. CD5, CD43, and cyclin D1 are consistently negative. Among DLBCLs of the leg, lymphomas with positivity for lymphocyte function antigen (LFA-1) have a more favorable course than those which are LFA-1-negative (Lair et al. 2000).

Genetics
More than 80% of large-B-cell lymphomas of the leg show a clonal Ig heavy-chain gene rearrangement. The translocation t(14;18) has never been observed, either in lymphoma of the leg or at other localizations. If the t(14;18) is detected in cutaneous DLBCL, it is a strong indication for a secondary cutaneous manifestation (Yang et al. 2000).

Differential Diagnosis
This is almost the same as described for nodal DLBCL. If the B-cell origin is ascertained by staining for CD20, and if based on the cytology and cellular composition the diagnosis of DLBCL is made, an indication should be given concerning the localization, differentiating those lymphomas localized on the leg. Sometimes there are clinical indications of Lyme disease. This does not exclude a DLBCL as these two events may occur at the same time (see Addendum).

In rare instances, SALT lymphoma may transform into DLBCL. In such tumors, remnants of the primary low-grade compartment are mostly visible. The blasts of secondary DLBCL from SALT have slightly smaller nuclei with inconspicuous nucleoli and mostly a small cytoplasmic rim.

Rarely, a DLBCL may develop in arms or legs with chronic lymphedema. In such patients with chronic edema, an angiosarcoma (Stewart-Treves syndrome) may develop after 20–30 years, which thus has to be differentiated from DLBCL (Vermeer et al. 1996; Torres-Paoli and Sanchez 2000).

TCRBCL is included in the differential diagnosis of lymphoid hyperplasia (pseudolymphoma) and pleomorphic T-cell lymphoma; however, the presence of CD20/CD79α-staining blasts diffusely distributed throughout the infiltrate and the lack of germinal centers are indicative of TCRBCL.

Occurrence
Cutaneous DLBCLs make up about one-third of cutaneous B-cell lymphomas. There is a clear female preponderance (3–5:1) (Liu et al. 2000; Vermeer et al. 1996). The median age for patients with primary localization on the leg is around 75 years, the other patients are about 10 years younger.

Clinical Presentation and Prognosis
Half of the patients present with solitary nodules, the other half with multiple nodules. In two-thirds of the patients, the tumor is primarily localized on the lower leg. These lymphomas constitute a distinct clinicopathological entity. In the remaining one-third of patients, there is a prevalence of nodules on the head and neck (Liu et al. 2000; Vermeer et al. 1996; Grange et al. 1999; Lair et al. 2000). B symptoms or increased LDH is nearly never observed. The 5-year survival rate is around 50% with polychemotherapy. Patients with leg localization seem to have poorer outcome than those with other localizations. Patients with a solitary lesion have a more favorable prognosis than those with multiple nodules or disseminated disease (Vermeer et al. 1996; Liu et al. 2000; Grange et al. 1999).

Patients with TCRBCL have an excellent prognosis, which is in contrast to those with nodal TCRBCL (Li et al. 2001).

Addendum: Infectious Diseases and Primary Cutaneous B-Cell Lymphomas

A number of different infectious agents are known to occur in association with several types of cutaneous B-cell lymphomas, i.e. *B. burgdorferi*, HCV, EBV, paramyxovirus, and molluscum contagiosum. Among these, *B. burgdorferi* is the most important one. This spirochete is the causative agent for Lyme disease. During the course of this disease different cutaneous disorders may occur, including erythema chronicum migrans, acrodermatitis chronica atrophicans, and lymphocytoma cutis.

Initially, it was thought that the detection of a positive antibody titer indicating a florid infection excluded the diagnosis of a CBCL automatically and instead implied diagnosis of a lymphoid hyperplasia (pseudolymphoma). This was substantiated by the observation that many cutaneous lesions disappeared after antibiotic therapy. During the last 10 years, however, increasing evidence has been presented that the two diseases may occur simultaneously, so that an infection does not rule out a CBCL. Using PCR techniques, the presence of *Borrelia* in some cutaneous lymphomas could be demonstrated. Cerroni reported *Borrelia*-specific genomic DNA in nearly 20% of CBCLs (Cerroni et al. 1997b). This posed the question whether infectious agents may be causative for some CBCLs. Different types of CBCL have been described, including MZBCL/SALT lymphoma, DLBCL, and follicular lymphoma (Fig. 6.99, 6.100). Goodland presented evidence for the development of a MZBCL from *Borrelia*-associated B-cell proliferation. This observation may indicate that a chronic stimulation of lymphoid tissue in the setting of a *Borrelia* infection can lead to an overt lymphoma. This situation is very similar to the association between gastric *H. pylori* infection and MALT lymphoma (Slater 2001). Thus we are faced with a similar problem in the morphological differential diagnosis. Independent of a possible *Borrelia* infection a lymphoid hyperplasia (pseudolymphoma) has to be differentiated from a CBCL, e.g. MZBCL or follicular lymphoma. In all of these doubtful cases, monoclonality has to be checked either by immunohistochemistry or, in negative tumors, by PCR for rearrangement of Ig heavy-chain genes.

Other associations between infectious agents and CBCL have been described, although this seems to be a very rare and sometimes doubtful event. Single cases associated with chronic hepatitis C, EBV, or HHV8 have been detailed (Nagore et al. 2000; McKiernan et al. 1999; Morand et al. 1999).

This indicates that the clinical status of the patient has to be taken into account; however, a morphologically based diagnosis including immunohistochemistry and molecular clonality studies is of independent value and thus should be carried out separately.

6.14.2 Cutaneous T-Cell Lymphoma

6.14.2.1 Mycosis Fungoides – Classical Type (ICD-O: 9700/3)

Synonyms

- Kiel: Small-cell cerebriform – mycosis fungoides
- REAL: Mycosis fungoides
- WHO: Mycosis fungoides

Definition

Mycosis fungoides (reviews: Kerl and Kresbach 1979; Sterry 1985; Slater 1987; Geerts 1988) is a T-lymphocytic lymphoma with primary manifestation in the skin. Here it manifests primarily as an epidermotropic

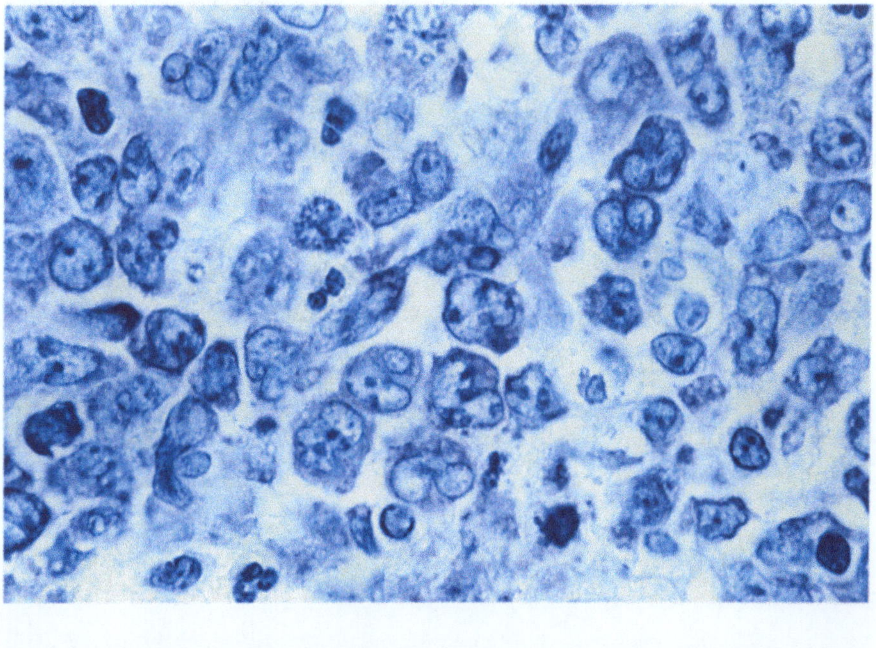

Fig. 6.100. Primary diffuse large-B-cell lymphoma of the skin with multiple multilobulated centroblasts in a case associated with borreliosis (Giemsa stain)

band-like infiltrate. Lymph nodes and other organs are not involved until later in the clinical course. The T-lymphocytes of mycosis fungoides have "cerebriform" nuclei (so-called Lutzner cells), i.e. nuclei with deep indentations resembling the sulci on the surface of the brain.

Histology

The histology of mycosis fungoides is reviewed in Matthews (1985). In the early phase, a band-shaped epidermotropic infiltrate is found in the *upper* papillary dermis, with only focal involvement of the lower epidermis (patch stage). Spongiosis is seen quite frequently, although it is not clear whether this is due to the neoplastic infiltrate or to an overlying dermatitis (Fig. 6.101a). The infiltrate consists of small to medium-sized pleomorphic cells and exceptionally large blasts (Fig. 6.101b). The cells have, in part, deeply indented gyriform nuclei with quite small nucleoli and

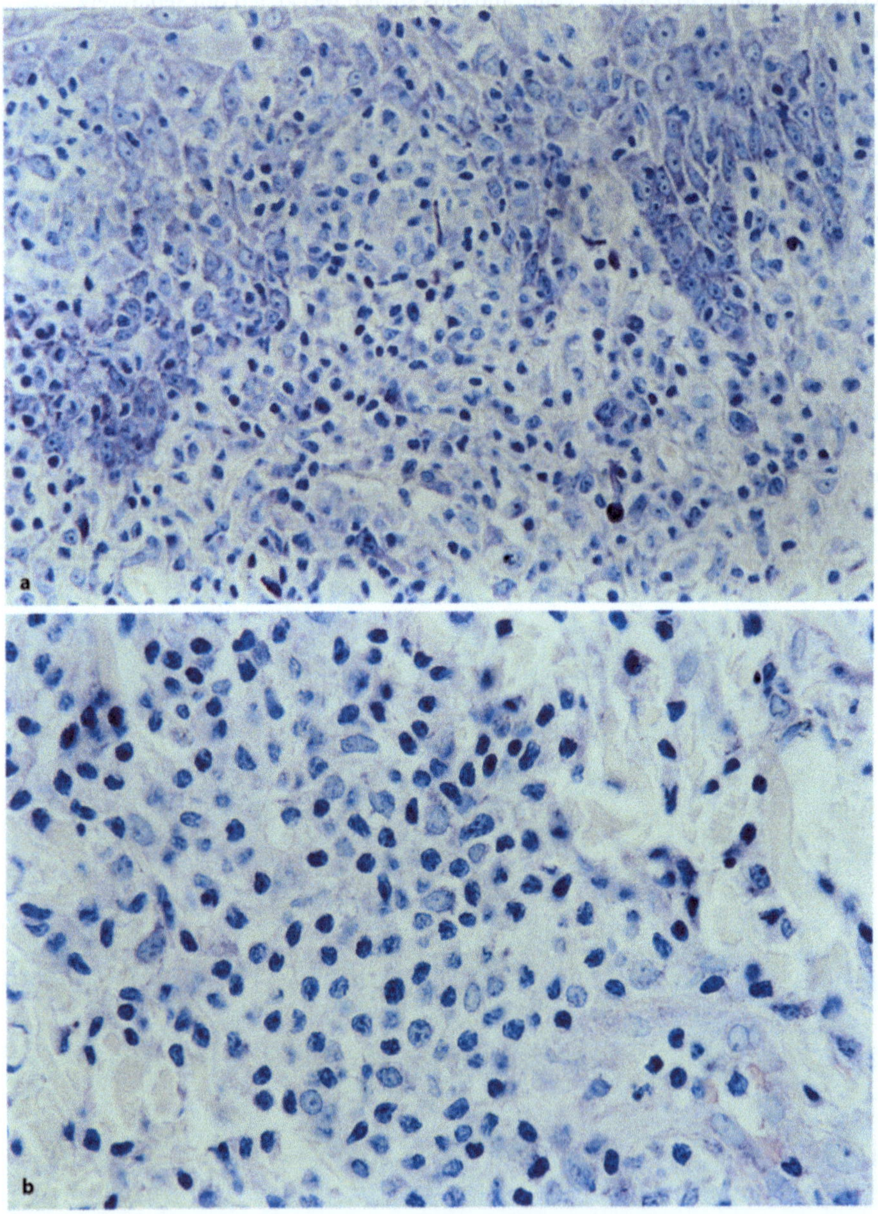

Fig. 6.101 a, b. Typical small-cell infiltrate in mycosis fungoides. Note the marked epidermotropism. **b** High-power magnification of **a**

a small cytoplasmic rim (MF cells) intermingled with a few inflammatory cells. Characteristic medium-sized cells with slightly hyperchromatic chromatin and remarkable (cerebriform) nuclear indentations (Fig. 6.102) are also present. Pautrier's microabscesses are highly characteristic of this type of lymphoma although they are found in only about 20–30 % of the tumors (Fig. 6.103).

The disease progresses over a period of years. This progression is histologically characterized by a more diffuse and denser infiltrate that also proliferates into the lower dermis (plaque stage). The epidermotropism

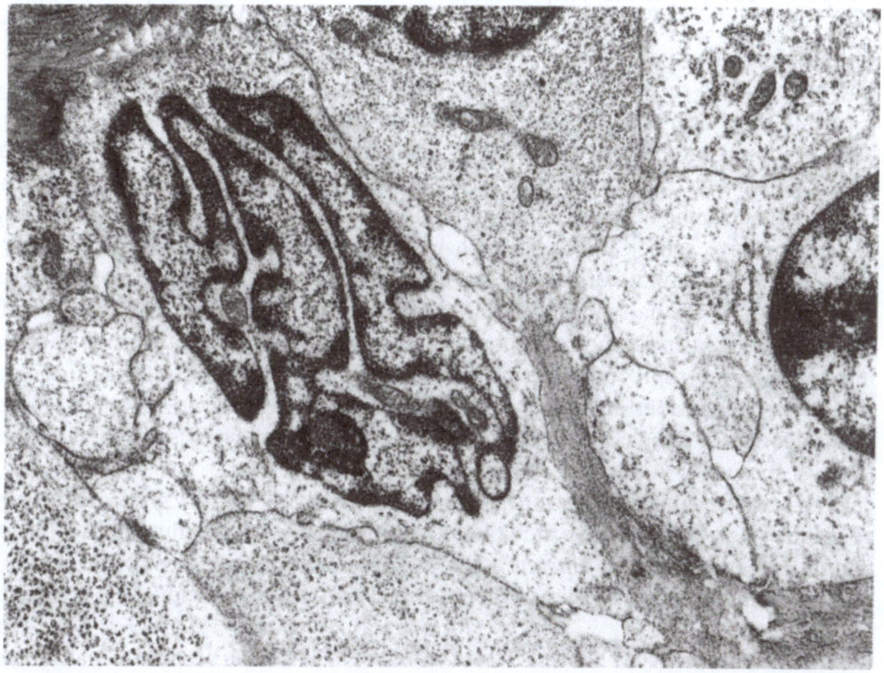

Fig. 6.102. Electron microscopy of a typical cerebriform cell in mycosis fungoides

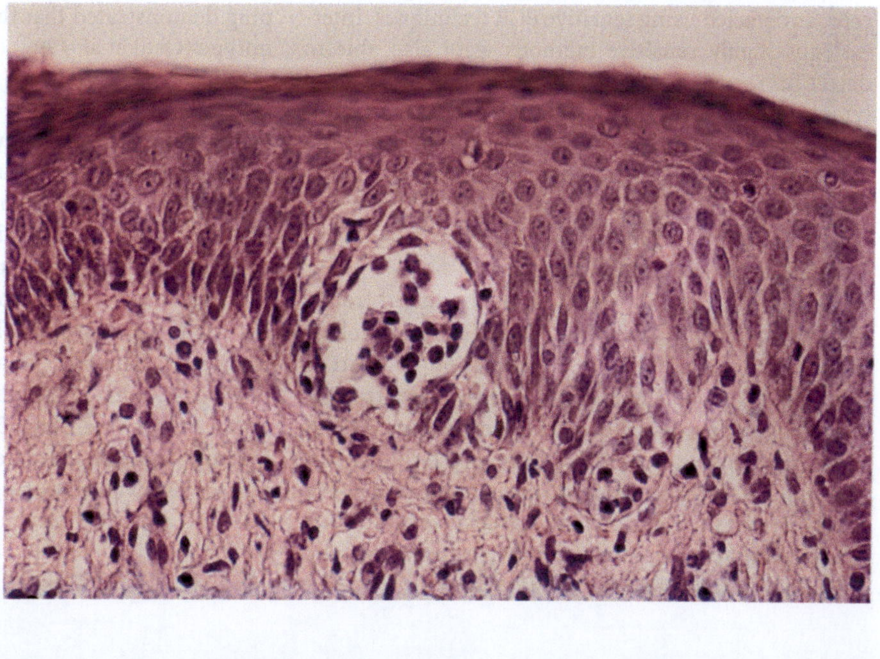

Fig. 6.103. Pautrier microabscess in mycosis fungoides (H and E stain)

is less intense. Mostly the tumor cells become larger and partly show a nuclear pleomorphism. The final step is described as the tumor-forming stage, in which there is a dense infiltrate of medium-sized to large cells with bizarre nuclei throughout the whole dermis. Some cells resemble Reed-Sternberg cells. This stage is difficult to differentiate from other primary CTCLs (pleomorphic T-cell lymphoma, unspecified).

Immunohistochemistry

The neoplastic T-cells show the phenotype of mature T-cells (CD2+, CD3+, CD5+, CD45RO+). In addition, they predominantly express CD4. The interspersed CD8-positive cells may be considered to be reactive. Only rarely does the neoplastic cell population consist of CD8-positive cells. CD8+ cells with a phenotype CD2–,CD7+ may have a worse prognosis than cells that are CD2+, CD7– (Agnarsson et al. 1990). CD103 is typically expressed in epidermotropic phases but is absent in non-epidermotropic tumor-forming stage (Dietz et al. 1996). The number of Ki-67-positive cells in skin infiltrates is less than 5%. In tumor-forming stages there is frequently a partial antigen loss; the tumor cells may also become CD30-positive. During the patch or plaque stage, in some cases only the intraepidermal lymphocytes show partial antigen loss – a phenomenon not found in reactive lesions (Michie et al. 1990).

Genetic Features

TCRβ and TCRγ are almost always rearranged in MF cells, as detected using sensitive PCR techniques. Interestingly, highly sensitive methods were also able to detect tumor cell clones in histologically non-involved lymph nodes and even in the blood and bone marrow (Veelken et al. 1995).

Consistent cytogenetic abnormalities have so far not been described.

Diagnosis and Differential Diagnosis

The patch stage cannot easily be distinguished from a reactive *inflammatory infiltrate* based on morphology alone. Highly suggestive is the detection of Pautrier microabscesses and a markedly diffuse infiltrate of pleomorphic lymphocytes into the epidermis. Otherwise, repeated biopsies and inclusion of the clinical history into the diagnosis are of great importance. The most relevant simulators of early mycosis fungoides are allergic contact dermatitis, plaque parapsoriasis, and lymphocytic infiltrates due to some drugs.

Large plaque parapsoriasis is histologically almost identical to the early patch phases of mycosis fungoides with an infiltrate of mature CD4+ T-cells. Thus it is also thought to be a precursor of mycosis fungoides. At least 10% of these patients progress or develop an overt mycosis fungoides.

Contact dermatitis can be another simulator of early mycosis fungoides. However, mostly it is accompanied by spongiosis and an edema in the papillary dermis (Ackerman et al. 1974).

The plaque and tumor stages have an easily detectable tumor cell clone with atypical, partly highly pleomorphic small and medium-sized lymphocytes intermingled with blasts resembling immunoblasts.

Advanced stages of mycosis fungoides have to be differentiated from *other primary cutaneous peripheral T-cell lymphomas* (pleomorphic medium-sized and large cells), unspecified. As this might be morphologically impossible, a detailed clinical history is essential. At the tumor stage, mycosis fungoides cells may even become CD30-positive and should thus not be confused with a primary CD30-positive lymphoma.

Sézary syndrome is very similar or identical to early mycosis fungoides infiltrates. The blood picture is conclusive (see Chap. 6.14.2.2).

Individual cases have been described as *epidermotropic cutaneous B-cell lymphomas*, in which the cutaneous infiltrate was almost indistinguishable by morphology from mycosis fungoides. Immunophenotyping demonstrated that the infiltrate had a B-cell phenotype (Chui et al. 1999).

Occurrence

Primary onset mostly occurs in adult life. A manifestation below 20 years is rare although it has occurred. There is a male preponderance of about 1.5–2:1. Mycosis fungoides comprises about 40–50% of all primary cutaneous lymphomas. Beside the typical mycosis fungoides, which makes up more than 90% of the cases within this group, follicular mucinosis is the most frequent variant with about 5%.

Mycosis fungoides may disseminate primarily to lymph nodes (see Chap. 5.2.2.3) followed by the bone marrow. Individual studies have shown that the bone marrow is involved during the clinical course in up to 25% of patients (Graham et al. 1993) (see Chap. 9.3.5.3).

Clinical Presentation and Prognosis

Mycosis fungoides is primarily an indolent disease that is stable over many years. When the disease reaches the tumor phase, the clinical course is more aggressive. About 50 % of the patients have palpable lymph nodes; however, this is mostly due to a dermatopathic lymphadenitis, which by conventional histology does not show tumor cell infiltrates. During this stage, the disease spreads to different organs (spleen, lung). This type of involvement can also be observed 2–5 years after treatment and remission of mycosis fungoides.

The prognosis strongly depends on the stage of the disease and the age of the patient at the time of disease onset. Patients with patch- or plaque-stage disease have a median survival of over 12 years. Lymph node manifestations or tumor-phase mycosis fungoides dramatically reduces the median survival rate to 3–6 years (Kim et al. 1995). Bone marrow involvement with atypical lymphoid cells is also indicative of a poor prognosis (Graham et al. 1993) and seems to be independent from the clinical stage. In some patients, the disease progresses after longer duration to the tumor stage with extensive nodular infiltrates.

During the clinical course, the typical patchy mycosis fungoides may evolve to a tumor phase, frequently disseminating to the organs.

Mycosis Fungoides: Variant Follicular Mucinosis

The primary infiltrate consists of atypical, medium-sized, sometimes cerebriform cells infiltrating around vessels and especially the hair follicles, primarily occurring in the head and neck region (van Dorn et al. 2002). If this disease is not accompanied by typical mycosis fungoides, it does not infiltrate the epithelium except the hair follicles. The follicles show a mucinous degeneration with possible subsequent disruption of the follicle (Fig. 6.104). Mostly, an inflammatory admixture of eosinophils, histiocytes, and sometimes plasma cells is seen. Such cases have to be distinguished from other peripheral T-cell lymphomas, unspecified. This can easily be done due to the typical mode of follicular infiltration with mucinous degeneration.

The immunophenotype is identical to that of mycosis fungoides.

This disease has been described as an indolent variant occurring especially in children and undergoing spontaneous regression; however, follicular mucinosis also occurs in association with typical mycosis fungoides or other malignant lymphomas. Molecular genetic studies have shown that follicular mucinosis is characterized by a monoclonal T-cell proliferation. The medium 5-year survival rate is around 70 % (van Dorn et al. 2003).

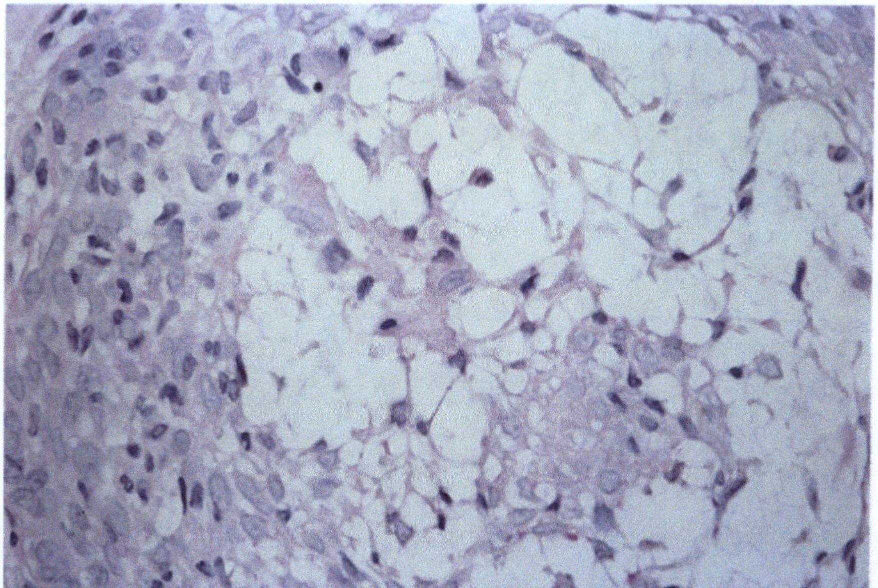

Fig. 6.104. Mycosis fungoides, variant follicular mucinosis. The mucin containing areas do not stain with H and E. Note the pleomorphic cerebriform nuclei of the neoplastic T-cells in between and surrounding the lesion

Mycosis Fungoides: Variant Pagetoid Reticulosis (Woringer-Kolopp Disease)

This variant is characterized by its localized, typical pagetoid infiltrate of the epidermal layer. The infiltrate consists of atypical medium-sized and large, sometimes pleomorphic cells and is accompanied by acanthosis, hyperkeratosis, and disaggregation of the epidermis. The underlying dermis may be infiltrated or spared (Fig. 6.105) (Braun-Falco et al. 1973; Deneau et al. 1984; Haghighi 1998; Dargent et al. 2001; Smoller et al. 1995).

Pagetoid reticulosis tumor cells have a mature T-cell phenotype and may be either CD4- or CD8-positive. Expression of CD30 has also been reported (Burns et al. 1995). By molecular genetics pagetoid reticulosis has been shown to be a monoclonal T-cell proliferation (Wood et al. 1988).

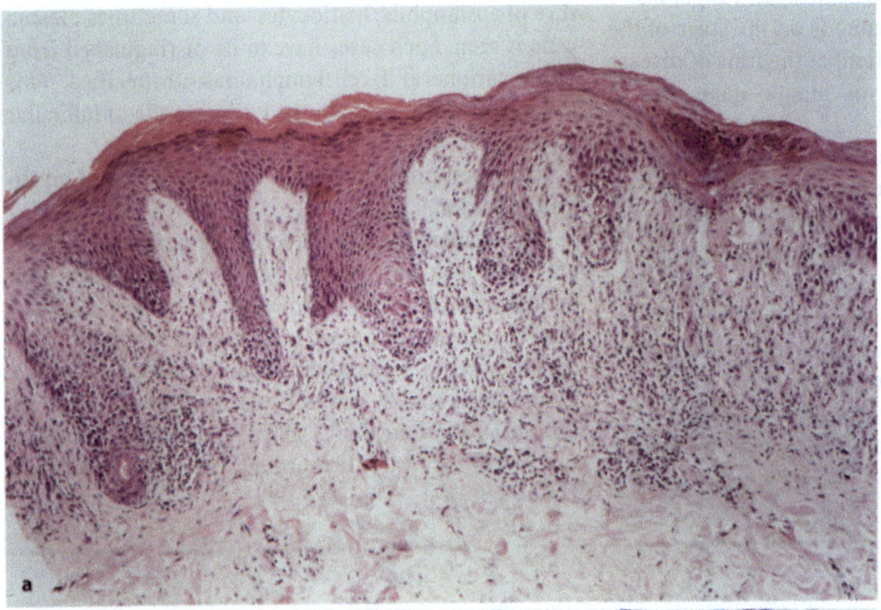

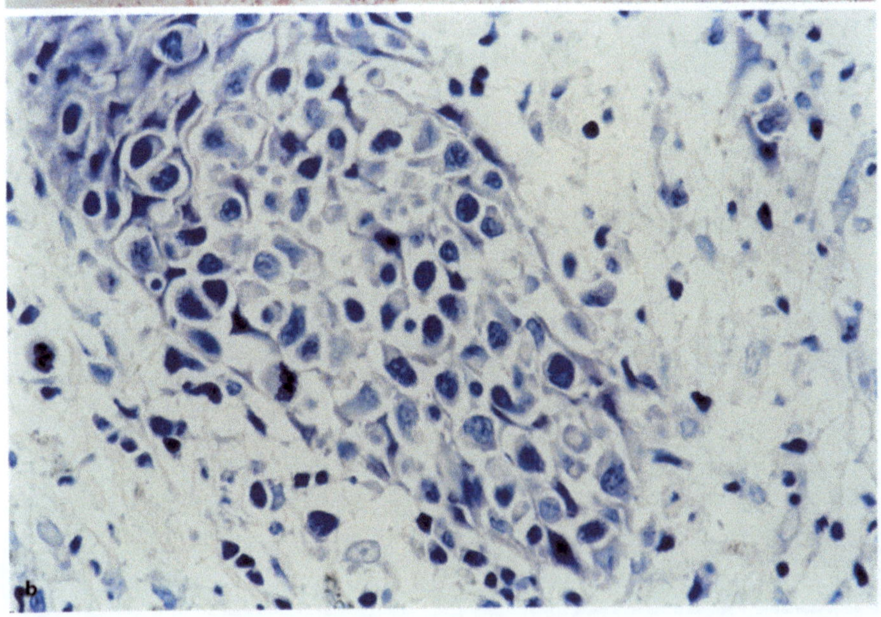

Fig. 6.105 a – c Mycosis fungoides, variant pagetoid reticulosis. **a** The main infiltrate is localized in the dermo-epidermal junction (H and E stain). **b** The neoplastic cells are seen in the basal layer of the epidermis (Giemsa stain). **c** Neoplastic cells are stained for CD8 (immunoperoxidase)

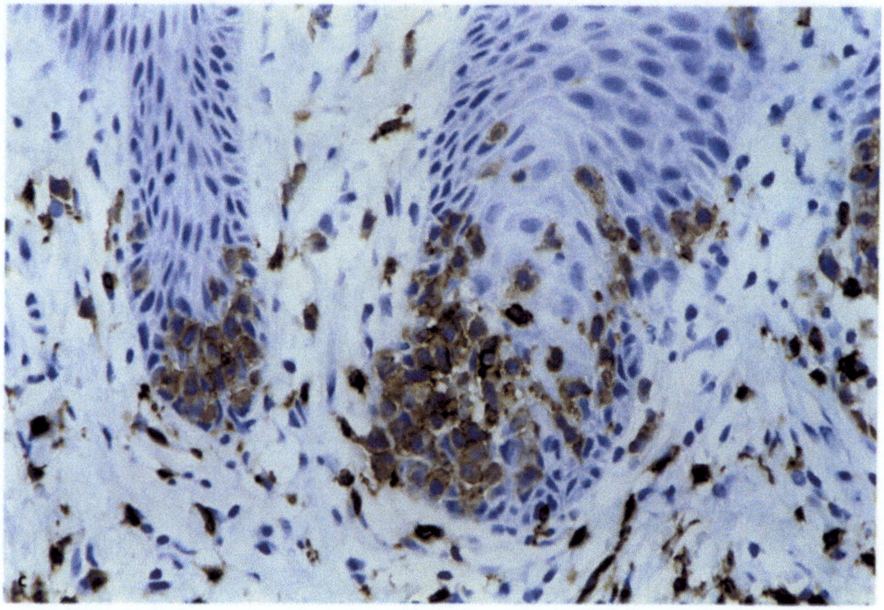

Fig. 6.105c

The lesions appear as single patches or plaques, are clinically slow-growing, and localized predominately to the distal limbs. The disease has an indolent course.

Mycosis fungoides: Variant Granulomatous Slack Skin Disease

This variant is a very rare disease which primarily becomes apparent due to the characteristic clinical picture of impressive skin folds in the intertriginous areas. Histologically, there is a dense infiltrate of atypical cells similar to that seen in mycosis fungoides. This infiltrate is intermingled with large, mostly multinucleated giant cells. Moreover, small granulomas can be seen. Elastic fibers are almost always absent and partly phagocytosed by the giant cells. The immunophenotype is identical to that of mycosis fungoides.

6.14.2.2 Sézary's Syndrome (ICD-O: 9701/3)

Synonyms

- Kiel: Small-cell cerebriform – Sézary's syndrome
- REAL: Sézary syndrome
- WHO: Sézary syndrome

The triad of erythroderma, generalized lymphadenopathy, and a leukemic blood picture, along with Lutzner cells in the peripheral blood, characterizes Sézary's syndrome.

The histological findings are very similar or identical to those of mycosis fungoides. However, the infiltrate may be more uniform in Sézary's syndrome, and epidermotropism may be absent (Fig. 6.106).

Beyond these findings the immunophenotype is identical to that of mycosis fungoides. The disease process involves a monoclonal T-cell proliferation.

The clinical picture is slightly more intensive than that of mycosis fungoides, with alopecia, generalized lymphadenopathy pruritus, and palmoplantar hyperkeratosis (Wieselthier and Koh 1990) (Fig. 6.107).

The clinical course is much worse than in mycosis fungoides. The medium survival after 5 years is between 10 and 20% (Kim et al. 1995).

6.14.2.3 Primary Cutaneous CD30+ T-Cell Lymphoproliferative Disorders

A spectrum of CD30+ primary cutaneous lymphoproliferative diseases (PCLD) with a relatively favorable prognosis has been identified (Kadin 1990; Willemze and Beljaards 1993). This group consists of lymphomatoid papulosis (LyP), anaplastic large-cell lymphoma (ALCL), and a group of lesions displaying histomorphological and often clinical features at the border between LyP and ALCL. Also, cases previously considered to be "regressing atypical histiocytosis" are now

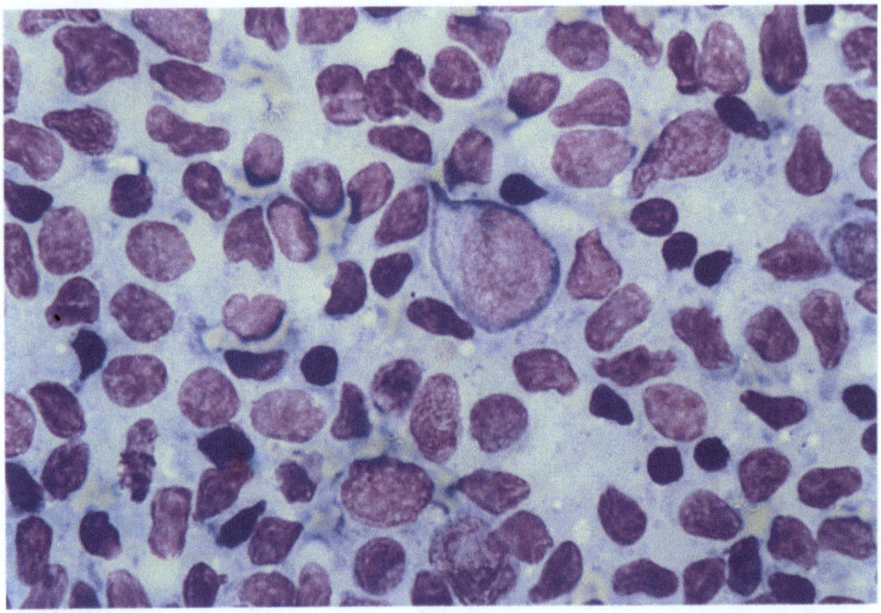

Fig. 6.106. Imprint of Sézary syndrome lesion. Note the typical slightly elongated cells with irregular nuclei and single blasts (Pappenheim stain)

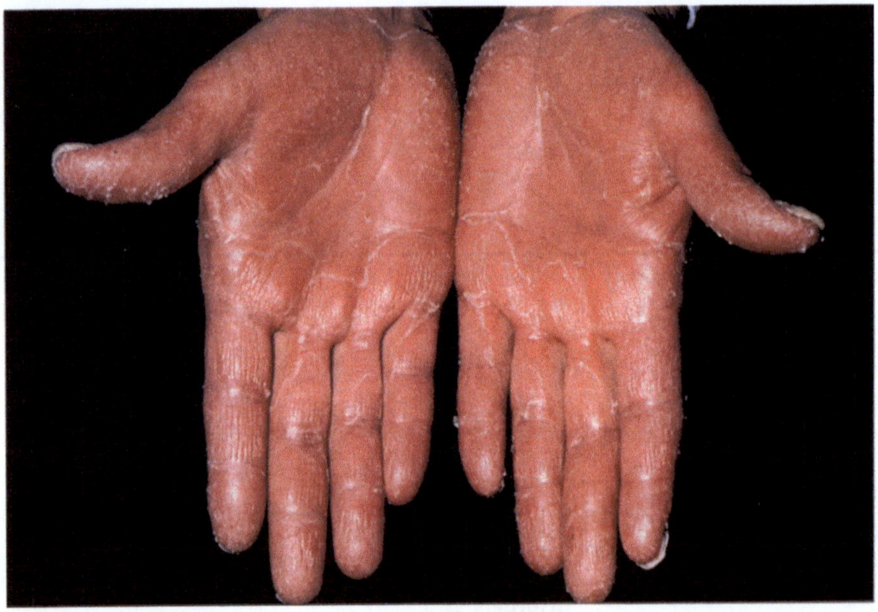

Fig. 6.107. Sézary syndrome with typical erythroderma and hyperkeratosis

classified as ALCL. All of these disorders have in common large atypical CD30+ (Stein et al. 1985) cells some of which morphologically resemble Hodgkin and Reed-Sternberg cells.

6.14.2.3.1 Lymphomatoid Papulosis (ICD-O: 9718/1)

Synonyms

- Kiel: Not listed
- REAL: Not listed
- WHO: Lymphomatoid papulosis

Definition

Lymphomatoid papulosis is a self-healing, episodic, paradoxical eruption histologically mimicking a malignant lymphoma, but which is clinically benign. LyP presents with recurrent crops of papulonodular lesions that regress spontaneously (within few weeks) leaving only a small scar or area of altered pigmentation (Macaulay 1968).

Morphology

Lymphomatoid papulosis lesions have a peculiar wedge-shaped pattern of dermal involvement with superficial and deep perivascular lymphoid infiltrates Fig. 6.108). In classic LyP, the cellular infiltrate is polymorphic and contains neutrophils, eosinophils, histiocytes, and two populations of atypical cells (Figs. 6.109, 6.110): (1) small to medium-sized T-lymphocytes with

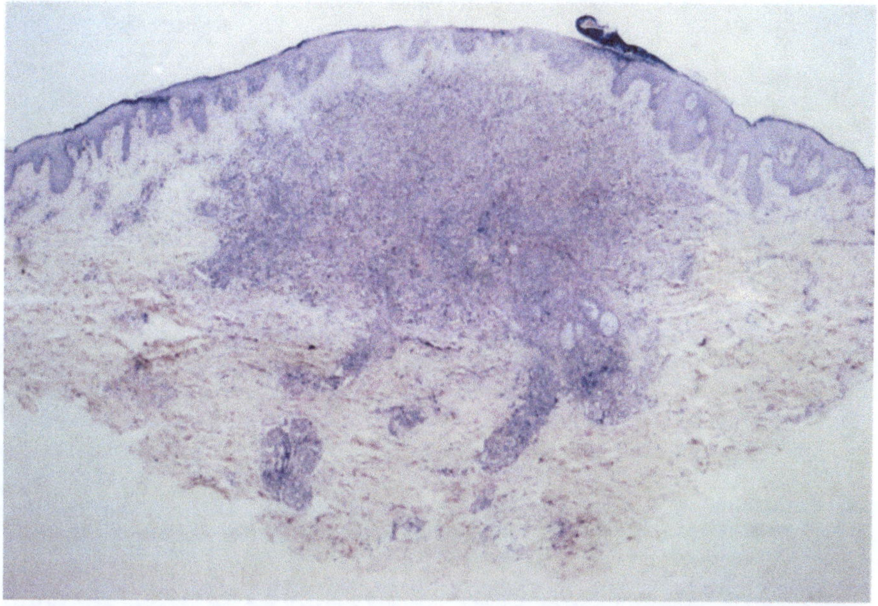

Fig. 6.108. Lymphomatoid papulosis with a typical wedge-shaped pattern of dermal infiltration (H and E stain)

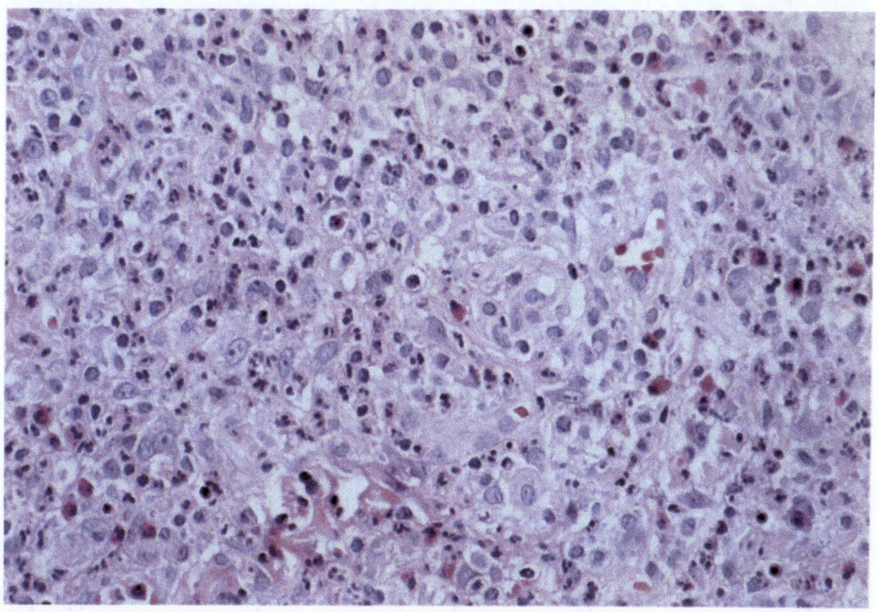

Fig. 6.109. Lymphomatoid papulosis with a mixed cellular infiltrate with scattered large atypical cells in a reactive cellular background (Giemsa stain)

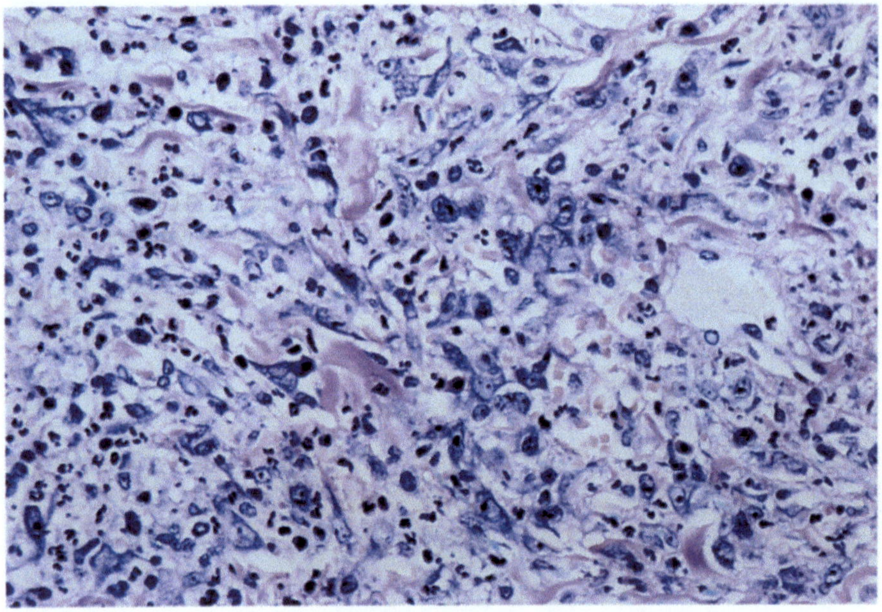

Fig. 6.110. Lymphomatoid papulosis with a mixed cellular infiltrate with scattered large atypical cells in a reactive cellular background (Giemsa stain)

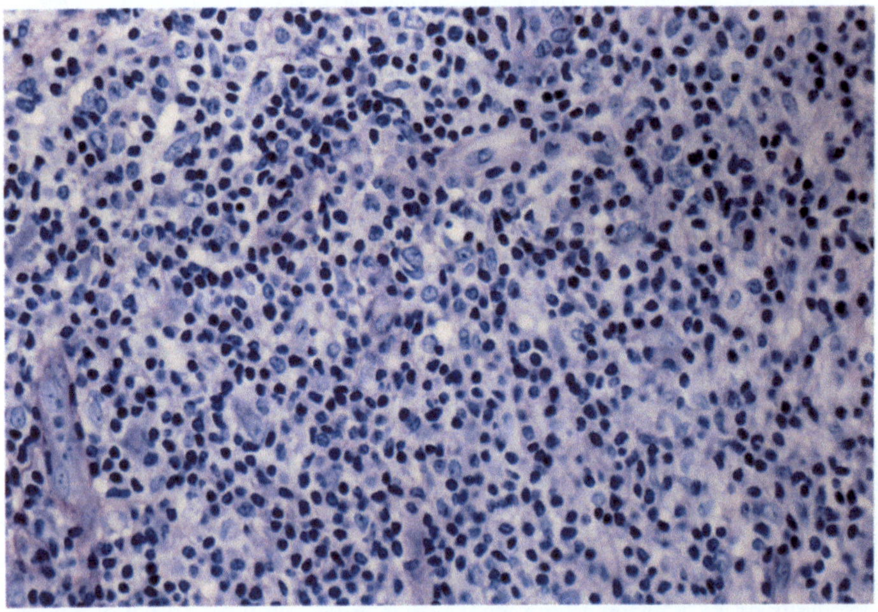

Fig. 6.111. Lymphomatoid papulosis, type B, with a predominant lymphocytic infiltrate consisting of only a few large cells (Giemsa stain)

irregular, cerebriform, hyperchromatic nuclei, and (2) large atypical cells resembling Hodgkin and Reed-Sternberg cells; these cells are usually few and sparse in distribution but rarely they form small clusters. These cytomorphological features correspond to the LyP type A of Willemze et al. (1982), who also described LyP type B (Willemze et al. 1982). The cellular infiltrate of LyP type B consists of atypical T-lymphocytes with cerebriform nuclei and a few inflammatory cells including eosinophils (Fig. 6.111); atypical large CD30+ Hodgkin and Reed-Sternberg cells are usually absent. Associated dermo-epidermal changes depend on the clinical stage of the individual lesion and may include parakeratosis as well as spongiosis, necrosis, ulceration, and a variable degree of epidermal pseudo-epitheliomatous hyperplasia (Willemze et al. 1982; Scarisbrick et al. 2001). LyP type C cannot be morphologically distinguished from ALCL and is thus discussed under borderline cases.

Immunohistochemistry

Atypical cells have a CD4 T-helper-cell phenotype (CD3+, CD4+, CD8–); often they express an aberrant phenotype with loss of one or the other T-cell antigens (i.e. CD2, CD5) (Ralfkiaer et al. 1985; Kadin et al. 1985). Positivity for CD30 and other activation antigens (CD25, HLA-DR, etc.) is confined to small clusters of atypical cells and scattered large Hodgkin- and Reed-Sternberg-like cells (Fig. 6.112) (Willemze and Beljaards 1993; Kadin et al. 1985). The cellular infiltrate in LyP type B is CD30-negative (Willemze and Beljaards 1993; Willemze et al. 1982). Cytotoxic-granule-associated proteins (i.e. TIA-1, perforin, granzyme B) are detectable in most cases (Boulland et al. 2000). Expression of CD15 antigen in the large-cell component may be sporadically observed (Kadin et al. 1985). The reaction for the ALK protein is always negative (Herbst et al. 1997).

Genetics

A clonal rearrangement of TCR genes can be detected in about 50% of the patients mostly those with LyP type B but rarely in those with classic LyP (type A) (Weiss et al. 1986; Whittaker et al. 1991). The detection of an identical clone of neoplastic T-lymphocytes has been demonstrated in one and the same patient with LyP and another associated lymphoma (Whittaker et al. 1991) in two distinct skin lesions.

Although nucleophosmin-anaplastic lymphoma kinase (NPM-ALK) fusions have been detected in a few patients with LyP by means of nested RT-PCR techniques (Beylot-Barry et al. 1996), numerous other studies did not confirm this finding (Wood et al. 1996; Beylot-Barry et al. 1998). However, to date, it is widely accepted that neither the translocation t(2;5) nor other specific cytogenetic abnormalities are associated with LyP (Stein et al. 2000).

EBV viral RNA and EBV gene products are absent in both LyP and ALCL (Kadin et al. 1993; Kempf et al. 2001); in addition, nested PCR showed that LyP is not associated with human herpes virus (HHV)-6, HHV-7, or HHV-8 (Kempf et al. 2001).

Differential Diagnosis

Classic (type A) LyP must be differentiated from others primary cutaneous lymphoproliferative disorders (ALCL and borderline lesions) and rare cases of primary or secondary cutaneous Hodgkin's lymphoma (Kadin 1990; Willemze and Beljaards 1993; Slater 1992); LyP type B also must be distinguished from mycosis fungoides and CD30-negative pleomorphic small-cell T-cell lymphoma (Willemze et al. 1982; Slat-

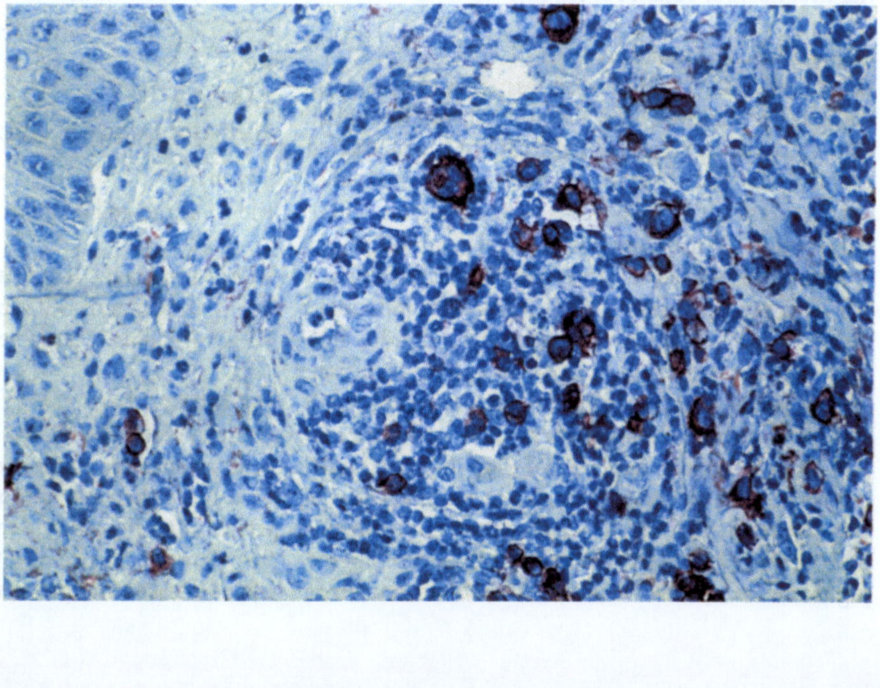

Fig. 6.112 Immunohistochemical staining for CD30 in a lymphomatoid papulosis, type A (alkaline phosphatase)

	Cutaneous CD30 + ALCL	Borderline lesions	LyP
Clinical criteria			
Extent of skin lesions	Solitary > regional > generalized	Regional	Regional/ generalized
Type of skin lesions	Nodule/tumor	Nodule/papulono-dular	Papule
Spontaneous regression	Rare	Frequent	Always
Extracutaneous disease	Possible	Rare	Never
Histological criteria			
Wedge-shaped infiltrate	Never	Sometimes	Regular
Large sheets of CD30+ cells	Always	Sometimes	Never
Infiltration of subcutis	Regular	Rare	Rare
Inflammatory infiltrate	Variable	Often conspicuous	Conspicuous

Table 6.4. Clinical and histological differences between primary cutaneous CD30+ ALCL, borderline lesions, and LyP

er 1992). A combined clinicopathological analysis is the *conditio sine qua non* to accurately discriminate between the various subtypes of primary cutaneous CD30+ lymphoproliferative disorders. Table 6.4 summarizes the major clinical and histological differences between LyP, primary cutaneous CD30+ ALCL, and borderline lesions. Regarding non-neoplastic conditions, differential diagnostic problems may include follicular lymphoid hyperplasia with a high content of "activated" T-CD30+ lymphocytes (Eckert et al. 1989) and cutaneous infection by parapoxvirus (i.e. milker's nodule), which induces CD30 expression in the cellular infiltrate of the lesion (Rose et al. 1999) (see Differential Diagnosis of cutaneous ALCL).

Clinical Features and Prognosis

LyP usually affects adults and less frequently elderly patients and children (Paulli et al. 1995; van Neer et al. 2001). Classic LyP (type A) consists of a generalized eruption of reddish-brown papules which spontaneously regress within 3–6 weeks (Willemze et al. 1982). Some patients may present with several eruptions within a short period of time, others may have only a few over several years. Clinical features of individual classic (type A) LyP lesion have been subdivided into four clinical stages according to the age of the lesion: stage I, early lesion (erythematous dermal papule); stage II, developing lesion (intermediate between I and III); stage III, fully developed lesion (hemorrhagic, ulceronecrotic, or crusted papular or nodular lesion); stage IV, resolving lesion (occasionally leaving a varioliform scar or, more frequently, a small area of altered pigmentation) (Willemze et al. 1982). The occurrence of lymphoma (mostly mycosis fungoides or Hodgkin's lymphoma) associated either before, after, or concurrent with LyP has been reported in up to 20% of LyP patients (Bejjaards and Willemze 1992) but only a minority of them develop extracutaneous disease (Bekkenk et al. 2000).

In spite of its postulated association with malignant lymphoma, numerous studies have confirmed that LyP has an excellent prognosis thereby sparing patients from unnecessary aggressive treatments (Paulli et al. 1995; Bekkenk et al. 2000; Vergier et al. 1998). For this reason, LyP may not be considered a lymphoma *sensu strictu* but, more carefully, a sometimes clonal, atypical T-cell lymphoproliferative disorder with a low risk of progression to lymphoma .

6.14.2.3.2 Anaplastic Large-Cell Lymphoma (ICD-O: 9718/3)

Synonyms

Kiel: Large-cell anaplastic lymphoma of T-cell type (Ki-1)
REAL: Anaplastic large-cell lymphoma (CD30+, T- and null-cell types)
WHO: Anaplastic large-cell lymphoma

Definition

Primary cutaneous CD30-positive ALCL usually presents as one to multiple medium-sized to large nodules or tumors that may temporarily regress initially, but which often persist; the mostly anaplastic tumor cells form large cohesive sheets. The ALCL category also includes cases that previously were clinically classified as regressing atypical histiocytosis (RAH) (Flynn et al. 1982; Headington et al. 1987).

Morphology

ALCL lesions usually show a grossly nodular and/or diffuse pattern of dermal involvement with frequent extension to the subcutis (Fig. 6.113). The dense lymphoma infiltrate contains large polygonal cells with pale cytoplasm (predominant population), Hodgkin and Reed-Sternberg-like cells, and scattered bizarre multinucleated cells (Figs. 6.114, 6.115). Lymphoma cells are usually grouped in large and confluent cohesive sheets. Exocytosis and transepidermal elimination of lymphoma cells may occur, particularly in those tumors previously classified as RAH (Flynn et al. 1982; Headington et al. 1987). The inflammatory cellular

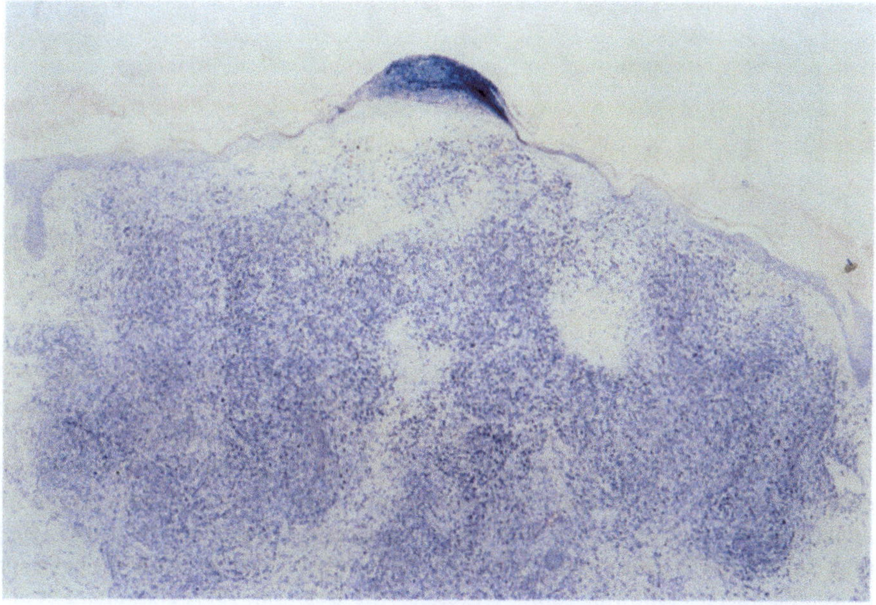

Fig. 6.113. Primary anaplastic large-cell lymphoma (ALCL). Note the blurred, demarcated nodular infiltrate (Giemsa stain)

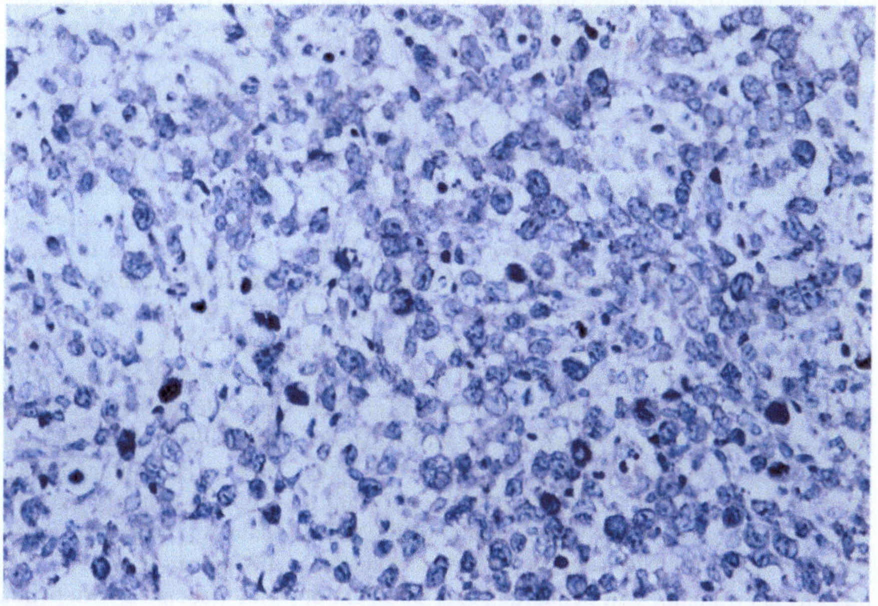

Fig. 6.114. Cytology of a primary cutaneous ALCL. Note the many large, bizarre atypical cells resembling Hodgkin and Reed-Sternberg cells (Giemsa stain)

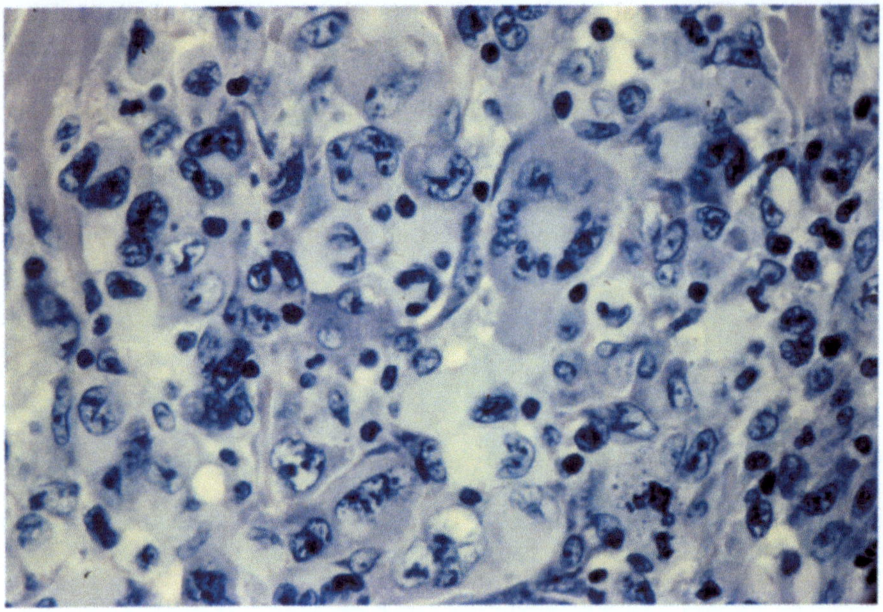

Fig. 6.115. Cytology of a primary cutaneous ALCL. Note the many large, bizarre atypical cells resembling Hodgkin and Reed-Sternberg cells (Giemsa stain)

background varies in amount: scanty and confined to the perimeter of the lesion in some cases, abundant and intermingled with the lymphoma population in others. Associated dermo-epidermal changes include spongiosis, parakeratosis, epidermal pseudoepitheliomatous hyperplasia, and often necrosis with epidermal ulceration. Subdermal fibrosis may be prominent in the larger lesions whereas following tumor regression the area of the lesion may show only increased vascularity and fibrosis with few to no lymphoma cells or inflammation.

Immunohistochemistry

Lymphoma cells usually express a CD4 T-helper-cell phenotype (CD3+, CD4+, CD8–). An aberrant phenotype with defective expression of some T-cell antigens (i.e. CD2, CD5, CD7) has been reported (Kadin 1990; Kaudewitz et al. 1989; Beljaards et al. 1993); tumor cells with a null(non-B non-T) phenotype are rare (Kadin 1990; Kaudewitz et al. 1989; De Bruin et al. 1993). CD30 and other activation antigens (CD25, HLA-DR, etc.) as well as cytotoxic-granule-associated proteins (granzyme B, perforin, TIA-1) are found in the majority (more than 80%) of the lymphoma cells (Boulland et al. 2000; Kummer et al. 1997; Beljaards et al. 1989). Some studies have indicated that, unlike in systemic (nodal) ALCL, EMA antigen is not expressed in the primary cutaneous forms (Willemze and Beljaards 1993; De Bruin et al. 1993). In contrast, we (M. Paulli, unpublished observations) and other authors (Vergier et al. 1998) have observed EMA positivity in primary cutaneous ALCL as well as in some borderline lesions. The reactions for both CD15 antigen and ALK protein are negative (Willemze and Beljaards 1993; Herbst et al. 1997). Expression of CD56 has been sporadically reported (Paulli et al. 1997; Natkunam et al. 2000) in primary cutaneous CD30+ ALCL but the biological relevance of these findings is still largely unknown.

Genetics

Clonally rearranged TCR genes are detected in most primary cutaneous ALCLs, including some of the rare lymphomas with a null immunophenotype (Banerjee et al. 1991). The presence of the translocation t(2; 5) (Willemze et al. 1982; or NPM-ALK fusion transcripts has been reported in rare cases of primary cutaneous CD30+ ALCL (Beylot-Barry et al. 1998) but numerous other studies have not confirmed these observations (Wood et al. 1996; Beylot-Barry et al. 1998; DeCoteau et al. 1996). It seems likely that most reported (Willemze et al. 1982; Willemze and Beljaards 1993) t(2;5)-positive cases of cutaneous ALCL represent skin manifestations of primary extracutaneous (nodal) disease. To date, it is widely accepted that the t(2;5) translocation (Willemze et al. 1982; Willemze and Beljaards 1993) is not associated with primary cutaneous ALCL (Stein et al. 2000). Recently, an allelic deletion at 9p21–22 was demonstrated in a small number of primary cutaneous ALCLs (Boni et al. 2000).

Differential Diagnosis

Primary cutaneous ALCL must be differentiated from both other CD30-positive cutaneous lymphoproliferative disorders and primary cutaneous but CD30-negative large-cell lymphoma (Willemze and Beljaards 1993; Slater 1992). Major clinicopathological differences between primary cutaneous CD30+ ALCL, LyP, and borderline lesions are listed in Table 6.4.

CD30 expression, coupled with indolent clinical behaviour, distinguishes primary cutaneous CD30+ ALCL from the clinically more aggressive CD30-negative cutaneous large-cell lymphoma (pleomorphic medium-sized/large-cell and immunoblastic subtypes) (Beljaards et al. 1994). It is of probable clinical relevance to differentiate primary cutaneous CD30+ ALCL from: (1) skin manifestation of a primary systemic form, and (2) CD30+ ALCL that has developed from another primary cutaneous lymphoma (Willemze and Beljaards 1993; Eckert et al. 1989). Careful clinical evaluation and clinical staging are crucial; immunostaining for ALK may be helpful, but ALK-negative primary systemic CD30+ALCL has also been reported, particularly affecting adults and elderly patients (Stein et al. 2000).

An aggressive clinical behaviour and the frequent finding of CD15 antigen expression by the large atypical CD30+ cells are the major features of CD30+ ALCL that has progressed from other, preexisting primary cutaneous lymphomas (usually mycosis fungoides) (Willemze and Beljaards 1993; Cerroni et al. 1992; Vergier et al. 2000).

Infection with parapoxvirus, which is causative for milker's nodule, may induce a CD30-positive cutaneous T-cell infiltrate. The infiltrate consists of lymphocytes, eosinophils, plasma cells, and large pleomorphic cells with prominent nucleoli. The lesion shows a superficial and deep infiltrate and is highly proliferative. The T-cells are almost all CD4-positive with small clusters of CD30-positive cells mostly in the upper dermis. The epidermis is hyperplastic with parakeratosis. Parapoxvirus particles can be found in keratinocytes by electron microscopy (Rose et al. 1999).

Beyond this a number of reactive lesions occurring in association with other diseases may sometimes contain a large number of CD30-positive cells, e.g., measles, drug-induced hypersensitivity, cutaneous lymphadenoma, and atopic dermatitis. These observations again indicate that clinical information is extremely helpful in doubtful cases.

Clinical Features and Prognosis

Primary cutaneous CD30+ ALCL usually affects adults and elderly patients, and less frequently children and adolescents (Paulli et al. 1995; Bekkenk et al. 2000). Most patients present with solitary or localized reddish-brown nodules or tumors that are often ulcerated (Paulli et al. 1995; Bekkenk et al. 2000). Complete or partial spontaneous regression of the lymphoma lesions has been reported in up to 25% of patients in certain series (Willemze et al. 1997). Extracutaneous disease progression is infrequent (less than 10% of patients) (Eckert et al. 1989), but regional lymph node involvement and skin relapses occur, respectively, in about 25% and 40% of patients (Eckert et al. 1989; van Neer et al. 2001). Visceral spread is rare (Kaudewitz et al. 1989; Beljaards et al. 1993).

Loco-regional lymph node involvement does not seem to affect prognosis, which remains favorable for most patients (Kempf et al. 2001; Eckert et al. 1989; Rose et al. 1999). To date, risk factors predicting possible lymphoma dissemination are unknown. Regional lymph node involvement may occur but. in contrast to primary cutaneous ALCL, skin localizations of primary extracutaneous (nodal) CD30+ ALCL are often associated with a poor clinical outcome (Eckert et al. 1989). The prognosis of patients who have a CD30+ ALCL that progressed from a preexistent cutaneous lymphoma (usually mycosis fungoides) is very poor (Willemze and Beljaards 1993; Paulli et al. 1997).

6.14.2.3.3 Borderline Lesions

Definition

Within the spectrum of primary cutaneous CD30+ lymphoproliferative disorders, the term borderline lesion identifies a group of diseases characterized by a discrepancy between the clinical features and the histological appearance of LyP and CD30+ ALCL (Willemze and Beljaards 1993; Paulli et al. 1995). As a consequence they cannot be readily distinguished from LyP or CD30+ ALCL. Usually, borderline lesions have a favorable clinical outcome similar to that of LyP (Paulli et al. 1995; Bekkenk et al. 2000; Vergier et al. 1998; Willemze et al. 1997).

Morphology

Borderline lesions have clinicopathological features at the border between LyP and cutaneous ALCL. Histologically, most of them show a nodular pattern of dermal involvement, sometimes with extension to the subcutis (Fig. 6.116).

The cellular infiltrate consists of atypical cells grouped in clusters and admixed with a variable amount of inflammatory cells. In some cases, large confluent sheets of atypical cells mimicking a lymphoma can be observed in the deeper part of the lesion, whereas in the upper dermis, the atypical cells are scattered or in small clusters admixed with an heavy inflammatory infiltrate (mainly granulocytes) (Fig. 6.117, 6.118). Apoptotic features may be frequent. In other cases, the atypical cells in the clusters are

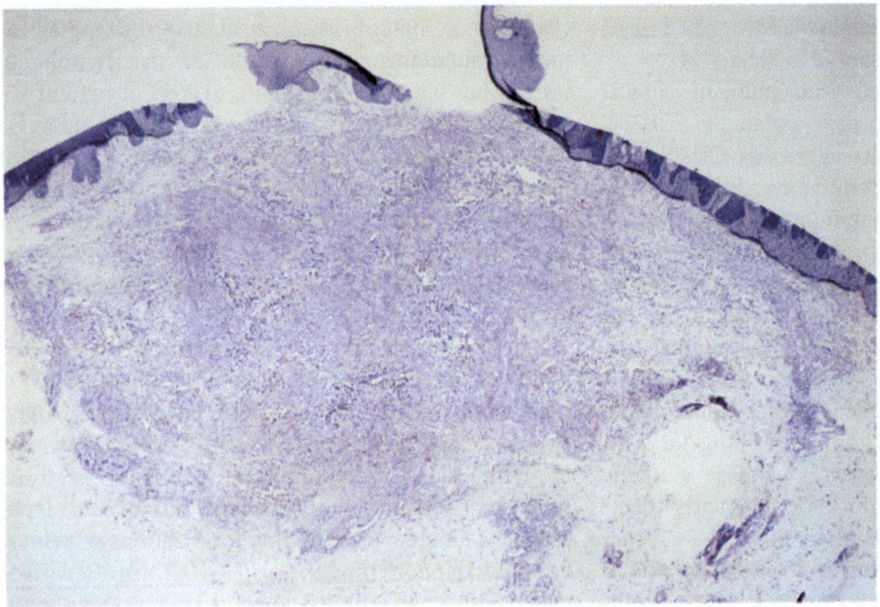

Fig. 6.116. Lymphomatoid papulosis, borderline lesion to anaplastic large-cell lymphoma. A grossly nodular infiltrate extends throughout the entire dermis (Giemsa stain)

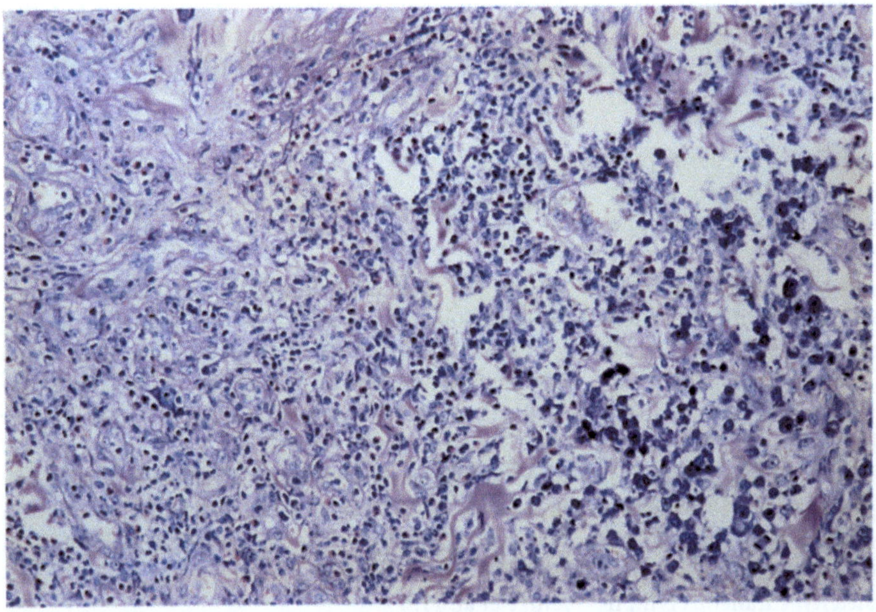

Fig. 6.117. Cellular infiltrate of a borderline lesion between lymphomatoid papulosis and ALCL. Note the accumulation of large atypical cells (Giemsa stain)

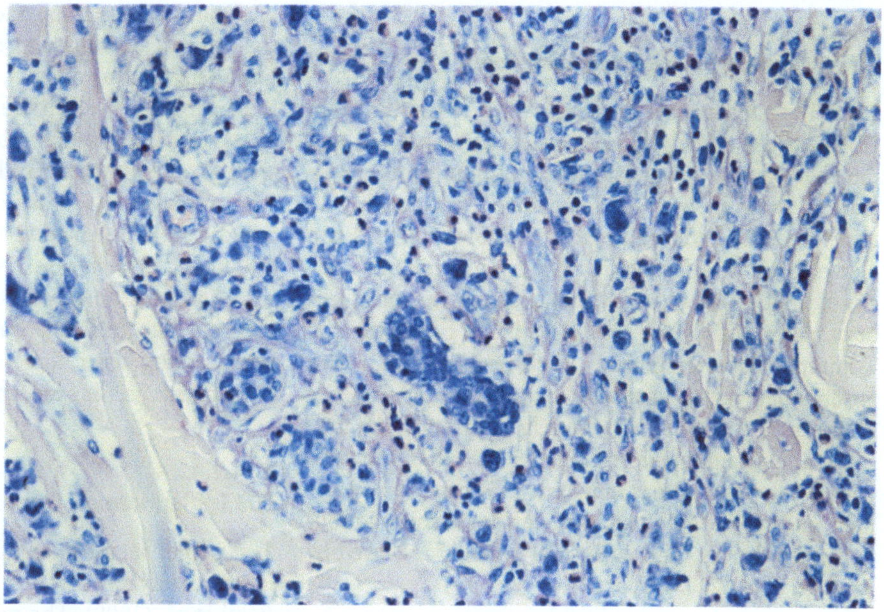

Fig. 6.118. Cellular infiltrate of a borderline lesion between lymphomatoid papulosis and ALCL. Note the accumulation of scattered large atypical cells (Giemsa stain)

smaller in size, resembling histologically the cellular infiltrate in LyP . Associated dermo-epidermal changes include a variable degree of spongiosis, parakeratosis, pseudoepitheliomatous hyperplasia and, often, necrosis and epidermal ulceration. Lesions with similar clinicopathological features were classified by Willemze as LyP type C or LyP diffuse type (Willemze and Beljaards 1993; Willemze et al. 1997). Other investigators have defined these lesions as "LyP-like ALCL". However, it seems preferable to refer to these lesions as borderline, at least until more data become available to clarify the exact biological relationship with LyP and ALCL.

Immunohistochemistry

Detailed descriptions of CD30+ cutaneous borderline lesions are sporadic, thus preventing an exhaustive report on their immunophenotypic, molecular, and cytogenetic features. Available (Willemze and Beljaards 1993; Paulli et al. 1995; Vergier et al. 1998; Willemze et al. 1997) and unpublished data therefore suggest that the atypical/neoplastic cells of borderline lesions closely resemble in their morphology as well as in their antigenic and molecular profiles the cellular infiltrates of LyP and ALCL.

Differential Diagnosis

The term "borderline lesions" describes conditions exhibiting clinicopathological features that cannot be readily distinguished from those of LyP or CD30+ ALCL. As a consequence, no definitive clinicopathological diagnostic criteria are available, but only guidelines (see Table 6.4). In general, patients with borderline lesions clinically present with nodular rather than papular lesions, but papular LyP-like lesions have been also described. Histologically, the clusters of atypical cells in borderline lesions have a less cohesive appearance than the confluent sheets of lymphoma cells in ALCL; this difference may be due to the conspicuous inflammatory cellular infiltrate and high apoptotic rate, both of which are common findings in borderline lesions.

Clinical Features and Prognosis

Patients with borderline lesions more often present with solitary nodular lesions that may spontaneously regress (Willemze and Beljaards 1993; Willemze et al. 1997; Paulli et al. 1995; Bekkenk et al. 2000); in other patients, the lesions clinically resemble LyP papular lesions. Reported cases of cutaneous CD30+ borderline lesions are few, thus preventing definitive conclusions to be drawn regarding the clinical outcome of these patients. Although it has been suggested that, compared to patients with LyP, there is an increased risk for development of a CD30+ ALCL , to date, most borderline lesions have a favorable prognosis, similar to that of LyP (Paulli et al. 1995, Bekkenk et al. 2000).

6.14.2.4
Primary Cutaneous NK/T-Cell Lymphoma

These lymphomas have in common that in most of them CD56 antigen and cytotoxic granules are expressed and they have a poor prognosis. Some tumors within these entities show an overlap, indicating a relationship to each other. The morphology is variable and thus not always diagnostically decisive. The lymphomas may consist of small, medium-sized, and large pleomorphic cells or of blasts, which even may resemble or be identical to T-immunoblasts. In imprints, some neoplastic cells have an abundant cytoplasm with cytoplasmic azurophilic granules. The number of these cells is variable, but they are an important diagnostic sign for the NK/T-cell category. These lymphomas may lack TCR gene rearrangement and express cytotoxic granules, as shown by immunohistochemistry. This entity was recently reviewed by Santucci et al. (2003).

6.14.2.4.1
Pleomorphic Small-Cell, Pleomorphic Medium- and Large-Cell

Synonyms

- Kiel: Pleomorphic small-cell, pleomorphic medium- and large-cell (in part)
- REAL: Peripheral T-cell lymphoma, unspecified (in part)
- WHO: Peripheral T-cell lymphoma, unspecified (in part)

This group comprises either predominately small, medium and/or large cells which have in part or in the majority pleomorphic nuclei. The cell size as well as the negativity or positivity for CD30 is of prognostic importance and thus have to be assessed and included in the final diagnosis. The large-cell type requires more than 30% large cells (double or more the size of the nucleus of a lymphocyte).

The detailed morphology is described in Chap. 5.2.2.2 (nodal lymphomas). As stressed above, these lymphomas can be CD30-positive or -negative. This cannot be predicted by morphology. Even if the cells are CD30-positive, the tumor should be distinguished from ALCL because of the different morphology; this should be indicated in the diagnosis.

In individual cases there might be an overlap with NK/T-cell lymphomas in that pleomorphic lymphomas also may express CD56 and cytotoxic granules without the other typical features of the NK/T cell lymphomas (necrosis, angiocentricity, etc.) described below.

Regarding the differential diagnosis, individual cases in children have been described in which a strongly pleomorphic infiltrate is found in association with molluscum contagiosum. T-cell monoclonality could not be detected. The molluscum lesion itself is diagnostic in such cases. All such lesions show spontaneous regression (Guitart and Hurt 1999). A similar pleomorphic infiltrate can be observed in varicella infection; however, the detection of an accompanying blister leads to the correct diagnosis.

6.14.2.4.2
CD8 Epidermotropic Cytotoxic T-Cell Lymphoma

This group seems to comprise a distinct clinicopathological entity and was first recognized and described by Berti et al. (1999). The patients present with generalized patches, plaques, and tumor nodules. There is a band-like infiltrate in the upper dermis with a marked epidermotropism and blistering. The neoplastic cells are of variable size, mostly with pleomorphic nuclei and intermingled with some blasts. They typically express CD3 and CD8 and contain cytotoxic granules.

The clinical course is aggressive, and most patients die within 2 years after onset. The neoplasm disseminates to unusual sites such as lung, CNS, and testis and thus shows some overlap with NK/T-cell lymphoma, nasal type.

6.14.2.4.3
Cutaneous NK/T-Cell Lymphoma, Nasal Type

This type of lymphoma is rare in Europe but more frequent in Asia, where an association with EBV is found. It is identical to those lymphomas described as primary nasal NK/T-cell lymphomas and may thus occur either primarily in the skin or together with a nasal localization or infiltrate the skin secondarily from a primary nasal localization. The immunophenotype is the same as in the primary nasal localization (CD56+, cCD3+, sCD3–, cytotoxic granules including TIA1, CD4– and CD8–). The tumor infiltrates the dermis and invades the subcutaneous fat and underlying muscle. Angioinvasion and angiodestruction with subsequent necrosis may be found. The cytology is similar to that of pleomorphic small-. medium-, and large-T-cell lym-

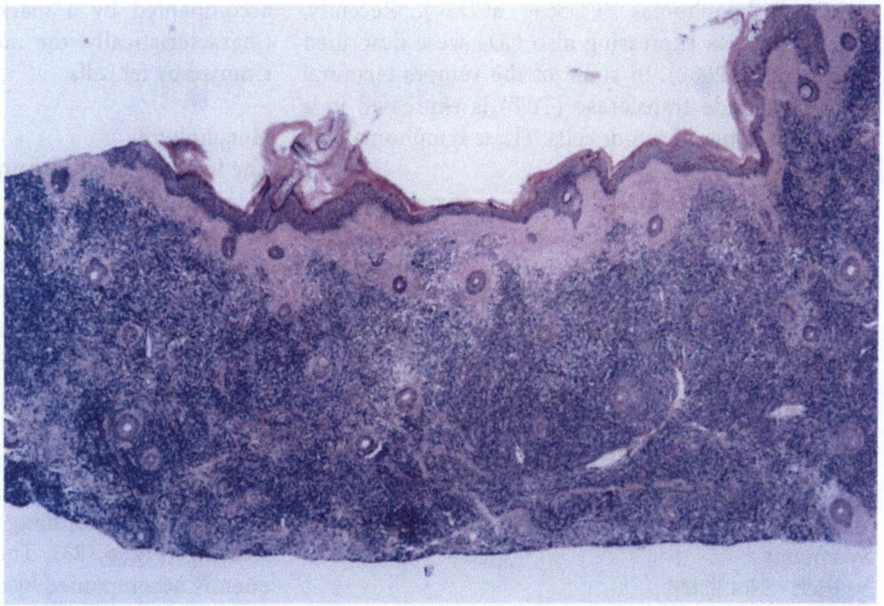

Fig. 6.119. Extended cutaneous infiltrate of a cutaneous NK/T-cell lymphoma, nasal type. Infiltrate of the dermis without epidermotropism (Giemsa stain)

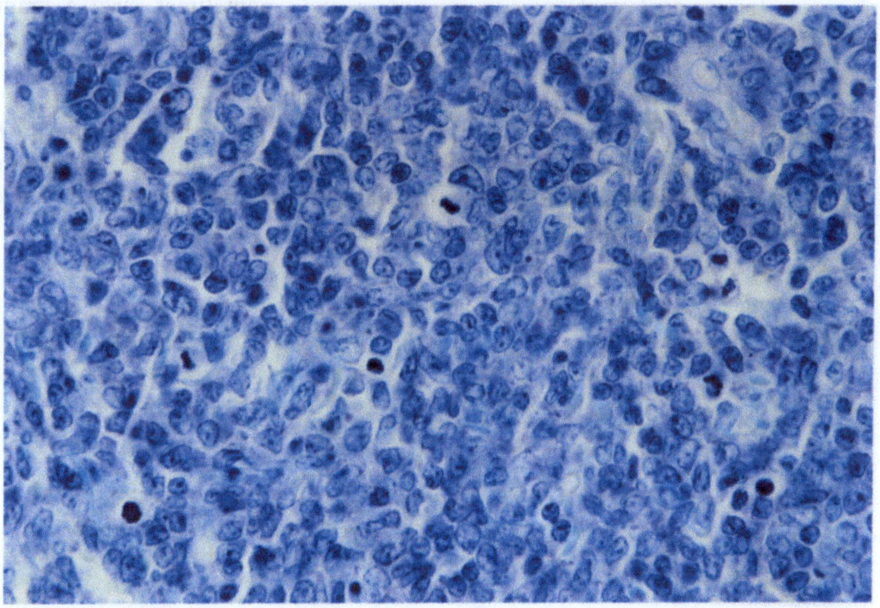

Fig. 6.120. Primary blastic NK/T-cell lymphoma. Diffuse infiltrate of medium to large pleomorphic, partly blastic-appearing cells with slight nuclear irregularity. The cells express cytotoxic granules and CD56 (not shown) (Giemsa stain)

phomas although there is a more intense admixture of inflammatory cells (Figs. 6.119, 6.120).

6.14.2.4.4 Blastic NK/T-Cell Lymphoma (ICD-O: 9727/3)

These lymphomas are extremely rare and consist of a quite monotonous infiltrate of medium-sized blasts with round, occasionally angular nuclei and fine chromatin. Sometimes the cells resemble lymphoblasts. Angioinvasion and angiodestruction are absent as are areas of necrosis. Blastic NK/T-cell lymphomas may be accompanied by a leukemic blood picture and usually disseminate rapidly. Some patients show signs of neurological involvement (Child et al. 2003).

The immunophenotype is similar to that of other

NK/T-cell lymphomas (CD56+, sCD3–). Recently, three leukemias expressing also CD4 were described (Falcao et al. 2002). In some of the tumors terminal deoxynucleotide transferase (TdT) is expressed in a variable number of tumor cells. These lymphomas are EBV-negative.

It is of major importance to differentiate this entity from a myelomonocytic infiltrate of an acute leukemia, which also may express CD56. Thus the tumor cells should always be stained additionally for myelomonocytic antigens (CD33, CD68, CD15, lysozyme) as well as for CD34.

6.14.2.4.5 Subcutaneous Panniculitis-Like T-Cell Lymphoma (ICD-O: 9708/3)

Synonyms

- Kiel: Not listed
- REAL: Subcutaneous panniculitis T-cell lymphoma (provisional type)
- WHO: Subcutaneous panniculitis-like T-cell lymphoma

Definition

Subcutaneous panniculitis-like T-cell lymphoma (SPLTCL) is primarily manifested in the subcutaneous fatty tissue with pleomorphic tumor cells mostly accompanied by a marked inflammatory infiltrate. Characteristically, the mostly CD8+ tumor cells are rimmed by fat cells.

Morphology

The infiltrate is predominately localized in the subcutaneous fat, although a secondary extension to the dermis can be observed (Fig. 6.121). Whereas the infiltrate is mostly diffuse in the subcutaneous fat, it is patchier and sometimes perivascularly accentuated in the dermis. The epidermis is almost always spared. The neoplastic cell infiltrate is highly variable, ranging from small to medium-sized cells as well as some large cells with mostly pleomorphic nuclei (Fig. 6.122). In some cases, the cells of the infiltrate have rounder nuclei similar to those of lymphoblasts. The neoplastic cells show a typical fat cell rimming best recognized by immunostaining (Fig. 6.123). The neoplastic infiltrate is frequently accompanied by a heavy admixture of inflammatory cells such as histiocytes and granulocytes. Sometimes even a granulomatous reaction can be found as well as erythrophagocytosis (Salhany et al. 1998) (Fig. 6.124). The destruction of the tissue leads to fat necrosis with areas of typical foamy macrophages. The lesions are mostly heavily proliferative, with a large number of apoptotic cells and karyorrhexis. Sometimes more extended areas of necrosis are found (Salhany et al. 1998).

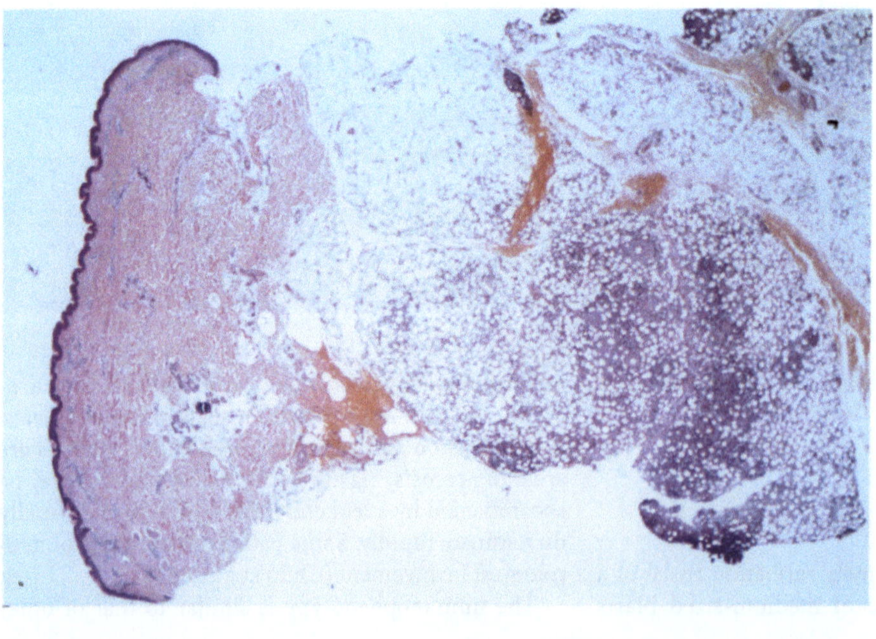

Fig. 6.121. Subcutaneous panniculitis-like T-cell lymphoma with an infiltrate sparing the cutis (H and E stain)

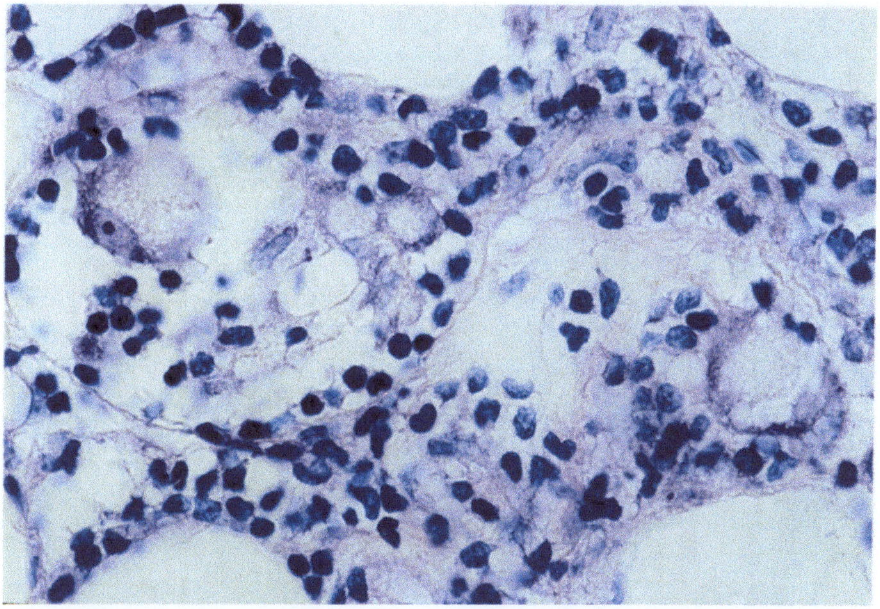

Fig. 6.122. Subcutaneous panniculitis-like T-cell lymphoma. Pleomorphic infiltrate in the subcutaneous fat. Note the presence of foamy cells (Giemsa stain)

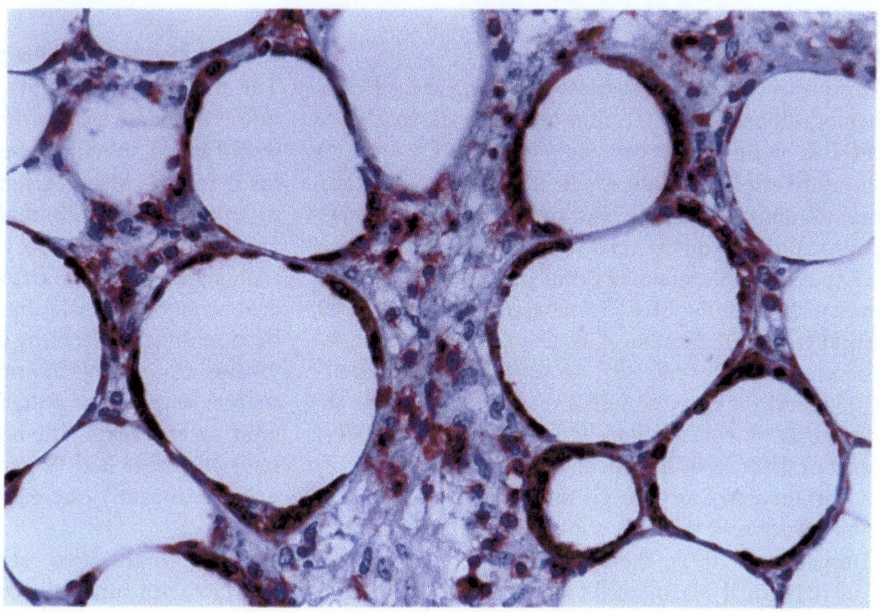

Fig. 6.123. Subcutaneous panniculitis-like T-cell lymphoma. Typical fat cell rimmed by neoplastic T-cells stained for CD2 (immunohistochemistry, alkaline phosphatase)

Immunohistochemistry

The neoplastic cells have a mature T-cell immunophenotype and express CD3, CD2, and less frequently CD5. Most SPLTCL cells express α/β-TCRs, the remaining $\gamma\delta$, and are positive for CD8, with more or less constant expression of cytotoxic granules (TIA1 and/or granzyme B, perforin). Some tumor cells are double-negative for CD8 and CD4 (Salhany et al. 1998) but more frequently express CD56, which is not found in all SPLTCLs. Most of these lymphomas are EBV-negative, although cases of EBV-positive SPLTCL have been found in Asia.

Genetic Features

Subcutaneous panniculitis-like T-cell lymphoma has a monoclonal TCR rearrangement. Characteristic cytogenetic abnormalities have not yet been described.

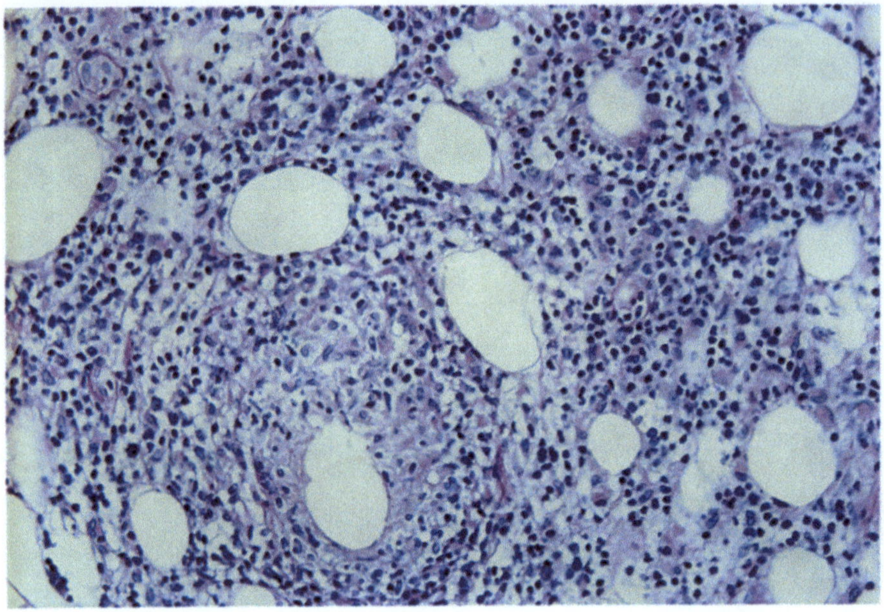

Fig. 6.124. Subcutaneous panniculitis-like T-cell lymphoma with a granulomatous reaction (Giemsa stain)

Differential Diagnosis

Various inflammatory diseases involving the subcutaneous adipose tissue and thus generally designated as reactive panniculitis can simulate SPLTCL. Among these are erythema induratum, after infection or trauma, α1-antitrypsin deficiency, cytophagic histiocytic panniculitis (Requena and Sanchez-Yus 2001). Nasal NK/T-cell lymphoma may occur primarily in the skin even with a panniculitis-like pattern (Chang et al. 2000; Ansai et al. 1997; Kojima et al. 2000). In such cases, the presence of angiocentricity, necrosis, the expression of CD56, and the detection of EBV very much favor the diagnosis of a nasal type lymphoma (Kinney 1999). Most of these cases have been described in Asia.

Variant cases of benign subcutaneous lymphoid hyperplasia have been described as simulating SPLTCL (Dargent et al. 2001). The detection of B-cell aggregates and polyclonal plasma cells may indicate the benign process. Monoclonality of the T-cells has to be excluded. In lymphomatoid granulomatosis, the skin is the most frequently involved site besides the lung. Some of these patients present with a panniculitis-like infiltrate mostly with lymphohistiocytic angiodestructive infiltrates. EBV-positive B-cells can be detected in some of these lesions (Beaty et al. 2001).

Clinical Features and Prognosis

The majority of patients have disseminated disease; however, single lesions do occur. The patients present with typical subcutaneous nodular infiltrates mostly involving the lower extremities and/or a hemophagocytic syndrome (HPS) together with fever, weight loss, and myalgias. HPS is recognized in 40–50% of patients with signs of bone marrow failure. The median age is around 40 years, and a slight female preponderance has been reported (Weeninig et al. 2001). The median survival is around 2 years, ranging from a few months to several years. Some patients are alive and disease-free after several years. The occurrence of HPS indicates a fatal outcome; if HPS is present, chemotherapy does not significantly increase survival (Marzano et al. 2000).

Interestingly, two recent papers indicate that patients with tumors of γ/δ phenotype have a poorer prognosis compared to patients with lesions of α/β phenotype (Hoque et al. 2003; Toro et al. 2003). This might explain some localized indolent cases which possibly express γ/δ-T-cell receptor.

6.15 Lymphoma of Soft Tissues

Malignant lymphomas occur only occasionally as a primary soft-tissue tumor (Salomao et al. 1996; Butori et al. 1997). They seem to be more frequent in patients with immunodeficiencies, particularly with HIV infection.

Secondary extension from a primary nodal or extranodal localization are more frequent, one of the best examples being primary large-B-cell lymphoma of the thymus extending to the soft tissue of the mediastinum (see Chap. 6.6.1).

Only primary soft-tissue lymphomas will be discussed here. They mostly develop either in peripheral muscle (Kandel et al. 1984; Grem et al. 1985; Schwalke et al. 1990; Buttori et al. 1997) or soft tissue (adipose and connective tissue) (Lanham et al. 1989; Salomao et al. 1996). They are observed in the upper or lower extremities (Travis et al. 1987), less frequently in the anterior or posterior torso.

Patients present with a soft-tissue mass measuring 2–8 cm in diameter (Salomao et al. 1996). In such primary tumors, there is no clinical or pathological evidence of direct extension of a tumor from skin or adjacent lymph nodes.

Diffuse large-B-cell lymphomas represent the most frequent type of soft-tissue lymphoma. In a series published by Salomao et al. (1996), 12 of 19 cases were DLBCL, most of them belonging to one of the centroblastic subtypes (monomorphic, polymorphic, multilobate)and two resembling a T-cell rich B-cell lymphomas (see Chap. 4.2.2.2). Immunoblastic lymphomas were not observed in this series (Salomao et al. 1996). Another type, *intravascular large-B-cell lymphoma*, has been reported to occur rarely in peripheral muscle as a primary disease manifestation (Fig. 6.125) (Stroup et al. 1990; Prayson 1996; Buttori et al. 1997) (see Chap. 6.18).

Burkitt's lymphomas and its variants represent the second most frequent morphological subtype, predominately found in HIV-positive patients and mostly with muscle and soft-tissue localizations (see Chap. 4.2.3).

Small-B-cell lymphomas (small lymphocytic and follicular lymphomas) and *NK/T-cell lymphomas* are mostly described as individual cases.

Soft-tissue lymphomas may be difficult to distinguish from other malignant neoplasias including undifferentiated carcinoma, sarcoma of the "small blue cell" tumor type (neuroblastoma, extraskeletal Ewing's

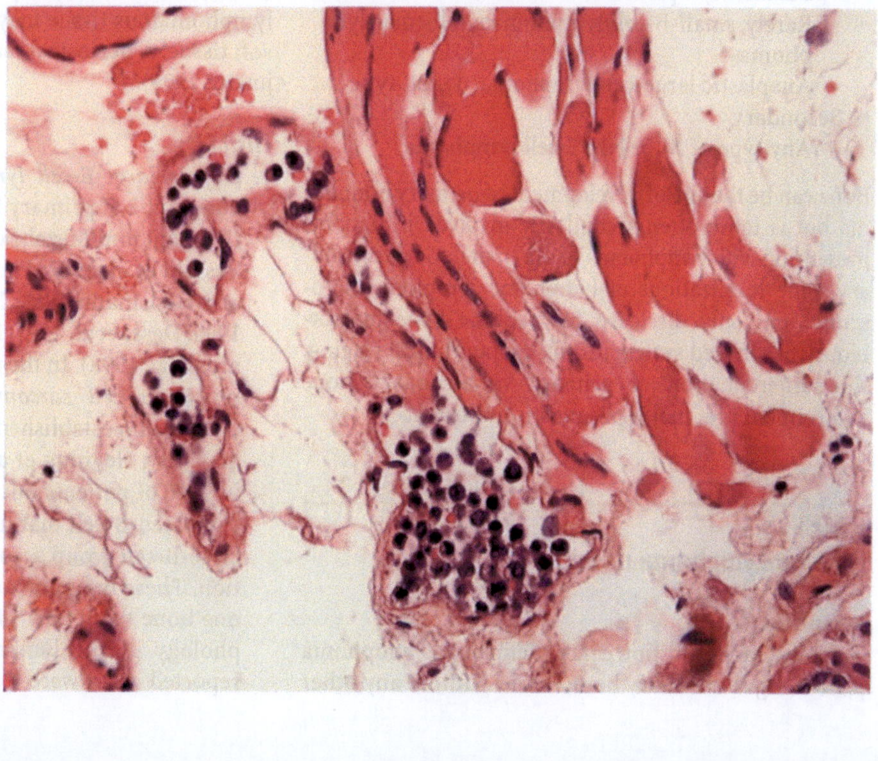

Fig. 6.125. Peripheral muscle biopsy. Large cells in a vessel demonstrate an intravascular large-B-cell lymphoma (H and E stain)

sarcoma, rhabdomyosarcoma, synovialosarcoma, primary neuroectodermal tumor, and myeloid (granulocytic) sarcoma). Immunohistochemistry and clinical data are mandatory for the differential diagnosis.

There is a slight male predominance and the majority of the patients are older than 60 years, even those with Burkitt's lymphoma.

These lymphomas present as solitary tumors with or without general symptoms.

Small-B-cell lymphomas of low stage occurring in soft tissue have the same good prognosis as when they occur in other, extranodal sites (Salomao et al. 1996).

The number of Burkitt's lymphomas is too few to draw final conclusion regarding the prognosis.

Large-B-cell lymphomas, by contrast, have a poor prognosis, with many patients belonging to high-risk groups in the International Prognosis Index (Salomao et al. 1996).

6.16 Lymphoma of the Bone

- Primary
  - Large-B-cell lymphomas (centroblastic, all subtypes; immunoblastic, both subtypes)
  - Burkitt's lymphoma
  - Rarely, small-B-cell lymphomas: follicular lymphoma
  - Anaplastic large-cell lymphoma, T/null type
- Secondary
  - Any type of B- or NK/T-cell lymphoma

Bone can be the site of development of primary lymphoma but is more often secondarily involved in patients presenting with lymphomas of other sites. Such secondary bone localizations of lymphoma are often microscopic and only disclosed by trephine bone marrow biopsy performed systematically during clinical staging. The differentiation of primary vs secondary bone involvement is of major prognostic importance.

6.16.1 Primary Lymphoma of Bone

Definition

This very rare condition can be defined as a lymphoma presenting as a solitary bone tumor without any other osseous or non-osseous localization within 6 months after the onset of symptoms but with possible extension to regional lymph nodes (Schajowicz 1994). With this definition, many of the bone lymphomas reported as primary in the older literature cannot be regarded as such.

Morphology

Macroscopy. This type of lymphoma may develop in any bone. The most common sites are in long tubular bones (50%), most often the femur, tibia and humerus and in the ilium (12%), the rachis (12%) and scapula (Huvos 1991; Schajowicz 1994; Baar et al. 1994; Heyning et al. 1999). Involvement of mandible (Pileri et al. 1990) and skull has also been described (Dahlin and Unni 1986). Lymphoma of the mandible represents 7.8% of primary NHLs of head and neck excluding the CNS (Economopoulos et al. 1998). The tumor can be unifocal or, less frequently, multifocal.

When the tumor affects a long tubular bone and is resected, a wide zone of destruction of bone in the diaphysis or metadiaphysis is recognized macroscopically. The cortical bone is thinned or distended. It may be perforated or totally destroyed by the tumorous tissue, which appears grayish or whitish with a fish-flesh consistency (Diebold 1997). Areas of hemorrhages (black) or of necrosis (yellow) can be observed. The lymphomatous tissue may extend into the periosseous soft tissue. A periosteal reaction is often lacking (Schajowicz 1994).

Histology

1. *Diffuse large-B-cell lymphomas* are the most frequent type of primary lymphoma observed in bone (Dumont and Mazabraud 1979; Clayton et al. 1987; Vassalo et al. 1987; Falini et al. 1988; Radaskiewicz and Hansmann 1988; Fiche et al. 1990; Pileri et al. 1990; Desai et al. 1991; Baar et al. 1994; Economopoulos et al. 1998). In the past, they were interpreted as *reticulum cell sarcoma* by Parker and Jackson (1939), who established primary bone lymphoma as an entity. Heyning et al. (1999) demonstrated that, in 92% of patients out of a series of 60, the tumors expressed B-cell markers and thus belonged to the large-B-cell group according to the REAL classification. These lymphomas cause diffuse infiltration in one bone or in part of a bone. Based on the morphology of the lymphomas, the majority of the reported cases were *centroblastic lymphoma* (Clay-

ton et al. 1987; Vassalo et al. 1987, 1988; Baar et al. 1994), either monomorphic, polymorphic, or multilobated (Pettit et al. 1990). Multilobated centroblastic represented 45 % of the series published by Heyning et al. (1999), an observation also made by Pettit et al. (1990). Other lymphomas corresponded to *B-immunoblastic lymphoma* with or without plasmacytoid differentiation (Fiche et al. 1990). These lymphomas appear as sheets of lymphomatous cells destroying the medullary adipose and hematopoietic tissues, as well as the bone trabeculae. Osteoclastic resorption and neo-osteogenesis are associated. Collagenous fibrosis surrounds these large sheets. A large number of reactive T-lymphocytes is often present, as well as dispersed macrophages and nests of reactive plasma cells.

2. *Burkitt's lymphoma* is responsible for facial bone involvement, particularly the inferior and superior maxilla, but only exceptionally with a primary bone lymphoma presentation (see Chap. 4.2.3).
3. Among the very rare *small-B-cell lymphomas,* only follicular lymphoma is responsible for primary bone lymphoma (Clayton et al. 1987; Vassalo et al. 1987, 1988; Baar et al. 1994). There are nodular infiltrates, often with a paratrabecular localization and sometimes associated with an interstitial or diffuse infiltrate. The infiltrate consists of a mixture of large cells (centroblasts) and of small and medium-sized cells (centrocytes). Extensive collagenous fibrosis is frequent, often infiltrated by reactive T-lymphocytes and plasma cells.
4. The majority of *precursor and peripheral NK/T-cell lymphomas* involve bone secondarily and are not responsible for a true primary bone lymphoma. Only *anaplastic large-cell lymphoma* with a T or null phenotype may develop as primary bone lymphoma. About 21 cases have been published at least (Chan et al. 1991; Ishizawa et al. 1995; Heyning et al. 1999; Nagasaka et al. 2000). Sheets of typical large anaplastic cells are recognized (see Chap. 5.2.2.4). At a distance from the tumor, there is intravascular or, rarely, interstitial dissemination of single cells.

Immunohistochemistry

The vast majority of primary bone lymphomas express CD20. The T-cell origin of some anaplastic large-cell lymphomas has been demonstrated (Nagasaka et al. 2000).

Differential Diagnosis

Primary bone large-B-cell lymphoma and anaplastic large-cell lymphoma of the bone should be distinguished from:

1. *Metastasis of carcinoma*: The diagnosis is based on the morphology and the size of the cells, their organization and immunohistochemistry (CD20, CD30, and CD45 negativity, cytokeratin positivity).
2. *Myeloid (granulocytic) sarcoma.* Such tumors are made up of myeloblasts or a mixture of myeloblasts and monoblasts and may develop as primary bone tumors mainly in the facial (particularly orbital) bones. Macroscopically, these tumors have a greenish color that disappears rapidly under the influence of light (chloroma). Again, the morphology of the cells (medium-sized, sometimes with eosinophilic or neutrophilic or azurophilic cytoplasmic granules), positivity for naphthol-ASD-chloracetate-esterase, and immunohistochemistry (negativity for B- and T-cell markers, but CD45, CD15, CD4 or CD68 positivity, lysozyme and myeloperoxidase positivity) are decisive for the differential diagnosis.
3. *Transformed multiple myeloma.* This disease is the most difficult to distinguish from immunoblastic lymphoma with plasmacytoid differentiation. The morphology of these two tumors is very similar. Therefore, the only possibility to make a correct diagnosis is to obtain precise information concerning the clinical presentation: presence or absence of typical multiple bone lesions on X-rays, presence of a serum monoclonal component: IgA, IgG, IgD or only κ- or λ-light-chains (see Chap. 7.1).
4. Due to intense proliferation of reactive fibroblasts, primary lymphoma of bone can be erroneously interpreted as *malignant fibrous histiocytoma* or *Ewing's sarcoma.* This latter neoplasia is mostly discussed in the differential diagnosis of some large-B-cell (centroblastic) lymphomas and Burkitt's lymphoma. The morphology of the cells, immunohistochemistry, and molecular genetics play an important role in diagnosing Ewing's sarcoma. The cells are medium-sized with a pale cytoplasm and indistinct borders; they contain PAS-positive granules that surround an ovoid nucleus which has a ground-glass appearance. Neuron-specific enolase is positive. In addition, specific genetics markers can be demonstrated by cytogenetic studies or PCR.

Occurrence
Primary lymphoma of the bone is an extremely rare type of extranodal lymphoma, representing about 3–7% of all malignant bone tumors (Dahlin and Unni 1986; Schajowicz 1994) and 1–3% of extranodal lymphomas (Dumont and Mazabraud 1979).

It may develop at any age, but seems to be more frequent in adults between 30 and 40 years; it remains rare before the age of 10 or 15 years (Furman et al. 1989; Schajowicz 1994). Both sexes can be affected but there is a male predominance (Dahlin and Unni 1986; Huvos 1991; Schajowicz 1994).

Clinical Presentation
Pain of variable intensity represents the most important symptom. Swelling often develops in the surrounding tissue. A palpable mass with local tenderness can be observed.

The onset of the disease is often slow and insidious. Neurological symptoms can occur in the case of vertebral localization. Spontaneous pathologic fractures can happen and are sometimes the primary clinical manifestation.

In the majority of patients, the lymphoma presents as a monostatic lesion with extension to the soft tissue (stage IEA). A regional lymph node extension can be disclosed corresponding to stage IIEA (Dahlin and Unni 1986; Clayton et al. 1987; Vassalo et al. 1987, 1988). In the series reported by Heyning et al. (1999), 40% of the patients had Ann Arbor stage I disease, 16% stage II, and 16% stage IV essentially due to multiple bone localizations; the stage was unknown in 20%.

LDH is often high in patients with large-B-cell lymphoma. X-rays, bone scan, gallium scan, and CT are very helpful in the diagnosis.

The prognosis for diffuse large-B-cell lymphomas depends more on local extension and the absence of dissemination than on histological type. In the series of Clayton et al. (1987), a 5-year survival was observed in 55% of patients with localized disease and in only 9% of patients with disseminated disease – pelvis and the vertebrae being localizations resulting in an inferior prognosis (Schajowicz 1994). In the series of Heyning et al. (1999), 61% of the patients had a 5-year overall survival and 46% were free of progression at 5 years. Patient age plays an important role. Those older than 60 years at presentation had a worse overall survival than the younger group (7% vs 57%) and worse progression-free disease (58% vs 28%). Histopathological subtypes were also important. For example, patients with immunoblastic type had a poorer survival than those with centroblastic monomorphic, or polymorphic, or multilobate.

Follicular lymphomas seems to have a more favorable outcome.

6.16.2 Secondary Bone Lymphoma

Any type of lymphoma occurring in any type of organ can be responsible for secondary bone involvement. Some are only detectable by trephine bone marrow biopsy (see Chap. 9), others present as osseous lesions that can be disclosed by imaging techniques. Secondary bone lymphomas can be classified into two groups based on the type of clinical presentation and the extent of the disease (Mary et al. 1986):

1. Lymphoma of the bone with simultaneous nodal and/or soft-tissue involvement (or development of these lesions within 6 months)
2. Lymphoma of bone diagnosed at least 6 months after an initial diagnosis of nodal or extranodal (soft-tissue) lymphoma

In secondary bone lymphomas, the site of involvement is more often the axial than the appendicular skeleton (Schajowicz 1994) including the skull with possible extradural and intracranial extensions (Dai et al. 2000).

The frequency of secondary bone involvement is not easy to appreciate due to the lack of precise information. The bone lesions develop during the course of the disease, often many months after the initial diagnosis.

Persistent bone pain is the most frequent symptom. Sometimes a spontaneous fracture may be the first symptom. Imaging discloses a solitary bone lesion due to osteolysis. Osteoporosis, osteocondensation, and necrosis can be sometimes associated. Disease evolution depends on the type of lymphoma.

6.17 Lymphoma of the Central Nervous System

During the last 15–20 years, a steady increase in the number of CNS lymphomas has been observed. Between 1975 and 1985, the frequency tripled. This is due almost exclusively to the increasing number of extranodal lymphomas in immunocompromised patients, primarily those with HIV (Hao et al. 1999; Schabet 1999). Thirty years ago about 50% of CNS lymphomas were diagnosed as lymphocytic or small-cell and the rest as lymphoblastic (Henry et al. 1974; Simon et al. 1987). Overall, it became clear that the vast majority of CNS lymphomas were primary CNS lymphomas. Today, about 90% of CNS lymphomas are high-grade or large-B-cell lymphomas, most of them are within the diffuse large-cell or Burkitt categories. However, many of these lymphomas do not really fit completely into these categories, especially those lymphomas occurring in immunocompromised patients (Eby et al. 1988; Grant and Isaacson 1992; Nuckols et al. 1999). Primary lymphocytic lymphomas and peripheral T-cell lymphomas are only occasionally noted in this location.

Synonyms

- Kiel: Centroblastic lymphoma, in part
- REAL: Diffuse large-B-cell lymphoma, in part
- WHO: Diffuse large-B cell lymphoma

Definition

Primary lymphomas of the CNS are mostly diffuse large-B-cell lymphoma or Burkitt's lymphoma/Burkitt's type. Most often, they start periventricularly in the hemispheres and rarely disseminate to other locations. An immunodeficiency should be excluded in such patients.

Individual cases of small-B-cell lymphoma may occur.

Morphology

The vast majority of these lymphomas are made up of blasts and are thus high-grade, or are DLBCLs . The infiltration pattern is diffuse with a frequent characteristic perivascular accentuation sometimes in a concentric pattern. Often, the adjacent ventricle walls and sometimes the meninges are infiltrated, especially in HIV-associated lymphomas. It is difficult to exactly describe the tumor margins within the brain parenchyma. The central areas of the infiltrate are dense whereas the margins are more sparsely populated and the perivascular growth more obvious. This marginal infiltrate induces an astrocytic gliosis that can be observed in stereotactic biopsies and which is of great importance for the differential diagnosis. The perivascular growth is characteristically accompanied by an increased amount of perivascular reticulin fibers, easily demonstrated by silver impregnation staining (Fig. 6.126).

In non-immunocompromised patients, DLBCLs dominate. The majority of these tumors can be classified as centroblastic. A small group has an immunoblastic morphology; some cannot be classified and have a morphology between that of immunoblastic lymphomas and Burkitt's-like or atypical Burkitt's lymphoma (Figs. 6.127–6.129).This latter type is quite character-

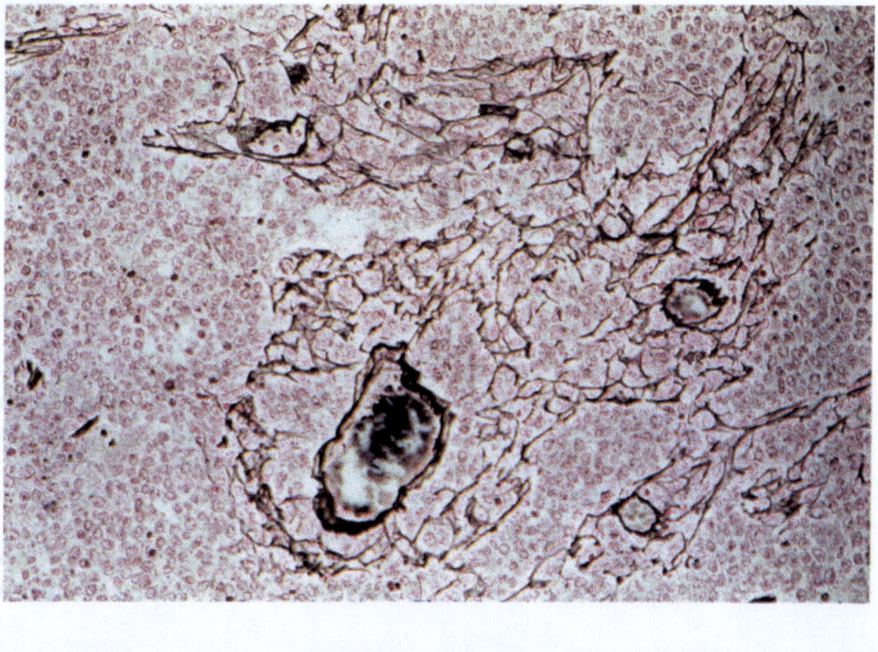

Fig. 6.126. DLBC-lymphoma of the CNS. Silver impregnation shows the increase in perivascular reticulin fibers (Gomori stain)

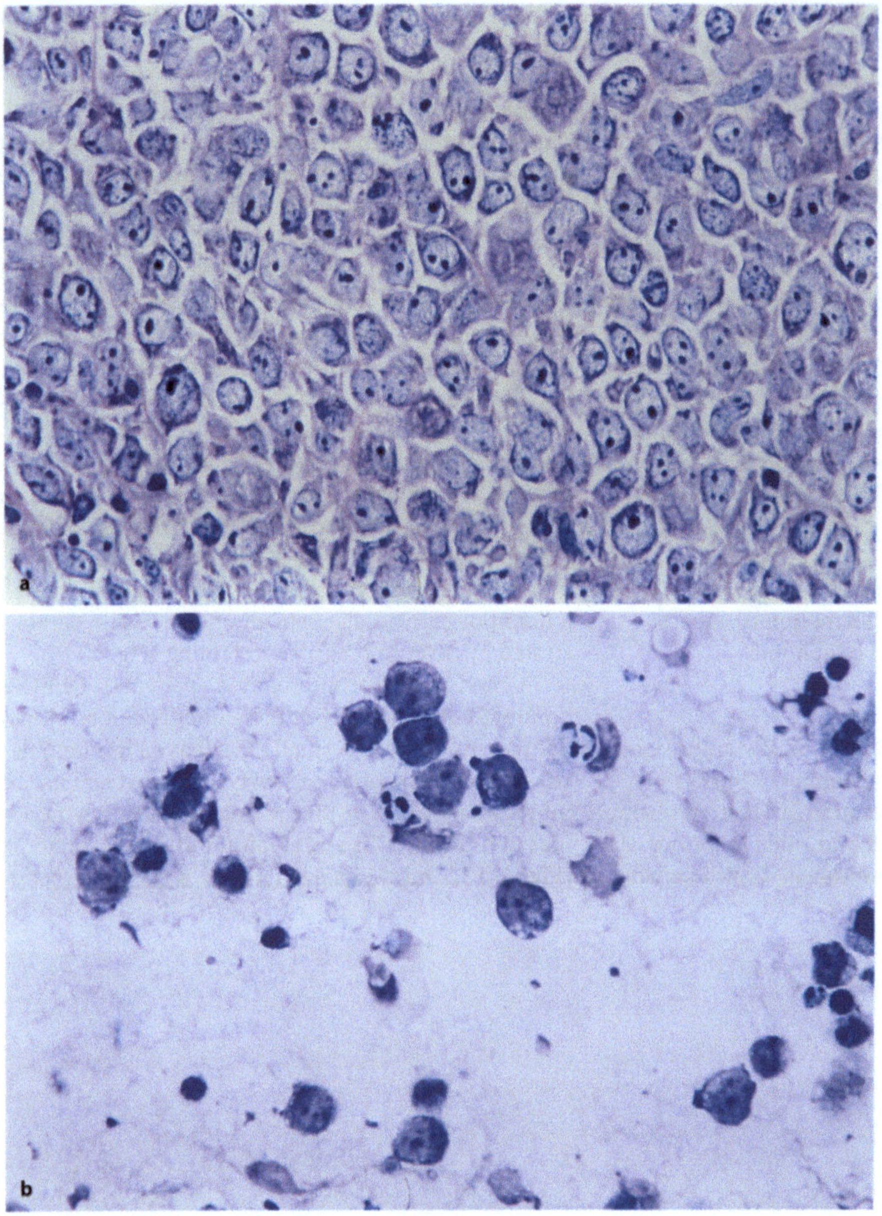

Fig. 6.127 a, b. Diffuse large B-cell lymphoma of the CNS. **a** Giemsa stained section shows large blastic cells with a broad cytoplasmic rim and multiple, in part prominent, nucleoli. Some of the cells resemble centroblasts. **b** Imprint of lymphoma in **a**. Note the vacuoles in the cytoplasm. In this imprint, the cells in part resemble those of a Burkitt's lymphoma (Giemsa stain)

istic in *immunocompromised patients*. The cells are smaller than typical centroblasts or immunoblasts, the cytoplasmic rim is small to medium-sized and frequently vacuolated. The nuclei are round with inconspicuous nucleoli. The chromatin is slightly coarser than in centroblastic or immunoblastic lymphoma cells. Typical immunoblasts are usually found within this infiltrate, but this should not lead to the diagnosis of an immunoblastic lymphoma (for definition see Chap. 4.2.2.2). The second most frequent type is B-immunoblastic lymphoma. Necrosis is frequent in lymphomas of immunocompromised patients. Lymphocytes are more frequently intermingled than in typical nodal DLBCL.

Small lymphocytic lymphomas are very rare as primary CNS lymphomas although they do exist. They

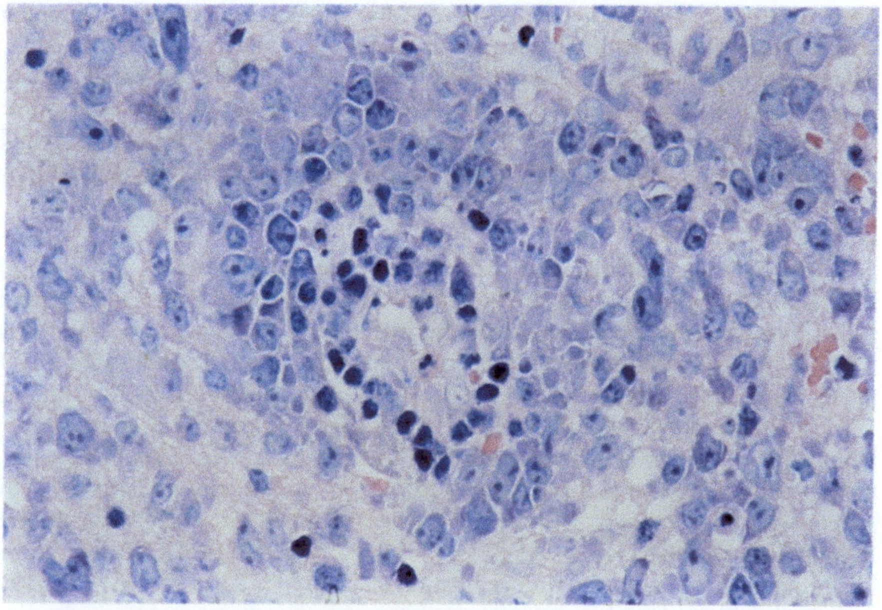

Fig. 6.128. Diffuse large B-cell lymphoma of the CNS, with typical perivascular growth. The cells with dark nuclei are reactive perivascular T-cells. The blasts are medium-sized. Some of the nuclei resemble those of immunoblasts, and some those of Burkitt's lymphoma (Giemsa)

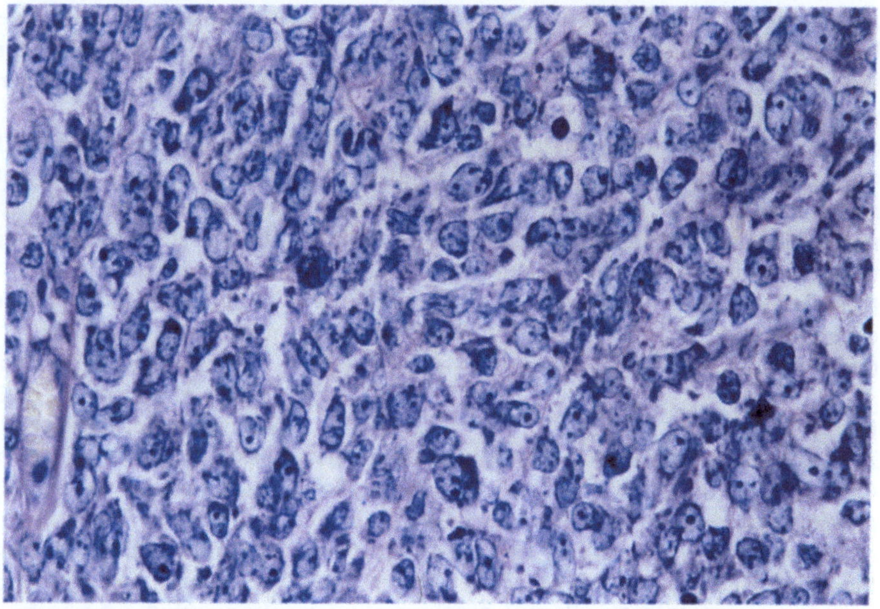

Fig. 6.129. Diffuse large B-cell lymphoma of the CNS. The nuclei are more pleomorphic and irregular than those in Fig. 6.127. This lymphoma closely resembles or is identical to a diffuse large-B-cell lymphoma, variant centroblastic (Giemsa stain)

consist predominately of small lymphocytes intermingled with plasmacytoid and plasmacytic lymphoid cells as well as prolymphocytes and a few paraimmunoblasts. Thus, most of these lymphomas have been designated as immunocytomas. They frequently involve the leptomeningeal tissues.

Follicular lymphomas with a follicular growth pattern have not been described so far.

About 30 cases have been described as primary T-cell lymphoma of the CNS. These lymphomas show an infiltration pattern similar to that of B-cell lymphoma. Some of them have been described as lymphocytic. In Japan and the Caribbean region, there seems to be an association with HTLV-1. In such cases, however, CNS involvement mostly is secondary. Some cases of primary ALCL of the CNS have also been described.

There is a clear association between primary CNS lymphomas and lymphomas of the eye, i.e. lymphomas of the retina and vitreous humor (Akpek et al. 1999b; Cassoux et al. 2000). This is especially true for HIV-associated lymphomas. Such primary CNS lymphomas disseminate to the vitreous humor (review by Jellinger and Paulus 1992; Grant and Isaacson 1992; Ellison and Wilkins 2001).

Due to clinical symptoms, some patients are pretreated with corticosteroids before lymphoma biopsy. Large areas of necrosis perhaps with only small remnants of a perivascular lymphocytic infiltrate renders the diagnosis much more difficult.

Most lymphomas secondarily involving the CNS are lymphocytic, sometimes in association with transformation into a diffuse large-B-cell lymphoma.

Immunohistochemistry
The profile is that of a DLBCL with expression of CD20 and CD79α. These lymphomas can be bcl-2-positive and in some cases CD10-positive. The expression of bcl-6 has been associated with a favorable prognosis. CD5 coexpression is not found in primary CNS lymphoma. T-cells are mostly few in number and may show a perivascular accentuation, which might be helpful in differentiating DLBCL from small-B-cell lymphocytic lymphoma. DLBCLs occurring in immunocompromised patients frequently express EBV-associated proteins. The proliferation index may be even higher in these latter cases than in primary CNS lymphoma occurring without underlying immunodeficiency (review Ellison and Wilkins 2001).

Genetics
Aneuploidy is detected in more than 50 % of the tumors. Chromosomal imbalances detected by comparative genomic hybridization have been described. Gains of chromosomes 12 and 18q and deletions of 6q have been found, similar to in DLBCLs at other sites (Rickert et al. 1999; Weber et al. 2000; Harada et al. 2001).

Differential Diagnosis
The differential diagnosis comprises especially *glioblastoma multiforme, primary neuroectodermal tumor, metastasis of an anaplastic carcinoma, metastasis of a malignant melanoma.* Immunohistochemistry is mandatory in doubtful cases. If frozen-section diagnosis is requested, an imprint is extremely helpful, especially to recognize cohesive (carcinoma, glioblastoma) or non-cohesive growth (lymphoma) as well as the chromatin pattern.

Reactive gliosis imitating astrocytoma in the margins of a lymphoma infiltrates may occur.

Pretreatment of lymphomas with corticosteroids leads to an inflammatory infiltrate and necrosis, which obscures the lymphoma.

Occurrence
In non-immunocompromised patients, the median age is around 60 years without a clear gender preponderance. Patients with AIDS-related primary CNS lymphoma are 5 – 10 years younger. A slight male predominance has been reported.

CNS lymphomas in non-immunocompromised patients account for 4 – 5 % of all extranodal NHLs and 1 – 2 % of all NHLs. Primary CNS lymphoma makes up about 2 % of all brain tumors.

AIDS-related primary CNS lymphoma has become as common as meningiomas. It is the most common cause of a mass lesion in HIV-infected children and the second most common cause after toxoplasmosis in adults (Krogh-Jensen et al. 1994; review: Ciacci et al. 1999).

Clinical Presentation and Prognosis
Most patients present with focal symptoms and or symptoms caused by increased intracranial pressure (headache). Symptoms can rapidly progress into a subacute process.

About 5 – 10 % of primary CNS lymphomas disseminate to other locations.

A primary complete response can be achieved in up to 90 % of patients by radiation therapy; however, the survival is between 1 and 2 years (Abrey et al. 1998, 2000). Therefore a combination of radiotherapy and chemotherapy has been suggested, although long-term neurotoxicity limits this procedure (DeAngelis 1999; Hollender et al. 2000). Prognosis of patients with T-cell lymphomas seems to be slightly more favorable than those with B-cell lymphomas (Gitjenbeek et al. 2001). However, experience regarding T-cell lymphomas is limited due to their rare occurrence.

Further Reading

Hollender A, Kvaloy S, Lote K, Nome O, Holte H (2000) Prognostic factors in 140 adult patients with non-Hodgkin's lymphoma with systemic central nervous system (CNS) involvement. A single centre analysis. Eur J Cancer 36:1762–1768

Jellinger KA, Paulus W (1995) Primary central nervous system lymphomas - new pathological developments. J Neuro Oncol 24:33–36

Kanavaros P, Mikol J, Nemeth J, Galian A, Dupont B, Thiebaut JB, Thurel C (1990) Stereotactic biopsy diagnosis of primary Non-Hodgkin's lymphoma of the central nervous system. A histological and immunohistochemical study. Pathol Res Pract 186:459–466

6.18 Intravascular Large-B-Cell Malignant Lymphoma (ICD-O: 9680/3)

Synonyms

- Kiel: Angio-endotheliotropic (intravascular) lymphoma
- REAL: Intravascular large-B-cell lymphoma
- WHO: Intravascular large-B-cell lymphoma
- Other: Neoplastic angio-endotheliosis
  Intravascular lymphomatosis
  Malignant angio-endotheliomatosis

Definition

In this very rare and very aggressive lymphoma, described in 1959 (Pfleger and Tappeiner 1959), large tumor cells expressing a B-cell immunophenotype (Bhawan et al. 1985; Domizio et al. 1989; Stroup et al. 1990; Demirer et al. 1994; Perniciaro et al. 1995; Dufau et al. 2000) accumulate in the lumen of vessels of the microcirculation (terminal arteries, small veins, capillaries, sinuses and sinusoids) of different organs and tissues, e.g. skin, liver, spleen, bone marrow, muscle (Fig. 6.125), peripheral nerves, brain, kidneys, adrenals, and lung.

The lymphoma cells are peripheral B-cells that probably abnormally express certain adhesion molecules and homing receptors.

Morphology

Large cells with the morphology of centroblasts, immunoblasts, or anaplastic cells are present in the lumen of small vessels (Figs. 6.130 – 132). The architecture of the tissue is preserved. In some cases, associated nodal or extranodal DLBCL has been observed. In some tissues, e.g. bone marrow (Fig. 6.130a), spleen (Fig. 6.131), liver, and lung (Fig. 6.132), erythrophagocytic histiocytosis may be associated (Cheng et al. 1997; Dufau et al. 2000). The association of erythrophagocytic histiocytosis with an activated macrophage syndrome and the discovery of an intravascular large-B-cell lymphoma originating in the bone marrow seems to represent a specific variant occurring mostly in Asian patients (Murase et al. 1997). Two cases reported in France in fact involved one patient born in China and living in the South Pacific and another born in the French West Indies and living in the Caribbean (Dufau et al. 2000).

Sometimes, blood coagulation occurs and the lymphoma cells are embedded in a fibrin clot (Fig. 6.133).

The diagnosis is often made on biopsy of the skin,

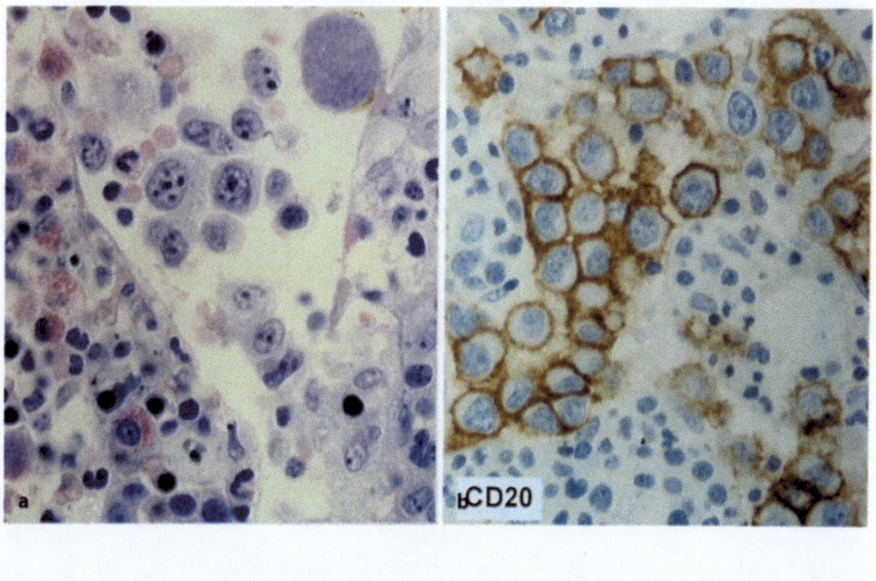

Fig. 6.130 a, b. Bone marrow biopsy. **a** Large cells in the lumen of the venous sinuses (Giemsa stain). **b** The intravascular lymphoma cells express CD20 (immunohistochemistry, peroxidase)

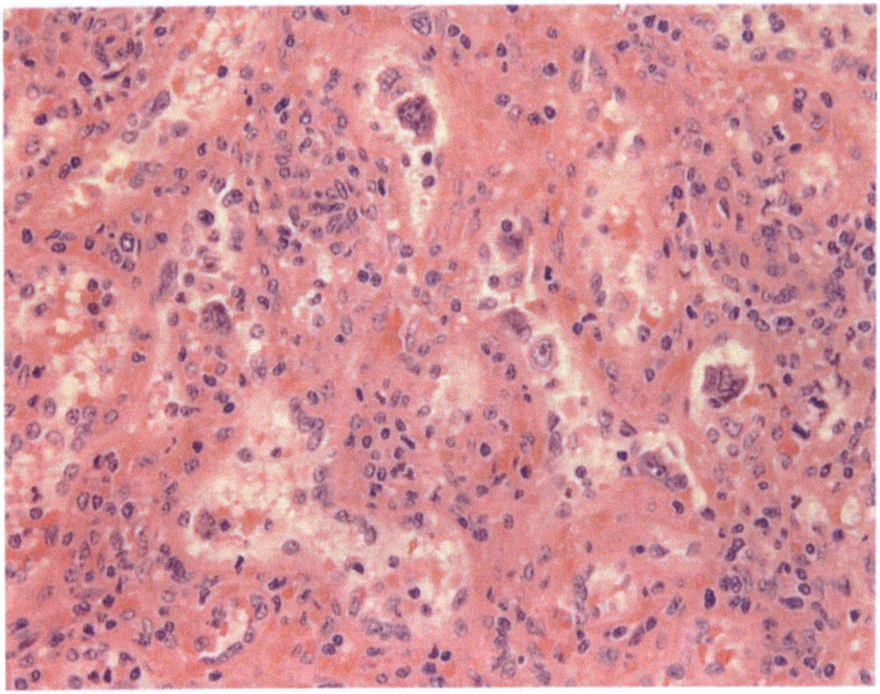

Fig. 6.131. Intravascular large-B-cell lymphoma discovered in a removed spleen. Note the groups of large cells in the lumen of sinuses in the red pulp (H and E stain)

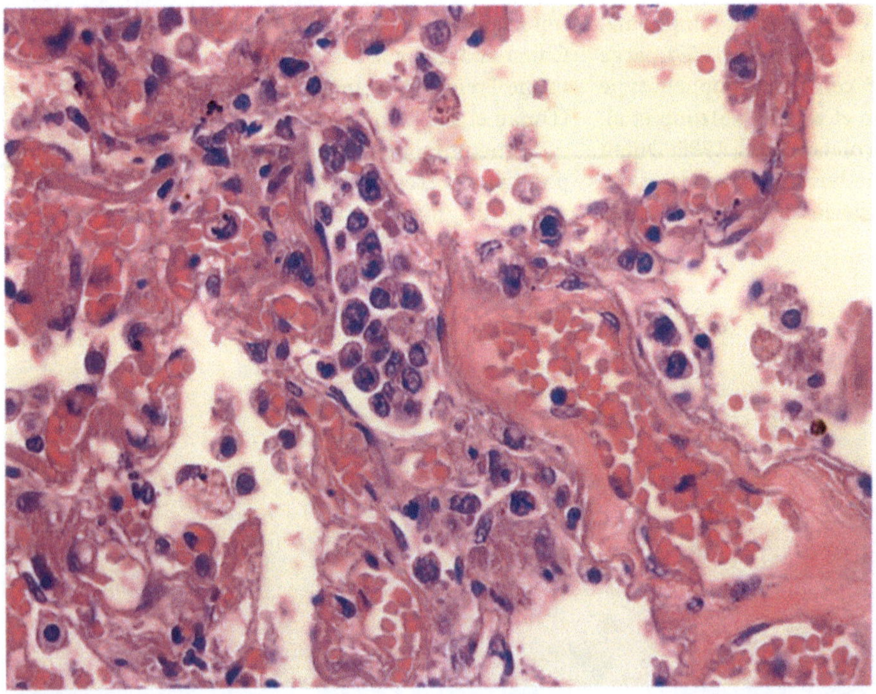

Fig. 6.132. Intravascular large-B-cell lymphoma. Lymphoma cells are present in the lumen of lung capillaries (H and E stain)

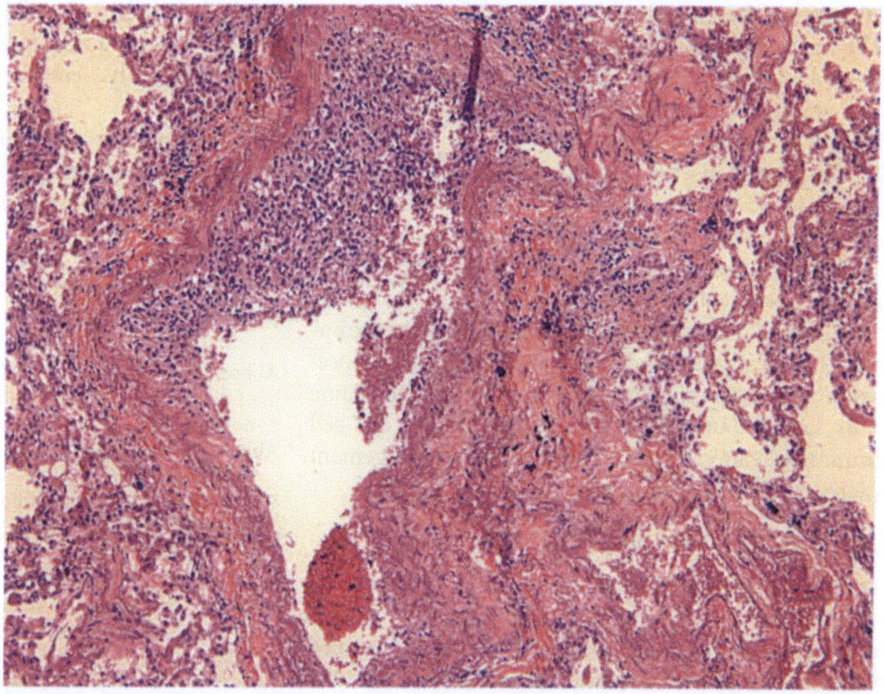

Fig. 6.133. Same patient as in Fig. 6.132. Note the mural thrombosis containing a large number of lymphoma cells in a pulmonary artery (H and E stain)

liver (sinusoidal infiltration), bone marrow (Fig. 6.130) (venous sinuses), spleen (Fig. 6.131), brain and muscle (Buttori et al. 1997), testis (Van Droogenbroeck et al. 2001), kidney (Cheng et al. 1997), and lung (capillaries) with interstitial disease (Fig. 6.132) (Ko et al. 1997; Walls et al. 1999). The intravascular infiltration can be very difficult to detect, for example, in bone marrow biopsies (Estalilla et al. 1999; Tucker et al. 1999; Dufau et al. 2000). Immunohistochemistry is mandatory (Molina et al. 1990; Estalilla et al. 1999). Sometimes, a large number of lymphoma cells are trapped in fibrin clots thereby forming mural thrombi in large vessels (Fig. 6.133).

On surgically resected organs or during autopsies, the areas with hemorrhage and necrosis should be studied at the microscopic level.

Immunohistochemistry

The common leukocyte antigen (CD45) and the B-cell associated antigens CD20 (Fig. 6.130b) and CD79α (Kanda et al. 1999; Dufau et al. 2000) are expressed by the large tumor cells. sIg and sometimes intracytoplasmic Ig can also be demonstrated. Some intravascular large-B-cell lymphomas are CD5- or CD10-positive (Khalidi et al. 1998; Estalilla et al. 1999). Erythrophagocytic macrophages may be associated and are CD68- and S100-protein-positive (Dufau et al. 2000). Passively absorbed factor VIII has occasionally been disclosed in tumor cells and in macrophages.

Immunohistochemistry has recently confirmed the hypothesis that intravascular large-B-cell lymphoma occurs secondary to a defect of homing receptors on tumor cells (Ferry et al. 1988; Domizio et al. 1989; Di Giuseppe et al. 1994). A recent study demonstrated a lack of β1-integrin (CD29) and ICAM-1 (CD54) in six patients (Ponzoni et al. 2000). Another study showed deficient expression of the homing receptor CD11a/CD18 or expression of the Hermes-3-defined homing receptor antigen but with a loss of receptor for peanut agglutinin (Ferry et al. 1988).

Genetics

Ig heavy genes are monoclonally rearranged (Di Giuseppe et al. 1994; Sleater et al. 1994). In the rare cases which have been studied using cytogenetics, non characteristic chromosomal abnormalities have been shown.

No evidence of latent EBV infection has been disclosed even in patients with erythrophagocytic histiocytosis.

Differential Diagnosis

The first disease to be included in the differential diagnosis is *carcinomatous infiltration* of the lymphatics and veins. Immunohistochemistry is helpful in showing positivity for cytokeratins.

The second disease in the differential diagnosis is intravascular dissemination of a classic diffuse large-cell lymphoma, e.g. *large-B-cell lymphoma* or *anaplastic large-cell lymphoma*. The existence of a solid tumor mass allows the diagnosis.

Finally, a third disease to be excluded is the exceptional *intravascular large-T-cell lymphoma*, which presents with the same clinical symptoms and the same morphology but with large cells expressing a T-cell immunophenotype and with TCR rearrangement (Sepp et al. 1990; Khalidi et al. 1998).

Occurrence

In 1993, a review of the literature recorded 114 patients described so far (Prayson 1996). Intravascular large-B-cell lymphoma has only been reported in adults and without sex predominance. The variant called the Asian type, characterized by the association of an intravascular large-B-cell lymphoma in the bone marrow with hemophagocytic histiocytosis has been reported only in Japanese patients with a negative HTLV-1 serology (Murase et al. 1997)and, more recently, in one patient from China and one from Caribbean (Dufau et al. 2000).

Clinical Presentation

One of the most common signs is the development of purpuric skin plaques (Chang et al. 1998) and nodules. Nonetheless, due to possible involvement of all organs and tissues, the clinical presentation is highly variable (Murase et al. 1997; Kanda et al. 1999). Neurological symptoms, such as dementia, epilepsy, hemiparesis, and hemiplegia (Glass et al. 1993; Waring et al. 1999), may occur either initially or during disease evolution.

Other patients present with pyrexia, breathlessness, hypertension, and nephrotic syndrome. Various hematologic disorders have also been described: autoimmune hemolytic anemia, leukopenia, pancytopenia, hypoalbuminemia. Some of these symptoms are explained by a disseminated intravascular coagulation or by an activated histiocytic (macrophage) syndrome with erythrophagocytosis (Murase et al. 1997; Dufau et al. 2000). Sometimes the diagnosis is only made at necropsy (Inooka et al. 1992).

Intravascular large B-cell lymphoma is very aggressive and the course rapidly fatal (less than 12 months). The response to polychemotherapy is poor (Di Giuseppe et al. 1994).

A few patients who were diagnosed early and who received combined chemotherapy have survived (Demirer et al. 1994; Di Giuseppe et al. 1994).

References

Abbondanzo SL, Wenig BM (1995) Non-Hodgkin's lymphoma of the sinonasal tract. A clinicopathologic and immunophenotypic study of 120 cases. Cancer 75:1281–1291

Abbondanzo SL, Seidman JD, Lefkowitz M, Tavassoli FA, Krishnan J (1996) Primary diffuse large B-cell lymphoma of the breast. A clinicopathologic study of 31 cases. Pathol Res Pract 192:37–43

Abrey LE, DeAngelis LM, Yahalom J (1998) Long-term survival in primary CNS lymphoma. J Clin Oncol 16:859–863

Abrey LE, Yahalom J, DeAngelis LM (2000) Treatment for primary CNS lymphoma: the next step. J Clin Oncol 18:3144–3150

Ackerman AB, Breza TS, Capland L (1974) Spongiotic simulants of mycosis fungoides. Arch Dermatol 109:218–220

Addis BJ, Isaacson PG (1986) Large cell lymphoma of the mediastinum: a B-cell tumour of probable thymic origin. Histopathology 10:379–390

Addis BJ, Hyjek E, Isaacson PG (1988) Primary pulmonary lymphoma: a re-appraisal of its histogenesis and its relationship to pseudolymphoma and lymphoid interstitial pneumonia. Histopathology 13:1–17

Agnarsson BA, Loughran TP, Starkebaum G, Kadin ME (1989) The pathology of large granular lymphocyte leukemia. Hum Pathol 20:643–651

Agnarsson BA, Vonderheid EC, Kadin ME (1990) Cutaneous T cell lymphoma with suppressor/cytotoxic (CD8) phenotype: identification of rapidly progressive and chronic subtypes. J Am Acad Dermatol 22:569–577

Ahmann DL, Kiely JM, Harrison EG, Payne WS (1966) Malignant lymphoma of the spleen. Cancer 19:461–489

Aiello A, Giardini T, Tondini C, Balzarotti M. Diss T, Peng H, Delia D, Pilotti S (1999) PCR-based clonality analysis: a reliable method for the diagnosis and follow-up monitoring of conservatively treated gastric B-cell MALT lymphomas? Histopathology 34:326–330

Akpek EK, Polcharoen W, Ferry JA, Foster CS (1999a) Conjunctival lymphoma masquerading as chronic conjunctivitis. Ophtalmology 106:757–760

Akpek EK, Ahmed I, Hochberg H, Soheilian M, Dryja TP, Jakobiec FA, Foster CS (1999b) Intraocular-central nervous system lymphoma. Ophthalmology 106:1805–1810

Albada J, Hordijk GJ, Van Unnik JAM, Dekker AW (1985) Non Hodgkin's lymphoma of Waldeyer's ring. Cancer 56:2911–2913

Alkan S, Ross CW, Hanson CA, Schnitzer B (1996) Follicular lymphoma with involvement of the splenic marginal zone: a pitfall in the differential diagnosis of splenic marginal zone cell lymphoma. Hum Pathol 27:503–506

Alonsozana EL, Stambert J, Kumar D, Jaffe ES, Medeiros LJ, Frantz C, Schiffer CA, O'Comvell BA, Kerman S, Stass SA, Abruzzo LV (1997) Isochromosome 7q: the primary cytogenetic abnormality in hepatosplenic gamma-delta T cell lymphoma. Leukemia 11:1367–1372

Alvarez A, Ortiz JA, Sacristan F (1997) Large B-cell lymphoma of the uterine corpus: case report with immunohistochemical and molecular study. Gynecol Oncol 65:534–538

Amin R (1985) Extramedullary plasmocytoma of the lung. Cancer 56:152–159

Andreola S, Audisio RA, Mazzaferro V, Doci R, Makowka L, Gennari L (1988) Primary lymphoma of the liver showing immunohistochemical evidence of T-cell origin. Successful management by right trisegmentectomy. Dig Dis Sci 33:1632–1636

Ansai SI, Maeda K, Yamakawa M, Matsuda M, Saitoh S, Suwa S, Saitoh H, Ohtsuka M, Iwatsuki K (1997) CD56-positive (nasal-type NK/T cell) lymphoma arising on the skin. J Cutan Pathol 24:468–476

Ansari MQ, Dawson DB, Nador R, Rutheford C, Schneider NR, Latimer MJ, Picker L, Knowles DM, McKenna RW (1996) Primary body cavity-based AIDS-related lymphomas. Am J Clin Pathol 105:221–229

Anscombe AM, Wright DH (1985) Primary malignant lymphoma of the thyroid: a tumour of mucosa-associated lymphoid tissue. Review of seventy-six cases. Histopathology 9:81–97

Anthony PP, Sarsfield P, Clarke T (1990) Primary lymphoma of the liver: clinical and pathological features of 10 patients. J Clin Pathol 43:1007–1013

Aozasa K, Inoue A, Tajima K, Miyauchi A, Matsuzuka F, Kuma K (1986a) Malignant lymphomas of the thyroid gland. Analysis of 79 patients with emphasis on histologic prognostic factors. Cancer 58:100–104

Aozasa K, Inoue A, Yoshimura H, Miyauchi H, Matsuzuka F, Kuma K (1986b) Plasmacytoma of the thyroid gland. Cancer 58:105–110

Aozasa K, Ohsawa M, Saeki K, Horiuchi K, Kawano K, Taguchi T (1992) Malignant lymphoma of the breast. Immunologic type and association with lymphocytic mastopathy. Am J Clin Pathol 97:699–704

Aozasa K, Mishima K, Ohsawa M (1993a) Primary malignant lymphoma of the liver. Leuk Lymph 10:353–357

Aozasa K, Saeki K, Ohsawa M, Horiuchi K, Mishima K, Tsujimoto M (1993b) Malignant lymphoma of the uterus. Report of seven cases with immunohistochemical study. Cancer 72:1959–1964

Aozasa K, Ueda T, Katagiri S, Matsuzuka F, Kuma K, Yonezawa T (1987) Immunologic and immunohistologic analylis of 27 cases with thyroid lymphomas. Cancer 60:969–973

Arber DA, Weiss LM, Albujar PF, Chen YY, Jaffe ES (1993) Nasal lymphomas in Peru. High incidence of T-cell immunophenotype and Epstein-Barr virus infection. Am J Surg Pathol 17-392-399

Arber DA, Simpson JF, Weiss LM, Rappaport H (1994) Non-Hodgkin's lymphoma involving the breast. Am J Surg Pathol 18:288–295

Arber DA, Rappaport H, Weiss LM (1997) Non-Hodgkin's lymphoproliferative disorders involving the spleen. Mod Pathol 10:18–32

Arends JE, Bot FJ, Gisbertz IAM, Schouten HC (1999) Expression of CD10, CD75 and CD43 in MALT lymphoma and their usefulness in discriminating MALT lymphoma from follicular lymphoma and chronic gastritis. Histopathology 35: 209–215

Armitage JA, Weisenburger DD for the Non-Hodgkin's Lymphoma Classification Project (1998) New approach to classifying non-Hodgkin's lymphomas: clinical features of the major histologic subtypes. J Clin Oncol 16:2780–2795

Arnulf B, Copie-Bergman C, Delfau-Larue MH, Lavergne-Slove A, Bosq J, Wechsler J, Wassef M, Matuchansky C, Epardeau B, Stern M, Bagot M, Reyes F, Gaulard P (1998) Non hepatosplenic $\gamma\delta$ T-cell lymphoma: a subset of cytotoxic lymphomas with mucosal or skin localization. Blood 91:1723–1731

Ascoli V, Lo Cocco F, Artini M et al (1998) Extranodal lymphomas associated with hepatitis C virus infection. Am J Clin Pathol 109:600–609

Ashton-Key M, Singh N, Pan LX, Smith ME (1996) HLA antigen expression in enteropathy associated T-cell lymphoma. J Clin Pathol 49:545–548

Ashton-Key M, Diss TC, Pan L, Du MQ, Isaacson PG (1997) Molecular analysis of T-cell clonality in ulcerative jejunitis and enteropathy-associated T-cell lymphoma. Am J Pathol 151:493–498

Audouin J, Diebold J, Schvartz H, Le Tourneau A, Bernadou A, Zittoun R (1988) Malignant lymphoplasmacytic lymphoma with prominent splenomegaly (primary lymphoma of the spleen). J Pathol 155:17–33

Audouin J, Le Tourneau A, Diebold J, Reynes M, Tabbah I, Bernadou A (1989) A primary intestinal lymphoma of Ki-1 large cell anaplastic type with mesenteric lymph node and spleen involvement in a renal transplant recipient. Hematol Oncol 7:441–449

Avlonitis VS, Linos D (1999) Primary hepatic lymphoma: a review. Eur J Surg 165:725–729

Axelsen RA, Laird PP, Horn M (1991) Case report: intravascular large cell lymphoma. Diagnosis on renal biopsy. Pathology 23:241–243

Baar J, Burkes RL, Bell R, Blackstein ME, Fernandes B, Langer F (1994) Primary non Hodgkin's lymphoma of bone. A clinicopathologic study. Cancer 73:1194–1199

Bagdi E, Diss TC, Munson P, Isaacson PG (1999) Mucosal intraepithelial lymphocytes in enteropathy-associated T-cell lymphoma, ulcerative jejunitis, and refractory celiac disease constitute a neoplastic population. Blood 94:260–264

Bailey EM, Ferry JA, Harris NL, Mihm MC, Jacobson JO, Duncan LM (1996) Marginal zone lymphoma (low-grade B-cell lymphoma of mucosa-associated lymphoid tissue type) of skin and subcutaneous tissue. Am J Surg Pathol 20:1011–1023

Bairey O, Kremer I, Rakowsky E, Hadar H, Shakiai M (1994) Orbital and adnexal involvement in systemic non-Hodgkin's lymphoma. Cancer 73:2395–2399

Baldassano MF, Bailey EM, Ferry JA, Harris NL, Duncan LM (1999) Cutaneous lymphoid hyperplasia and cutaneous marginal zone lymphoma. Am J Surg Pathol 23:88–96

Banerjee SS, Heald J, Harris M (1991) Twelve cases of Ki-positive large cell lymphoma of skin. J Clin Pathol 44:119–125

Barth TFE, Leithäuser F, Döhner H, Bentz M, Pawlita M, Schmid U, Möller P (2000) Primary gastric apoptosis-rich T-cell lymphoma co-expressing CD4, CD8 and cytotoxic molecules. Virchows Arch 436:357–364

Barth TFE, Leithäuser F, Möller P (2001) Mediastinal B-cell lymphoma, a lymphoma type with several characteristics unique among diffuse large B-cell lymphomas. Ann Hematol 80:B49–B53

Barton JH, Osborne BM, Butler JJ et al (1984) Non Hodgkin's lymphoma of the tonsil. A clinicopathologic study of 55 cases. Cancer 53:86–95

Baschinsky DY, Weidner N, Baker PB, Frankel WL (2001) Primary hepatic anaplastic large-cell lymphoma of T-cell phenotype in acquired immunodeficiency syndrome: a report of an autopsy case and review of the literature. Am J Gastroenterol 96:227–232

Bates AW, Norton AJ, Baithun SI (2000) Malignant lymphoma of the urinary bladder: a clinicopathological study of 11 cases. J Clin Pathol 53:458–461

Beaty MW, Kumar S, Sorbara L, Miller K, Raffeld M, Jaffe ES (1999) A biophenotypic human herpesvirus 8-associated primary bowel lymphoma. Am J Surg Pathol 23:992–994

Beaty MW, Toro J, Sorbara L, Stern JB, Pittaluga S, Raffeld M, Wilson WH, Jaffe ES (2001) Cutaneous lymphomatoid granulomatosis. Correlation of clinical and biologic features. Am J Surg Pathol 25:1111–1120

Bekkenk MW, Geelen FAM, van Voorst Vader PC, Heule F, Geerts ML, Van Vloten WA, Meijer JLM, Willemze R (2000) Primary and secondary cutaneous lymphoproliferative disorders: a report from the Dutch Cutaneous Lymphoma Group on the long-term follow-up data of 219 patients and guidelines for diagnosis and treatment. Blood 95:3653–3661

Beljaards RC, Willemze R (1992) The prognosis of patients with lymphomatoid papulosis associated with malignant lymphomas. Br J Dermatol 126:596–602

Beljaards RC, Meijer CJLM, Scheffer E, Toonstra J, van Vloten WA, van der Putte SCJ, Geerts ML, Willemze R (1989) Prognostic significance of CD30 (Ki-1/Ber-H2) expression of primary cutaneous large-cell lymphomas of T-cell origin. A clinicopathologic and immunohistochemical study in 20 patients. Am J Pathol 135:1169–1178

Belijaards RC, Kaudewitz P, Berti E, Gianotti R, Neumann C, Rosso R, Paulli M, Meijer CJLM, Willemze R (1993) Primary cutaneous CD30-positive large cell lymphoma: definition of a new type of cutaneous lymphoma with a favorable prognosis. A European multicenter study on 47 cases. Cancer 71:2097–2104

Beljaards RC, Meijer CJLM, van der Putte SCJ, Hollema H, Geerts ML, Bezemer PD, Willemze R (1994) Primary cutaneous T-cell lymphomas. Clinicopathologic features and prognostic parameters of 35 cases other than mycosis fungoides and CD30-positive large cell lymphoma. J Pathol 172:53–60

Bell CR, Napier MP, Morgan RJ, Dick R, Jarmulowicz M, Jones AL (1995) Primary non-Hodgkin's lymphoma of the prostate gland: case report and review of the literature. Clin Oncol (R Coll Radiol) 7:409–410

Bennett SR, Greer JP, Stein RS, Glick AD, Cousar JB, Collins RB (1984) Death due to splenic rupture in suppressor cell mycosis fungoides: a case report. Am J Clin Pathol 82:104–109

Bentz M, Barth TFE, Brüderlein S, Bock D, Schwerer MJ, Baudis M, Joos S, Viardot A, Feller AC, Müller-Hermelink HK, Lichter P, Döhner H, Möller P (2001) Gain of chromosome arm 9p is characteristic of primary mediastinal B-cell lymphoma (MBL) – a comprehensive molecular cytogenetic analysis and presentation of a novel cell line. Genes Chromosome Cancer 30:393–401

Berger F, Felman P, Thieblemont C, Pradier T, Baseggio L, Bryon PA, Salles G, Gallet-Bauchu E, Coiffier B (2000) Non-MALT marginal zone B-cell lymphomas: a description of clinical presentation and outcome in 124 patients. Blood 95:1950–1956

Bergman R, Kurtin PJ, Gibson LE, Hull PR, Kimlinger TK, Schroeter AL (2001) Clinicopathologic, immunophenotypic, and molecular characterization of primary cutaneous follicular B-cell lymphoma. Arch Dermatol 137:432–439

Berkman N, Breuer R (1993) Pulmonary involvement in lymphoma. Respir Med 87:85–92

Berkman N, Breuer R, Kramer MR, Polliack A (1996) Pulmonary involvement in lymphoma. Leuk Lymph 20:229–237

Berti E, Gianotti R, Alessi E, Caputo R (1990) Primary cutaneous follicular center cell lymphoma: immunophenotypical and immunogenotypical aspects. Curr Probl Dermatol 19:196–202

Berti E, Tomasini D, Vermeer MH, Meijer CJ, Alessi E, Willemze R (1999) Primary cutaneous CD8-positive epidermotropic cytotoxic T cell lymphomas. A distinct clinicopathological entity with an aggressive clinical behavior. Am J Pathol 155:483–492

Bertoncelli C, Airoldi G, Zigrossi P, Catania E, Ramponi A, Monteverde A (1993) Parenchymal renal involvement in 3 cases of non-Hodgkin lymphomas: clinical and pathological features. Haematologica 78:58–60

Beylot-Barry M, Lamant L, Vergier B, de Muret A, Fraitag S, Delord B, Dubus P, Vaillant L, Delaunay M, MacGrogan G, Beylot C, de Mascarel A, Delsol G, Merlio JP (1996) Detection of t (2;5) (p23;q35) translocation by reverse transcriptase polymerase chain reaction and in situ hybridization in CD30-positive primary cutaneous lymphoma and lymphomatoid papulosis. Am J Pathol 149:483–492

Beylot-Barry M, Groppi A, Vergier B, Pulford K, Merlio JP (1998) Characterization of t(2;5) reciprocal transcripts and genomic breakpoints in CD30+ cutaneous lymphoproliferations. Blood 91:4668–4676

Bhawan J, Wolff SM, Ucci AA, Bhan AK (1985) Malignant lymphoma and malignant angioendotheliomatosis: one disease. Cancer 55:570–576

Bienenstock J (1973) Bronchus-associated lymphoid tissue. In: Bienenstock J (ed) Immunology of the lung and upper respiratory tract, vol 1. McGraw-Hill, New York, pp 96–118

Bienenstock J, Johnston N (1976) A morphologic study of rabbit bronchial lymphoid aggregates and lymphoepithelium. Lab Invest 35:343–348

Binet JL, Leporrier M, Dighierro G, Charron D, D'Athis P, Vaugier G, Merle-Beral H, Natali JC, Raphael M, Nizet MG, Follezou JY (1977) A clinical staging system for chronic lymphocytic leukemia: prognostic significance. Cancer 40:855–863

Binet JL, Auquier A, Dighierro G et al (1981) A view prognostic classification of chronic lymphocytic leukemia derived from a multivariate survival analysis. Cancer 48:198

Bishop PC, Wilson WH, Pearson D, Janik J, Jaffe ES, Elwood PC (1999) CNS involvement in primary mediastinal large B-cell lymphoma. J Clin Oncol 17:2479–2485

Bjorn-Hansen R (1973) Primary plasmocytoma of the spleen. Am J Roentg Radiol Ther Nucl Med CXVII:81–83

Blakolmer K, Vesely M, Kummer JA, Jurecka W, Mannhalter C, Chott A (2000) Immunoreactivity of B-cell markers (CD791, L26) in rare cases of extranodal cytotoxic peripheral T- (NK/T) cell lymphomas. Mod Pathol 13:766–772

Bobrow LG, Richards MA, Happerfield LC, Diss TC, Isaacson PG, Lammie GA, Millis RR (1993) Breast lymphoma: a clinicopathologic review. Hum Pathol 24:274–278

Boni R, Xin H, Kamarashev J, Utzinger E, Dummer R, Kempft W, Kutzner H, Burg G (2000) Allelic deletion at 9p21–22 in primary cutaneous CD30+ large cell lymphoma. J Invest Dermatol 115:1104–1107

Borgonovo G, d'Oiron R, Amato A, Leger-Ravet MB, Iseni MC, Smadja C, Lemaigre G, Franco D (1995) Primary lymphoplasmacytic lymphoma of the liver associated with a serum monoclonal peak of IgG kappa. Am J Gastroenterol 90:137–140

Bosch F, Campo E, Jares P, Pittaluga S, Munoz J, Nayach I, Piris MA, De Wolf-Peeters C, Jaffe ES, Rozman C, Montserrat E, Cardesa A (1995) Increased expression of the PRAD-1/CCND1 gene in hairy cell leukemia. Br J Hematol 91:1025–1030

Bostwick DG, Mann RB (1985) Malignant lymphomas involving the prostate. A study of 13 cases. Cancer 56:2932–2938

Bostwick DG, Iczkowski KA, Amin MB, Discigil G, Osborne B (1998) Malignant lymphoma involving the prostate: report of 62 cases. Cancer 83:732–738

Boulland ML, Kanavaros P, Wechsler J, Casiraghi O, Gaulard P (1997) Cytotoxic protein expression in natural killer cell lymphomas and in αβ and γδ peripheral T-cell lymphomas. J Pathol 183:432–439

Boulland ML,Wechsler J, Bagot M, Pulford K, Kanavaros P, Gaulard P.(2000) Primary CD30-positive cutaneous T-cell lymphomas and lymphomatoid papulosis frequently express cytotoxic proteins. Histopathology 36:136–144

Bouroncle BA (1994) Thirty-five years in the progress of hairy cell leukaemia. Leuk Lymph 14 [Suppl 1]:1–12

Bowman SJ, Levison DA, Cotter FE, Kingsley GH (1994) Primary T-cell lymphoma of the liver in a patient with Felty syndrome. Br J Rheumatol 33:157–160

Brady SP, Magro CM, Diaz-Cano SJ, Wolfe HJ (1999) Analysis of clonality of atypical cutaneous lymphoid infiltrates associated with drug therapy by PCR/DGGE. Hum Pathol 30:130–136

Brandter LB, Smith CI, Hammerström L, Lindemalm C, Christensson B (1989) Clonal immunoglobulin gene rearrangements in primary mediastinal clear cell lymphomas. Leukemia 3:122–129

Braun-Falco O, Marghescu S, Wolff HH (1973) Pagetoide Reticulose: Morbus Woringer-Kolopp. Hautarzt 24:11–21

Breslin NP, Urbanski SJ, Shaffer EA (1999) Mucosa-associated lymphoid tissue (MALT) lymphoma manifesting as multiple lymphomatosis polyposis of the gastrointestinal tract. Am J Gastroenterol 94:2540–2545

Brooks HL, Downing J, McClure JA, Engel HM (1984) Orbital Burkitt's lymphoma in a homosexual man with acquired immunodeficiency. Arch Ophtalmol 102:1533–1537

Brouet JC, Sasportes M, Flandrin G, Preud'Homme JL, Seligmann M (1975) Chronic lymphocytic leukaemia of T-cell origin. Immunological and clinical evaluation in eleven patients. Lancet 2:890–893

Brouland JP, Meeus F, Rossert J, Hernigou A, Gentric D, Jacquot C, Diebold J, Nochy D (1994) Primary bilateral B-cell renal lymphoma: a case report and review of the literature. Am J Kidney Dis 24:586–589

Buck DS, Peterson MS, Borogovitz D et al (1992) Non-Hodgkin lymphoma of the ureter: CT demonstration with pathologic correlation. Urol Radiol 14:183–187

Burke JS (1981) Surgical pathology of the spleen: an approach to the differential diagnosis of splenic lymphomas and leukemias, part 1. Disease of the white pulp. Am J Surg Pathol 5:551–563

Burke JS (1985) The diagnosis of lymphoma and lymphoid proliferations in the spleen. In: Jaffe ES (ed) Surgical pathology of the lymph nodes and related organs. Saunders, Philadelphia, pp 249–281

Burke JS, Rappaport H (1984) The diagnosis and differential diagnosis of hairy cell leukemia in bone marrow and spleen. Semin Oncol 11:334–346

Burke JS, Byrne GE, Rappaport H (1974a) Hairy cell leukemia (leukemic reticuloendotheliosis). I. A clinicopathologic study of 21 patients. Cancer 33:1399–1410

Burke JS, MacKay B, Rappaport H (1974b) Hairy cell leukemia (leukemic reticuloendotheliosis). II. Ultrastructure of the spleen. Cancer 37:2267–2274

Burns MK, Chan LS, Cooper KD (1995) Woringer-Kolopp disease (localized pagetoid reticulosis) or unilesional mycosis fungoides? (Letter to the editor.) Arch Dermatol 131:325

Buttori C, Perrin C, Chevallier A, Taillan B, Michiels JF, Diebold J, Hofman P (1997) Diagnostic d'un lymphome intravasculaire sur une biopsie musculaire. Ann Pathol 17:340–342

Caccamo D, Pervez NK, Marchevsky A (1986) Primary lymphoma of the liver in the acquired immunodeficiency syndrome. Arch Pathol Lab Med 110:553–555

Cairns P, Butany J, Fulop J, Rakowski H, Hassaram S (1987) Cardiac presentation of non-Hodgkin's lymphoma. Arch Pathol Lab Med 111:80–83

Camitta BM, Casper JT, Kun LE, Lauer SJ, Starshak RJ, Oechler HW (1986) Isolated bilateral T-cell renal lymphoblastic lymphoma. Am J Pediatr Hematol Oncol 8:8–12

Capello D, Vitolo U, Pasqualucci L et al (2000) Distribution and pattern of BCL-6 mutations throughout the spectrum of B-cell neoplasia. Blood 95:651–659

Capron F, Audouin J, Diebold J, Ameille J, Lebeau B, Rochemaure J (1985) Pulmonary polymorphic centroblastic type malignant lymphoma in a patient with lymphomatoid granulomatosis, Sjögren syndrome and other manifestations of a dysimmune state. Pathol Res Pract 179:656–665

Carbonnel F, Grollet-Brioul L, Brouet JC, Teilhac MF, Cosnes J, Angonin R, Deschaseaux M, Chatelet FP, Gendre JP, Sigaux F (1998) Are complicated forms of celiac disease cryptic T-cell lymphomas? Blood 92:3879–3886

Carey RW, Harris N, Kliman B (1987) Addison's disease secondary to lymphomatous infiltration of the adrenal glands: recovery of adrenocortical function after chemotherapy. Cancer 59:1087–1090

Carter DK, Batts KP, de Groen PC, Kurtin PJ (1996) Angiotropic large cell lymphoma (intravascular lymphomatosis) occurring after follicular small cleaved cell lymphoma. Mayo Clin Proc 71:869–873
Cassoux N, Merle-Beral H, Leblond V, Bodaghi B, Milea D, Gerber S, Fardeau C, Reux I, Xuan KH, Chan CC, LeHoang P (2000) Ocular and central nervous system lymphoma: clinical features and diaganosis. Occ Immunol Inflamm 8:243–250
Castroagudin JF, Gonzalez-Quintela A, Fraga M, Forteza J, Barrio E (1999) Presentation of T-cell-rich B-cell lymphoma mimicking acute hepatitis. Hepatogastroenterology 46: 1710–1713
Cazals-Hatem D, Lepage E, Brice P, Ferrant A, d'Agay MF, Baumelou E, Brière J, Blanc M, Gaulard P, Biron P, Schlaifer D, Diebold J, Audouin J (1996) Primary mediastinal large B-cell lymphoma. A clinicopathologic study of 141 cases compared with 916 nonmediastinal large B-cell lymphomas. A GELA ("Groupe d'Etude des Lymphomes de l'Adulte") study. Am J Surg Pathol 20:877–888
Cellier C, Delabesse E, Helmer C, Patey N, Matuchansky C, Jabri B, Macintyre E, Cerf-Bensussan N, Brousse N (2000) Refractory sprue, coeliac disease, and enteropathy-associated T-cell lymphoma. French Coeliac Disease Study Group. Lancet 356:203–208
Cerroni L, Rieger E, Hodl S, Kerl H (1992) Clinicopathologic and immunologic features associated with transformation of mycosis fungoides to large-cell lymphoma. Am J Surg Pathol 16:543–552
Cerroni L, Volkenandt M, Rieger E, Soyer HP, Kerl H (1994) bcl-2 protein expression and correlation with the interchromosomal 14;18 translocation in cutaneous lymphomas and pseudolymphomas. J Invest Dermatol 102:231–235
Cerroni L, Signoretti S, Höfler G, Annessi G, Pütz B, Lackinger E, Metze D, Giannetti A, Kerl H (1997a) Primary cutaneous marginal zone B-cell lymphoma: a recently described entity of low-grade malignant cutaneous B-cell lymphoma. Am J Surg Pathol 21:1307–1315
Cerroni L, Zochling N, Putz B, Kerl H (1997b) Infection by Borrelia burgdorferi and cutaneous B-cell lymphoma. J Cutan Pathol 24:457–461
Cerroni L, Arzberger E, Putz B, Hofler G, Metze D, Sander CA, Rose C, Wolf P, Rutten A, McNiff JM, Kerl H (2000) Primary cutaneous follicle center cell lymphoma with follicular growth pattern. Blood 95:3922–3928
Cesarman E, Chang Y, Moore PS, Said JW, Knowles DM (1995) Kaposi's sarcoma-associated herpesvirus-like DNA sequences in AIDS-related body-cavity-based lymphomas. N Engl J Med 332:1186–1191
Cesarman E, Nador RG, Aozasa K, Delsol G, Said JW, Knowles DM (1996) Kaposi's sarcoma-associated herpesvirus in non-AIDS related lymphomas occurring in body cavities. Am J Pathol 149:53–57
Chadburn A, Frizzera G (1999) Mediastinal large B-cell lymphoma vs classic Hodgkin lymphoma. Am J Clin Pathol 112:155–158
Chan AC, Ho JW, Chiang AK, Srivastava G (1999) Phenotypic and cytotoxic characteristics of peripheral T-cell and NK-cell lymphomas in relation to Epstein-Barr virus association. Histopathology 34:16–24
Chan JK, Ng CS, Lau WH, Lo ST (1987a) Most nasal/nasopharyngeal lymphomas are peripheral T-cell neoplasms. Am J Surg Pathol 11:418–429
Chan JK, Ng CS, Lo STH (1987b) Immunohistological characterization of malignant lymphomas of the Waldeyer's ring other than the nasopharynx. Histopathology 11:885–899
Chan JK, Ng CS, Isaacson PG (1990) Relationship between high-grade lymphoma and low-grade B-cell mucosa-associated lymphoid tissue lymphoma (MALToma) of the stomach. Am J Pathol 136:1153–1164
Chan JK, Ng CS, Hui P et al (1991) Anaplastic large cell Ki-1 lymphoma of bone. Cancer 68:2186–2191
Chan WC, Link S, Mawle A, Check I, Brynes RK, Winton EF (1986) Heterogeneity of large granular lymphocyte proliferations: delineation of two major subtypes. Blood 68:1142–1153
Chan WC, Catovsky D, Foucar K, Montserrat E (2001) T-cell large granular lymphocyte leukaemia. In: Jaffe ES, Harris NL, Stein H, Vardiman JW (eds) World Health Organization Classification of Tumours. Pathology and genetics of tumours of haematopoietic and lymphoid tissues. IARC Press, Lyon
Chang A, Zic JA, Boyd AS (1998) Intravascular large cell lymphoma: a patient with asymptomatic purpuric patches and a chronic clinical course. J Am Acad Dermatol 39:318–321
Chang SE, Huh J, Choi JH, Sung KJ, Moon KC, Koh JK (2000) Clinicopathological features of CD56+ nasal-type T/natural killer cell lymphomas with lobular panniculitis. Br J Dermatol 142:924–930
Charton-Bain MC, Brousset P, Bouabdallal R, Gaulard P, Merlio JP, Dubus P, Rostaing L, de Roux C, Weiller PJ, Hassoun J, Xerri L (2000a) Variation in the histological pattern of nodal involvement by gamma/delta T-cell lymphoma. Histopathology 36:233–239
Charton-Bain MC, Lelong B, Bouabdallah R, Dubus P, Merlio JP, Hassoun J, Xerri L (2000b) Hepatic MALT lymphoma disclosing a nodal extension. Ann Pathol 20:137–141
Chen F, Ike O, Wada H, Hitomi S (2000) Pulmonary mucosa-associated lymphoid tissue lymphoma 8 years after resection of the same type of lymphoma of the liver. Jpn J Thorac Cardiovasc Surg 48:233–235
Cheng FY, Tsui WM, Yeung WT et al (1997) Intravascular lymphomatosis: a case presenting with encephalomyelitis and reactive haemophagocytic syndrome diagnosed by renal biopsy. Histopathology 31:552–554
Cheung MM, Chan JK, Lau WH, Foo W, Chan PT, NG CS, Ngan RK (1998) Primary non-Hodgkin's lymphoma of the nose and nasopharynx: clinical features, tumor immunophenotype, and treatment outcome in 113 patients. J Clin Oncol 16:70–77
Child FJ, Mitchell TJ, Whittaker SJ, Calonje E, Spittle M, Crokker J, Russel-Jones R (2003) Blastic natural killer cell and extranodal natural killer cell-like T-cell lymphoma presenting in the skin: report of six cases from the U.K. Br J Dermatol 148:507–15
Child FJ, Russel-Jones R, Woolford AJ, Calonje E, Photiou A, Orchard G, Whittaker SJ (2001) Absence of the t(14;18) chromosomal translocation in primary cutaneous B-cell lymphoma. Br J Dermatol 144:735–744
Chim CS, Chan AC, Kwong YL, Liang R (1997) Primary cardiac lymphoma. Am J Hematol 54:79–83

Chorlton I, Norris HJ, King FM (1974) Malignant reticuloendothelial disease involving the ovary as a primary manifestation: a series of 19 lymphomas and 1 granulocytic sarcoma. Cancer 34:397–407

Chott A, Dragosics B, Radaszkiewicz T (1992) Peripheral T-cell lymphomas of the intestine. Am J Pathol 141

Chott A, Haedicke W, Mosberger I, Födinger M, Winkler K, Mannhalter C, Müller-Hermelink HK (1998) Most CD56+ intestinal lymphomas are CD8+CD5- T-cell lymphomas of monomorphic small to medium size histology. Am J Pathol 153:1483–1490

Chowla A, Malhi-Chowla N, Chidambaram A, Surick B (1999) Primary hepatic lymphoma in hepatitis C: case report and review of the literature. Am Surg 65:881–883

Chui CT, Hoppe RT, Kohler S, Kim YH (1999) Epidermotropic cutaneous B-cell lymphoma mimicking mycosis fungoides. J Am Acad Dermatol 41:271–274

Ciacci JD, Tellez C, VonRoenn J, Levy RM (1999) Lymphoma of the central nervous system in AIDS. Semin Neurol 19:213–221

Clayton F, Butler JJ, Ayala AG, Ro J, Zornoza J (1987) Non-Hodgkin's lymphoma in bone: pathologic and radiologic features with clinical correlates. Cancer 60:2494–2501

Cleary KR, Batsakis JG (1994) Sinonasal lymphomas. Ann Otol Rhinol Laryngol 103:911–914

Close PM, Macrae MB, Hammond JM et al (1993) Anaplastic large cell Ki-1 lymphoma. Pulmonary presentation mimicking miliary tuberculosis. Am J Clin Pathol 94:631–636

Cogliatti SB, Schmid U, Schumacher U, Eckert F, Hansmann ML, Hedderich J, Takahashi H, Lennert K (1991) Primary B-cell gastric lymphma: a cliniopathological study of 145 patients. Gastroenterology 101:1159–7170

Cohen PL, Brooks JJ (1991) Lymphomas of the breast: a clinicopathologic and immunohistochemical study of primary and secondary cases. Cancer 67:1359–1369

Collins MH, Orazi A, Bauman M, Vik T, West K, Herema NA, Klatt, Neiman RS (1993) Primary hepatic B-cell lymphoma in a child. Am J Surg Pathol 17:1182–1186

Colomo L, Lopez-Guillermo A, Perales M, Rives S, Martinez A, Bosch F, Colomer D, Falini B, Montserrat E, Campo E (2003) Clinical impact of the differentiation profile assessed by immunophenotyping in patients with diffuse large B-cell lymphoma. Blood 101:78–84

Colwill R, Dube I, Scott JG, Bailey D, Deharven E, Carstairs K, Pantalony D (1990) Isochromosome 7q as the role abnormality in an unusual case of T-cell lineage malignancy. Hematol Pathol 4:53–58

Connors JM, Klimo P, Voss N et al (1988) Testicular lymphoma: improved outcome with early brief chemotherapy. J Clin Oncol 6:776–781

Cooke CB, Krenacs L, Stetler STE, Venson M, Greiner TC, Raffeld M, Hingma DW, Abruzzo L, Frantz C, Kaviani M, Jaffe ES (1996) Hepatosplenic T-cell lymphoma: a distinct clinicopathologic entity of cytotoxic gamma delta T-cell origin. Blood 88:4265–4274

Copie-Bergman C, Niedobitek G, Mangham DC, Selves J, Baloch K, Diss TC, Knowles DN, Delsol G, Isaacson PG (1997) Epstein-Barr virus in B-cell lymphomas associated with chronic suppurative inflammation. J Pathol 183:287–292

Copie-Bergman C, Wotherspoon AC, Norton AJ, Diss TC, Isaacson PG (1998) True histiocytic lymphoma: a morphologic, immunohistochemical, and molecular genetic study of 13 cases. Am J Surg Pathol 22:1386–1392

Copie-Bergman C, Gaulard P, Maouche-Chrétien L, Brière J, Haioun C, Alonso MA, Romeo PH, Leroy K (1999) The MAL gene is expressed in primary mediastinal large B-cell lymphoma. Blood 94:3567–3575

Corcoran MM, Mould ST, Orchard JA et al (1999) Dysregulation of cyclin dependent kinase 6 expression in splenic marginal zone lymphoma through chromosome 7q translocation. Oncogene 18:6271–6277

Coupland SE, Foss HD, Hidayat AA, Cockerham GC, Hummel M, Stein H (2002) Extranodal marginal zone B cell lymphoma of the uvea: an analysis of 13 cases. J Pathol 197:333–40

Coupland SE, Foss HD, Assaf C, Auw-Haedrich C, Anastassiou G, Anagnostopoulos I, Hummel M, Karesh JW, Lee WR, Stein H (1999) T-cell and T/natural killer-cell lymphomas involving ocular and ocular adnexal tissues: a clinicopathologic, immunohistochemical, and molecular study of seven cases. Ophtalmology 106:2109–2120

Cualing H, Steele P, Zellner D (2000) Blastic transformation of splenic marginal zone B-cell lymphoma. Arch Pathol Lab Med 124:748–752

Dahlin DC, Unni KK (1986) Bone tumors: general aspects and data on 8542 cases. Thomas, Springfield

Dai MS, Ho CL, Chen CY, Chen TM, Yu CP, Chau TY (2000) Lymphoma of bone with initial presentation as a calvarial mass. Ann Hematol 79:700–702

Damaj G, Verkarre V, Delmer A, Solal-Celigny P, Yakoub-Agha I, Cellier C, Maurschhauser F, Bouabdallah R, Leblond V, Lefrere F, Bouscary D, Audouin J, Coiffier B, Varet B, Molina T, Broussa N, Hermine O (2003) Primary follicular lymphoma of the gastrointestinal tract: a study of 25 cases and a literature review. Ann Oncol 14:623–629

D'Amore F, Brincker H, Christensen BE, Thorling K, Pedersen M, Nielsen JL, Sandberg E, Pedersen NT, Sorensen E (1992) Non-Hodgkin's lymphoma in the elderly. A study of 602 patients aged 70 or older from a Danish population-based registry. The Danish LYEO-Study Group. Ann Oncol 3:379–386

Daniel MT, Tigaud I, Flexor MA et al (1995) Leukaemic non-Hodgkin's lymphomas with hyperdiploid cells and t(11;14)(q13;q32): a subtype of mantle cell lymphoma? Br J Haematol 90:77–84

Daniele RP (1990) Immunoglobulin secretion in the airways. Annu Rev Physiol 52:177–195

Dargent JL, De Wolf-Peeters C (1998) Liver involvement by lymphoma: identification of a distinct pattern of infiltration related to T-cell/histiocyte-rich B-cell lymphoma. Ann Diagn Pathol 2:363–369

Dargent JL, Diedhiou A, Lothaire P, Demunter A, Lespagnard L, de Wolf-Peeters C (2001) Subcutaneous lymphoid hyperplasia arising at site of ethnic scarifications and mimicking subcutaneous panniculitis-like T-cell lymphoma. Virchows Arch 438:298–301

Das DK, Gupta SK, Ayyagari S et al (1987) Pleural effusions in non-Hodgkin's lymphoma. Acta Cytol 31:119–124

Daum S, Weiss D, Hummel M, Ullrich R, Heise W, Stein H, Riecken EO, Foss HD, Intestinal Lymphoma Study Group

(2001) Frequency of clonal intraepithelial T lymphocyte proliferations in enteropathy-type intestinal T cell lymphoma, coeliac disease, and refractory sprue. GUT 49:804–812

DeAngelis LM (1999) Primary CNS lymphoma: treatment with combined chemotherapy and radiotherapy. J Neurooncol 43:249–257

DeCoteau JF, Butmarc JR, Kinney MC, Kadin ME (1996) The t(2;5) chromosomal translocation is not anaplastic large cell lymphoma of nodal origin. Blood 87:3437–3441

De Bruin PC, Beljaards RC, van Heerde P, van der Valk P, Noorduyn LA, van Krieken JHJM, Kluin-Nelemans JC, Willemze R, Meijer CJLM (1993) Differences in clinical behaviour and immunophenotype between primary cutaneous and primary nodal anaplastic large cell lymphoma of T-cell or null cell phenotype. Histopathology 23:127–135

De Bruyne R, Peters O, Goossens A, Braekman J, Denis LJ (1987) Primary IgG-lambda immunocytoma of the urinary bladder. Eur J Surg Oncol 13:361–364

De Girolami U, Henin D, Girard B, Katlama C, Le Hoang P, Hauw JJ (1989) Etude pathologique de l'œil et du système nerveux central dans 25 cas de SIDA. Rev Neurol 145:819–828

De Jong D, Boot H, can Heerde P, Hart GA, Taal BG (1997) Histological grading in gastric lymphoma: pretreatment criteria and clinical relevance. Gastroenterology 112:1466–1474

De Jong D, Vyth-Dreese F, Dellemijn T, Verra N, Ruskone-Fourmestraux A, Lavergne-Slove A, Hart G, Boot H (2001) Histological and immunological parameters to predict treatment outcome of Helicobacter pylori eradication in low-grade gastric MALT lymphoma. J Pathol 193: 318–324

Delafaye C, Gin H, Morlat P, Ragnaud JM, Aubertin J (1990) Lymphome non hodgkinien bilateral primitif et isolé des glandes surrénales. Semin Hôp Paris 66:1473–1475

De la Fouchardiere A, Balme B, Chouvet B, Sebban C, Perrot H, Claudy A, Bryon PA, Coiffier B, Berger F (1999) Primary cutaneous marginal zone B-cell lymphoma: a report of 9 cases. J Am Acad Dermatol 41: 181–188

De Leval L, Ferry JA, Falini B, Shipp M, Harris NL (2001) Expression of bcl-6 and CD10 in primary mediastinal large B-cell lymphoma. Evidence for derivation from germinal center B-cells? Am J Surg Pathol 25:1277–1282

Delventhal S, Brandis A, Ostertag H, Pabst R (1992) Low incidence of bronchus-associated lymphoid tissue (BALT) in chronically inflamed human lungs. Virchows Archiv B Cell Pathol 62:271–274

De Mascarel A, Merlio JP, Coindre JM, Goussot JF, Broustet A (1989) Gastric large cell lymphoma expressing cytokeratin but no leukocyte common antigen: a diagnostic dilemna. Am J Clin Pathol 91:478–480

De Ment SH, Mann RB, Staal SP, Kuhajda FP, Boitnott JK (1987) Primary lymphomas of the liver. Report of six cases and review of the literature. Am J Clin Pathol 88:255–263

Demirer T, Dail D, Aboulafia D (1994) Four varied cases of intravascular lymphomatosis and the literature review. Cancer 73:1738–1745

Demirhan B, Sokmensuer C, Karakayali H, Gungen Y, Dogan A, Haberal M (1997) Primary extramedullary plasmacytoma of the liver. J Clin Pathol 50:74–76

Deneau DG, Wood GS, Beckstead J, Hoppe RT, Price N (1984) Woringer-Kolopp disease (pagetoid reticulosis). Four cases with histopathologic, ultrastructural, and immunohistologic observations. Arch Dermatol 120:1045–1051

Desai S, Jambhekar NA, Soman CS, Advani SH (1991) Primary lymphoma of bone. A clinico-pathologic study of 25 cases reported over 10 years. J Surg Oncol 46:265–269

Devine RM, Edis AJ, Banks PM (1981) Primary lymphoma of the thyroid. A review of the Mayo Clinic experience through 1978. World J Surg 5:33–38

Diebold J (1989) Tumeurs spleniques conjonctives et hématopoïétiques. Lymphomes malins. In: Delaitre B, Baret B (eds) La Rate. Springer, Berlin Heidelberg New York, pp 271–290

Diebold J (1997) Primary lymphoma of bone. In: Forest M, Tomeno B, Vanel D (eds) Orthopedic surgical pathology. Churchill Livingstone, Edinburgh, pp 467–475

Diebold J, Chomette G, Tricot G, Reynès M (1977) La rate dans la leucémie à tricholeucocytes. Virchows Arch A Anat Pathol 372:325–336

Diebold J, Reynès M, Tricot G, Zafrani E, Weill B, Dao C, Zittoun R, James JM, de Carbonière C, Bilski-Pasquier G (1978) Sarcomes lympho-plasmocytaires spléniques découverts par laparotomie exploratrice au cours de 2 cas de maladie chronique des agglutinines froides. Sem Hop Paris 54:1325–1330

Diebold J, Kanavaros P, Audouin J, Bernadou A, Zittoun R (1987) Les lymphomes malins centroblastiques centrocytiques et centroblastiques à prédominance splénique (ou primitifs de la rate). Etude anatomo-clinique de 17 cas. Bull Cancer 74:437–453

Diebold J, Audouin J, Viry B, Ghandour C, Betti P, D'Ornano G (1990) Primary lymphoplasmacytic lymphoma of the larynx: a rare localization of MALT lymphoma. Ann Otol Rhinol Laryngol 99:577–580

Diebold J, Raphaël M, Prévot S, Audouin J (1997) Lymphomas associated with HIV infection. In: Wotherspoon WC (ed) Lymphoma cancer surveys series, vol 30. Cold Spring Harbor Laboratory Press, Cold Spring Harbor, pp 263–294

Dierlamm J, Pittaluga S, Wlodarska I et al (1996) Marginal zone B-cell lymphomas of different sites share similar cytogenetic and morphologic features. Blood 87:299–307

Dierlamm J, Pittaluga S, Stul M, Wlodarska I, Michaux L, Thomas J, Verhoef G, Verhest A, Depardieu C, Cassiman JJ, Hagemeijer A, De Wolf-Peeters C, Van Den Berghe H (1997) Bcl-6 gene rearrangements also occur in marginal zone B-cell lymphoma. Br J Haematol 98:719–725

Dierlamm J, Wlodarska I, Michaux L, Stefanova M, Hinz K, van den Berghe H, Hagemeijer A, Hossfeld DK (2000) Genetic abnormalities in marginal zone B-cell lymphoma. Hematol Oncol 18:1–13

Dietz SB, Whitaker-Menezes D, Lessin SR (1996) The role of alpha E beta 7 integrin (CD103) and E-cadherin in epidermotropismin cutaneous T-cell lymphoma. J Cutan Pathol 23:312–318

Dighiero G, Charron D, Debré P, Leporrier VG, Follezou JV, Degos L, Jacquillat CI, Buret JL (1979) Identification of a pure splenic form of chronic lymphocytic leukemia. Br J Haematol 41:169–176

DiGiuseppe JA, Nelson WG, Seifter EJ, Boitnott JK, Mann RB (1994) Intravascular lymphomatosis: a clinicopathologic study of 10 cases and assessment of response to chemotherapy. J Clin Oncol 12:2573–2579

Dixon JM, Lumsden AB, Krajewski A, Elton RA, Anderson TJ (1987) Primary lymphoma of the breast. Brit J Surg 74:241–247

Domizio P, Hall PA, Cotter F, Amiel S, Tucker J, Besser GM, et al (1989) Angiotropic large cell lymphoma (ALCL): morphological, immunohistochemical and genotypic studies with analysis of previous reports. Hematol Oncol 7:195–206

Domizio P, Owen RA, Shepherd NA, Talbot IC, Norton AJ (1993) Primary lymphoma of the small intestine. A clinicopathological study of 119 cases. Am J Surg Pathol 17:429–442

Donnadieu J, Patte C, Kalifa C, Lemerle J (1992) Diagnostic and therapeutic problems posed by malignant non-Hodgkin lymphoma of renal origin in children. A proposal of 7 cases. Arch Fr Pediatr 49:699–704

Drut R, Drut RM (2001) Primary angiocentric T-cell intestinal lymphoma with Epstein-Barr virus in a 5-year-old boy. Int J Surg Pathol 9:163–68

Du MQ, Peng HZ, Dogan A, Diss TC, Liu H, Pan LX, Moseley RP, Briskin MJ, Chan JKC, Isaacson PG (1997) Preferential dissemination of B-cell gastric mucosa-associated lymphoid tissue (MALT) lymphoma to the splenic marginal zone. Blood 90:4071–4077

Du MQ, Diss TC, Dogan A, Ye HT, Aiello A, Wotherspoon AC, Pan LX, Isaacson PG (2000) Clone-specific PCR reveals wide dissemination of gastric MALT lymphoma to the gastric mucosa. J Pathol 192:488–493

Dufau JP, Le Tourneau A, Molina T, Le Houcq M, Claessens YE, Rio B, Delmer A, Diebold J (2000) Intravascular large B-cell lymphoma with bone marrow involvement at presentation and haemophagocytic syndrome: two Western cases in favour of a specific variant. Histopathology 37:509–512

Duggan MJ, Weisenburger DD, Le YL et al (1990) Mantle zone lymphoma: a clinicopathologic study of 22 cases. Cancer 66:522–529

Dumont J, Mazabraud A (1979) Primary lymphomas of bone (so-called "Parker and Jackson's reticulum cell sarcoma"). Histological review of 75 cases according to the new classifications of non-Hodgkin's lymphomas. Biomedicine 31:271–275

Duncan LM, LeBoit PE (1997) Are primary cutaneous immunocytoma and marginal zone lymphoma the same disease? Am J Surg Pathol 21:1368–1372

Dunn-Walters DK, Boursier L, Spencer J, Isaacson PG (1998) Analysis of immunoglobulin genes in splenic marginal zone lymphoma suggests ongoing mutation. Hum Pathol 29:585–593

Dunphy CH, Bee C, McDonald JW, Grosso LE (1998) Incidental early detection of a splenic marginal zone lymphoma by polymerase chain reaction analysis of paraffin-embedded tissue. Arch Pathol Lab Med 122:84–86

Dunphy CH, Oza YV, Skelly ME (1999) An otherwise typical case of non-Japanese hairy cell leukemia with CD10 and CDW75 expression. Response to cladaribine phosphate therapy. J Clin Lab Anat 13:141–144

Duong Van Huyen JP, Molina T, Delmer A, Audouin J, Le Tourneau A, Zittoun R, Bernadou A, Diebold J (2000) Splenic marginal zone lymphoma with or without plasmacytic differentiation. Am J Surg Pathol 24:1581–1592

Eby NL, Grufferman S, Flannelly CM, Schold SC Jr, Vogel FS, Burger PC (1988) Increasing incidence of primary brain lymphoma in the US. Cancer 62:2461–2465

Eckert F, Schmid U, Kaudewitz P, Burg G, Braun-Falco O (1989) Follicular lymphoid hyperplasia of the skin with high content of Ki-1 positive lymphocytes. Am J Dermatopathol 11:345–352

Economopoulos T, Fountzilas G, Kostourou A, Daniilidis J, Pavlidis N, Andreopoulos H et al (1998) Primary extranodal non-Hodgkin's lymphoma of the head and neck in adults: a clinicopathological comparaison beetween tonsillar and non-tonsillar lymphomas. Anticancer Res 18:4655–4660

Edelson RL (1980) Cutaneous T cell lymphoma: mycosis fungoides, Sézary syndrome, and other variants. A Am Acad Dermatol 2:89–106

Egawa N, Fukayama M, Kawaguchi K et al (1995) Relapsing oral and colonic ulcers with monoclonal T-cell infiltration. A low grade mucosal T-lymphoproliferative disease of the digestive tract. Cancer 75:1728–1733

Elenitoba-Johnson KS, Zarate-Osorno A, Meneses A, Krenacs L, Kingma DW, Raffeld M, Jaffe ES (1998) Cytotoxic granular protein expression, Epstein-Barr virus stain type, and latent membrane protein-1 oncogene deletions in nasal T-lymphocyte/natural killer cell lymphomas from Mexico. Mod Pathol 11:754–761

Ellis GL, Auclair PL (1996) Malignant lymphomas of the major salivary glands. Tumors of the salivary glands. Atlas of tumor pathology, 3rd ser, fasc 17. Armed Forces Institute of Pathology, Washington DC

Ellis JH, Banks PM, Campbell RJ, Liesegang TJ (1985) Lymphoid tumors of the ocular adnexa. Clinical correlation with the working formulation classification and immunoperoxidase staining of paraffin sections. Opthalmology 92:1311–1324

Ellison DW, Wilkins BS (2001) Lymphoma and the nervous system. Neuropathol 95:239–265

Enno A, Catovsky D, O'Brien M, Cherchi M, Kumarran TO, Galton DAG (1979) "Prolymphocytoid" transformation of chronic lymphocytic leukaemia. Br J Haematol 41:9–18

Epstein EH Jr, Levin DL, Croft JD Jr, Lutzner MA (1972) Mycosis fungoides. Survival, prognostic features, response to therapy, and autopsy findings. Medicine (Baltimore) 51:61–72

Estalilla OC, Koo CH, Brynes RK, Medeiros LJ (1999) Intravascular large B-cell lymphoma. A report of five cases initially diagnosed by bone marrow biopsy. Am J Clin Pathol 112:248–255

Fairley NH, Mackie FP (1937) Clinical and biochemical syndrome in lymphadenoma and allied diseases involving mesenteric lymph glands. Br Med J 1: 973–980

Falcao RP, Garcia AB, Marques MG, Simoes BP, Fonseca BA, Rodrigues ML, Foss NT (2002) Blastic CD4 NK cell leukemia/lymphoma: a distinct clinical entity. Leuk Res 26:803–7

Falini B, Binazzi R, Pileri S et al (1988) Large cell lymphoma of bone: a report of 3 cases of B-cell origin. Histopathology 12:177–190

Falini B, Pileri S, Flenghi L et al (1990) Selection of a panel of monoclonal antibodies for monitoring residual disease in peripheral blood and bone marrow of interferon-treated hairy cell leukemia patients. Br J Haematol 76:460–468

Falini B, Venturi S, Martelli M et al (1995) Mediastinal large B-cell lymphoma: clinical and immunohistological findings of 18 patients with two different third generation regimens. Br J Haematol 89:780–789

Falini B, Fizzotti M, Pucciarini A, Bigerna B, Marafioti T, Gambacorta M, Pacini R, Alunni C, Natali-Tanci L, Ugolini B, Sebastiani C, Cattoretti G, Pileri S, Dalla-Favera R, Stein H (2000) A monoclonal antibody (MUM1p) detects expression of the MUM1/IRF4 protein in a subset of germinal center B cells, plasma cells, and activated T cells. Blood 95:2084–2092

Falk S, Karhoff M, Takeshita M, Stutte HS (1990) Primary pleomorphic T-cell lymphoma of the spleen. Histopathology 16:191–192

Farcet JP, Gaulard P, Marolleau JP, Henni T, Gourdin MF, Divine M, Haioun C, Zafrani S, Goossens M, Hercend T, Reyes F (1990) Hepatosplenic T cell lymphoma: sinusal-sinusoidal localization of malignant cells expressing the T cell receptor gamma-delta. Blood 75:2213–2219

Fauci AS, Haynes BF, Costa J, Katz P, Wolff SM (1982) Lymphomatoid granulomatosis. Prospective clinical and therapeutic experience over 10 years. N Engl J Med 306:68–74

Fellbaum C, Hansmann ML, Lennert K (1989) Malignant lymphomas of the nasal cavity and paranasal sinuses. Virchows Arch A 414:399–405

Ferry JA, Young RH (1991) Malignant lymphoma, pseudolymphoma and hematopoietic disorders of the female genital tract. Pathol Annu 62:227–263

Ferry JA, Harris NL, Pickel LJ (1988) Intravascular lymphomatosis (malignant angioendotheliomatosis). A B-cell neoplasm expressing surface homing receptors. Modern Pathol 1:44–52

Ferry JA, Harris NL, Young RH, Coen J, Zietman A, Scully RE (1994) Malignant lymphoma of the testis, epididymis, and spermatic cord. A clinicopathologic study of 69 cases with immunophenotypic analysis. Am J Surg Pathol 18:376–390

Ferry JA, Harris NL, Papanicolaou N, Young RH (1995) Lymphoma of the kidney. A report of 11 cases. Am J Surg Pathol 19:134–144

Ferry JA, Yang WI, Zukerberg LR, Wotherspoon AC, Arnold A, Harris NL (1996) CD5+ extranodal marginal zone B-cell (MALT) lymphoma. A low grade neoplasma with a propensity for bone marrow involvement and relapse. Am J Clin Pathol 105:31–37

Fiche M, Le Tourneau A, Audouin J, Touzard RC, Diebold J (1990) A case of primary osseous malignant immunoblastic B cell lymphoma with intracytoplasmic μ-lambda immunoglobulin inclusions. Histopathology 16:167–172

Fiche M, Capron F, Berger F, Galateau F, Cordier JF, Loire R, Diebold J (1995) Primary pulmonary non-Hodgkin's lymphomas. Histopathology 26:529–537

Fidias P, Wright C, Harris NL, Urba W, Grossbard ML (1996) Primary tracheal non-Hodgkin's lymphoma. A case report and review of the literature. Cancer 77:2332–2338

Fischbach W, Kestel W, Kirchner T, Mossner J, Wilms K (1992) Malignant lymphomas of the upper gastrointestinal tract. Results of a prospective study in 103 patients. Cancer 70:1075–1080

Flynn KJ, Dehner LP, Gajl-Peczalska KJ, Dahl MV, Ramsay N, Wang N (1982) Regressing Atypical Histiocytosis: a cutaneous proliferation of atypical neoplastic histiocytes with unexpectedly indolent biologic behavior. Cancer 49:959–970

Fraga M, Lloret E, Sanchez-Verde L, Orradre JL, Campo E, Bosch F, Piris MA (1995) Mucosal mantle cell (centrocytic) lymphomas. Histopathology 26:413–422

Franco V, Florena AM, Iannitto E (2003) Splenic marginal zone lymphoma. Blood 101:2464–72

François A, Lesesve JF, Stamatoullas A, Comoz F, Lenormand B, Etienne I, Mendel I, Hemet J, Bastard C, Tilly H (1997) Hepatosplenic γδ T-cell lymphoma: a report of two cases in immunocompromised patients, associated with isochromosome 7q. Am J Surg Pathol 21:781–790

Fraternali-Orcioni G, Falini B, Quaini F, Campo E, Piccioli M, Gamberi B, Pasquinelli G, Poggi S, Ascani S, Sabattini E, Pileri SA (1999) Beta-HCG aberrant expression in primary mediastinal large B-cell lymphoma. Am J Surg Pathol 23:717–721

Freeman C, Berg JW, Cotler SJ (1972) Occurrence and prognosis of extranodal lymphomas. Cancer 29:252–260

Freeman HJ, Anderson ME, Gascogne RD (1997) Clinical, pathological and molecular genetic findings in small intestinal follicle centre cell lymphoma. Can J Gastroenterol 11:31–34

Frierson HF Jr, Mills SE, Innes DJ Jr (1984) Non-Hodgkin's lymphomas of the sinonasal region: histologic types and their clinicopathologic features. Am J Clin Pathol 81:721–727

Fukayama M, Hayashi Y, Ooba T, Funata N, Ibura T, Koike M, Hebisawa H, Kurasawa A, Fukayama M, Nakahiro K, Kudoh S (1995) Pyothorax-associated lymphoma: development of Epstein-Barr virus-associated lymphoma within the inflammatory cavity. Pathol Intern 45:825–831

Furman WL, Fitch S, Hustu O, Callihan T, Murphy SB (1989) Primary lymphoma of bone in children. J Clin Oncol 7:1275–1280

Gale J, Simmonds PD, Mead GM, Sweetenham JW, Wright DH (2000) Enteropathy-type intestinal T-cell lymphoma; clinical features and treatment of 31 patients in a single center. J Clin Oncol 18:795–803

Gamelin E, Beldent V, Rousselet MC, Rieux D, Rohmer V, Ifrah N, Boasson M, Bigorgne JC (1992) Non-Hodgkin's lymphoma presenting with primary adrenal insufficiency. A disease with an under estimated frequency? Cancer 69:2333–2336

Ganem G, Gisselbrecht C, Jouault H, Tricot G, Martin M, Boiron M (1985) Lymphomes malins du testicule. Presse Med 14:1739–1742

Gassel AM, Westphal E, Hansmann ML, Leimenstoll G, Gassel HJ (1991) Malignant lymphoma of donor origin after renal transplantation. A case report. Hum Pathol 22:1291–1293

Gaulard P, Zafrani ES, Mavier P, Rocha D, Farcet JP, Divine M, Haioun C, Pinaudeau Y (1986) Peripheral T-cell lymphoma presenting as predominant liver disease. A report of 3 cases. Hepatology 6:864–868

Gaulard P, Bourquelot P, Kanavaros P et al (1990) Expression of the αβ and γδ T-cell receptors in 57 cases of peripheral T-cell lymphomas. Identification of a subset of γδ T-cell lymphomas. Am J Pathol 137:617–628

Gaulard P, Kanavaros P, Farcet JP, Rocha FD, Haioun C, Divine M, Reyes F, Zafrani ES (1991) Bone marrow histologic and immunohistochemical findings in peripheral T-cell lymphomas. A study of 38 cases. Hum Pathol 22: 331–338

Geelen F, Vermeer MH, Meijer C, Van der Putte S, Kerkhof E, Kluin PM, Willemze R (1998) BCL-2 protein expression in primary cutaneous large B-cell lymphoma is site-related. J Clin Oncol 16:2080–2085

Geerts M-L (1988) Mycosis fungoides. Een morfologische studie. Proefschrift tot het verkrijgen van de graad van Geaggregeerde voor het Hoger Onderwijs. Rijksuniversiteit, Afd. Huidziekten, Gent

Gentile TC, Uner AH, Hutchison RE, Wright J, Ben Ezra J, Russell EC, Loughran TP Jr (1994) CD3+, CD56+ aggressive variant of large granular lymphocyte leukemia. Blood 84:2315–2321

Giardini R, Piccolo C, Rilke F (1992) Primary non-Hodgkin's lymphomas of the female breast. Cancer 69:725–736

Gitjenbeek JM, Rosenblum MK, DeAngelis LM (2001) Primary central nervous system T-cell lymphoma. Neurology 57:716–718

Givler RL (1969) Testicular involvement in leukemia and lymphoma. Cancer 23:1290–1295

Glass J, Hochberg FH, Miller DC (1993) Intravascular lymphomatosis. A systemic disease with neurologic manifestations. Cancer 71:3156–3164

Gleeson MJ, Bennett MH, Cawson RA (1986) Lymphomas of salivary glands. Cancer 58:699–704

Goodlad JR, Davidson MM, Hollowood D, Batstone P, Ho-Yen DO (2000a) Borrelia burgdorferi-associated cutaneous marginal zone lymphoma: a clinicopathological study of two cases illustrating the temporal progression of B. burgdorferi-associated B-cell proliferation in the skin. Histopathology 37:501–508

Goodlad JR, Davidson MM, Hollowood K, Ling C, MacKenzie C, Christie I, Batstone PJ, Ho-Yen DO (2000b) Primary cutaneous B-cell lymphoma and Borrelia burgdorferi infection in patients from the Highlands of Scotland. Am J Surg Pathol 24:1279–1285

Graham SJ, Sharpe RW, Steinberg SM, Cotelingam JD, Sausville EA, Foss FM (1993) Prognostic implications of a bone marrow histopathologic classification system in mycosis fungoides and the Sézary syndrome. Cancer 72:726–734

Grange F, Hedelin G, Joly P, Beylot-Barry M, D'Incan M, Delaunay M, Vaillant L, Avril MF, Bosq J, Wechsler J, Dalac S, Grosieux C, Franck N, Esteve E, Michel C, Bodemer C, Vergier B, Laroche L, Bagot M (1999) Prognostic factors in primary cutaneous lymphomas other than mycosis fungoides and the Sézary-syndrome. The French Study Group on Cutaneous Lymphomas. Blood 93:3637–3642

Grant JW, Isaacson PG (1992) Primary central nervous system lymphoma. Brain Pathol 2:97–109

Green I, Espiritu E, Ladanyi M, Chaponda R, Wieczorek R, Gall L, Feiner H (1995) Primary lymphomatous effusions in AIDS: a morphological, immunophenotypic and molecular study. Mod Pathol 8:39–45

Grem JL, Neville AJ, Smith SC, Gould HR, Love RR, Trump DL (1985) Massive skeletal muscle invasion by lymphoma. Arch Intern Med 145:1818–1822

Griffin CA, Zehnbauer BA, Beschorner WE, Ambinder R, Mann R (1992) t(11;18)(q21;q21) is a recurrent chromosome abnormality in small lymphocytic lymphoma. Genes Chromosomes Cancer 4:153–157

Gronbaek K, Möller PH, Nedergaard T, Thomsen K, Baadsgaard O, Hou-Jensen K, Zeuthen J, Guldberg P, Ralkfiaer E (2000) Primary cutaneous B-cell lymphoma: a clinical, histological, phenotypic and genotypic study of 21 cases. Br J Dermatol 142:913–923

Guarner J, Brynes RK, Chan WC (1987) Primary non-Hodgkin's lymphoma of the heart in two patients with the acquired immunodeficiency syndrome. Arch Pathol Lab Med 111:254–256

Guinee D Jr, Jaffe E, Kingma D, Fishback N, Walberg K, Krishnan J, Frizzera G, Travis W, Koss M (1994) Pulmonary lymphomatoid granulomatosis. Evidence for a proliferation of Epstein-Barr virus infected B-lymphocytes with a prominent T-cell component and vasculitis. Am J Surg Pathol 18:753–764

Guitart J, Hurt MA (1999) Pleomorphic T-cell infiltrate associated with molluscum contagiosum. Am J Dermatopathol 21:178–180

Haghighi B, Smoller BR, LeBoit PE, Warnke RA, Sander CA, Kohle S (2000) Pagetoid reticulosis (Woringer-Kolopp disease): an immunophenotypic, molecular, and clinicopathologic study. Mod Pathol 13: 502–10

Haglund U, Juliusson G, Stellan B, Gahrton G (1994) Hairy cell leukemia is characterized by clonal chromosome abnormalities clustered to specific regions. Blood 83:2637–2645

Hammer RD, Glick AD, Greer JP et al (1996) Splenic marginal zone lymphoma. A distinct B-cell neoplasm. Am J Surg Pathol 20:613–626

Hansen TG, Ottesen GL, Pedersen NT, Andersen JA (1992) Primary non-Hodgkin's lymphoma of the breast. A clinicopathological study of seven cases. APMIS 100:1089–1096

Hao D, DiFrancesco LM, Brasher PMA, deMetz C, Fulton DS, DeAngelis LM, Forsyth PAJ (1999) Is primary CNS lymphoma really becoming more common? A population-based study of incidence, clinicopathological features and outcomes in Alberta from 1975 to 1996. Ann Oncol 10:65–70

Haque AK, Myers JL, Hudnall SD, Gelman BB, Lloyd RV, Payne D, Borucki M (1998) Pulmonary lymphomatoid granulomatosis in acquired immunodeficiency syndrome: lesions with Epstein-Barr virus infection. Mod Pathol 11:347–356

Hara K, Ito M, Shimizu K, Matsumoto T, Suchi T, Lijima S (1985) Three cases of primary splenic lymphoma. Case report and review of the Japanese literature. Acta Pathol Jpn 35:419–435

Harada K, Nishizaki T, Kubota H, Harada K, Suzuki M, Sasaki K (2001) Distinct primary central nervous system lymphoma defined by comparative genomic hybridization and laser scanning cytometry. Cancer Gen Cytogen 125:147–150

Harris NL, Scully RE (1984) Malignant lymphoma and granulocytic sarcoma of the uterus and vagina. A clinicopathologic analysis of 27 cases. Cancer 53:2530–2545

Harris NL, Aisenberg AC, Meyer JE, Ellman L, Elman A (1984) Diffuse large cell lymphoma of the spleen. Clinical and pathologic characteristics of ten cases. Cancer 54:2460–2467

Harrison NR, Twelves C, Addis BJ, Newman-Taylor AJ, Souhami RL, Isaacson PG (1988) Peripheral T-cell lymphoma presenting with angioedema and diffuse pulmonary infiltrates. Am Rev Respir Dis 138:976–980

Hashimoto Y, Nakamura N, Kuze T, Ono N, Abe M (1999) Multiple lymphomatous polyposis of the gastrointestinal tract is a heterogenous group that includes mantle cell lymphoma and follicular lymphoma: analysis of somatic mutation of immunoglobulin heavy chain gene variable region. Hum Pathol 30:581–587

Headington JT, Roth MS, Schnitzer B (1987) Regressing atypical histiocytosis: a review and critical appraisal. Semin Diagn Pathol 4: 28–37

Heimann R, Vannineuse A, De Sloover C, Dor P (1978) Malignant lymphomas and undifferentiated small cell carcinoma of the thyroid: a clinicopathological review in the light of the Kiel classification for malignant lymphomas. Histopathology 2:201–203

Henry JM, Heffner RR, Dillard SH, Earle KM, Davis RL (1974) Primary malignant lymphomas of the central nervous system. Cancer 34:1293–1302

Herbst H, Sander C, Tronnier M, Kutzner H, Hügel H, Kaudewitz P (1997) Absence of anaplastic lymphoma kinase (ALK) and Epstein-Barr virus gene products in primary cutaneous anaplastic large-cell lymphoma and lymphomatoid papulosis. Br J Dermatol 137:680–686

Heyning FH, Hogendoorn PC, Kramer MH, Hermans J, Kluin-Nelemans JC, Noordijk EM, Kluin PM (1999) Primary non-Hodgkin's lymphoma of bone: a clinicopathological investigation of 60 cases. Leukemia 13:2094–2098

Higgins JP, Warnke RA (1999) CD30 expression is common in mediastinal large B-cell lymphoma. Am J Clin Pathol 112:241–247

Higgins JP, Warnke RA (2000) Large B-cell lymphoma of thyroid. Two cases with a marginal zone distribution of the neoplastic cells. Am J Clin Pathol 114:264–270

Hirakawa K, Fuchigami T, Nakamura S, Daimaru Y, Ohshima K, Sakai Y, Ichimaru T (1996) Primary Gastrointestinal T-Cell Lymphoma Resembling Multiple Lymphomatous Polyposis. Gastroenterology 111:778–782

Höffkes HG, Schumann A, Uppenkamp M, Teschendorf C, Schindler AE, Parwaresch R, Brittinger G (1995) Primary non-Hodgkin's lymphoma of the vagina. Case report and review of the literature. Ann Hematol 70:273–276

Hofman P, Le Tourneau A, Negre F, Michiels JF, Diebold J (1992) Primary uveal B immunoblastic lymphoma in a patient with AIDS. Br J Ophtalmol 76:700–702

Hoppe RT, Burke JS, Glatstein E, Kaplan HS (1978) Non Hodgkin's lymphomas: involvement of Waldeyer's ring. Cancer 42:1096–1104

Hoque SR, Child FJ, Whittaker SJ, Ferreira S, Orchard G, Jenner K, Spittle M, Russel-Jones R (2003) Subcutaneous panniculitis-like T-cell lymphoma: a clinicopathological, immunophenotypic and molecular analysis of six patients. Br J Dermatol 148:516–25

Horenstein MG, Nador RG, Chadburn A, Hyjek EM, Inghirami G, Knowles DM, Cesarman E (1997) Epstein-Barr virus latent gene expression in primary effusion lymphomas containing Kaposi's sarcoma-associated herpesvirus/human herpesvirus-8. Blood 90:1186–1191

Horny HP, Kaiserling E (1995) Involvement of the larynx by hematopoietic neoplasms. An investigation of autopsy cases and review of the literature. Pathol Res Pract 191:130–138

Hoshida Y, Kusakabe H, Furukawa H, Kasugai T, Miwa H, Ishiguro S, Aozasa K (1997) Reassessment of gastric lymphoma in light of the concept of mucosa-associated lymphoid tissue lymphoma: analysis of 53 patients. Cancer 80:1151–1159

Hounieu H, Shashikant C, Saati T et al (1992) Hairy cell leukemia: diagnosis of bone marrow involvement in paraffin-embedded sections with monoclonal antibody DBA-44. Am J Clin Pathol 28:26–33

Hoyer JD, Li CY, Yam LT, Hanson CA, Kurtin PJ (1997) Immunohistochemical demonstration of acid phosphatase isoenzyme 5 (tartrate-resistant) in paraffin sections of hairy cell leukemia and other hematologic disorders. Am J Clin Pathol 108:308–315

Hsiao CH, Lee WI, Chang SL, Su IJ (1996) Angiocentric T-cell lymphoma of the intestine: a distinct etiology of ischemic bowel disease. Gastroenterology 110: 985–90

Hsu SM, Yang K, Jaffe ES (1983) Hairy cell leukemia: a B-cell neoplasm with a unique antigenic profile. Am J Clin Pathol 80:421

Huang JZ, Sanger WG, Greiner TC, Staudt LM, Weisenburger DD, Pickering DL, Lynch JC, Armitage JO, Warnke RA, Alizadeh AA, Lossos IS, Levy R, Chan WC (2002) The t(14;18) defines a unique subset of diffuse large B-cell lymphoma with a germinal center B-cell gene expression profile. Blood 99:2285-90

Huang CB, Eng HL, Chuang JH, Cheng YF, Chen WJ (1997) Primary Burkitt's lymphoma of the liver: report of a case with long-term survival after surgical resection and combination chemotherapy. J Pediatr Hematol Oncol 19:135–138

Hugh JC, Jackson FI, Hanson J, Poppema S (1990) Primary breast lymphoma. An immunohistologic study of 20 new cases. Cancer 66:2602–2611

Huminer D, Garty M, Lapidot M, Leiba S, Boronov H, Rosenfeld JR (1988) Lymphoma presenting with adrenal insufficiency. Am J Med 84:169–172

Huvos AG (1991) Skeletal manifestations of malignant lymphomas and leukemias. In: Huvos AG (ed) Bone tumors, diagnosis, treatment and prognosis. 2nd edn. Saunders, Philadelphia

Hyjek E, Isaacson PG (1988) Primary B-cell lymphoma of the thyroid and its relation to Hashimoto thyroiditis. Hum Pathol 19:1315–1326

Ibuka T, Fukayama M, Hayashi Y, Funata N, Koike M, Ikeda T, Mizutani S (1994) Pyothorax-associated pleural lymphoma. A case evolving from T-cell-rich lymphoid infiltration to overt B-cell lymphoma in association with Epstein-Barr virus. Cancer 73:738–744

Inooka G, Ishikawa S, Saito T, Saito K, Kamoshida T, Kuzuya T (1992) An autopsy case of intravascular lymphomatosis (neoplastic angioendotheliomatosis) accompanied by high fever, hypertension and without focal sign. Intern Med 31:666–670

International Lymphoma Study Group (1997) The Non-Hodgkin's Lymphoma Classification Project 1997. A clinical evaluation of the International Lymphoma Study Group classification of non-Hodgkin's lymphoma. The Non-Hodgkin's Lymphoma Classification Project. Blood 89:3909–3918

Isaacson PG (1996) Splenic marginal zone lymphoma. Blood 88:751–752

Isaacson PG (1999a) Mucosa-associated lymphoid tissue lymphoma. Semin Hematol 36:139–147

Isaacson PG (1999b) Gastrointestinal lymphomas of T- and B-Cell Types. Mod Pathol 12:151–158

Isaacson PG, Norton AJ (1994) Extranodal lymhomas. Churchill Livingstone, Edinburgh

Isaacson PG, Spencer J (1987) Malignant lymphoma of mucosa-associated lymphoid tissue. Histopathology 11:445–462

Isacson PG, Wright DH (1978) Malignant histiocytosis of the intestine. Its relationship to malabsorption and ulcerative jejunitis. Hum Pathol 9:661–677

Isaacson PG, Wright DH (1984) Extranodal malignant lymphoma arising from mucosa-associated lymphoid tissue. Cancer 53:2515–2524

Isaacson PG, Norton AJ, Addis BJ (1987) The human thymus contains a novel population of B lymphocytes. Lancet 2:1488–1491

Isaacson PG, Spencer J, Wright DH (1988) Classifying primary gut lymphomas. Lancet ii:1148–1149

Isaacson PG, Wotherspoon AC, Diss T, Pan LX (1991) Follicular colonization in B-cell lymphoma of mucosa-associated lymphoid tissue. Am J Surg Pathol 15:819–828

Isaacson PG, Chan JK, Tang C, Addis BJ (1990) Low-grade B-cell lymphoma of mucosa-associated lymphoid tissue arising in the thymus. A thymic lymphoma mimicking myoepithelial sialodenitis. Am J Surg Pathol 14:342–351

Isaacson PG, Matutes E, Burke M et al (1994) The histopathology of splenic lymphoma with villous lymphocytes. Blood 84:3828–3834

Isaacson PG, Banks PM, Best PV, McLure SP, Muller-Hermelink HK, Wyatt JL (1995) Primary low-grade hepatic B-cell lymphoma of mucosa-associated lymphoid tissue (MALT)-type. Am J Surg Pathol 19:571–575

Isaacson PG, Diss TC, Wotherspoon AC, Barbazza R, De Boni M, Doglioni C (1999) Long-term follow-up of gastric MALT lymphoma treated by eradication of H. pylori with antibiotics. Gastroenterology 117:750–751

Ishida F, Kitano K, Ichikawa N et al (1999) Hairy cell leukemia with translocation (11;20)(q13;q11) and overexpression of cyclin D1. Leuk Res 23:763–765

Ishizawa M, Okabe H, Matsumoto K, Hukuda S, Hodohara K, Ota S (1995) Anaplastic large cell Ki1 lymphoma with bone involvement. Report of 2 cases. Virchows Arch 427:105–110

Ito M, Nakagawsa A, Tsuzuki T, Yokoi T, Yamashita Y, Asai J (1996) Primary cardiac lymphoma. No evidence for an etiologic association with Epstein-Barr virus. Arch Pathol Lab Med 120:555–559

Iuchi K, Aozasa K, Yamamoto S et al (1989) Non-Hodgkin's lymphoma of the pleural cavity developing from long-standing pyothorax. Summary of clinical and pathological findings in 37 cases. Jpn J Clin Oncol 19:249–257

Jaffe ES (1996) Primary body cavity-based AIDS-related lymphomas. Evolution of a new disease entity (editorial). Am J Clin Pathol 109:141–143

Jaffe ES (1999) Nasal / nasal type NK/T cell lymphoma (angiocentric lymphoma) and lymphomatoid granulomatosis. In: Mason DY, Harris NL (eds) Human lymphoma: clinical implications of the REAL classification. Springer, Berlin Heidelberg New York

Jaffe ES, Wilson WH (1997) Lymphomatoid granulomatosis: pathogenesis, pathology and clinical implications. Cancer Surv 30:233–248

Jaffe ES, Harris NL, Stein H, Vardiman JW (eds) (2001) WHO classification of tumours: pathology and genetics of tumours of haematopoietic and lymphoid tissues. IARC Press, Lyon

Jaffe ES, Zarate-Osorno A, Medeiros LJ (1992) The interrelationship of Hodgkin's disease and non-Hodgkin's lymphomas – lessons learned from composite and sequential malignancies. Semin Diagn Pathol 9:297–303

Janin A, Morel P, Quiquandon I et al (1992) Non-Hodgkin's lymphoma and Sjögren's syndrome. An immunopathological study of 113 patients. Clin Exp Rheumatol 10:565–570

Jelic S, Filipovic-Ljeskovic I (1999) Positive serology for lyme disease borrelias in primary cutaneous B-cell lymphoma: a study in 22 patients; is it a fortuitous finding? Hematol Oncol 17:107–116

Jellinger KA, Paulus W (1992) Primary central nervous system lymphomas – an update. J Cancer Res Clin Oncol 119:7–27

Jenkins C, Rose GE, Bunce C, Wright JE, Cree IA, Plowman N, Lightman s, Moseley I, Norton A (2000) Histological features of ocular adnexal lymphoma (REAL classification) and their association with patient morbidity and survival. Br J Ophthalmol 84:907–913

Jeon HJ, Akagi T, Hoshida Y, Hayashi K, Yoshino T, Tanaka T, Ito J, Kamei T, Kawabata K (1992) Primary non-Hodgkin malignant lymphoma of the breast. An immunohistochemical study of 7 patients and literature review of 152 patients with breast lymphoma in Japan. Cancer 70:2451–2459

Johnsson A, Brun E, Akerman M, Cavallin-Stahl E (1992) Primary gastric non-Hodgkin's lymphoma. A retrospective clinico-pathological study. Acta Oncol 31:525–531

Jones RE, Willis S, Innes DJ, Wanebo HJ (1988) Primary gastric lymphoma. Problems in staging and management. Am J Surg 155:118–123

Joos S, Otanos-Joos MI, Ziegler S, Brüderlein S, du Manoir S, Bentz M, Möller P, Lichter P (1996) Primary mediastinal (thymic) B-cell lymphoma is characterized by gains of chromosomal material including 9p and amplification of the REL gene. Blood 87:1571–1578

Joseph G, Pandit M, Korfhage L (1993) Primary pulmonary plasmacytoma. Cancer 71:721–724

Juliusson G, Lenkei R, Liliemark J (1994) Flow cytometry of blood and bone marrow cells from patients with hairy cell leukemia: phenotype of hairy cells and lymphocyte subsets after treatment with 2-chlorodeoxyadenosine. Blood 83:3672–3681

Kadin ME (1990) The spectrum of Ki-1+ cutaneous lymphomas. Curr Probl Dermatol 19:132–143

Kadin ME, Nasu K, Sako D, Said J, Vonderheid EC.(1985) Lymphomatoid papulosis: a cutaneous proliferation of activated helper T cells expressing Hodgkin's disease-associated antigens. Am J Pathol 119:315–325

Kadin ME, Vonderheid EC, Weiss LM (1993) Absence of Epstein-Barr viral RNA in lymphomatoid papulosis. J Pathol

Kampmeier P, Spielberger R, Dickstein J, Mick R, Golomb H, Vardiman JW (1994) Increased incidence of second neoplasms in patients treated with interferon α 2b for hairy cell leukemia: a clinicopathologic assessment. Blood 83:2931–2938

Kanavaros P, Farcet JP, Gaulard P, Haioun C, Divine M, Le Couedic JP, Le Franc MP, Reyes F (1991) Recombinative events of the T-cell antigen receptor δ gene in peripheral T-cell lymphomas. J Clin Invest 87:666–672

Kanavaros P, Lescs MC, Brière J, Divine M, Galateau F, Joab I, Bosq J, Farcet JP, Reyès F, Gaulard P (1993) Nasal T-cell lymphoma: a clinicopathologic entity associated with peculiar phenotype and with Epstein-Barr virus. Blood 81:2688–2695

Kanda M, Suzumiya J, Ohshima K et al (1999) Intravascular large cell lymphoma: clinicopathological, immuno-histochemical and molecular genetic studies. Leuk Lymph 34:569–580

Kandel LB, McCulough DL, Harrison LH, Woodruff RD, An LE Jr, Munitz HA (1987) Primary renal lymphoma. Does it exist? Cancer 60:386–391

Kandel RA, Bedard YC, Pritzker KP et al (1984) Lymphoma presenting as an intramuscular small cell malignant tumor. Cancer 53:1586–1589

Kanehira K, Braylan RC, Lauwers GY (2001) Early phase of intestinal mantle cell lymphoma: a report of two cases associated with advanced colonic adenocarcinoma. Mod Pathol 14:811–817

Kaplan MA, Pettit CL, Zukerberg LR, Harris NL (1992) Primary lymphoma of the trachea with morphologic and immunophenotypic characteristics of low-grade B-cell lymphoma of mucosa-associated lymphoid tissue. Am J Surg Pathol 16:71–75

Katoh A, Ohshima K, Kanda M, Haraoka S, Sugihara M, Suzumiya J, Kawasaki C, Shimazaki K, Ikeda S, Kikuchi M (2000) Gastrointestinal T cell lymphoma: predominant cytotoxic phenotypes, including alpha/beta, gamma/delta T cell and natural killer cells. Leuk Lymphoma 39: 97–111

Katzenstein AL, Carrington CB, Liebow AA (1979) Lymphomatoid granulomatosis: a clinicopathologic study of 152 cases. Cancer 43:360–373

Kaudewitz P, Stein H, Dallenbach F (1989) Primary and secondary Ki-1+ (CD30+) anaplastic large cell lymphomas. Am J Pathol 135:359–367

Kellie SJ, Pui CH, Murphy SB (1989) Childhood non-Hodgkin's lymphoma involving the testis: clinical features and treatment outcome. J Clin Oncol 7:1066–1070

Kempf W, Kadin ME, Kutzner H, Lord CL, Burg G, Letwin NL, Koralnik IJ (2001) Lymphomatoid papulosis and human herpesviruses. A PCR-based evaluation for the presence of human herpesvirus 6, 7 and 8 and related herpesviruses. J Cutan Pathol 28:29–33

Kennedy J, Nathwani B, Burke J et al (1985) Pulmonary lymphomas and other pulmonary lymphoid lesions. A clinicopathologic and immunologic study of 64 patients. Cancer 56:539–552

Kerl H, Cerroni L (1997) Primary B-cell lymphomas of the skin. Ann Oncol 8:29–32

Kerl H, Kresbach H (1979) Lymphoreticuläre Hyperplasien und Neoplasien der Haut. In: Schnyder UW (ed) Histopathologie der Haut, 2nd edn, part 2. Stoffwechselkrankheiten und Tumoren. Springer, Berlin Heidelberg New York, pp 351–480 (Spezielle pathologische Anatomie, vol 7/2)

Khalidi HS, Brynes RK, Browne P, Koo CH, Battifora H, Medeiros LJ (1998) Intravascular large B-cell lymphoma: the CD5 antigen is expressed by a subset of cases. Mod Pathol 11:983–988

Khan WA, Yu L, Eisenbrey AB, Crisan D, Al Saadi A, Davis BH, Hankin RC, Mattson JC (2001) Hepatosplenic gamma/delta T-cell lymphoma in immunocompromised patients. Report of two cases and review of the literature. Am J Clin Pathol 116:41–50

Kim BK, Surti U, Pandya AG, Swerdlow SH (2003) Primary and Secondary Cutaneous Diffuse Large B-Cell Lymphomas: A Multiparameter Analysis of 25 Cases Including Fluorescence In Situ Hybridization for t(14; 18) Translocation. Am J Surg Pathol 27:356–64

Kim H, Dorfman RF, Rosenberg SA (1976) Pathology of malignant lymphomas in the liver: application in staging. In: Popper H, Schaffner F (eds) Progress in liver diseases, vol V. Grune and Stratton, New York, pp 683–698

Kim HS, Ko YH, Ree HJ (2000a) A case report of primary T-cell lymphoma of the liver. J Korean Med Sci 15:240–242

Kim JH, Kim HY, Kang I, Kim YB, Park CK, Yoo JY, Kim ST (2000b) A case of primary hepatic lymphoma with hepatitis C liver cirrhosis. Am J Gastroenterol 95:2377–2380

Kim YH, Bishop K, Varghese A, Hoppe RT (1995) Prognostic factors in erythrodermic mycosis fungoides and the Sézary syndrome. Arch Dermatol 131:1003–1008

Kinney MC (1999) The role of morphologic features, phenotype, genotype, and anatomic site in defining extranodal T-cell or NK-cell neoplasms. Am J Clin Pathol 111 [Suppl 1]:S104–S118

Kirk CM, Lewin D, Lazarchick J (1999) Primary hepatic B-cell lymphoma of mucosa-associated lymphoid tissue. Arch Pathol Lab Med 132:716–719

Kluin-Nelemans HC, Beuerstock GC, Mollevanger P, Wessels HW, Hoogendoorn E, Willemze R, Falkenburg JHF (1994) Proliferation and cytogenetic analysis of hairy cell leukemia upon stimulation via the CD40 antigen. Blood 84:3134–3141

Knowles DM (1992) Lymphoblastic lymphoma. In: Knowles DM (ed) Neoplastic hematopathology. Williams and Wilkins, Baltimore, pp 715–747

Knowles DM (1999) Morphologic, immunologic and genetic features of lymphoproliferative disorders associated with immunodeficiency. In: Mason DY, Harris NL (eds) Human lymphoma: clinical implications of the REAL classification. Springer, Berlin Heidelberg New York

Knowles DM, Chamulak JA, Subar M (1988) Lymphoid neoplasia associated with the acquired immunodeficiency syndrome (AIDS). Ann Intern Med 108:744–753

Knowles DM, Jakobiec FA, McNally L, Burke JS (1990) Lymphoid hyperplasia and malignant lymphoma occurring in the ocular adnexa (orbit, conjunctiva, and eyelids): a prospective multiparametric analysis of 108 cases during 1977 to 1987. Hum Pathol 21:959–973

Ko YH, Han JH, Go JH et al (1997) Intravascular lymphomatosis: a clinicopathological study of two cases presenting as an interstitial lung disease. Histopathology 31:555–562

Koch P, Grothaus-Pinke B, Hiddemann W, Willich N, Reers B, del Valle F, Bodenstein H, Pfreundschuh M, Moller E, Kocik J, Parwaresch R, Tiemann M (1997) Primary lymphoma of the stomach: three-year results of a prospective multicenter study. The German Multicenter Study Group on GI-NHL. Ann Oncol 8 [Suppl 1]:85–88

Koh PK, Horsman JM, Radstone CR, Hancock H, Goepel JR, Hancock BW (2001) Localised extranodal non-Hodgkin's lymphoma of the gastrointestinal tract: Sheffield Lymphoma Group experience (1989–1998). Intern J Oncol 18:743–748

Kojima M, Tamaki Y, Nakamura S, Hosomura Y, Kurabayashi Y, Itoh H, Yoshida K, Niibe H, Suchi T, Johshita T (1993) Malignant lymphoma of Waldeyer's ring. A histological and immunohistochemical study. APMIS 101:537–544

Kojima H, Mukai HY, Shinagawa A, Yoshida C, Kamoshita M, Komeno T, Hasegawa Y, Yamashita Y, Mori N, Nagasawa T (2000) Clinicopathological analyses of 5 Japanese patients with CD56+ primary cutaneous lymphomas. Int J Hematol 72:477–483

Korsmeyer S, Greene W, Cossman J (1983) Rearrangement and expression of immunoglobulin genes and expression of Tac antigen in hairy cell leukemia. Proc Natl Acad Sci USA 80:4522–4528

Kosaka M, Tsuchihashi N, Takishita M, Miyamoto Y, Okagawa K, Gotoh T, Saito S, Komaki M, Morimoto T, Sano T (1992) Primary adult T-cell lymphoma of the breast. Acta Haematol 87:202–205

Koss M, Hochholzer I, Nichols P et al (1985) Primary non-Hodgkin's lymphoma and pseudolymphoma of lung. A study of 161 patients. Hum Pathol 14:1024–1038

Koss MN, Hochholzer L, Langloss JM, Wehunt WD, Lazarus AA, Nichols PW (1986) Lymphomatoid granulomatosis: a clinicopathologic study of 42 patients. Pathology 18:283–288

Koss MN, Hochholzer L, Moran CA, Frizzera G (1998) Pulmonary plasmacytomas: a clinicopathologic and immunohistochemical study of five cases. Ann Diagn Pathol 2:1–11

Krogh-Jensen M, d'Amore F, Jensen MK, Christensen BE, Thorling K, Pedersen M, Johansen P, Boesen AM, Andersen E (1994) Incidence, clinicopathological features and outcome of primary central nervous system lymphomas. Ann Oncol 5:349–354

Kumar S, Krenacs L, Otsuki T, Kumar D, Harris CA, Wellman A, Jaffe ES, Raffeld M (1996) Bcl-1 rearrangement and cyclin D1 protein expression in multiple lymphomatous polyposis. Am J Clin Pathol 105:737–743

Kumar S, Fend F, Quintanilla-Martinez L, Kingma DW, Sorbara L, Raffeld L, Banks PM, Jaffe ES (2000) Epstein-Barr virus-positive primary gastrointestinal Hodgkin's disease: association with inflammatory bowel disease and immunosuppression. Am J Surg Pathol 24:66–73

Kummer JA, Vermeer MH, Dukers D, Meijer CJLM, Willemze R (1997) Most primary cutaneous CD30-positive lymphoproliferative disorders have a CD4-positive cytotoxic T-cell phenotype. J Invest Dermatol 109:636–640

Kwong YL, Chan AC, Liang R, Chiang AK, Chim CS, Chan TK, Todd D, Ho FC (1997) CD56+ NK lymphomas: clinicopathological features and prognosis. Br J Haematol 97:821–829

Lai R, Larratt LM, Etches W, Mortimer ST, Jewell LD, Dabbadh L, Coupland RW (2000) Hepatosplenic T-cell lymphoma of alpha beta lineage in a 16-years-old boy presenting with hemolytic anemia and thrombocytopenia. Am J Surg Pathol 24:459–463

Lair G, Parant E, Tessier MH, Jumbou O, Dreno B (2000) Primary cutaneous B-cell lymphomas of the lower limbs: a study of integrin expression in 11 cases. Acta Derm Venereol 80:367–369

Lam KY, Dickens P, Chan AC (1993) Tumors of the heart. A 20-year experience with a review of 12,485 consecutive autopsies. Arch Pathol Lab Med 117:1027–1031

Lamovec J, Jancar J (1987) Primary malignant lymphoma of the breast. Lymphoma of the mucosa-associated lymphoid tissue. Cancer 60:3033–3041

Lamy T, Loughran TP Jr (1999) Current concepts: large granular lymphocyte leukemia. Blood Rev 13:230–240

Lanham GR, Weiss SW, Enzinger FM (1989) Malignant lymphoma: a study of 75 cases presenting in soft tissue. Am J Surg Pathol 13:1–10

Latteri MA, Cipolla C, Gebbia V, Lampasona G, Amato C, Gebbia N (1995) Primary extranodal non-Hodgkin lymphomas of the uterus and the breast: report of three cases. Eur J Surg Oncol 21:432–434

Lavergne A, Brouland JP, Launay E, Nemeth J, Ruskone-Fourmestraux A, Galian A (1994) Multiple lymphomatous polyposis of the gastrointestinal tract. An extensive histopathologic and immunohistochemical study of 12 cases. Cancer 74:3042–3050

Lavergne A, Brocheriou I, Delfau MH, Copie-Bergmann C, Houdart R, Gaulard PH (1998) Primary intestinal gamma-delta T-cell lymphoma with evidence of Epstein-Barr virus. Histopathology 32:271–276

Lawnicke LC, Weisenburger DD, Aoun P, Chan WC, Wickert RS, Greiner TC (2002) The t(14;18) and bcl-2 expression are present in a subset of primary cutaneous follicular lymphoma: association with low grade. Am J Clin Pathol 118:765–72

Lazzarino M, Morra E, Rossi R et al (1985) Clinicopathologic and immunologic characteristics of non-Hodgkin's lymphomas presenting in the orbit. A report of eight cases. Cancer 55:1907–1912

Lazzarino M, Orlandi E, Paulli M, Strater J, Klersy C, Gianelli U, Gargantini L, Rousset MT, Gambacorta M, Marra E, Lavabre-Bertrand T, Magrini U, Manegold C, Bernasconi C, Moller P (1997) Treatment outcome and prognostic factors for primary mediastinal (thymic) B-cell lymphoma: a multicenter study of 106 patients. J Clin Oncol 15:1646–1653

Leff SR, Shields JA, Augsburger JJ, Miller RV, Liberatore B (1985) Unilateral eyelid, conjunctival, and choroidal tumours as initial presentation of diffuse large-cell lymphoma. Br Ophtalmol 69:861–864

Lei KI, Chow JH, Johnson PJ (1995) Aggressive primary hepatic lymphoma in Chinese patients. Presentation, pathologic features, and outcome. Cancer 76:1336–1343

Leidenix MJ, Mamalis N, Olson RJ, McLeish WM, Anderson RL (1993) Primary T-cell immunoblastic lymphoma of the orbit in a pediatric patient. Ophtalmology 100:998–1002

Leithäuser F, Bäuerle M, Huynh MQ, Möller P (2001) Isotype-switched immunoglobin genes with a high load of somatic hypermutation and lack of ongoing mutational activity are prevalent in mediastinal B-cell lymphoma. Blood 98:2762–2770

Lennert K, Schmid U (1983) Prelymphoma, early lymphoma, and manifest lymphoma in immunosialadenitis (Sjögren's syndrome): a model of lymphogenesis. Hämatol Bluttransfus 28:418–422

Le Pessot F, Courville P, Moguelet P, Lemoine JP, Duval C (2001) Lymphome du MALT primitif du sein. A propos d'une observation. Ann Pathol 21:59–62

Le Tourneau A, Audouin J, Garbe L, Capron F, Servais B, Manges G, Payan H, Diebold J (1983) Primary pulmonary malignant lymphoma. Clinical and pathological findings, immunocytochemical and ultrastructural studies in 15 cases. Haematol Oncol 1:49–60

Levaltier X, Troussard X, Fournier L, Reznick Y, Reman O, Mahoude J, Leporrier M (1994) Primary adrenal lymphoma. Report of a case. Presse Med 23:372–374

Levine PH, Kamaraja LS, Connelly RR et al (1982) The American Burkitt's Lymphoma Registry: eight years's experience. Cancer 49:1016–1022

Levison DA, Shepherd NA (1986) Gastric lymphomas and smooth muscle tumours. In: Preece PE, Cushieri A, Wellwood JM (eds) Gastric tumours. Grum and Stratton, London

Lewin KJ, Appelman HD (1995) Tumors of the esophagus and stomach. Atlas of tumor pathology, 3rd ser, no 18. Armed Forces Institute of Pathology, Washington DC

Lewin KJ, Ranchod M, Dorfman RF (1978) Lymphomas of the gastrointestinal tract: a study of 117 cases presenting with gastrointestinal disease. Cancer 42:693–707

L'Hoste RJ, Filippa DA, Lieberman PH, Bretsky S (1984) Primary pulmonary lymphomas. Cancer 54:1397–1406

Li G, Hansmann ML, Zwingers T, Lennert K (1990) Primary lymphomas of lung. Morphological immunohistochemical and clinical features. Histopathology 16:519–531

Li S, Griffin CA, Mann RB, Borowitz MJ (2001) Primary cutaneous T-cell-rich B-cell lymphoma: clinically distinct from its nodal counterpart? Mod Pathol 14:10–13

Liang R, Chan WP, Kwong YL, Xu WS, Srivastava G, Ho FC (1997a) High incidence of BCL-6 gene rearrangement in diffuse large B-cell lymphoma of primary gastric origin. Cancer Genet Cytogenet 97:114–118

Liang R, Chan WP, Kwong YL, Chan AC, Xu WS, Au WY, Srivastava G, Ho FC (1997b) Bcl-6 gene hypermutations in diffuse large B-cell lymphoma of primary gastric origin. Br J Haematol 99:668–670

Liebow A (1973) Pulmonary angiitis and granulomatosis. Am Rev Respir Dis 108:1–15

Liebow A, Carrington C, Friedman P (1972) Lymphomatoid granulomatosis. Hum Pathol 3:457–558

Lipford E, Wright JJ, Urba W, Whang-Peng J, Kirsch IR, Raffeld M, Cossman J, Longo DL, Bakhshi A, Korsmeyer SJ (1987) Refinement of lymphoma cytogenetics by the chromosome 18q21 major breakpoint region. Blood 70:1816–1823

Lipford EH Jr, Margolick JB, Longo DL, Fauci AS, Jaffe ES (1988) Angiocentric immunoproliferative lesions: a clinicopathologic spectrum of post-thymic T-cell proliferations. Blood 72:1674–1681

Liu Q, Ohshima K, Kikuchi M (2000) Primary cutaneous B-cell lymphoma in Japanese patients. Pathlog Int 50:960–966

Lloret E, Mollejo M, Mateo MS, Villuendas R, Algara P, Martinez P, Piris MA (1999) Splenic marginal zone lymphoma with increased number of blasts: an aggressive variant? Hum Pathol 30:1153–1160

Long JC, Mihm MC (1974) Mycosis fungoides with extracutaneous dissemination: a distinct clinico-pathologic entity. Cancer 34:1745–1755

Lorsbach RB, Pinkus GS, Shahsafaei A, Dorfman DM (2000) Primary marginal zone lymphoma of the thymus. Am J Clin Pathol 113:784–791

Loughran TP Jr (1993) Clonal diseases of large granular lymphocytes. Blood 82:1–14

Loughran TP, Jr, Kadin ME, Starkebaum G, Abkowitz JL, Clark EA, Disteche C, Lum LG, Slichter SJ (1985) Leukemia of large granular lymphocytes: association with clonal chromosomal abnormalities and autoimmune neutropenia, thrombocytopenia, and hemolytic anemia. Ann Intern Med 102:169–175

Loughran TP Jr, Starkebaum G, Aprile JA (1988) Rearrangement and expression of T-cell receptor genes in large granular lymphocyte leukemia. Blood 71:822–824

Luppi M, Longo G, Ferrari MG, Ferrara L, Marasca R, Barozzi P, Morselli M, Emilia G, Torelli G (1996) Additional neoplasms and HCV infection in low-grade lymphoma of MALT. Br J Haematol 94:373–375

Lynch SA, Brugge JS, Fromowitz F, Glantz L, Wang P, Caruso R, Viola MV (1993) Increased expression of the src proto-oncogene in hairy cell leukemia and a subgroup of B-cell lymphomas. Leukemia 7:1416–1422

Macaulay WL (1968) Lymphomatoid papulosis: A continuing self-healing eruption, clinically benign-histologically malignant. Arch Dermatol 97:23–30

MacIntosh FR, Colby TV, Podolsky WJ et al (1982) Central nervous system involvement in non-Hodgkin's lymphoma. An analysis of 105 cases. Cancer 49:589–595

Macon WR, Levy NB, Kurtin PJ, Salhany KE, Elkhalifa MY, Casey TT, Craig FE, Vnencak-Jones CL, Gulley ML, Park JP, Cousar JB (2001) Hepatosplenic alpha beta T-cell lymphomas: a report of 14 cases and comparison with hepatosplenic gamma delta T-cell lymphomas. Am J Surg Pathol 25:285–296

Maes M, Depardieu C, Dargent JL, Hermans M, Verhaeghe JL, Dela J, Pittaluga S, Troufleau P, Verhest A, De Wolf-Peeters C (1997) Primary low-grade B-cell lymphoma of MALT occurring in the liver: a study of two cases. J Hepatol 27:922–927

Marchevsky A, Padilla M, Kaneko M et al (1983) Localized lymphoid nodules of lung. A reappraisal of the lymphoma versus pseudolymphoma dilemma. Cancer 51:2070–2077

Martenson JA, Buskirk SJ, Ilstrup DM et al (1988) Patterns of failure in primary testicular non-Hodgkin's lymphoma. J Clin Oncol 6:297–303

Martin A, Capron F, Liguory-Brunaud MD, Frejacques C, Pluot M, Diebold J (1994) Epstein-Barr virus-associated primary malignant lymphomas of the pleural cavity occurring in long-standing pleural chronic inflammation. Hum Pathol 25:1314–1318

Mary LO, Krishnan KU, Peter MB, Thomas CS, Richard GE, Michael JO, William FF (1986) Malignant lymphoma of bone. Cancer 58:2646–2655

Marzano AV, Berti E, Paulli M, Caputo R (2000) Cytophagic histiocytic panniculitis and subcutaneous panniculitis-like T-cell lymphoma. Arch Dermatol 136:889–896

Mastovich S, Ratech H, Ware RE, Moope JO, Borowitz MJ (1994) Hepatosplenic T-cell lymphoma: an unusual case of a gamma delta T-cell lymphoma with a blast-like terminal transformation. Hum Pathol 25:102–108

Matano S, Nakamura S, Annen Y, Hattori N, Kiyohara K, Kakuta K, Kyoda K, Sugimoto T (1998) Primary hepatic lymphoma in a patient with chronic hepatitis B. Am J Gastroenterol 93:2301–2302

Mateo M, Mollejo M, Villvendas R et al (1999) 7q31–32 allelic loss is a frequent finding in splenic marginal zone lymphoma. Am J Pathol 154:1583–1589

Matsuyama T, Tsukamoto N, Kaku T, Matsukuma K, Hirakawa T (1989) Primary malignant lymphoma of the uterine corpus and cervix. Report of a case with immunocytochemical analysis. Acta Cytol 33:228–232

Matsuzuka F, Miyauchi A, Katayama S et al (1993) Clinical aspects of primary thyroid lymphoma: diagnosis and treatment based on our experience of 119 cases. Thyroid 2:101–108

Matthews MJ (1985) Surgical pathology of mycosis fungoides and Sézary syndrome. In: Jaffe ES (ed) Surgical pathology of the lymph nodes and related organs. Saunders, Philadelphia, pp 329–356 (Major problems in pathology, vol 16)

Mattia AR, Ferry JA, Harris NL (1993) Breast lymphoma. A B-cell spectrum including the low grade B-cell lymphoma of mucosa-associated lymphoid tissue. Am J Surg Pathol 17:574–587

Matutes E, Morilla R, Owusu-Ankomah K, Houliham A, Meeus P, Catovsky D (1994) The immunophenotype of hairy cell leukemia (HCL). Proposal for a scoring system to distinguish HCL from B-cell disorders with hairy or villous lymphocytes. Leuk Lymphoma 14 Suppl 1:57–61

McAllister HA, Fenoglio JJ (1978) Tumors of the cardiovascular system, 2nd ser, fasc 15, Atlas of tumor pathology. Armed Forces Institute of Pathology, Washington DC, pp 99–100

McDermott MB, O'Briain DS, Shiels OM et al (1995) Malignant lymphoma of the epididymis. A case report of bilateral involvement by a follicular large cell lymphoma. Cancer 75:2174–2179

McDonnell PJ, Mann RB, Buckley BH (1982) Involvement of the heart by malignant lymphoma. Cancer 49:944–951

McKenna RW, Parkin J, Kersey JH, Gajl-Peczalska KJ, Peterson L, Brunning RD (1977) Chronic lymphoproliferative disorder with unusual clinical, morphologic, ultrastructural and membrane surface marker characteristics. Am J Med 62:588–596

McKiernan S, Pilkington R, Ramsay B, Walsh A, Sweeney E, Kelleher D (1999) Primary cutaneous B-cell lymphoma: an association of chronic hepatitis C infection. Eur J Gastroenterol Hepatol 11:669–672

McNiff JM, Cooper D, Howe G, Crotty PL, Tallini G, Crouch J, Eisen RN (1996) Lymphomatoid granulomatosis of the skin and lung. An angiocentric T-cell-rich B-cell lymphoproliferative disorder. Arch Dermatol 132:1464–1470

Medeiros LJ, Harris NL (1989) Lymphoid infiltrates of the orbit and conjunctiva. A morphologic and immunophenotypic study of 99 cases. Am J Surg Pathol 13:459–471

Medeiros LJ, Peiper SC, Elwood L, Yano T, Raffeld M, Jaffe ES (1991) Angiocentric immunoproliferative lesions: a molecular analysis of eight cases. Hum Pathol 22:1150–1157

Melo JV, Robinson DSF, Gregory C et al (1987a) Splenic B-cell lymphoma with "villous" lymphocytes in the peripheral blood: a disorder distinct from hairy cell leukemia. Leukemia 1:294–299

Melo JV, Hedge U, Parreire A, Thompson I, Lampert IA, Catovsky D (1987b) Splenic B-cell lymphoma with circulating villous lymphocytes: differential diagnosis of B-cell leukaemias with large spleens. J Clin Pathol 40:642–651

Menarguez J, Mollejo M, Carrion R et al (1994) Waldeyer ring lymphomas. A clinicopathological study of 79 cases. Histopathology 24:13–22

Mercieca J, Puga M, Matutes E, Moskovic E, Salim S, Catovsky D (1994) Incidence and significance of abdominal lymphadenopathy in hairy cell leukaemia. Leuk Lymph 14 [Suppl 1]:79–83

Meuge C, Hoerni B, de Mascarel A (1972) Non Hodgkin's malignant lymphomas. Clinico-pathologic correlations with the Kiel classification. Retrospective analysis of a series of 274 cases. Eur J Cancer 14:587–592

Meulders Q, Viron B, Michel C et al (1993) Burkitt's lymphoma of the kidney presenting as acute renal failure in AIDS. Nephrol Dial Transplant 8:458–460

Michie SA, Abel EA, Hoppe RT, Warnke RA, Wood GS (1990) Discordant expression of antigens between intraepidermal and intradermal T cells in mycosis fungoides. Am J Pathol 137:1447–1451

Mills SE, Gaffey MJ, Frierson HF Jr (2000) Tumors of the upper aerodigestive tract and ear. Atlas of tumor pathology, 3rd ser, fasc 26. Armed Forces Institute of Pathology, Washington DC

Mittal K, Neri A, Feiner H, Schinella R, Alfonso F (1990) Lymphomatoid granulomatosis in the acquired immunodeficiency syndrome. Evidence of Epstein-Barr virus infection and B-cell clonal selection without myc rearrangement. Cancer 65:1345–1349

Miyake JS, Fitterer S, Houghton DC (1990) Diagnosis and characterization of non-Hodgkin's lymphoma in a patient with acute renal failure. Am J Kidney Dis 16:262–263

Miyamura T, Obama K, Takahira H et al (1993) A case of primary non-Hodgkin lymphoma of the adrenal gland presenting with Addison's disease. Rinsmo Ketsuki 34:882–884

Mizorogi F, Hiramoto J, Nozato A, Takekuma Y, Nagayama K, Tana T, Takagi K (2000) Hepatitis C virus infection in patients with B-cell non-Hodgkin's lymphoma. Intern Med 39:112–117

Mizukami Y, Matsubara F, Hashimoto T et al (1987) Primary T-cell lymphoma of the thyroid. Acta Pathol Jpn 37:1987–1995

Moertel CL, Watterson J, McCormick SR, Simonton SG (1995) Follicular large cell lymphoma of the testis. Cancer 75:1182–1186

Mohler M, Gutzler F, Kallinowski B, Goeser T, Stremmel W (1997) Primary hepatic high-grade non-Hodgkin's lymphoma and chronic hepatitis C infection. Dig Dis Sci 42:2241–2245

Moldenhauer G, Mielke B, Dorken B, Schwartz-Albiez R, Moller P (1990) Identity of HML-1 antigen on intestinal intraepithelial T-cells and of B-ly7 antigen on hairy cell leukaemia. Scand J Immunol 32:77–82

Molina A, Lombard C, Donlon T, Bangs CD, Dorfman RF (1990) Immunohistochemical and cytogenetic studies indicate that malignant angioendotheliomatosis is a primary intravascular (angiotropic) lymphoma. [published erratum appears in Cancer 1990, 15:66:683] Cancer 66:474–479

Molina TJ, Delmer A, Cymbalista F, Le Tourneau A, Perrot JY, Ramond S, Marie JP, Audouin J, Zittoun R, Diebold J (2000) Mantle cell lymphoma in leukaemic phase with prominent splenomegaly. A report of eight cases with similar clinical presentation and aggressive outcome. Virchows Arch 437: 591–598

Moliniè V, Pouchot J, Navratil E, Aubert F, Vinceneux P, Barge J (1996) Primary Epstein-Barr virus-related non-Hodgkin's lymphoma of the pleural cavity following long-standing tuberculosis empyema. Arch Pathol Lab Med 120:288–291

Mollejo M, Menarguez J, Lloret E et al (1995) Splenic marginal zone lymphoma: a distinctive type of low grade B-cell lymphoma. A clinicopathological study of 13 cases. Am J Surg Pathol 19:1146–1157

Moller MB, d'Amore F, Christensen BE (1994) Testicular lymphoma: A population-based study. Eur J Cancer 30A:1760–1764

Möller P, Lammler B, Eberlein-Gonska M, Feichter GE, Hofmann WJ, Schmitteckert H, Otto HF (1986) Primary mediastinal clear cell lymphoma of B-cell type. Virchows Arch A Pathol Anat Histopathol 409:79–92

Möller P, Moldenhauer G, Momburg F, Lammler B, Eberlein-Gonska M, Kiesel S, Dorken B (1987) Mediastinal lymphoma of clear cell type is a tumor corresponding to terminal steps of B-cell differentiation. Blood 69:1087–1095

Möller P, Mielke B, Moldenhauer G (1990) Monoclonal antibody HML-1, a marker for intraepithelial T-cells and lymphomas derived thereof, also recognizes hairy cell leukemia and some B-cell lymphomas. Am J Pathol 136:509–512

Montalban C, Castrillo JM, Abraira V, Serrano M, Bellas C, Piris MA, Carrion R, Cruz MA, Larana JG, Menarguez J et al (1995) Gastric B-cell mucosa-associated lymphoid tissue (MALT) lymphoma. Clinicopathological study and evaluation of the prognostic factors in 143 patients. Ann Oncol 6:355–362.

Monterroso V, Jaffe ES, Merino MS, Medeiros LJ (1993) Malignant lymphomas involving the ovary. A clinicopathologic analysis of 39 cases. Am J Surg Pathol 17:154–170

Morand P, Buisson M, Collandre H, Chanzy B, Genoulaz O, Bourgeat MJ, Pinel N, Leclercq P, Leroux D, Marechal V, Fritsch L, Ruigrok R, Seigneurin JM (1999) Human herpesvirus 8 and Epstein Barr-virus in a cutaneous B-cell lymphoma and a malignant cell line established from the blood of an AIDS patient. Leuk Lymph 35:379–387

Morel P, Dupriez B, Herbrecht R et al (1994) Aggressive lymphomas with renal involvement: a study of 48 patients treated with the LNH-84 and LNH-87 regimens. Br J Cancer 70:154–159

Morgan K, MacLennan KA, Narula A, Bradley PJ, Morgan DA (1989) Non-Hodgkin's lymphoma of the larynx (stage 1E). Cancer 64:1123–1127

Mori N, Yatabe Y, Oka K, Yokose T, Ishido T, Kikuchi M, Asai J (1994) Primary gastric Ki-1 positive anaplastic large cell lymphoma: a report of two cases. Pathol Intern 44:164–169

Mori N, Yatabe Y, Narita M, Kobayashi T, Asai J (1996) Pyothorax-associated lymphoma. An unusual case with biphenotypic character of T and B cells. Am J Surg Pathol 20:760–766

Moriginaga S, Watanabe H, Gemma A et al (1987) Plasmocytoma of the lung associated with nodular deposits of immunoglobulin. Am J Surg Pathol 11:989–994

Morson BC, Dawson IMP (1990) Gastrointestinal pathology, 3rd edn. Blackwell Scientific, Boston

Mossad SB, Tomford JW, Avery RK, Hussein MA, Vaughn KW (2000) Isolated primary hepatic lymphoma in a patient with acquired immunodeficiency syndrome. Int J Infect Dis 4:57–58

Mounedji-Boudiaf L, Culine S, Devoldere G et al (1994) Lymphome B de grande malignité primitif de la prostate. A propos d'un cas avec revue de la literature. Bull Cancer 81:334–337

Moynihan MJ, Bast MA, Chan WC, Delabie J, Wickert RS, Wu G, Weisenburger DD (1996) Lymphomatous polyposis. A neoplasm of either follicular mantle or germinal center cell origin. Am J Surg Pathol 20:442–452

Mullaney BP, Ng VL, Herndier BG, McGrath MS, Pallavicini MG (2000) Comparative genomic analysis of primary effusion lymphoma. Arch Pathol Lab Med 124:824–826

Mulligan SP, Matutes E, Dearden C, Catovsky D (1991) Splenic lymphoma with villous lymphocytes: natural history and response to therapy in 50 cases. Br J Haematol 78:206–209

Muntz HG, Ferry JA, Flynn D, Fuller AF Jr, Tarraza HM (1991) Stage IE primary malignant lymphoma of the uterine cervix. Cancer 68:2023–2032

Murakami H, Irisawa H, Saitoh T, Matsushima T, Tamura J, Sawamura M, Karasawa M, Hosomura Y, Kojima M (1997) Immunological abnormalities in splenic marginal zone cell lymphoma. Am J Hematol 56:173–178

Murase T, Nakamurra S, Tashiro K et al (1997) Malignant histiocytosis-like B-cell lymphoma. A distinct pathologic variant of intravascular lymphomatosis: a report of five cases and review of the literature. Br J Haematol 99:656–664

Muscardin LM, Pulsoni A, Cerroni L (2000) Primary cutaneous plasmacytoma: report of a case with review of the literature. J Am Acad Dermatol 43:962–965

Myers JL, Kurtin PJ, Katzenstein AL, Tazelaar HD, Colby TV, Strickler JG, Lloyd RV, Isaacson PG (1995) Lymphomatoid granulomatosis. Evidence of immunophenotypic diversity and relationship to Epstein-Barr virus infection. Am J Surg Pathol 19:1300–1312

Myszor MF, Record CO (1990) Primary and secondary malignant disease of the liver and fulminant hepatic failure. J Clin Gastroenterol 12:441–446

Nador RG, Cesarman E, Chadburn A, Dawson DB, Ansari MQ, Said J, Knowles DM (1996) Primary effusion lymphoma: a distinct clinicopathologic entity associated with the Kaposi's sarcoma-associated herpes virus. Blood 88:645–656

Nagamine K, Noda H (1990) Two cases of primary cardiac lymphoma presenting with pericardial effusion and cardiac tamponade. Jpn Circ J 54:1158–1164

Nagasaka T, Nakamura S, Medeiros LJ, Juco J, Lai R (2000) Anaplastic large cell lymphomas presented as bone lesions: a clinicopathologic study of six cases and review of the literature. Mod Pathol 13:1143–1149

Nagore E, Ledesma E, Collado C, Oliver V, Perez-Perez A, Aliaga A (2000) Detection of Epstein-Barr virus and human herpesvirus 7 and 8 genomes in primary cutaneous T- and B-cell lymphomas. Br J Dermatol 143:320–323

Nakatsuka S, Yao M, Hoshida Y, Yamamoto S, Iuchi K, Aozasa K (2002) Pyothorax-associated lymphoma: a review of 106 cases. J Clin Oncol 20:4255–4260

Nalesnik MA, Jaffe R, Starzl TE et al (1988) The pathology of posttransplant lymphoproliferative disorders occurring in the setting of cyclosporine A-prednisone immunosuppression. Am J Pathol 133:173–192

Nanba K, Soban EJ, Bowling MC, Berard CW (1977) Splenic pseudosinuses and hepatic angiomatous lesions. Distinctive features of hairy cell leukemia. Am J Clin Pathol 67:415–426

Nand S, Mullen M, Lonchyna A, Moncada R (1991) Primary lymphoma of the heart. Prolonged survival with early systemic therapy in a patient. Cancer 68:2289–2292

Narang S, Wolf BC, Neiman RS (1985) Malignant lymphoma presenting with prominent splenomegaly. A clinicopathologic study with special reference to intermediate cell lymphoma. Cancer 55:1948–1957

Natkunam Y, Warnke RA, Haghighi B, Su LD, Le Boit PE, Kim YH, Kohler S. (2000) Co-expression of CD56 and CD30 in lymphoma with primary presentation in the skin. Clinicopathologic, immunohistochemical and molecular analysis of seven cases. J Cutan Pathol 27:392–329

Nazeer T, Burkart P, Dunn H, Jennings TA, Wolf B (1997) Blastic transformation of hairy cell leukemia. Arch Pathol Lab Med 121:707–713

Neri A, Fracchiolla NS, Roscetti E, Garatti S, Trecca D, Boletini A, Perletti L, Baldini L, Maiolo AT, Berti E (1995) Molecular analysis of cutaneous B- and T-cell lymphomas. Blood 86:3160–3172

Newton R, Ferlay J, Beral V, Devesa SS (1997) The epidemiology of non-Hodgkin's lymphoma: comparison of nodal and extra-nodal sites. Int J Cancer 923–930

Ng CS, Lo ST, Chan JK (1999) Peripheral T and putative natural killer cell lymphomas commonly coexpress CD95 andCD95 ligand. Hum Pathol 30:48–53

Nicholson A, Wotherspoon A, Diss T et al (1995) Pulmonary B-cell non-Hodgkin's lymphomas. The value of immunohistochemistry and gene analysis in diagnosis. Histopathology 26:395–403

Nicholson AG, Wotherspoon AC, Diss TC, Singh N, Butcher DN, Pan LX, Isaacson PG, Corrin B (1996) Lymphomatoid granulomatosis: evidence that some cases represent Epstein-Barr virus-associated B-cell lymphoma. Histopathology 29:317–324

Nonomura N, Aozasa K, Ueda T et al (1989) Malignant lymphoma of the testis: histological and immuno-histological study of 28 cases. J Urol 141:1368–1371

Nuckols JD, Liu K, Burchette JL, McLendon RE, Traweek ST. (1999) Primary central nervous system lymphomas: a 30-year experience at a single institution. Mod Pathol 12:1167–1173

O'Farelly C, Feighery C; O'Brian DS, Stevens F, Connolly CE, McCarthy C, Weir DG (1986) Humoral response to wheat protein in patients with coeliac disease and enteropathy associated T cell lymphoma. Br Med J 293:908–910

Ogawa A, Fukushima N, Satoh T, Kishikawa M, Miyazaki K, Tokunaga O (2000) Primary intestinal T-cell lymphoma resembling lymphomatous polyposis: report of a case. Virchows Arch 437:450–453

Ohsawa M, Aozasa K, Horiuchi K, Kataoka M, Hida J, Shimada H, Oka K, Wakata Y (1992) Malignant lymphoma of the liver. Report of five cases and review of the literature. Dig Dis Sci 37:1105–1109

Ohsawa M, Aozasa K, Horiuchi K et al (1993) Malignant lymphoma of bladder. Cancer 72:1969–1974

Ohsawa M, Tomita Y, Kanno H, Iuchi K, Kawabata Y, Nakajima Y, Komatsu H, Mukai K, Shimoyama M, Aozasa K (1995) Role of Epstein-Barr virus in pleural lymphomagenesis. Mod Pathol 8:848–853

Ohsawa M, Tomita Y, Hashimoto M, Yasunaga Y, Kanno H, Aozasa K (1996) Malignant lymphoma of the adrenal gland: its possible correlation with the Epstein-Barr virus. Mod Pathol 9:534–543

Oinonen R, Franssila K, Elonen E (1997) Spontaneous splenic rupture in two patients with a blastoid variant of mantle cell lymphoma. Ann Hematol 74:33–35

Okada Y, Nakanishi I, Nomura H, Takeda R, Nonomura A, Takekun K (1994) Angiotropic B-cell lymphoma with hemophagocytic syndrome. Pathol Res Pract 190:718–724

Okuno SH, Hoyer JD, Ristow K, Witzig TE (1995) Primary renal non-Hodgkin's lymphoma. An unusual extranodal site. Cancer 75:2258–2261

Osborne BM, Robboy SJ (1983) Lymphomas or leukemia presenting as ovarian tumors. An analysis of 42 cases. Cancer 52:1933–1943

Osborne BM, Butler JJ, Guarda LA (1985) Primary lymphoma of the liver. Ten cases and a review of the literature. Cancer 56:2902–2910

Osborne BM, Brenner M, Weitzner S, Butler JJ (1987) Malignant lymphoma presenting as a renal mass: four cases. Am J Surg Pathol 11:375–382

Oshimi K, Yamada O, Kaneko T, Nishinarita S, Iizuka Y, Urabe A, Inamori T, Asano S, Takahashi S, Hattori M (1993) Laboratory findings and clinical courses of 33 patients with granular lymphocyte-proliferative disorders. Leukemia 7:782–788

Ostronoff M, Soussain C, Zambron E et al (1995) Localized stage non-Hodgkin's lymphoma of the testis: a retrospective study of 16 cases. Nouv Rev Fr Hematol 37:267–272

Pabst R (1992) Is BALT a major component of the human lung immune system? Immunol Today 13:119–122

Paladugu RR, Bearman RM, Rappaport H (1980) Malignant lymphoma with primary manifestation in the gonad: a clinicopathologic study of 38 patients. Cancer 45:561–571

Paling MR, Williamson BRJ (1983) Adrenal involvement in non-Hodgkin lymphoma. AJR 141:303–305

Pandolfi F, Loughran TP Jr, Starkebaum G, Chisesi T, Barbui T, Chan WC, Brouet JC, De Rossi G, McKenna RW, Salsano F (1990) Clinical course and prognosis of the lymphoproliferative disease of granular lymphocytes. A multicenter study. Cancer 65:341–348

Parry-Jones N, Matutes E, Gruszka-Westwood AM, Swansbury GJ, Wotherspoon AC, Catovsky D (2003) Prognostic features of splenic lymphoma with villous lymphocytes: a report on 129 patients. Br J Haematol 120:759–64

Parveen T, Navarro-Roman L, Medeiros LJ, Raffeld M, Jaffe ES (1993) Low grade B-cell lymphoma of mucosa-associated lymphoid tissue arising in the kidney. Arch Pathol Lab Med 117:780–783

Patey-Mariaud De Serre N, Cellier C, Jabri B, Delabesse E, Verkarre V, Roche B, Lavergne A, Brière J, Mauvieux L, Leborgne M, Barbier JP, Modigliani R, Matuchansky C, Macintyre E, Cerf-Benussan N, Brousse N (2000) Distinction between celiac disease and refractory sprue: a simple immunohistochemical method. Histopathology 37:70–77

Paulli M, Berti E, Rosso R, Boveri E, Kindl S, Klersy C, Lazzarino M, Borroni G, Menestrina F, Santucci M, Gambini C, Vassallo G, Magrini U, Sterry W, Burg G, Geerts ML, Meijer CJLM, Willemze R, Feller AC, Muller-Hermelink HK, Kadin ME (1995) CD30/Ki-1-positive lymphoproliferative disorders of the skin. Clinicopathologic correlation and statistical analysis of 86 cases: a multicentric study from the European Organization for Research and Treatment of Cancer utaneous Lymphoma Project Group. J Clin Oncol 13:1343–1354

Paulli M, Boveri E, Rosso R, Arico' M, Kindl S, Viglio A, Berti E, Leithauser F, Locatelli F, Gianelli U, Beluffi G, Feller AC,

Borroni G, Magrini U (1997) CD56/Neural Cell Adhesion Molecule expression in primary extranodal Ki-1/CD30+ lymphoma. Report of a pediatric case with a simultaneous cutaneous and bone localization. Am J Dermatopathol 19:384–390

Paulli M, Strater J, Gianelli U, Rousset MT, Gambacorta M, Orlandi E, Klersy C, Lavabre-Bertrand T, Morra E, Manegold C, Lazzarino M, Magrini U, Moller P (1999) Mediastinal B-cell lymphoma: a study of its histomorphologic spectrum based on 109 cases. Hum Pathol 30:178–187

Paulli M, Viglio A, Vivenza D, Capello D, Rossi D, Riboni R, Lucioni M, Incardona P, Boveri E, Bellosta M, Orlandi E, Borroni G, Lazzarino M, Berti E, Alessi E, Magrini U, Gaidano G (2002) Primary cutaneous large B-cell lymphoma of the leg: histogenetic analysis of a controversial clinicopathologic entity. Hum Pathol 33:937–943

Paulsen J, Lennert K (1994) Low-grade B-cell lymphoma of mucosa-associated lymphoid tissue type in Waldeyer's ring. Histopathology 24:1–11

Pawade J, Banerjee SS, Harris M, Isaacson P, Wright D (1993) Lymphomas of mucosa-associated lymphoid tissue arising in the urinary bladder. Histopathology 23:147–151

Pawade J, Wilkins BS, Wright DH (1995) Low-grade B-cell lymphomas of the splenic marginal zone: a clinicopathological and immunohistochemical study of 14 cases. Histopathology 27:129–137

Pedersen RK, Pedersen NT (1996) Primary non-Hodgkin's lymphoma of the thyroid gland: a population based study. Histopathology 28:25–32

Perniciaro C, Winkelmann RK, Daoud MS, Su WP (1995) Malignant angioendotheliomatosis is an angiotropic intravascular lymphoma. Immunohistochemical ultrastructural, and molecular genetics studies. Am J Dermatopathol 17:242–248

Perren T, Farrant M, McCarthy K, Harper P, Wiltshaw E (1992) Lymphomas of the cervix and upper vagina: a report of five cases and a review of the literature. Gynecol Oncol 44:87–95

Perrier E, Gargin JM, Chanudet X, Pujol A, Gros P, Voog E, Larroque P (1994) Lymphome primitif des surrénales. Presse Med 23:1541

Pescovitz MD, Snover DC, Orchard P, Neglia JP, Najarian JS, Payne WD (1990) Primary hepatic lymphoma in an adolescent treated with hepatic lobectomy and chemotherapy. Cancer 65:2222–2226

Petersen CD, Robinson WA, Kurnick JE (1976) Involvement of the heart and pericardium in the malignant lymphomas. Am J Med Sci 272:161–165

Peterson H, Snider H, Yam L et al (1985) Primary pulmonary lymphoma. A clinical and immunohistochemical study of six cases. Cancer 56:805–813

Petrella T, Delfau-Larue MH, Caillot D, Morcillo JL, Casasnovas O, Portier H, Gaulard P, Farcet JP, Arnould L (1996) Nasopharyngeal lymphomas further evidence for a natural killer cell origin. Hum Pathol 27:827–833

Pettinato G, Manivel JC, Petrella G, De Chiara A (1991) Primary multilobated T-cell lymphoma of the breast diagnosed by fine needle aspiration cytology and immunocytochemistry. Acta Cytol 35:294–299

Pettit AR, Zuzel M, Cawley JC (1999) Hairy cell leukaemia: biology and management. Br J Haematol 106:2–8

Pettit CK, Zukerberg LR, Gray MH, Ferry JA, Rosenberg AE, Harmon DC, Harris NL (1990) Primary lymphoma of bone. A B-cell neoplasm with a high frequency of multilobated cells. Am J Surg Pathol 14:329–334

Pfleger L, Tappeiner J (1959) Zur Kenntnis der systemisierten Endotheliomatose der cutanen Blutgefäße. Hautarzt 10:359–363

Pileri SA, Montanari M, Falini B, Poggi S, Sabattini E, Baglioni P et al (1990) Malignant lymphoma involving the mandible. Clinical, morphologic, and immunohistochemical study of 17 cases. Am J Surg Pathol 14:652–659

Pimpinelli N, Santucci M, Carli P, Paglierani M, Bosi A, Moretti S, Giannotti B (1990) Primary cutaneous follicular center cell lymphoma: clinical and histological aspects. Curr Probl Dermatol 19:203–220

Piris MA, Isaacson PG (1998) Splenic marginal zone lymphoma and its differential diagnosis. Pathology of the spleen: report of the workshop of the VIIIth meeting of the European Association for Haematopathology, Paris 1996. Histopathology 32:172–174

Piris MA, Mollejo M, Campo E, Menarguez J, Floresti T, Isaacson P (1998) A marginal zone pattern may be found in different varieties of non-Hodgkin's lymphoma: the morphology and immunohistology of splenic involvement by B-cell lymphomas simulating splenic marginal zone lymphoma. Histopathology 33:230–239

Piro L, Carrera C, Carson D, Beutler E (1990) Lasting remissions in hairy cell leukemia induced by a single infusion of 2'-chlorodeoxyadenosine. Cancer 332:1117–1121

Piura B, Bar-David J, Glezerman M, Zirkin HJ (1986) Bilateral ovarian involvement as the only manifestation of malignant lymphoma. J Surg Oncol 33:126–128

Pombo de Oliviera MS, Jaffe ES, Catovsky D (1989) Leukaemic phase of mantle cell lymphoma (intermediate): its characterization in 11 cases. J Clin Pathol 89:962–972

Ponzoni M, Arrigoni G, Gould VE, Del Curto B, Maggioni M, Scapinello A et al (2000) Lack of CD29 (beta 1 integrin) and CD54 (ICAM-1) adhesion molecules in intravascular lymphomatosis. Hum Pathol 31:220–226

Prabhu RM, Medeiros LJ, Kumar D, Drachenberg CI, Papadimitriou JC, Appelman HD, Johnson LB, Laurin J, Heyman M, Abruzzo LV (1998) Primary hepatic low-grade B-cell lymphoma of mucosa-associated lymphoid tissue (MALT) associated with primary biliary cirrhosis. Mod Pathol 11:404–410

Prayson RA (1996) Angiotropic large cell lymphoma: simultaneous peripheral nerve and skeletal muscle involvement. Pathology 28:25–27

Prévot S, Hugol D, Le Tourneau A, Audouin J, Diebold J (1990) Lymphomes malins non hodgkiniens primitifs mammaires. Diagnostic anatomo-pathologique de 14 ans. Bull Cancer 77:123–136

Prévot S, Hugol D, Audouin J, Truc JB, Decroix Y, Poitout P, Diebold J (1992) Primary non-Hodgkin's malignant lymphoma of the vagina. Report of 3 cases with review of the literature. Pathol Res Pract 188:78–85

Przybylski G, Wu H, Macon WR, Finan J, Leonard DGB, Felgar RE, DiGiuseppe JA, Nowell PC, Swerdlow SH, Kadin ME, Wasik MA, Salhani KE (2000) Hepatosplenic and subcutaneous panniculitis-like γ/δ T-cell lymphomas are derived from different Vδ subsets of γ/δ T-lymphocytes. J Mol Diag 2:11–19

Quintanilla-Martinez L, Lome-Maldonade C, Ott G, Gschwendtner A, Gredler E, Angeles-Angeles A, Fend F (1997) Primary non-Hodgkin's lymphoma of the intestine: high prevalence of Epstein-Barr virus in Mexican lymphomas as compared with European cases. Blood 89:644–651

Quintanilla-Martinez L, Franklion JL, Guerrero I, Krenacs L, Naresh KN, Rama-Rao C, Bhatia K, Raffeld M, Magrath IT (1999) Histological and immunophenotypic profile of nasal NK/T-cell lymphoma from Peru: high prevalence of p53 overexpression. Hum Pathol 30:849–855

Radaszkiewicz T, Hansmann ML (1988) Primary high grade malignant lymphomas of bone. Virchows Arch A Pathol Anat Histopathol 413:269–274

Rai KR, Sawitsky A, Cronkite EP et al (1975) Clinical staging of chronic lymphocytic leukemia. Blood 46:219

Ralfkiaer E, Stein H, Wantzin GL, Thomsen K, Ralfkiaer N, Mason DY (1985) Lymphomatoid papulosis. Characterization of skin infiltrates by monoclonal antibodies. Am J Clin Pathol 84:587–593

Rambaldi A, Pelicci PG, Allavena P, Knowles DM, Rossini S, Bassan R, Barbui T, Dalla-Favera R, Mantovani A (1985) T- cell receptor beta chain gene rearrangements in lymphoproliferative disorders of large granular lymphocytes/natural killer cells. J Exp Med 162:2156–2162

Raphaël M, Gentilhomme O, Tulliez M, Byron PA, Diebold J and the French Study Group of Pathology for Human Immunodeficiency Virus-Associated Tumors (1991) Histopathologic features of high-grade non-Hodgkin's lymphomas in acquired immunodeficiency syndrome. Arch Pathol Lab Med 115:15–20

Rappaport H, Thomas TB (1974) Mycosis fungoides: the pathology of extracutaneous involvement. Cancer 34:1198–1229

Redondo C, Martin L, Cano AL, Cabellon P, Vazquez JM, Collantes J (1987) Primary lymphoma of the liver treated with hepatic lobectomy and chemotherapy. Cancer 60:736–740

Ree HJ, Rege VB, Knisley RE et al (1980) Malignant lymphoma of Waldeyer's ring following gastrointestinal lymphoma. Cancer 46:1528–1535

Reichert CM, O'Leary TJ, Levens DL, Simrell CR, Macher AM (1983) Autopsy pathology in the acquired immune deficiency syndrome. Am J Pathol 112:357–382

Reiser M, Josting A, Diehl V, Engert A (2001) Primary lymphoma of the conjunctiva – a rare manifestation of indolent non-Hodgkin's lymphoma. Ann Hematol 80:311–313

Reman O, Troussard X, Dao T, Gallet B, Gallet E, Leporrier M (1990) Primary malignant lymphoma of the liver. Report of two cases and review of the literature. Acta Gastroenterol Belg 53:34–41

Remberger K, Nawrath-Koll I, Gokel JM, Haider M (1987) Systemic angioendotheliomatosis of the lung. Pathol Res Pract 182:265–270

Remstein ED, James CD, Kurtin PJ (2000) Incidence and subtype specificity of AP12-MALT 1 fusion translocation in extranodal, nodal and splenic marginal zone lymphomas. Am J Pathol 156:1183–1188

Renno SI, Moreland WS, Pettenati MJ, Beaty MW, Keung YK (2002) Primary malignant lymphoma of uterine corpus: case report and review of Literature. Ann Hematol 81:44–47

Requena L, Sanchez-Yus E (2001) Panniculitis, part II. Mostly lobular panniculitis. J Am Acad Dermatol 45: 325–361

Reyes F, Belhadj K, Tilly F, Charlotte F, Leblond V, Duval C, Angonin E, Deconink E, Tulliez M, Perot C, Pico JS, Zafrani ES, Farcet JP, Gaulard P (1997) Hepatosplenic gd T-cell lymphoma: a recently recognized entity which is fatal. Blood 90 [10 Suppl 1]:338a

Richards MA, Mootoosamy I, Reznek RH, Webb JAW, Lister TA. (1990) Renal involvement in patients with non-Hodgkin's lymphoma: clinical and pathological features of 23 cases. Hematol Oncol 8:105–110

Rickert CH, Dockhorn-Dworniczak B, Simon R, Paulus W (1999) Chromosomal imbalances in primary lymphomas of the central nervous system. Am J Pathol 155:1445–1451

Rijlaarsdam U, Bakels V, van Oostveen JW, Gordijn RJL, Geerts ML, Meijer CJ, Willemze R (1992) Demonstration of clonal immunoglobulin gene rearrangements in cutaneous B-cell lymphomas and pseudo-B-cell lymphomas: differential diagnostic and pathogenetic aspects. J Invest Dermatol 99:749–754

Risdall R, Hoppe RT, Warnke R (1979) Non-Hodgkin's lymphoma: a study of the evolution of the disease based upon 92 autopsied cases. Cancer 44:529–542

Robbins BA, Ellison DJ, Spinosa JC, Carey CA, Lukes RJ, Poppema S, Saven A, Piro LD (1993) Diagnostic application of two-color flow cytometry in 161 cases of hairy cell leukemia. Blood 82:1277–1287

Rooney N, Snead D, Goodman S, Webb AJ (1994) Primary breast lymphoma with skin involvement arising in lymphocytic lobulitis. Histopathology 24:81–84

Root M, Wang TY, Hescock H, Parker M, Hudson P, Balducci L (1990) Burkitt's lymphoma of the testicle: report of 2 cases occurring in elderly patients. J Urol 144:1239–1241

Rosaï J, Carcangiu ML, Delellis RA (1992) Tumors of the thyroid gland. Atlas of tumor pathology, 3rd ser, fasc 5. Armed Forces Institute of Pathology, Washington DC

Rose C, Staroatik P, Brocker EB (1999) Infection with parapoxvirus induces CD30-positive cutaneous infiltrates in humans. J Cutan Pathol 26:520–522

Rosenberg SA, Diamond HD, Jaslavitz B, Craver LF (1961) Lymphosarcoma: a review of 1269 cases. Medicine (Baltimore) 40:31–84

Rosenberg SA, Ribas-Munddo M, Goffinet DR (1978) Staging in adult non Hogkin's lymphoma. Rec Res Cancer Res 65:51–57

Ross CW, Hanson CA, Schnitzer B (1992) CD30 (Ki-1)-anaplastic large cell lymphoma mimicking gastrointestinal carcinoma. Cancer 70:2517–2523

Ross CW, Schnitzer B, Sheldon S, Braun DK, Hanson CA (1994) Gamma/delta T-cell posttransplantation lymphoproliferative disorder primarily in the spleen. Am J Clin Pathol 102:310–315

Rosso R, Neiman RS, Paulli M et al (1995) Splenic marginal zone cell lymphoma: report of an indolent variant without massive splenomegaly presumably representing an early phase of the disease. Hum Pathol 26:39–46

Rotmensch J, Woodruff JD (1982) Lymphoma of the ovary: report of 20 new cases and update of previous series. Am J Obstet Gynecol 143:870–875

Rousselet MC, Gardembas-Pain M, Renier G et al (1992) Splenic lymphoma with circulating villous lymphocytes. Report of a case with immunologic and ultrastructural studies. Am J Clin Pathol 97:147–152

Rubbia-Brandt L, Brundler MA, Kerl K, Negro F, Nador RG, Scherr A, Kurt AM, Mentha G, Borisch B (1999) Primary hepatic diffuse large B-cell lymphoma in a patient with chronic hepatitis C. Am J Surg Pathol 23:1124–1130

Rubin J, Johnson JT, Killeen R, Barnes L (1990) Extramedullary plasmacytomas of the thyroid associated with a serum monoclonal gammopathy. Arch Otolaryngol Head Neck Surg 116:855–859

Rush WL, Andriko JA, Taubenberger JK, Nelson AM, Abbondanzo SL, Travis WD, Koss MN (2000) Primary anaplastic large cell lymphoma of the lung: a clinicopathologic study of five patients. Mod Pathol 13:1285–1292

Ruskone-Fourmestraux A (2000) Gastrointestinal lymphomas: the French experience of the Groupe D'Étude des Lymphomes Digestif (GELD). Rec Res Cancer Res 156:99–103

Said W, Chien K, Takeuchi S, Tasaka T, Asou H, Cho SK, de Vos S, Cesarman E, Knowles DM, Koeffler HP (1996a) Kaposi's sarcoma-associated herpesvirus (KSHV or HHV8) in primary effusion lymphoma: ultrastructural demonstration of herpesvirus in lymphoma cells. Blood 87:4937–4943

Said JW, Tasaka T, Takeuchi S, Hiroya A, de Vos S, Cesarman E, Knowles DM, Koeffler HP (1996b) Primary effusion lymphoma in women: report of two cases of Kaposi's sarcoma Herpes virus-associated effusion-based lymphoma in tumour immunodeficiency virus-negative women. Blood 88:3124–3128

Salhany KE, Macon WR, Choi JK, Elenitsas R, Lessin SR, Felgar RE, Wilson DM, Przybylski GK, Lister J, Wasik MA, Swerdlow SH (1998) Subcutaneous panniculitis-like T-cell lymphoma. Clinicopathologic, immunophenotypic, and genotypic analysis of alpha/beta and gamma/delta subtypes. Am J Surg Pathol 22:881–893

Salles G, Herbrecht R, Tilly H et al (1991) Aggressive primary gastrointestinal lymphomas: review of 91 patients treated with the LNH-84 regimen. A study of the Groupe d'Etude des Lymphomes Agressifs. Am J Med 90:77–84

Salomao DR, Nascimento AG, Lloyd RV, Chen MG, Habermann TM, Strickler JG (1996) Lymphoma in soft tissue. A clinicopathologic study of 19 cases. Hum Pathol 27:253–257

Santucci M, Pimpinelli N, Massi D, Kadin ME, Meijer CJ, Muller-Hermelink HK, Paulli M, Wechsler J, Willemze R, Audring H, Bernengo MG, Corroni L, Chimenti S, Chott A, Diaz-Perez JL, Dipp E, Duncan LM, Feller AC, Geerts ML, Hallermann C, Kempf W, Russel-Jones R, Sander C, Berti E; EORTC Cutaneous Lymphoma Task Force (2003) Cytotoxic/natural killer cell cutaneous lymphomas. Report of EORTC Cutaneous Lymphoma Task Force Workshop

Sarlis NJ, Knight RA, Sarlis I, Papadimitriou K, Kehayas P (1993) Primary non-Hodgkin lymphoma of the prostate gland. Int Urol Nephrol 25:163–168

Sasajima Y, Yamabe H, Kobashi Y et al (1993) High expression of the Epstein-Barr virus latent protein EB nuclear antigen-2 on pyothorax associated lymphomas. Am J Pathol 143:1280–1285

Satoh T, Yamada T, Nakano S, Tokunaga O, Huramochi S, Kanai T, Ishikawa H, Ogihara T (1997) The relationship between primary splenic malignant lymphoma and chronic liver disease associated with hepatitis C virus infection. Cancer 80:1981–1988

Saul SH, Kapadia SB (1985) Primary lymphoma of Waldeyer's ring. Clinicopathologic study of 68 cases. Cancer 56:157–166

Savilo E, Campo E, Mollejo M et al (1998) Absence of cyclin D-1 protein expression in splenic marginal zone lymphoma. Mod Pathol 11:601–606

Savio A, Franzin G, Wotherspoon AC, Zamboni G, Negrini R, Buffoli F, Diss TC, Pan L, Isaacson PG (1996) Diagnosis and posttreatment follow-up of helicobacter pylori-positive gastric lymphoma of mucosa-associated lymphoid tissue: histology, polymerase chain reaction, or both? Blood 87:1255–1260

Scarisbrick JJ, Calonje E, Orchard G, Child FJ, Russell-Jones R (2001) Pseudocarcinomatous change in lymphomatoid papulosis and primary cutaneous CD30+ lymphoma: a clinicopathologic and immunohistochemical study of 6 patients. J Am Acad Dermatol 44:239–247

Scarpa A, Borgato L, Chilosi M et al (1991) Evidence of c-myc gene abnormalities in mediastinal large B-cell lymphoma of young adult age. Blood 78:780–788

Scerpella EG, Villareal AA, Casanova PF, Moreno JN (1996) Primary lymphoma of the liver in AIDS. Report of one new case and review of the literature. J Clin Gastroenterol 22:51–53

Schabet M (1999) Epidemiology of primary CNS lymphoma. J Neurooncol 43:199–201

Schajowicz F (1994) Tumors and tumorlike lesions of bone, 2nd edn. Springer, Berlin Heidelberg New York

Schmid U, Helbron D, Lennert K (1982a) Primary malignant lymphomas localized in salivary glands. Histopathology 6:673–687

Schmid U, Helbron D, Lennert K (1982b) Development of malignant lymphoma in myoepithelial sialadenitis (Sjögren's syndrome). Virchows Arch A 395:11–43

Schmid U, Lennert K, Gloor F (1989) Immunosialadenitis (Sjögren's syndrome) and lymphoproliferation. Clin Exp Rheumatol 7:175–180

Schmid U, Kirkham N, Diss T et al (1992) Splenic marginal zone cell lymphoma. Am J Surg Pathol 16:455–466

Schwalke MA, Rodil JV, Vezeridis MP (1990) Primary lymphoma arising in skeletal muscle. Eur J Surg Oncol 16:70–73

Schweiger F, Shinder R, Rubin S (2000) Primary lymphoma of the liver: a case report and review. Can J Gastroenterol 14:955–957

Scoazec JY, Brousse N (1991) Localisations hépatiques des lymphomes non hodgkiniens. In: Solal-Céligny P, Brousse N, Reyes F, Gisselbrecht C, Coiffier B (eds) Lymphomes non hodgkiniens. Frison-Roche, Paris, pp 267–272

Scoazec JY, Degott C, Brousse N, Barge J, Molas G, Potet F, Benhamou JP (1991) Non-Hodgkin's lymphoma presenting as a primary tumor of the liver: presentation, diagnosis and outcome in eight patients. Hepatology 13:870–875

Semenzato G, Zambello R, Starkebaum G, Oshimi K, Loughran TP, Jr (1997) The lymphoproliferative disease of granular lymphocytes: updated criteria for diagnosis. Blood 89:256–260

Sepp N, Schuler G, Romani N, Geissler D, Gattringer C, Burg G et al (1990) Intravascular lymphomatosis (angioendotheliomatosis): evidence for a T-cell origin in two cases. Hum Pathol 21:1051–1058

Servitje O, Gallardo F, Estrach T, Pujol RM, Blanco A, Fernandez-Sevilla A, Petriz L, Peyri J, Romagosa V (2002) Primary cutaneous marginal zone B-cell lymphoma: a clinical, histopathological, immunophenotypic and molecular genetic study of 22 cases. Br J Dermatol 147:1147–58

Servitje O, Limon A, Blanco A, Carmona M, Serrano T, Romagosa V, Gallardo F, Garcia J, Peyri J (1999) Cardiac involvement and molecular staging in a fatal case of mycosis fungoides. Br J Dermatol 141:531–535

Sharifi S, Murphy M, Loda M, Pinkus GS, Khettry U (1999) Nodular lymphoid lesion of the liver: an immune-mediated disorder mimicking low-grade malignant lymphoma. Am J Surg Pathol 23:302–308

Shepherd NA, Hall PA, Coates PJ, Levison DA (1988) Primary malignant lymphoma of colon and rectum. A histopathological and immunohistochemical analysis of 45 cases with clinicopathologic correlation. Histopathology 12:235–252

Shima N, Kobashi Y, Tsutsui K, Ogawa K, Maetani S, Nakashima Y, Ichijima K, Yamabe H (1990) Extranodal non-Hodgkin's lymphoma of the head and neck. A clinicopathologic study of the Kyoto-Nara area of Japan. Cancer 66:1190–1197

Shimaoka K, Sokal JE, Pickren JW (1962) Metastatic neoplasms of the thyroid gland. Cancer 15:557–565

Shimosato Y, Mukai K (1997) Atypical hyperplastic lymphoepithelial lesion and mucosa-associated lymphoid tissue (MALT) lymphoma. Tumor of the mediastinum. Atlas of tumor pathology, 3rd ser, fasc 21. Armed Forces Institute of Pathology, Washington DC, pp 221–227

Shirato H, Tsuth H, Arimoto T et al (1986) Early stage head and neck non-Hodgkin's lymphoma. The effect of tumor burden on prognosis. Cancer 58:2312–2319

Siegel RJ, Napoli VM (1991) Malignant lymphoma of the urinary bladder. A case with signet-ring cells simulating urachal adenocarcinoma. Arch Pathol Lab Med 115:635–637

Signoretti S, Murphy M, Puddu P, DeCoteau JF, Faraggiana T, Kadin ME, Loda M (1999) Clonality of cutaneous B-cell infiltrates determined by microdissection and immunoglobulin gene rearrangement. Diagn Mol Pathol 8:176–182

Simon J, Jones EL, Trumper MM, Salmon MV (1987) Malignant lymphomas involving the central nervous system – a morphological and immunohistochemical study of 32 cases. Histopathology 11:335–349

Skacel M, Ross CW, Hsi ED (2000) A reassessment of primary thyroid lymphoma: high-grade MALT lymphoma as a distinct subtype of diffuse large B-cell lymphoma. Histopathology 37:10–18

Skodras G, Fields V, Kragel PJ (1994) Ovarian lymphoma and serous carcinoma of low malignant potential arising in the same ovary. A case report with literature review of 14 primary ovarian lymphomas. Arch Pathol Lab Med 118:647–650

Slater DN (1987) Recent developments in cutaneous lymphoproliferative disorders. J Pathol 153:5–19

Slater DN (1992) Diagnostic difficulties in "non-mycotic" cutaneous lymphoproliferative disorders. Histopathology 21:203–213

Slater DN (2001) Borrelia burgdorferi-associated primary cutaneous B-cell lymphoma. Histopathology 38:73–77

Sleater JP, Segal GH, Scott MD, Masih AS (1994) Intravascular (angiotropic) large cell lymphoma: determination of monoclonality by polymerase chain reaction on paraffin-embedded tissues. Mod Pathol 7:593–598

Sminia T, van deer Brugge-Gamelkoorn GJ (1989) Structure and function of bronchus-associated lymphoid tissue (BALT). Crit Rev Immunol 9:119–150

Smoller BR, Bishop K, Glusac E, Kim KH, Hendrickson M (1995) Reassessment of histologic parameters in the diagnosis of mycosis fungoides. Am J Surg Pathol 19:1423–1430

Snyder L, Harmon K, Estensen R (1989) Intravascular lymphomatosis (malignant angioendotheliomatosis) presenting as pulmonary hypertension. Chest 96:1199–1203

Sole B, Salaun V, Ballet JJ, Troussard X (1999a) Transcriptional and post-transcriptional mechanisms induce cyclin-D1 overexpression in B-chronic lymphoproliferative disorders. Int J Cancer 83:230–234

Sole F, Woessner S, Florensa L et al (1999b) Cytogenetic findings in five patients with hairy cell leukemia. Cancer Genet Cytogenet 110:41–43

Solomides CC, Miller AS, Christman RA, Talwar J, Simpkins H (2002) Lymphomas of the oral cavity: histology, immunologic type, and incidence of Epstein-Barr virus infection. Hum Pathol 33:153–157

Solves P, de la Rubia J, Jarque I, Cervera J, Sanz GF, Vera-Semperre, Sanz MA (1999) Liver disease as primary manifestation of multiple myeloma in young man. Leuk Res 23:103–405

Sordillo PP, Epremian B, Koziner B, Lacher M, Lieberman P (1982) Lymphomatoid granulomatosis: an analysis of clinical and immunologic characteristics. Cancer 49:2070–2076

Spier C, Kjeldsberg C, Eyre H, Behm F (1985) Malignant lymphoma with primary presentation in the spleen. Arch Pathol Lab Med 109:1076–1080

Spiers A, Moore D, Cassileth P et al (1987) Remissions in hairy-cell leukemia with pentostatin (2'-Deoxycoformycin). N Engl J Med 316:825–830

Srinisava NS, McGovern CH, Soler K, Poppema S, Halloran PF (1990) Progressive renal failure due to renal invasion and parenchymal destruction of adult T-cell lymphoma. Am J Kidney Dis 16:70–72

Stavem P, Hjort PF, Elgio K, Sommerschild H (1970) Solitary plasmacytoma of the spleen with marked polyclonal increase of gamma G normalized after splenectomy. Acta Med Scand 188:115–118

Stein H, Mason DY, Gerdes J, O'Connor N, Wainscoat J, Pallesen G, Gatter K, Falini B, Delsol G, Lemke H et al (1985) The expression of the Hodgkin's disease associated antigen Ki-1 in reactive and neoplastic lymphoid tissue: evidence that Reed-Sternberg cells and histiocytic malignancies are derived from activated lymphoid cells. Blood 66:848–858

Stein H, Foss HD, Durkop H, Marafioti T, Delsol G, Pulford K, Pileri S, Falini B (2000) CD30+ anaplastic large cell lymphoma: a review of its histopathologic, genetic, and clinical features. Blood 96:3681–3695

Sterry W (1985) Mycosis fungoides. Curr Top Pathol 74:167–223

Stockley et al (1990) Cellular and humoral mechanisms. In: Brevis RAL,Gibson GJ, Geddes DM (eds) Respiratory medicine. Bailliere Tindall, London, pp 189–203

Stone CW, Slease RB, Brubaker D, Fabian C, Grozea PN (1986) Thyroid lymphoma with gastrointestinal involvement. Report of 3 cases. Am J Hematol 21:357–365

Strauchen JA, Hauser AD, Burnstein D, Jimenez R, Moore PS, Chang Y (1996) Body cavity-based malignant lymphoma containing Kaposi sarcoma-associated herpes virus in an HIV-negative man with previous Kaposi sarcoma. Ann Intern Med 125:822–825

Strauss DJ, Filippa DA, Lieberman PH et al (1983) The non-Hodgkin's lymhomas. A retrospective clinical and pathologic analysis of 499 cases diagnosed between 1958 and 1969. Cancer 51:101–109

Stroup R, Sheibani K, Moncada A, Purdy J, Battifora H (1990) Angiotropic (intravascular) large cell lymphoma. A clinicopathologic study of seven cases with unique clinical presentation. Cancer 66:1781–1788

Suarez F, Wlodarska I, Rigal-Huguet F, Mempel M, Martin-Garcia N, Farcet JP, Delsol G, Gaulard P (2000) Hepatosplenic $\alpha\beta$ T-cell lymphoma: an unusual case with clinical, histologic and cytogenetic features of $\gamma\delta$ hepatosplenic T-cell lymphoma. Am J Surg Pathol 24:1027–1032

Suriawinata A, Ye MQ, Emre S, Strauchen J, Thung SN (2000) Hepatocellular carcinoma and non-Hodgkin lymphoma in a patient with chronic hepatitis C and cirrhosis. Arch Pathol Lab Med 124:1532–1534

Swerdlow SH (1992) Post-transplant lymphoproliferative disorders: a morphologic, phenotypic and genotypic spectrum of disease. Histopathology 20:373–385

Swerdlow SH, Williams ME (1993) Centrocytic lymphoma: a distinct clinicopathologic, immunophenotypic, and genotypic entity. Pathol Annu 28:171–197

Takagi N, Nakamura S, Yamamoto K et al (1992) Malignant lymphoma of mucosa-associated lymphoid tissue arising in the thymus of a patient with Sjögren's syndrome. A morphologic, phenotypic and genotypic study. Cancer 69:1347–1355

Takahashi H, Cheng J, Fujita S et al (1992) Primary malignant lymphoma of the salivary gland: a tumor of mucosa-associated lymphoid tissue. J Oral Pathol Med 21:318–325

Takahashi H, Fujita S, Okabe H, Tsuda N, Tezuka F (1993) Immunophenotypic analysis of extranodal non-Hodgkin's lymphomas in the oral cavity. Pathol Res Pract 189:300–311

Taketomi A, Takenaka K, Shirabe K, Matsumata T, Maeda T, Shima M, Ishibashi H, Sugimachi K (1996) Surgically resected primary malignant lymphoma of the liver. Hepatogastroenterology 43:651–657

Tan TB, Spaander PJ, Blaisse M, Gerritzen FM (1988) Angiotropic large cell lymphoma presenting as interstitial lung disease. Thorax 43:578–579

Taniere P, Thivolet-Bejui F, Vitrey D, Isaac S, Loire R, Cordier JF, Berger F (1998) Lymphomatoid granulomatosis – a report on four cases: evidence for B-phenotype of the tumoral cells. Eur Respir J 12:102–106

Tefferi A, Hanson CA, Kurtin PJ, Katzmann JA, Dalton RJ, Nichols WL (1997) Acquired von Willebrand's disease due to aberrant expression of platelet glycoprotein Ib by marginal zone lymphoma cells. Br J Haematol 96:850–853

Teruya-Feldstein J, Zauber P, Setsuda JE, Berman EL, Sorbara L, Raffeld M, Tosato G, Jaffe ES (1998) Expression of human herpesvirus-8 oncogene and cytokine homologues in an HIV-seronegative patient with multicentric Castleman's disease and primary effusion lymphoma. Lab Invest 78:11637–11642

Thieblemont C, Felman P, Callet-Bouchu E, Traverse-Glehen A, Salles G, Berger F, Coiffier B (2003) Splenic marginal-zone lymphoma: a distinct clinical and pathological entity. Lancet Oncol 4:95–103

Thieblemont C, Berger F, Dumontet C, Moullet I, Bouafia F, Felman P, Salles G, Coiffier B (2000) Mucosa-associated lymphoid tissue lymphoma is a disseminated disease in one third of 158 patients analyzed. Blood 95:802–806

Tierens A, Delabie J, Pittaluga S, Driessen A, De Wolf-Peeters C (1998) Mutation analysis of the rearranged immunoglobulin heavy chain genes of marginal zone cell lymphomas indicates an origin from different marginal zone B lymphocyte subsets. Blood 91:2381–2386

Torlakovic E, Cherwitz DL, Jessurun J, Scholes J, McGlennen R (1997) B-cell gene rearrangement in benign and malignant lymphoid proliferations of mucosa-associated lymphoid tissue and lymph nodes. Hum Pathol 28:166–173

Toro JR, Liewehr DJ, Pabby N, Sorbara L, Raffeld M, Steinberg SM, Jaffe ES (2003) Gamma delta T-cell phenothype is associated with significantly decreased survival in cutaneous T-cell lymphoma. Blood 101:3407–3412

Torres-Paoli D, Sanchez JL (2000) Primary cutaneous B-cell lymphoma of the leg in a chronic lymphadematous extremity. Am J Dermatopathology 22:257–260

Travis WD, Banks PM, Reiman HM (1987) Primary extranodal soft tissue lymphoma of the extremities. Am J Surg Pathol 11:359–366

Trojani M, Mongodin B, Seniuta P, Eghbali H, de Mascarel I, Coindre JM (1990) Lymphomes malins non hodgkiniens primitifs du sein. Etude de cinq cas. Ann Pathol 10:28–33

Troussard X, Valensi F, Duchayne E, Garand R, Felman P, Tulliez M, Henri-Amar M, Bryon PA, Flandrin G (1996) Splenic lymphoma with villous lymphocytes: clinical presentation, biology and prognostic factors in a series of 100 patients. Br J Haematol 93:731–736

Trudeau M, Sheperd FA, Blackstein ME (1988) Intraocular lymphomas: report of three cases and review of literature. Am J Clin Oncol 11:126–130

Tsang K, Kneafsey P, Gill MJ (1993) Primary lymphoma of the kidney in the acquired immunodeficiency syndrome. Arch Pathol Lab Med 117:541–543

Tsang P, Cesarman E, Chadburn A, Liu Y, Knowles DM (1996) Molecular characterization of primary mediastinal B-cell lymphoma. Am J Pathol 148:2017–2025

Tucker TJ, Bardales RH, Miranda RN (1999) Intravascular lymphomatosis with bone marrow involvement. Arch Pathol Lab Med 123:952–956

Turner RR, Colby TV, MacIntosh FR (1981) Testicular lymphomas: a clinico-pathologic study of 35 cases. Cancer 48:2095–2102

Ueda G, Oka K, Matsumoto T, Yatabe Y, Yamanaka K, Suyama M, Ariyama J, Futagawa S, Mori N (1996) Primary hepatic marginal zone B-cell lymphoma with mantle cell lymphoma phenotype. Virchows Arch 428:311–314

Ullrich A, Fischbach W, Blettner M (2002) Incidence of gastric B-cell lymphomas: a population-based study in Germany. Ann Oncol 13:1120–1127

Usha L, Bradlow B, Stock W, Platanias LC (2000) CD5+ immunophenotype in the bone marrow but not in the peripheral blood in a patient with hairy cell leukaemia. Acta Haematol 103:210–213

Utsunomiya M, Takatera H, Itoh H, Tsujimura T, Itatani H (1992) Bilateral primary non-Hodgkin's lymphoma of the adrenal glands with adrenal insufficiency: a case report. Hinyokika Kiyo 38:311–314

Vadlamudi G, Lionetti KA, Greenberg S, Mehta K (1996) Leukemic phase of mantle cell lymphoma. Two cases report and review of the literature. Arch Pathol Lab Med 120:35–40

Vallianatou K, Brito-Babapulle V, Matutes E, Atkinson S, Catovsky D (1999) p53 gene deletion and trisomy 12 in hairy cell leukemia and its variant. Leuk Res 23:1041–1045

Van Droogenbroeck J, Altintas S, Pollefliet C, Schroyens W, Berneman Z (2001) Intravascular large B-cell lymphoma or intravascular lymphomatosis: report of a case diagnosed by testicle biopsy. Ann Hematol 80:316–318

van Doorn R, Scheffer E, Willemze R (2002) Follicular mycosis fungoides, a distinct disease entity with or without associated follicular mucinosis: a clinicopathologic and follow-up study of 51 patients. Arch Dermatol 138: 191–198

Van Gelder T, Michiels JJ, Mulder AH, Klooswijk AL, Schalekamp MA (1992) Renal insufficiency due to bilateral primary renal lymphoma. Nephron 60:108–110

Van Gorp J, Weiping L, Jacobse K, Liu YH, Li FY, De Weger RA, Li G (1994) Epstein-Barr virus in nasal T-cell lymphomas (polymorphic reticulosis-midline malignant reticulosis) in western China. J Pathol 173:81–87

Van Krieken JHJM (1990) Histopathology of the spleen in non-Hodgkin's lymphoma. Histol Histopath 5:113–122

Van Krieken JH, Otter R, Hermans J et al (1989) Malignant lymphoma of the gastrointestinal tract and mesentery: a clinicopathologic study of the significance of histologic classification. Am J Pathol 135:281–289

Van Krieken JH, Medeiros LJ, Pals ST, Raffeld M, Kluin PM (1992) Diffuse aggressive B-cell lymphomas of the gastrointestinal tract and mesentery. An immunophenotypic and gene rearrangement analysis of 22 cases. Am J Clin Pathol 97:170–178

Van Neer FJ, Toonstra J, Van Voorst Vader PC, Willemze R, Van Vloten WA (2001) Lymphomatoid papulosis in children: a study of 10 children registered by the Dutch Cutaneous Lymphoma Working Group. Br J Dermatol 144:351–354

Vang R, Silva EG, Medeiros LJ, Deavers M (2000) Endometrial carcinoma and non-Hodgkin's lymphoma involving the female genital tract: a report of three cases. Int J Gynecol Pathol 19:133–138

Vassalo J, Roessner A, Vollmer E, Grundmann E (1987) Malignant lymphomas with primary bone manifestations. Pathol Res Pract 182:381–389

Vassalo J, Assuncao MCGA, Machado JC (1988) Primitive malignant lymphomas of bone. Study of 14 cases. Ann Pathol 8:44–48

Veelken H, Wood GS, Sklar J (1995) Molecular staging of cutaneous T-cell lymphoma: evidence for systemic involvement in early disease. J Invest Dermatol 104:889–894

Vega F, Medeiros LJ, Bueso-Ramos C, Jones D, Lai R, Luthra R, Abruzzo LV (2001) Hepatosplenic gamma/delta T-cell lymphoma in bone marrow. A sinusoidal neoplasm with blastic cytologic features. Am J Clin Pathol 116:410–419

Vergier B, Beylot-Barry M, Pulford K, Michel P, Bosq J, de Muret A, Beylot C, Delaunay MM, Avril MF, Dalac S, Bodemer C, Joly P, Groppi A, de Mascarel A, Bagot M, Mason DY, Wechsler J, Merlio JP. (1998) Statistical evaluation of diagnostic and prognostic features of CD30+ cutaneous lymphoproliferative disorders. Am J Surg Pathol 22:1192–1202

Vergier B, de Muret A, Beylot-Barry M, Vaillant L, Ekouevi D, Chene G, Carlotti A, Frack N, Dechelotte P, Souteyrand P, Courville P, Joly P, Delaunay M, Bagot M, Grange F, Fraitag S, Bosq J, Petrella T, Durlach A, de Mascarel A, Merlio JP, Wechsler J (2000) Transformation of mycosis fungoides: clinicopathological and prognostic features of 45 cases. French Study Group of Cutaneous Lymphomas. Blood 95:2212–2218

Vermeer MH, Geelen FA, van Haselen CW, van Voorst Vader PC, Geerts ML, van Vloten WA, Willemze R (1996) Primary cutaneous large B-cell lymphomas of the legs. A distinct type of cutaneous B-cell lymphoma with an intermediate prognosis. Arch Dermatol 132:1304–1308

Vie H, Chevalier S, Garand R, Moisan JP, Praloran V, Devilder MC, Moreau JF, Soulillou JP (1989) Clonal expansion of lymphocytes bearing the gamma delta T-cell receptor in a patient with large granular lymphocyte disorder. Blood 74:285–290

Visser L, Shaw A, Slupsky J, Vos H, Poppema S (1989) Monoclonal antibodies reactive with hairy cell leukemia. Blood 74:320–325

Wagner SD, Martinelli V, Luzzatto L (1994) Similar patterns of Vk gene usage but different degrees of somatic mutation in hairy cell leukemia, prolymphocytic leukemia, Waldenström's macroglobulinemia, and myeloma. Blood 83:3647–3653

Walls JG, Gia Hong Y, Cox JE et al (1999) Pulmonary intravascular lymphomatosis. Chest 115:1207–1210

Walz-Mattmuller R, Horny JP, Ruck P, Kaiserling E (1998) Incidence and pattern of liver involvement in haematological malignancies. Pathol Res Pract 194:781–789

Wang CC, Tien HF, Lin MT, Su IT, Wang CH, Chuang SM, Shen MC, Liiu CH (1995) Consistent presence of isochromosome 7q in hepatosplenic T-γ/δ-lymphoma: a new cytogenetic clinicopathologic entity. Genes Chromosomes Cancer 12:161–164

Wargotz ES, Jannotta ES, Nochomowitz LE (1987) Primary cardiac non-Hodgkin's lymphoma. Arch Pathol Lab Med 111:894–895

Waring WS, Wharton SB, Grant R, McIntyre M (1999) Angiotropic large B-cell lymphoma with clinical features resembling subacute combined degeneration of the cord. Clin Neurol Neurosurg 101:275–279

Weber RG, Pietsch T, von Schweinitz D, Lichter P (2000) Characterization of genomic alterations in hepatoblastomas. A role for gains on chromosomes 8q and 20 as predictors of poor outcome.Am J Pathol 157:571–578

Weening RH, Ng CS, Perniciaro C (2001) Subcutaneous panniculitis-like T-cell lymphoma. An elusive case presenting as lipomembranous panniculitis and a review of 72 cases in the literature. Am J Dermatopathol 23:206–215

Weichhold W, Labouyrie E, Merlio JP, Masson B, de Mascarel A (1995) Primary extramedullary plasmacytoma of the liver. A case report. Am J Surg Pathol 19:1197–1202

Weidmann E (2000) Hepatosplenic T-cell lymphoma. A review on 45 cases since first report describing the disease as a distinct lymphoma entity in 1990. Leukemia 14:991–997

Weisenburger DD, Nathwani BN, Diamond LW, Winberg CD, Rappaport H (1981) Malignant lymphoma, intermediate lymphocytic type: a clinicopathologic study of 42 cases. Cancer 48:1415–1425

Weiss LM, Wood GS, Trela M, Warnke RA, Sklar J (1986) Clonal T-cell populations in lymphomatoid papulosis. Evidence of a lymphoproliferative origin for a clinically benign disease. N Engl J Med 315:475–479

Wentzell RA, Berkheise R (1995) Malignant lymphomatosis of the kidneys. J Urol 74:177–185

Whitcup SM, de Smet MD, Rubin BI, Palestine AG, Martin DF, Burnier M Jr, CHAN CC, Nussenbaum RB (1993) Intraocular lymphoma. Clinical and histopathologic diagnosis. Ophthalmol. 100:1399–1406

Whittaker S, Smith N, Jones RR, Luzzatto L (1991) Analysis of beta, gamma and delta T-cell receptor genes in lymphomatoid papulosis: cellular basis of two distinct histologic subsets. J Invest Dermatol 96:786–791

Wieselthier JS, Koh HK (1990) Sézary-syndrome: diagnosis, prognosis, and critical review of treatment options. J Am Acad Dermatol 22:381–401

Willemze R, Beljaards RC (1993) Spectrum of primary cutaneous CD30 (Ki-1)-positive lymphoproliferative disorders. A proposal for classification and guidelines for management and treatment. J Am Acad Dermatol 973–980

Willemze R, Meijer CJ (1999) EORTC classification for primary cutaneous lymphomas: the best guide to good clinical management. Am J Dermatopathol 21:265–273

Willemze R, Meijer CJLM (1998) Classification of cutaneous lymphomas: crosstalk between pathologist and clinician. Curr Diagn Pathol 5:23–33

Willemze R, Meijer CJLM (2000) EORTC classification for primary cutaneous lymphomas: a comparison with the R.E.A.L. classification and the proposed WHO classification. Ann Oncol 11 [Suppl 1]:11–15

Willemze R, Beljaards RC, Meijer CJLM (1994) Classification of primary cutaneous T-cell lymphomas. Histopathology 24:405–415

Willemze R, Kerl H, Sterry W, Berti E, Cerroni L, Chimenti S, Diaz-Peréz JL, Geerts ML, Goos M, Knobler R, Ralfkiaer E, Santucci M, Smith N, Wechsler J, von Vloten WA, Meijer CJ (1997) EORTC classification for primary cutaneous lymphomas: a proposal from the cutaneous lymphoma study group of the European Organization for Research and Treatment of Cancer. Blood 90:345–371

Willemze R, Meijer CJLM, van Vloten WA, Scheffer E (1982) The clinical and histological spectrum of lymphomatoid papulosis. Br J Dermatol 107:131–144

Wilson WH, Kingma DW, Raffeld M, Wittes RE, Jaffe ES (1996) Association of lymphomatoid granulomatosis with Epstein-Barr viral infection of B-lymphocytes and response to Interferon-2b. Blood 87:4531–4537

Wolf BC, Neiman RS (1989) Disorders of the spleen. Saunders, Philadelphia

Wong KF, Chan JKC, Li LPK, Yau TK, Lee AWM (1994) Primary cutaneous plasmacytoma – report of two cases and review of the literature. Am J Dermatolpathol 16:392–397

Wong KF, Chan JKC, Matutes E et al (1995) Hepatosplenic γδT-cell lymphoma. A distinctive aggressive lymphoma type. Am J Surg Pathol 19:718–726

Wood GS, Weiss LM, Hu CH, Abel EA, Hoppe RT, Warnke RA, Sklar J (1988) T-cell antigen deficiencies and clonal rearrangements of T-cell receptor genes in pagetoid reticulosis (Woringer-Kolopp disease). N Engl J Med 318:164–167

Wood GS, Ngan BY, Tung R, Hoffman TE, Abel EA, Hoppe RT, Warnke RA, Gleary ML, Sklar J (1989) Clonal rearrangements of immunoglobulin genes and progression to B-cell lymphoma in cutaneous lymphoid hyperplasia. Am J Pathol 135:13–19

Wood GS, Hardman DL, Boni R, Dummer R, Kim YH, Smoller BR, Takeshita M, Kikuchi M, Burg G (1996) Lack of the t(2;5) or other mutations resulting in expression of anaplastic lymphoma kinase catalytic domain in CD30+ primary cutaneous lymphoproliferative disorders and Hodgkin's disease. Blood 88:1765–1770

Woodruff JD, Noli Castillo RD, Novak ER (1963) Lymphoma of the ovary; a study of 35 cases from the Ovarian Tumor Registry of the American Gynecological Society. Am J Obstet Gynecol 85:912–918

Wong KF, Zhang YM, Chan JK (1999) Cytogenetic abnormalities in natural killer cell lymphoma/leukaemia: is there a consistent pattern? Leuk Lymphoma 34:241–250

Wotherspoon AC (1998) Helicobacter pylori infection and gastric lymphoma. Br Med Bull 54:79–85

Wotherspoon AC (2000) A critical review of the effect of Helicobacter pylori eradication on gastric MALT lymphoma. Curr Gastroenterol Rep 2:494–498

Wotherspoon AC, Ortiz-Hidalgo C, Falzon MR, Isaacson PG (1991) *Heliobacter pylori*-associated gastritis and primary B-cell gastric lymphoma. Lancet 338:1175–1176

Wotherspoon AC, Pan LX, Diss TC, Isaacson PG (1992) Cytogenetic study of B-cell lymphoma of mucosa-associated lymphoid tissue. Cancer Genet Cytogenet 58:35–38

Wotherspoon AC, Diss TC, Pan LX, Schmid C, Kerr-Muir MG, Lea SH, Isaacson PG (1993a) Primary low-grade B-cell lymphoma of the conjunctiva: a mucosa-associated lymphoid tissue type lymphoma. Histopathology 23:417–424

Wotherspoon AC, Doglioni C, Diss TC, Pan L, Moshini A, de Boni M, Isaacson PG (1993b) Regression of primary low-grade B-cell gastric lymphoma of mucosa-associated lymphoid tissue type after eradication of Helicobacter pylori. Lancet 342:575–577

Wotherspoon AC, Finn TM, Isaacson PG (1995) Trisomy 3 in low-grade B-cell lymphomas of mucosa-associated lymphoid tissue. Blood 85:2000–2004

Wright DH (1979) Involvement of the liver by lymphoreticular disease. In: Wright R, Alberti KGMM, Karran S et al (eds) Liver and biliary disease: pathophysiology, diagnosis, management. Saunders, London, pp 926–940

Wright DH (1994) Lymphomas of Waldeyer's ring. Histopathology 24:97–99

Wu CD, Jackson CL, Medieros LJ (1996) Splenic marginal zone cell lymphoma. An immunophenotypic and molecular study of five cases. Am J Clin Pathol 105:277–285

Yamane T, Kirimoto K, Fujita M et al (1989) Ovarian involvement as an initial manifestation of malignant lymphoma. Jpn J Clin Oncol 19:163–166

Yang B, Tubs RR, Finn W, Carlson A, Pettay J, Hsi ED (2000) Clinicopathologic reassessment of primary cutaneous B-cell lymphomas with immunophenotypic and molecular genetic characterization. Am J Surg Pathol 24:694–702

Ye MQ, Suriawinata A, Black C, Min AD, Strauchen J, Thung SN (2000) Primary hepatic marginal zone B-cell lymphoma of mucosa-associated lymphoid tissue type in a patient with primary biliary cirrhosis. Arch Pathol Lab Med 124:604–608
Yoshino T, Miyake K, Ichimura K, Mannami T, Ohara N, Hamazaki S, Akagi T (2000a) Increased incidence of follicular lymphoma in the duodenum. Am J Surg Pathol 24:688–693
Yoshino T, Omonishi K, Kobayashi K, Mannami T, Okada H, Mizuno M, Yamadori I, Kondo E, Akagi T (2000b) Clinicopathological features of gastric mucosa associated lymphoid tissue (MALT) lymphomas: high grade transformation and comparison with diffuse large B-cell lymphomas without MALT lymphoma features. J Clin Pathol 53:187–190
Yousem SA, Colby TV (1990) Intravascular lymphomatosis presenting in the lung. Cancer 65:349–353
Zafrani ES, Gaulard P (1993) Primary lymphoma of the liver. Liver 13:57–61
Zafrani ES, Leclercq B, Vernant JP, Pinaudeau Y, Chomette G, Dhumeaux D (1983) Massive blastic infiltration of the liver: a cause of fulminant hepatic failure. Hepatology 3:428–432
Zettl A, Ott G, Makulik A, Katzenberger T, Starostik P, Eichler T, Puppe B, Bentz M, Muller-Hermelink HK, Chott A (2002) Chromosomal gains at 9q characterize enteropathy-type T-cell lymphoma. Am J Pathol 161: 1635–45
Zhu D, Oscier DG, Stevenson FK (1995) Splenic lymphoma with villous lymphocytes involves B cells with extensively mutated Ig heavy chain variable region genes. Blood 85: 1603–1607
Zucca E, Conconi A, Mughal TI, Sarris AH, Seymour JF, Vitolo U, Klasa R, Ozsahin M, Mead GM, Gianni MA, Cortelazzo S, Ferreri AJ, Ambrosetti A, Martelli M, Thieblemont C, Moreno HG, Pinotti G, Martinelli G, Mozzana R, Grisanti S, Provencio M, Balzarotti M, Laveder F, Oltean G, Callea V, Roy P, Cavalli F, Gospodarowicz MK; International Extranodal Lymphoma Study Group (2003) Patterns of outcome and prognostic factors in primary large-cell lymphoma of the testis in a survey by the International Extranodal Lymphoma Study Group. J Clin Oncol 21:20–27

7 Plasma Cell Proliferations

7.1 Plasma Cell Myeloma/Bone Marrow Plasmacytoma (ICD-O: 9732/3)

Synonyms

- KIEL: Plasmacytic lymphoma (plasmacytoma)
- REAL: Plasmacytoma /plasma cell myeloma
- WHO: Plasma cell myeloma
- Other: Multiple myeloma, Kahler's disease

Definition

This neoplastic proliferation consists of a unique diagnostic triad of osteolytic bone lesions, marrow infiltration by atypical plasma cells, and serum monoclonal gammopathy (Kyle 1992; Schajowicz 1994; Malpas et al. 1995; Grogan et al. 2001).

Morphology

Macroscopy. The neoplasia is responsible for the development of nodules in the bone marrow that consist of soft grayish or yellowish homogeneous tissue and measure about 1 cm in diameter. These nodules transform into large polycyclic masses that destroy not only the bone architecture of the medulla but also the cortex with extension to the surrounding soft tissues. These bone lesions cause collapse of the vertebral bodies and fracture of tubular bones.

Histology. The diagnosis of plasma cell myeloma is based on the type of bone marrow infiltration, the quantity of neoplastic cells, and the morphology of the cells (Reed et al. 1981; Kyle 1992; Bartl et al. 1982, 1995; Sailer et al. 1995).

Early lesions are made up of small nests of neoplastic cells that are dispersed between adipose cells, more or less intermingled with hematopoietic cells, and at a distance from the arterioles (Fig. 7.1). This localized interstitial involvement can be difficult to diagnose. The presence of large plasma cells, blastic or pleomorphic variants, is useful in making the diagnosis.

The presence of aggregate of about 25 plasma cells (Grogan et al. 2001) as well as of more diffuse interstitial infiltrates (Fig. 7.2) favors the diagnosis of plasma cell myeloma. Some of the aggregate may develop along the bone trabeculae (Fig. 7.3).

In more advanced cases, sheets of plasma cells form nodules or strands destroying and replacing the hematopoietic tissue. Finally, densely packed plasma cells lead to massive involvement of the medullary spaces. Collagen bands can develop around vessels and bone trabeculae (Fig. 7.3). Destruction of bone trabeculae by osteoclastic hyperplasia is often observed, mostly in advanced disease.

The neoplastic cells exhibit a variety of morphologies that either predominate or are variably associated.

One of the most frequent neoplastic cell types is that of *mature plasma cells* (Fig. 7.1), Marschalko type; these cells have an eccentric nucleus with dense chromatin ("cartwheel" pattern), no or only one small nucleolus, a large ovoid or triangular basophilic cytoplasm, and a clear juxtanuclear halo (extremely large Golgi apparatus). Giant forms can be observed.

Another neoplastic cell type is *lymphoid plasma cells.* These are smaller than Marschalko type cells, with scanty cytoplasm surrounding a round nucleus with dense chromatin blocks. They seem to often be associated with IgD production (Reed et al. 1981).

Proplasma cells are larger, with a pale nucleus containing a central medium-sized nucleolus (Fig. 7.4). Other types of plasma cells have an irregular, "cleaved" or "notched" nucleus. Large cells with the morphology of *immunoblasts, plasmablasts* (Fig. 7.5), or even *giant multinucleated cells* mimicking Sternberg-Reed cells are also observed. Vacuoles may be located in the cyto-

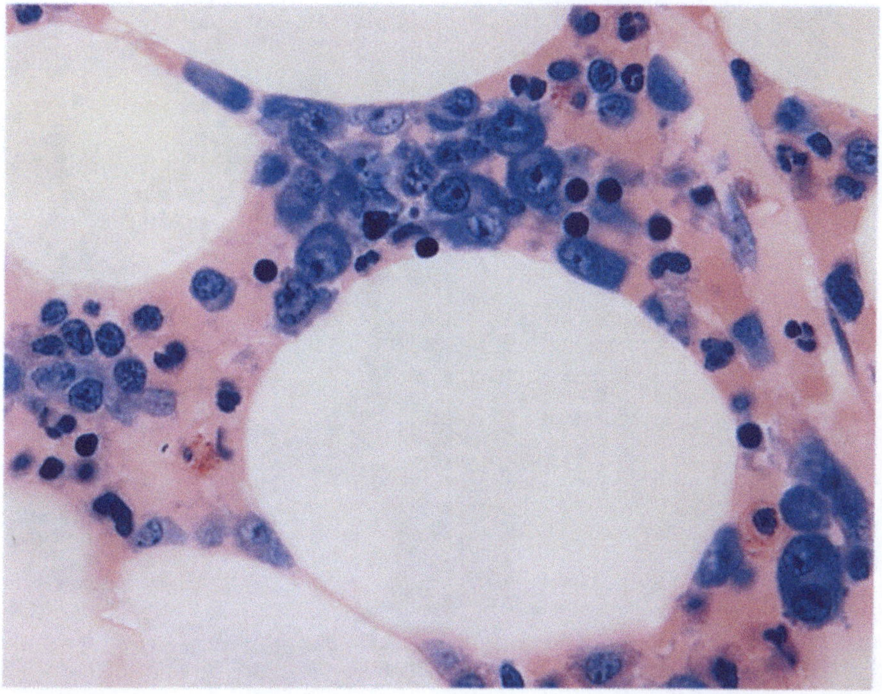

Fig. 7.1. Plasma cell myeloma. Early infiltration by dispersed small nests of mature plasma cells (Marschalko type), at a distance from capillaries and arterioles (Giemsa stain)

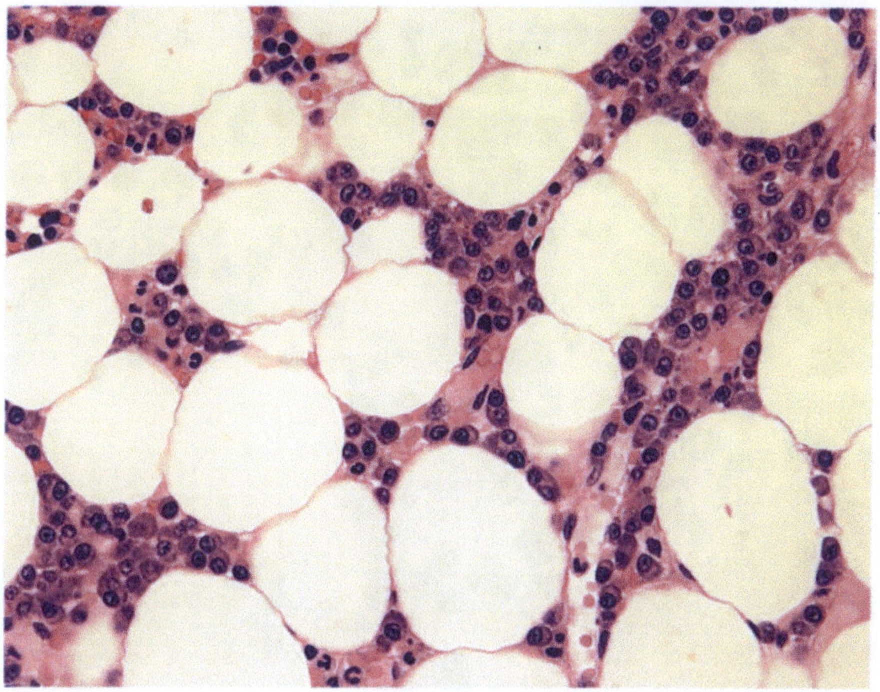

Fig. 7.2. Plasma cell myeloma. Interstitial infiltrate by plasma cells replaces the normal hematopoietic cells (H and E stain)

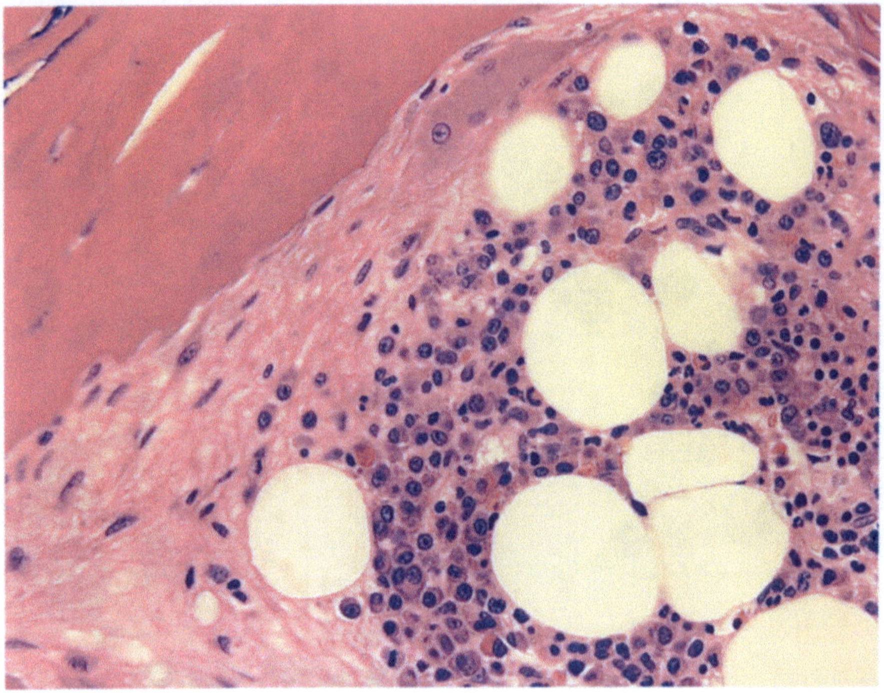

Fig. 7.3. Plasma cell myeloma. Large sheet of plasma cells near a bone trabeculae surrounded by collagenous fibrosis. Note an osteoclast, responsible for bone resorption, near the upper border (H and E stain)

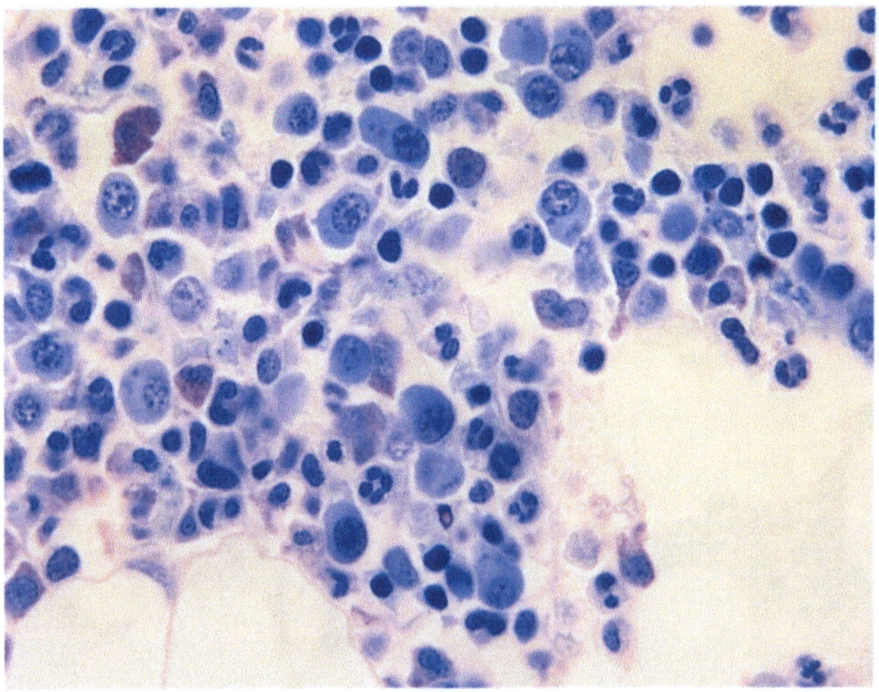

Fig. 7.4. Plasma cell myeloma. Interstitial infiltrate comprising mostly proplasma cells (Giemsa stain)

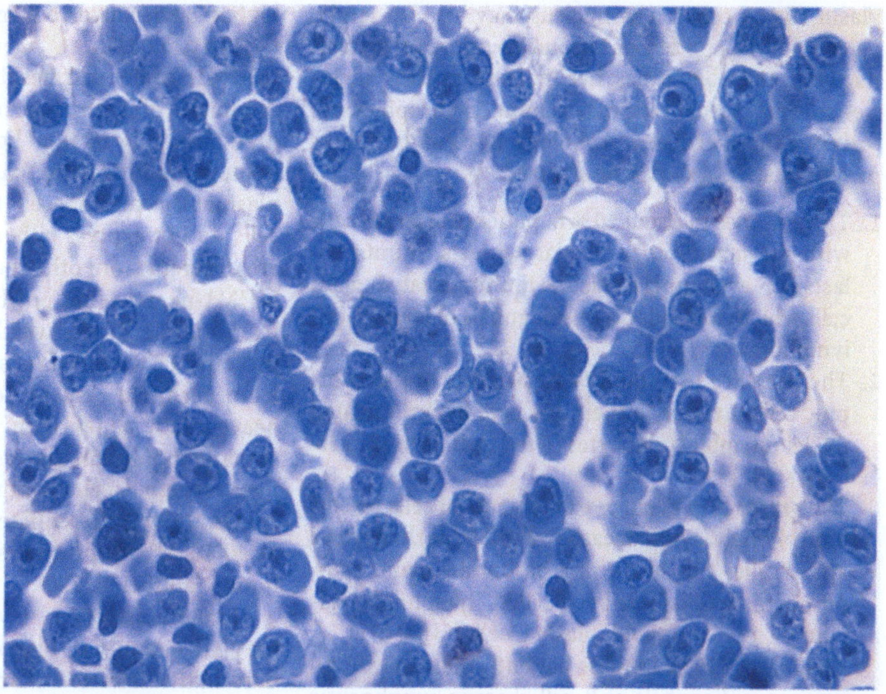

Fig. 7.5. Plasma cell myeloma. Massive involvement of large cells with the morphology of plasmablasts and immunoblasts (Giemsa stain)

plasm or in the nuclei. Proplasma cells are PAS-positive when they contain IgA. Immunoglobulin crystals may be seen in the cytoplasm of tumor cells, particularly in IgD myeloma (Gabriel et al. 1985). In some plasma cell myelomas, histiocytes accumulate around and between the tumor cells and may contain numerous immunoglobulin crystals (Gabriel et al. 1985).

A histological staging system of prognostic value that is based on the amount of tumor cells in the bone biopsy has been proposed (Bartl et al. 1982, 1987, 1995; Sailer et al. 1995):

- Stage I: less than 10% of the bone marrow is involved
- Stage II: 20–50% of the bone marrow is involved
- Stage III: More than 50% of the bone marrow is involved

A classification system dividing plasma cell myeloma into four types (mature, intermediate, immature, and plasmablastic) based on the morphology of the tumor cells (Bartl et al. 1982, 1987, 1995; Sukpanichnant et al. 1994; Sailer et al. 1995) and having prognostic value has also been proposed.

Angiogenesis was recently demonstrated in bone marrow biopsies from multiple myeloma patients (Moehler et al. 2001b) and seems to be of prognostic significance. Angiogenesis and mast cell density increase simultaneously with progression of multiple myeloma (Ribatti et al. 1999). It appears that myelofibrosis develops simultaneously.

Cytology. Plasma cell myeloma can be diagnosed from smears obtained either by sternal puncture or by puncture of a bone tumor. While the diagnosis is based on the presence of more than 10% plasma cells, the average plasma cell content is not enough. Severe plasmacytosis can be observed, for example, in infectious diseases (pneumonia, septicemia) as well as in dysimmune diseases, particularly Castleman's disease (Molina et al. 1996). Therefore, the increased number of plasma cells should be between 20 and 40% (Kyle 1992; Reed et al. 1981; Brunning and McKenna 1994) and associated with an atypical morphology. The neoplastic cells mostly resemble mature plasma cells (Marschalko type), but they may be larger and some may exhibit various changes (Brunning and McKenna 1994; Diebold 1997): fraying of the cytoplasmic borders, cytoplasmic shedding, presence of hyaline inclusions, granules (Mott cells), vacuoles, crystalline inclusions of various size, multiple Russell bodies, and a deep-red cytoplasm (flame cells). The nucleus may also be larger, paler, with less condensed chromatin, more prominent nucleoli, and sometimes hyaline intranuclear inclusions. Some plasma cells may exhibit erythrophagocytosis or a Gaucher-like morphology. Beyond that, three peculiar patterns should be stressed:

1. The presence in about 10 % of patients of larger cells with the morphology of plasmablasts, immunoblasts, or even unclassifiable multinucleated giant cells which can lead to a misdiagnosis of large-B-cell lymphoma.
2. The presence in about 2 % of patients of pleomorphic cells that due to their notched, hyperlobulated nuclei resemble monocytes (Reed et al. 1981; Zukerberg et al. 1990).
3. The presence in about 5 % of patients of cells resembling lymphocytes because of their dark nucleus and smaller size but with a basophilic ovoid cytoplasm; these cells have been called "lymphoplasmacytoid" or "lymphoid plasma cells" (Bartl et al. 1982, 1987, 1995). In these patients, there may be an erroneous diagnosis of B-cell chronic lymphocytic leukemia (B-CLL) with lymphoplasmacytoid differentiation or of lymphoplasmacytic lymphoma.

Immunohistochemistry is mandatory even on smears (see Chap. 4.2.1).

Immunohistochemistry

Plasma cell myeloma consists of mature B-cells expressing CD79α and the plasma-cell-associated antigens CD38 and CD138 (syndecan-1). The other B-cell-associated antigens, particularly CD20, are mostly negative. CD138 is an adhesion molecule and neoplastic plasma cells express other adhesion molecules such as CD56 and CD58, explaining perhaps the predominant settlement of the bone marrow (Ridley et al. 1993; Grogan et al. 2001). CD10 is sometimes also expressed (Van Riet et al. 1998) as well as cyclin D1.

Demonstration of intracytoplasmic immunoglobulin secretion with a light-chain restriction plays an important role in the diagnosis. Usually, the heavy-chain type is IgG, sometimes IgA, very rarely IgD, IgE, or IgM. About 85 % of plasma cell myelomas produce a complete Ig with heavy- and light-chains. In 15 % of these tumors, only one light-chain is produced by the neoplastic plasma cells (Bence Jones myeloma) (Grogan et al. 2001).

MUM1/IRF4 protein is the product of a homologous gene involved in the myeloma-associated t(6;14)(p25;q32). A new monoclonal antibody (MUM1p) demonstrates the presence of the protein in the nuclei of normal germinal center B-cells located predominantly in the "light zone" and with a morphology ranging from that of a centrocyte to that of a plasmablast/plasma cell (Falini et al. 2000). These cells do not express either Bcl-6 protein or Ki67 and are different from other germinal center cells that are MUM1-negative but positive for Bcl-6 and Ki67, and from mantle B-cells which are negative for all three proteins. PCR analysis of single MUM1+ cells isolated from germinal centers demonstrated rearranged Ig heavy-chain genes with a varying number of V_H somatic mutations, suggesting that these centrocytes may represent cells committed to exit the germinal center and to differentiate into plasma cells (Falini et al. 2000). MUM1 protein is strongly expressed in myeloma (Falini et al. 2000).

Immunohistochemistry using anti-CD34, anti-factor-VIII, or anti-CD31 is considered to be the gold standard in the detection of angiogenesis in bone marrow biopsies, but the permeability of the blood vessels cannot be determined (Mangi and Newland 2000; Moehler et al. 2001b). Vascular endothelial growth factor (VEGF) and interleukin-6 has also been used to demonstrate angiogenesis (Dankbar et al. 2000).

Genetic Features

Different types of genetic abnormalities have been disclosed (translocations, deletions, mutations) and are responsible for alteration of oncogenes and/or suppressor genes (Dewald et al. 1985). Chromosomes 1, 11, and 14 are most frequently involved. Translocation t(11;14) is common (Dewald et al. 1985). Three genes are present on chromosome 11 which play a role in disease evolution: (1) the neuronal-cell adhesion molecule (N-CAM) gene, located on 11q23; (2) the cyclin D1 gene, activated by the translocation near the IgH γ-switch region (Chesi et al. 1996); (3) the H-ras gene (p21), which has an effect on patient survival (Tsuchiya et al. 1988). Three other chromosomes may be involved: (1) the association of an abnormal chromosome 6 with increased secretion of tumor necrosis factor (TNF) which in turn is responsible for osteoclastic stimulation (Barlogie et al. 1989), (2) a deletion of the long arm of chromosome 7, associated with alteration of the multidrug resistance gene (drug resistance phenotype), (3) alteration of the PAX-5 gene on chromosome 9 resulting in the loss of CD19 expression (Mahmoud et al. 1996).

Chromosomal abnormalities have been disclosed in 18% of recently diagnosed patients and in 63% of patients with progressive disease (Barlogie et al. 1989). Fluorescent in situ hybridization (FISH) has recently been used to demonstrate the allelic loss of p53, predictive of an unfavorable evolution (Drach et al. 1998).

Immunoglobulin gene rearrangements are observed. In addition to monoclonal rearrangement, other rare types of rearrangement are compatible with oligoclonal or biclonal tumor development (Tsuchiya et al. 1988). Ig somatic mutations are frequently observed and are consistent with derivation of the tumor from a post-germinal-center B-cell. Patients with a light-chain restriction lose JH segments and/or parts of chromosome 14.

In some plasma cell myelomas, a γ-T-cell-receptor (TCR) gene rearrangement has been demonstrated.

Differential Diagnosis

In the majority of the cases, the diagnosis of plasma cell myeloma is easy, based on clinical presentation, cytology, histopathological pattern, and immunohistochemistry.

A severe *plasma cell hyperplasia*, representing 20–40% of the cells in the bone marrow, can be described in only a few non-neoplastic diseases. This reactive plasmacytosis has been described in patients with severe infections, for example, septicemia and pneumonitis, or in those with localized or multicentric Castleman's disease (Molina et al. 1996). Only mature polytypic plasma cells are present. The absence of atypical cells and the polytypic immunoglobulins represent the two criteria that allow this reactive plasmacytosis to be distinguished from plasma cell myeloma.

In early lesions of plasma cell myeloma, plasma cells may constitute less than 10% of the bone marrow hematopoietic cells. The diagnosis of plasma cell myeloma is based on the development of small nests of plasma cells at a distance from the capillaries and dispersed between adipose and the hematopoietic cells; on the existence of giant plasma cells, plasma cell precursors, and other atypical cells; and on the demonstration of monotypic cytoplasmic immunoglobulin in all these cells, contrasting with the polytypic pattern of the reactive plasma cells surrounding capillaries (Diebold 1997).

Another condition also raises difficult problems. *Massive osseous or juxtaosseous tumors consisting predominately of immunoblasts or plasmablasts* are very difficult to classify. There are almost no morphological or immunohistochemical criteria to distinguish between a large-B-cell lymphoma arising in a lymph node or in the soft tissue and extending into an adjacent bone or an extraosseous extension from a plasma cell myeloma transforming into an immunoblastic or plasmablastic variant. Only the clinical presentation may allow the distinction.

Occurrence

The sex ratio shows a male predominance of 3:2. The disease develops in adults over 35 years of age; the incidence increases with age.

Plasma cell myeloma accounts for 20–50% of primary bone tumors (Schajowicz 1994) and represents 1% of all malignant tumors (Kyle 1992). In the USA, the incidence is 2–3.9 cases per 100,000 people (Kyle 1992; Ries et al. 1991), representing 15% of all hematopoietic malignancies (Devesa et al. 1988). There is a higher incidence among black Americans (Schajowicz 1994), with myeloma being the most common lymphoid neoplasia in this population and the second most common in the white population (Devasa et al. 1988).

The incidence varies from one part of the world to the other, but in general increased to 45% from 1940 to the 1970s (Devesa et al. 1988). An increased risk of myeloma is observed after exposure to radiation, petroleum-derived pesticides, asbestos, rubber, plastic, and sawdust, and in response to chronic infection or persistent antigenic stimulation. Viral diseases may also play a role, for example, HIV and/or human herpes virus 8 (HHV8), which have been disclosed in bone marrow biopsy samples (Said et al. 1997). A "two-hit" hypothesis has been postulated in the pathogenesis of plasma cell myeloma, The disease probably develops from an end-stage B-cell, post-germinal-center, mature plasma cell (Hallek et al. 1998).

Clinical Presentation

Approximately 80% of the patients complain of localized or diffuse bone pain. In cases of vertebral localizations, sciatica or crural pain may be noted.

The first symptom in about 10% of the patients is a bone tumor in the ribs, sternum, or head.

Spontaneous fracture occurs as the presenting feature in about 5% of the patients.

Some patients also present with fever and weight loss.

Additional symptoms may be due to hyperviscosity syndrome, hypercalcemia, anemia, or amyloidosis.

Radiography of the skeleton discloses multiple round osteolytic lesions without sclerotic margins (Diebold 1997). These increase in size and coalesce, destroying the bone and the cortex which may appear very thin in the long bones, sternum, rib, and pelvis. Pathological fractures are observed in different bones, e.g. ribs or vertebrae with collapse of the vertebral bodies.

The bones involved are bone containing red marrow and with an active hematopoiesis, for example, vertebrae, ribs, skull, and pelvis in about 60% of patients, and long bones, scapular, sternum, and mandible in about 40% (Schajowicz 1994).

Immunoelectrophoresis shows a monoclonal gammopathy (IgG in 50–60%, IgA in 20–35%, rarely (2%) IgD or IgE) in 99% of the patients (Salmon and Cassady 1988), and a biclonal gammopathy with a light-chain restriction in 1%. Monoclonal light-chain (Bence Jones protein) is disclosed in the serum of 15% of patients and in the urine of 75% (Salmon and Cassady 1988).

During disease evolution, renal insufficiency and recurrent bacterial infections are common.

Plasma cell myeloma is an incurable disease (Grogan et al. 2001). A great majority of the patients die after a median survival of 3 years. Only about 10% survive at 10 years (Grogan et al. 2001). Increased tumor mass and poor renal function are associated with a shorter survival time.

A staging scheme was proposed by the WHO Classification 2001, based on tumor mass, renal function, hemoglobin level, serum calcium, assessment of lytic lesions, amount of M-component, and serum level of β2-microglobulin (poor survival in patients with a high level) (Rajkumar and Greipp 1999).

In addition, the percentage of infiltration of the bone marrow, classified in three stages, is of prognostic value (see Histopathology) (Bartl et al. 1982). Patients with immunoblastic or plasmablastic variants have a poor prognosis (Bartl et al. 1982; Greipp et al. 1998).

Recently, the increased amount of blood vessels due to angiogenesis in the bone marrow simultaneous with the growth of a neoplastic infiltrate has been studied by contrast-enhanced dynamic magnetic resonance imaging (Moehler et al. 2001a) and immunohistochemistry. Angiogenesis seems to be of prognostic value (Rajkumar et al. 2000; Moehler et al. 2001b).

7.1.1 Clinical Variants

Plasma cell myeloma presents with many variants.

7.1.1.1 Diffuse Decalcifying Myelomatosis

This variant is due to a diffuse infiltration of bone by plasma cells with severe bone rarefaction (osteoporosis).

It is characterized by the absence of lytic lesions on bone radiography; instead, there is diffuse decalcification (Kyle 1992; Bartl et al. 1982, 1987, 1995; Schajowicz 1994).

7.1.1.2 Osteosclerotic Myeloma

This variant is characterized by the development of large strands of collagen fibrosis that destroy the hematopoietic tissue of the bone marrow and by surrounding nests of plasma cells. Thickened bone trabeculae are surrounded by peritrabecular fibrosis with neo-osteogenesis (Miralles et al. 1992). These lesions develop focally, either in one bone or in multiple sites. At a distance, plasma cell nests with atypical large cells may be present, but often only a few mature plasma cells are observed.

The plasma cells may produce either IgA or IgG, even sometimes IgM, with a high incidence (about 90% of the tumors) of λ-light-chain restriction (Miralles et al. 1992).

In the differential diagnosis, all etiologies of osteomyelofibrosis have to be discussed: metastatic carcinoma, idiopathic myelofibrosis, myelofibrosis secondary to other chronic myeloproliferative disorders. The best criterion for diagnosing osteosclerotic myeloma is the discovery of monotypic (as determined by immunohistochemistry) plasma cell clusters in or between collagen bands.

Patients are often younger than those with typical plasma cell myeloma, and there is a male predominance. Anemia is rarely observed, in contrast to the occurrence of erythrocytosis and thrombocytosis. This type of myeloma is often associated with the so-called POEMS syndrome and/or with a pattern of lymphadenopathy typical of that in Castleman's disease (Miralles et al. 1992; Rolon et al. 1989).

7.1.1.3
Nonsecretory Myeloma

This variant of plasma cell myeloma can be defined as a myeloma without monoclonal immunoglobulin in the blood and urine (Bosman et al. 1996; Bourantas 1996).

The histopathological lesions are identical to those of typical plasma cell myeloma.

In the majority of these tumors, monotypic intracytoplasmic immunoglobulins can be demonstrated in the plasma cells. In very exceptional cases, it is impossible to disclose such immunoglobulin synthesis and the diagnosis can only be made based on morphology.

The patients present with the same clinical features as those with typical plasma cell myeloma but without any monoclonal component, due to the lack of excretion of the Ig synthesized by the plasma cells.

7.1.1.4
Solitary Myeloma (ICD-O: 9731/3*)

This type of plasma cell proliferation is responsible for a single bone tumor destroying either the central part of a short bone (vertebrae, rib) or of a long bone (Kyle 1992; Bataille and Sany 1981; Bacci et al. 1982; Bartl et al. 1982, 1987, 1995; Brunning and McKenna 1994; Guida et al. 1994; Schajowicz 1994).

Macroscopic study reveals that the cortex is thinned, but mostly without extension in the surrounding tissue. All of the histopathological patterns described for typical multiple myeloma can be observed; the immunohistochemistry is also identical to that of multiple myeloma.

Patients present with a single bone tumor, pain, and sometimes spontaneous fracture. In some patients, there is no monoclonal component in the blood or urine. Other patients may present with a low serum level of M-component.

Treatment of the tumor may be followed by complete remission with disappearance of the serum monoclonal component if present (Leibross et al. 1998). The risk of transformation into typical multiple plasma cell myeloma is high, occurring in about 55 % of the patients after 10 years of follow-up. Local recurrence is observed in about 10 % of the patients. Only 35 % seem to achieve complete remission (Kyle 1992).

* Given for solitary myeloma of the bone

7.1.1.5
Plasma Cell Leukemia

This type of leukemia can be detected before, or may be associated with bone manifestations (Kyle et al. 1974; Kyle 1992; Brunning and McKenna 1994; Dimopoulos et al. 1994; Garcia-Sanz et al. 1999).

Patients present with hepatosplenomegaly, thrombocytopenia, and a high level of LDH. The peripheral blood contains more than 20 % neoplastic plasma cells, which are hypodiploid with complex cytogenetic abnormalities (Garcia-Sanz et al. 1999).

The bone marrow is diffusely infiltrated. Liver biopsy reveals plasma cells in the lumen of hepatic sinuses.

Prompt chemotherapy is required. The median survival is about 20 months (Dimopoulos et al. 1994).

7.1.1.6
Variants with Peculiar Clinical Behavior

Plasma cell proliferations in fact comprise a broad spectrum of diseases, from the *monoclonal gammopathy of undetermined significance* (MGUS) (serum M-component less than the levels in myeloma, bone marrow plasmacytosis less than 10 % and no clinical signs or lytic bone lesions), which is often an incidental finding, to typical plasma cell myeloma with multiple lesions. Two clinical variants should be listed that fulfill some of the criteria for plasma cell myeloma but which are asymptomatic (Grogan et al. 2001). In *smoldering myeloma*, the serum M-component is at myeloma levels, there is a marrow plasmacytosis of 10 – 30 %, but no clinical or radiologic signs. In *indolent myeloma*, the serum M-component is at intermediate levels, marrow plasmacytosis is 10 – 30 %, there are up to three lytic bone lesions, but no other clinical or biological signs. Neither smoldering nor indolent myeloma requires immediate treatment..

7.2
Extraosseous (Extramedullary) Plasmacytoma (ICD-O: 9734/3)

Definition

Extraosseous (extramedullary) plasmacytoma is a neoplastic plasma cell proliferation developing outside the bone marrow, in the absence of a plasma cell myeloma.

Histology
These tumors are characterized by sheets of plasma cells infiltrating, destroying, and replacing normal tissue. The neoplastic cells show the morphology of mature plasma cells sometimes with giant plasma cells. In some cases, a variable number of proplasma cells, plasmablasts, or immunoblasts is recognized.

Immunohistochemistry and Genetic Features
Identical to those of plasma cell myeloma.

Differential Diagnosis
In all the localizations, plasmacytomas should be distinguished from chronic inflammatory diseases rich in plasma cells. The most important criterion is the demonstration of polytypic or monotypic immunoglobulin production.

In some sites (lymph node, spleen, tonsil, gastrointestinal tract, lung, skin, etc.), plasmacytomas should be distinguished from marginal zone lymphoma with a plasmacytic component and from lymphoplasmacytic lymphoma. The monoclonal immunoglobulin in these types of lymphomas is often IgM.

Clinical Features
Clinical presentation depends on the site. Extraosseous (extramedullary) plasmacytoma can arise in the upper respiratory tract (80% of the cases), gastrointestinal tract, lung, breast, thyroid, parotid gland, skin, testis, urinary bladder, central nervous system, as well as in lymphoid tissue (lymph node, spleen). There are no localizations in the bone marrow and no signs of plasma cell myeloma. A few patients only have a serum monoclonal component. Prognosis after radiotherapy in mostly good. There are local recurrences in about 25% of the patients, but transformation into a plasma cell multiple myeloma seems to be rare (Alexiou et al. 1999).

For more details, see the chapters on organ lymphomas.

7.3 Associated Diseases

7.3.1 Castleman's Disease

This peculiar disease of the lymph nodes may be either uni- or multicentric, the two subtypes of presentation probably corresponding to two different diseases.

Both subtypes have been observed in association with plasma cell myeloma, primary solitary bone plasmacytoma, and/or POEMS syndrome (Rolon et al. 1989). Some reported cases were associated with an HHV8 infection, particularly the multicentric variant occurring in HIV-positive patients.

7.3.2 POEMS Syndrome

The name of this syndrome is an acronym of the initials of the symptoms: *p*olyneuropathy, *o*rganomegaly (hepatomegaly, splenomegaly), *e*ndocrine disease (hypothyroidy, gynecomastia), *m*onoclonal immunoglobulin component in the blood, *s*kin lesions (thickening, hyperpigmentation, hypertrichosis).

The syndrome may be associated with Castleman's disease and/or with plasma cell myeloma often of the osteosclerotic variant (Miralles et al. 1992; Rolon et al. 1989).

This syndrome is probably due to the hyperproduction of cytokines (Klein 1995).

7.3.3 Primary Amyloidosis

Definition
Primary amyloidosis is characterized by the deposition in different tissues of a fibrillary protein (AL) with a β-pleated-sheet structure and consisting of immunoglobulin-light-chain (Kyle and Gertz 1990, 1995). Systemic AL amyloidosis involves the digestive tract, subcutaneous fat, and bone marrow, which are the sites that should be biopsied for the diagnosis. Numerous other organs or tissue can be involved: kidney, liver, spleen, heart, tongue, nerves.

Histology

The deposits are amorphous, eosinophilic (pink), acellular. They mostly predominate in the blood vessel walls, which are thickened, and on basement membranes. Perivascular and/or interstitial deposits can be observed and increase with progression. AL deposits stain with Kongo red showing green birefringence by polarization.

Differential Diagnosis

Systemic primary AL amyloidosis should be distinguished from other diseases caused by monoclonal immunoglobulin deposition; light-chain (mostly κ, i.e. Randall's syndrome), heavy-chain, or both light- and heavy-chains (de Lajarte-Thirouard et al. 1999).

These diseases are either associated with MGUS or with plasma cell myeloma. Deposits occur on basement membrane (glomerules, liver and spleen sinuses, bone marrow) or in joints. They are Congo-red-negative but can be characterized by immunohistochemistry (Preud'homme et al. 1994; Kambham et al. 1999).

Occurrence

AL amyloidosis occurs often in association with a plasma cell myeloma or an immunocytoma. About 20% of patients with AL amyloidosis have a plasma cell myeloma and 15% with plasma cell myeloma have primary AL amyloidosis.

Clinical Features

In some patients, systemic amyloidosis is disclosed fortuitously during the histological study of a biopsy, for example, a bone marrow biopsy.

Other patients present with symptoms that are unusual for a plasma cell myeloma: macroglossia, hepatosplenomegaly, congestive heart failure, malabsorption, peripheral neuropathy, bleeding, or nephrotic syndrome.

The suspected diagnosis should be confirmed by histolopathological evaluation of biopsies.

Myeloma patients with amyloidosis have a shorter survival (Kyle and Gertz 1990).

7.3.4 Light- and/or Heavy-Chain Deposition Diseases

Synonyms

- Randall disease

Definition

These diseases are characterized by a plasma cell proliferation associated with the deposition of a nonfibrillary amorphous material comprising immunoglobulin light-chains, heavy-chains, or both (Kambham et al. 1999).

These deposits are monoclonal, with a κ-light-chain predominance.

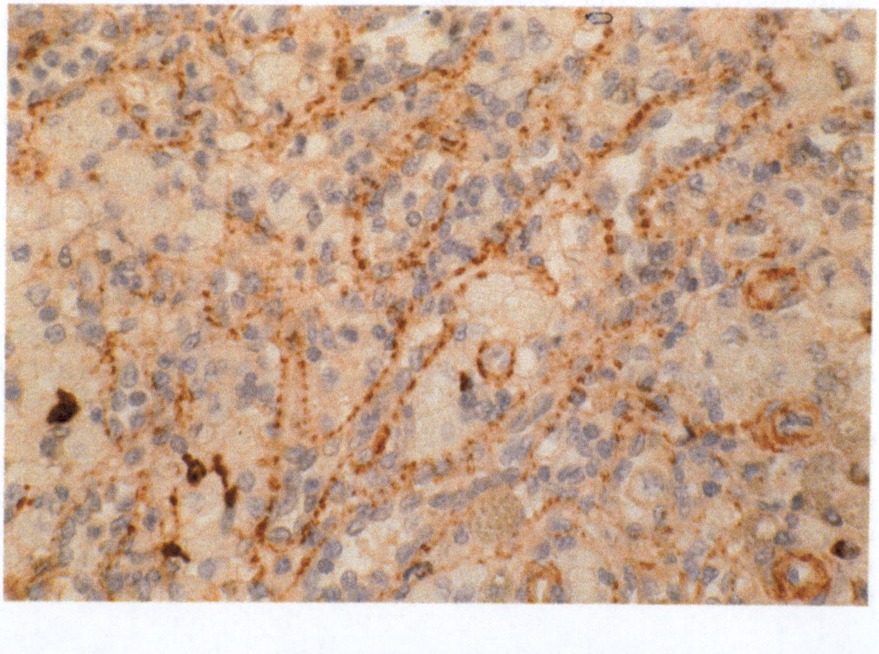

Fig. 7.6. Light-chain deposition disease. Deposition of immunoglobulin λ-light-chain on the basement membrane of the sinuses of the splenic red pulp

In contrast to the AL deposits of amyloidosis, these deposits do not have a β-pleated-sheet configuration.

Histology
These diseases are characterized by the deposition of an amorphous, eosinophilic, Congo-red-negative material on basement membranes of variable tissues: glomerules and tubules in the kidney (Preud'homme et al. 1994); sinusoids in the liver, spleen (Fig. 7.6) (De Lajarte et al. 1999), and bone marrow; nerves, heart, joints, and small vessels – the latter leading to vascular occlusion or microaneurysms.

Mostly, there are no plasma cells or only a few near the sites of deposition; however, the bone marrow is infiltrated by mature plasma cells, sometimes up to 60%.

Immunohistochemistry
The depositions are made of κ-light-chain in about 80% of the cases. In a few cases, heavy-chain is associated, mostly μ or γ. Sometimes only heavy-chain can be demonstrated. The cytoplasm of plasma cells in the bone marrow also has a light-chain restriction or a light-chain predominance (Kambham et al. 1999).

Genetic Features
The monoclonal immunoglobulin produced by the plasma cells shows structural changes due to deletions or mutations (Preud'homme et al. 1994). These changes are responsible for the deposition.

Differential Diagnosis
The most important disease to consider in the differential diagnosis is *primary amyloidosis.* In amyloidosis, the deposits are Congo-red- and thioflavin-positive, while these reactions are negative in monoclonal light-/heavy-chain deposition diseases.

Occurrence
This disease remains very rare. It occurs in adults between 30 and 80 years of age and without sex predominance (Grogan et al. 2001).

Clinical Presentation
The symptoms vary according to the main site of deposition: hepatomegaly, splenomegaly (De Lajarte-Thirouard et al. 1999), congestive heart failure, or often nephrotic syndrome and renal failure (Preud'homme et al. 1994). A monoclonal gammopathy is present in 85% of the patients, corresponding either to MGUS or sometimes to a typical myeloma (Kambham et al. 1999). Coagulopathy and hypocomplementemia have been observed.

The disease is rapidly fatal, survival being less than 2 years (Grogan et al. 2001) mostly due to variable visceral dysfunction, rarely to the plasma cell proliferation.

7.4 Heavy-Chain Diseases

Definition
These diseases are lymphoplasmacytic lymphomas in which only abnormal immunoglobulin heavy-chain is secreted.

μ-Heavy-Chain Disease. Bone marrow and lymph nodes show a diffuse infiltrate resembling that of B-CLL (Fig. 7.7). In association with small lymphocytes, it is possible to recognize plasma cells, often with a vacuolated cytoplasm. Macrophages containing PAS-positive material, sometimes crystallized, are dispersed between the lymphoid cells (Fig. 7.8)

The lymphoid cells express B-associated antigens (CD20, CD79α) and CD43 but are negative for CD5, CD10, and CD23. The plasma cells express CD38 and contain intracytoplasmic μ-heavy-chain, but light-chains cannot be demonstrated.

It is very difficult to distinguish μ-heavy-chain disease from B-CLL. The most important criterion is the discovery of typical vacuolated plasma cells.

Patients with this very rare lymphoma present with hepatosplenomegaly without adenopathy. The presence of μ-heavy-chain can be disclosed in the blood, but not in the urine, by immunoelectrophoresis. Light-chains (mostly κ) are found in the urine (Wahner-Roedler and Kyle 1992).

γ-Heavy-Chain Disease. Bone marrow and lymph node are diffusely infiltrated by an association of lymphocytes, lymphoplasmacytoid cells, mature plasma cells, a variable number of large cells with the morphology of immunoblasts, and some eosinophils. This pattern resembles lymphoplasmacytic lymphoma more than B-CLL.

Immunohistochemistry is identical to μ-heavy-chain disease with the exception of the γ-chain expression.

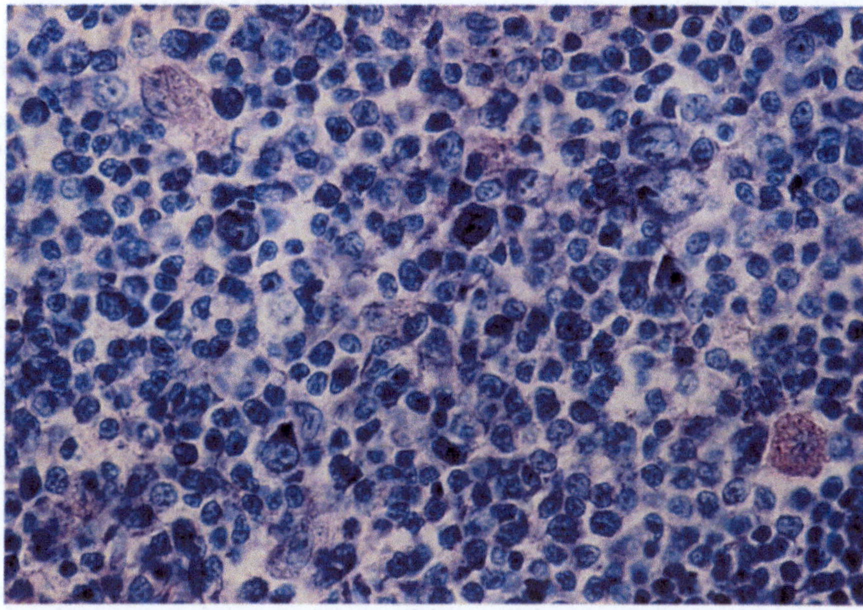

Fig. 7.7. μ-Heavy-chain disease. There is a diffuse infiltrate consisting of lymphocytes, lymphoplasmacytic cells, and plasma cells producing only μ-heavy chain without any light-chain. Rare dispersed immunoblasts and some histiocytes are seen (Giemsa stain)

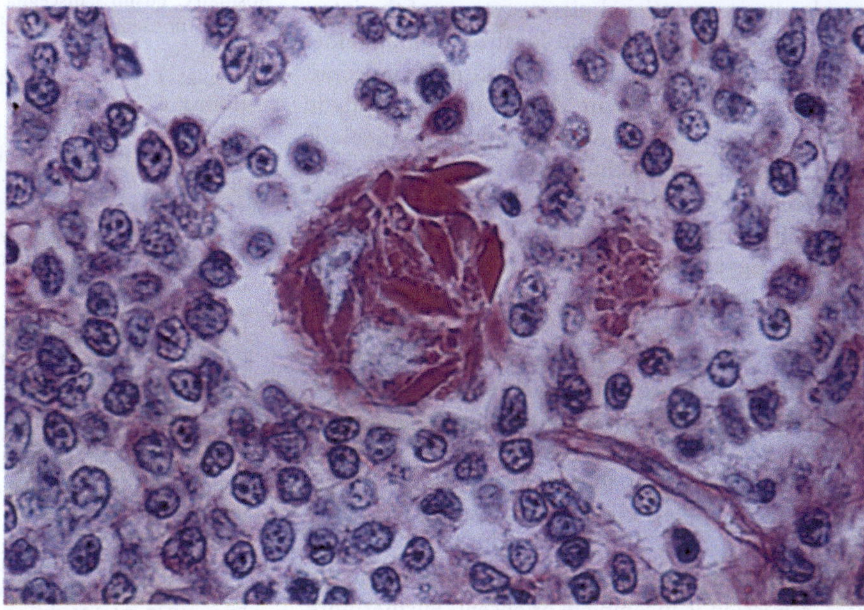

Fig. 7.8. Same patient as in Fig. 7.7. The histiocytes contain PAS-positive crystallized IgM (PAS stain)

It is difficult to distinguish γ-heavy-chain disease from lymphoplasmacytic lymphoma or, rarely, from B-CLL. Immunohistochemistry and peripheral blood immunoelectrophoresis are mandatory for the diagnosis.

This very rare disease occurs in adults with a median age of 60 years. Patients complain of anorexia, weight loss, and fever and present with peripheral adenopathies and hepatosplenomegaly. Involvement of Waldeyer's ring is very characteristic. Often, infections occur. Peripheral blood lymphocytosis mimics that of B-CLL. Immunofixation discloses the presence of γ-heavy-chain in the blood. Disease evolution is variable from patient to patient; in some there is an indolent course, while in others progression is very rapid and aggressive (Franklin et al. 1979; Fernand and Brouet 1999).

α-Heavy-Chain Disease. The lamina propria of the small intestine is diffusely and massively infiltrated by mature plasma cells associated with small lymphocytes. This infiltrate is responsible for the atrophy of the glands and villi (Galian et al. 1972). Lymph nodes may be infiltrated in untreated patients. Transformation into a more aggressive lymphoma consisting of plasmablasts, immunoblasts, or even giant cells with a Reed-Sternberg-like morphology has been observed. This type of transformation is responsible for the development of localized tumor along the intestine and of voluminous mesenteric adenopathies (Galian et al. 1972). A very few cases have been described in which the disease involves the respiratory tract.

The immunohistochemistry is identical to that of other heavy-chain diseases except for the presence of α-chain.

This disease represents a variant of MALT lymphoma, a mucosae-associated marginal zone lymphoma. The most difficult aspect of the differential diagnosis is to rule out an exceptional plasmacytoma of the intestine in which there is a solid localized tumor rather than the characteristic diffuse infiltrate of the mucosae.

This type of heavy-chain disease occurs mostly in children, adolescents, and young adults, particularly those living in the Mediterranean area under poor socioeconomic conditions.

It is interesting to note that in countries such as Lebanon, Egypt, Saudi Arabia, and North Africa this disease has more or less disappeared (personal experience).

Patients complain of abdominal pain, fever, diarrhea with steatorrhea, and malabsorption. α-Heavy-chain is present in gut secretions and in the peripheral blood.

Antibiotics given at the beginning of the disease results in a complete clinical and histological remission.

In patients treated later on in the course of the disease, remission is incomplete or absent. Furthermore, there is a risk of transformation of the disease into an aggressive lymphoma of immunoblastic type with plasmacytoid differentiation or of plasmablastic type, both of which have a rapid fatal evolution (Seligman 1975; Fernand and Brouet 1999).

References

Alexiou C, Kau RJ, Dietzfelbinger H et al (1999) Extramedullary plasmacytoma: tumor occurrence and therapeutic concepts. Cancer 85:2305–2314

Bacci G, Calderoni P, Cervellati C, Zambaldi A (1982) Solitary plasmacytoma of bone: a report of 19 cases. Ital J Orthop Traumatol 8:469–478

Barlogie B, Epstein J, Selvanayagam P, Alexanian R (1989) Plasma cell myeloma – new biological insights and advances in therapy. Blood 73:865–879.25

Bartl R, Frisch B, Burkhardt R et al (1982) Bone marrow histology in myeloma: its importance in diagnosis, prognosis, classification and staging. Br J Haematol 51:361–375

Bartl R, Frisch B, Fateh-Moghadam A, Kettner G, Jaeger K, Sommerfeld W (1987) Histologic classification and staging of multiple myeloma. A retrospective and prospective study of 674 cases. Am J Clin Pathol 87:342–355

Bartl R, Frisch B, Wilmanns N (1995) Morphology of multiple myeloma. In: Malpas JS, Bergsagel DE, Kyle RA (eds) Myeloma: biology and management. Oxford University Press, Oxford, pp 82–123

Bataille R, Sany J (1981) Solitary myeloma: clinical and progostic features of a review of 114 cases. Cancer 48:845–851

Bosman C, Fusilli S, Bisceglia M, Musto P, Corsi A (1996) Oncocytic nonsecretory multiple myeloma. Acta Haematol 96:50–56

Bourantas K (1996) Nonsecretory multiple myeloma. Eur J Haematol 56:109–111

Brunning RD, McKenna RW (1994) Tumors of the bone marrow. Atlas of tumor pathology. AFIP, Washington DC, pp 323–350

Chesi M, Bergsagel L, Brents L, Smith C, Gerhard D, Kuehl W (1996) Dysregulation of cyclin D1 by translocation into an IgH gamma switch region in two multiple myeloma cell lines. Blood 88:647–681

Dankbar B, Padro T, Leo R, Feldmann B, Kropff M, Mesters RM, Serve H, Berdel WE, Kienast J (2000) Vascular endothelial growth factor and interleukin-6 in paracrine tumor-stromal cell interactions in multiple myeloma. Blood 95:2630–2636

De Lajarte-Thirouard AS, Molina T, Audouin J, Le Tourneau A, Leduc F, Rose C, Diebold J (1999) Spleen localization of light-chain deposition disease associated with sea-blue histiocytosis revealed by spontaneous rupture. Virchows Arch 434:463–465

Devesa SS, Silverman DT, Young JL Jr et al (1988) Cancer incidence and mortality trends among whites in the United States 1947–84. J Natl Cancer Inst 79:701–770

Dewald GW, Kyle RA, Hicks GA, Greipp PR (1985) The clinical significance of cytogenetic studies in 100 patients with multiple myeloma, plasma cell leukemia, or amyloidosis. Blood 66:380–390

Diebold J (1997) Myeloma. In: Forrest M, Tomeno B, Vanel D (eds) Orthopedic surgical pathology. Churchill Livingstone, Edinburgh, pp 491–500

Dimopoulos MA, Palumbo A, Delasalle KB, Alexanian R (1994) Primary plasma cell leukemia. Br J Haematol 88:754–759

Drach J, Ackermann J, Fritz E et al (1998) Presence of a p53 gene deletion in patients with multiple myeloma predicts for short survival after conventional-dose chemotherapy. Blood 92:802–809

Falini B, Fizzotti M, Pucciarini A, Bigerna B, Marafioti T, Gambacorta M, Pacini R, Alunni C, Natali-Tanci L, Ugolini B, Sebastiani C, Cattoretti G, Pileri S, Dalla-Favera R, Stein H (2000) A monoclonal antibody (MUM1p) detects expression of the MUM1/IRF4 protein in a subset of germinal center B-cells, plasma cells and activated T cells. Blood 95:2084–2092

Fernand JP, Brouet JC (1999) Heavy-chain diseases. Hematol Oncol Clin North Am 13:1281–1294

Franklin EC, Kyle R, Seligmann M, Frangiona B (1979) Correlation of protein structure and immunoglobulin gene organization in the light of two new deleted heavy chain disease proteins. Mod Immunol 16:919–921

Galian A, Lecestre MJ, Scotto J, Bognel C, Matuchansky C, Rambaud JC (1972) Pathological study of alpha chain disease with special emphasis on evolution. Cancer 39:2081–2101

Garcia-Sanz R, Orfao A, Gonzalez M et al (1999) Primary plasma cell leukemia: clinical, immunophenotypic, DNA ploidy, and cytogenetic characteristics. Blood 93:1032–1037

Gabriel L, Escribano L, Perales J, Bellas C, Odriozola J, Navarro JL (1985) Multiple myeloma with crystalline inclusions in most hematopoietic cells. Am J Hematol 18:405–411

Greipp PR, Leong T, Bennett JM et al (1998) Plasmablastic morphology and independent prognostic factor with clinical and laboratory correlates: Eastern Cooperative Oncology Group (ECOG) myeloma trial E9486 report by the ECOG Myeloma Laboratory Group. Blood 91:2501–2507

Grogan TM, Van Camp B, Kyle RA, Müller-Hermelink HK, Harris NL (2001) Plasma cell neoplasms. In: Jaffe JS, Harris NL, Stein H, Vardiman JW, (eds) World Health Organization Classification of Tumors. Pathology and genetics of tumors of hematopoietic and lymphoid tissues. IARC Press, Lyon

Guida M, Casamassima A, Abbate I et al (1994) Solitary plasmacytoma of bone and extramedullary plasmacytoma: 2 different nosological entities? Tumori 80:370–377

Hallek M, Bergsagel PL, Anderson KC (1998) Multiple myeloma: increasing evidence for a multistep transformation process. Blood 91:3–21

Kambham N, Markowitz G, Appel G et al (1999) Heavy chain deposition disease: the disease spectrum. Am J Kidney Dis 33:954–962

Klein B (1995) Cytokine, cytokine receptors, transduction signals, and oncogenes in human multiple myeloma. Semin Hematol 32:4–19

Kyle RA (1992) Diagnostic criteria of multiple myeloma. Hematol Oncol Clin North Am 6:347–358

Kyle RA, Gertz MA (1990) Systemic amyloidosis. Crit Rev Oncol Hematol 10:49–87

Kyle RA, Gertz MA (1995) Primary systemic amyloidosis: clinical and laboratory features in 474 cases. Semin Hematol 32:45–59

Kyle RA, Maldonado JE, Bayrd ED (1974) Plasma cell leukemia. Report of 17 cases. Arch Intern Med 133:813–818

Leibross RH, Ha CS, Cox JD, Weber D, Delasalle K, Alexanian R (1998) Solitary bone plasmacytoma: outcome and prognostic factors following radiotherapy. Int J Radiat Oncol Biol Phys 41:1063–1067

Mahmoud M, Huang N, Nobuyoshi M, Lisuov I, Tanake H, Kawano M (1996) Altered expression of PAX-5 gene in human myeloma cells. Blood 87:4311–4315

Malpas JS, Bergsagel DE, Kyle RA (eds) (1995) Myeloma: biology and management. Oxford University Press, Oxford

Mangi MH, Newland A (2000) Angiogenesis and angiogenic mediators in haematological malignancies. Br J Haematol 111:43–51

Miralles GD, O'Fallon KR, Talley NJ (1992) Plasma-cell dyscrasia with polyneuropathy. The spectrum of POEMS syndrome. N Engl J Med 327:1919–1923

Moehler TM, Hawighorst H, Neben K, Egerer G, Max R, van Kaick G, Ho AD, Goldschmidt H (2001a) Bone marrow microcirculation analysis in multiple myeloma by contrast-enhanced dynamic magnetic resonance imaging. Int J Cancer 93:862–868

Moehler TM, Neben K, Ho AD, Goldschmidt H (2001b) Angiogenesis in hematologic malignancies. Ann Hematol 80:695–705

Molina T, Brouland JP, Bigorgne C, Le Tourneau A, Delmer A, Audouin J, Diebold J (1996) Plasmocytose médullaire pseudo-myélomateuse au cours d'une maladie de Castleman multicentrique. A propos d'une observation. Ann Pathol 16:133–136

Preud'homme J, Aucouturrier P, Touchard G et al (1994) Monoclonal immunoglobulin deposition disease (Randall type). Relationship with structural abnormalities of immunoglobulin chains. Kidney Int 46:965–972

Rajkumar SV, Greipp PR (1999) Prognostic factors in multiple myeloma. Hematol Oncol Clin North Am 13:1295–1314

Rajkumar SV, Leong T, Roche PC, Fonseca R, Dispenzieri A, Lacy MQ, Lust JA, Witzig TE, Kyle RA, Gertz MA, Greipp PR (2000) Prognostic value of bone marrow angiogenesis in multiple myeloma. Clin Cancer Res 6:3111–3116

Reed M, McKenna RW, Bridges R, Parkins J, Frizzera G, Brunning RD (1981) Morphologic manifestations of monoclonal gammopathies. Am J Clin Pathol 76:8–23

Ribatti D, Vacca A, Nico B, Quondamatteo F, Ria R, Minischetti M, Marzullo A, Herken R, Roncali L, Dammacco F (1999) Bone marrow angiogenesis and mast cell density increase simultaneously with progression of human multiple myeloma. Br J Cancer 79:451–455

Ridley R, Xiao H, Hata H et al (1993) Expression of syndecan regulates human myeloma plasma cell adhesion to type 1 collagen. Blood 81:767–774

Ries LA, Hankey BF, Miller BA, Hartman AM, Edwards BK (1991) Cancer statistics review 1973–1988. National Cancer Institute NIH Publ 91:2789

Rolon PG, Audouin J, Diebold J, Rolon PA, Gonzalez A (1989) Multicentric angiofollicular lymph node hyperplasia associated with a solitary osteolytic costal IgG lambda myeloma. POEMS syndrome in a South American (Paraguayan) patient. Pathol Res Pract 185:468–475

Said J, Rettig M, Heppner K et al (1997) Localization of Kaposi's-associated herpes virus in bone marrow biopsy samples from patients with multiple myeloma. Blood 90:4278–4282

Sailer M, Vykoupil KF, Peest D, Cordewey R, Deicher H, Georgii A (1995) Prognostic relevance of a histologic classification system applied in bone marrow biopsies from patients with multiple myeloma. A histopathological evaluation of biopsies from 153 untreated patients. Eur J Haematol 54:137–146

Salmon SE, Cassady JR (1988) Plasma cell neoplasms, chap 54. In: DeVita VT, Hellman S, Rosenberg S (eds) Cancer, principles and practice of oncology. Lippincott, Philadelphia

Schajowicz F (1994) Tumors and tumorlike lesions of bone, 2nd edn. Springer, Berlin Heidelberg New York

Seligmann M (1975) Immunochemical, clinical, and pathological features of alpha-heavy chain disease. Arch Intern Med 135:78–82

Sukpanichnant S, Cousar JB, Leesasiri A, Graber SE, Greer JP, Collins RD (1994) Diagnostic criteria and histologic grading in multiple myeloma: histologic and immunohistologic analysis of 176 cases with clinical correlation. Hum Pathol 25:308–318

Tsuchiya H, Epstein J, Selvanayagam P et al (1988) Correlated flow cytometric analysis of H-ras p21 and nuclear DNA in multiple myeloma. Blood 72:796–800

Van Riet I, Vanderkerken K, De Greef C, Van Camp B (1998) Homing behaviour of the malignant cell clone in multiple myeloma. Med Oncol 15:1554–1564

Wahner-Roedler DL, Kyle RA (1992) Mu-heavy chain disease: presentation as a benign monoclonal gammopathy. Am J Hematol 40:56–60

Zukerberg IR, Ferry JA, Conlon M, Harris NL (1990) Plasma cell myeloma with cleaved multilobated and monocytoid nuclei. Am J Clin Pathol 93:657–661

CHAPTER 8

Lymphoma Occurring in a Setting of Immunodeficiency

8

Lymphoma and lymphoproliferative disorders (LPDs), either congenital or acquired, that mimic and/or lead to lymphoma can occur in patients with immunodeficiencies. Each type of immunodeficiency has its own risk factors and is associated with a particular type of LPD or lymphoma. Two important points should be immediately stressed. First, evidence of clonality, demonstrated by immunohistochemistry or molecular biology, is not associated necessarily with an aggressive course and can regress if the immunological deficiency is cured. Second, Epstein-Barr virus (EBV) is often associated with the development of lymphoma and LPDs.

8.1 Lymphoproliferative Disorders Associated with Congenital Immunodeficiencies

Definition

Lymphomas and LPDs mimicking and/or leading to malignant lymphomas can occur in the following types of congenital immunodeficiencies (Rosen et al. 1992; Elenitoba-Johnson and Jaffe 1997): ataxia-telangiectasia (AT), Wiskott-Aldrich syndrome (WAS), common variable immunodeficiency (CVID), severe combined immunodeficiency (SCID), X-linked lymphoproliferative disorder (XLPD), hyper-IgM syndrome.

These disease are genetically determined and are manifested during the first year of life, mostly due to the development of recurrent infections.

Morphology

The lymphoid modifications corresponding to LPDs comprise a wide spectrum of histopathological lesions, ranging from non-specific reactive hyperplasia, often nodular, to atypical lymphoid hyperplasia and malignant lymphoma (Frizzera et al. 1980). These lesions, including lymphomas, develop more frequently at extranodal sites, for example, the central nervous system and gastrointestinal tract (Elenitoba-Johnson and Jaffe 1997).

The different types of lymphoid modifications will be described according to the type of congenital immunodeficiency.

Occurrence

LPDs represent a group of disorders, including lymphomas, that arise in patients with primary congenital immunodeficiencies. These disorders explain, in part, the mortality due to cancer in children with primary immunodeficiency, which is 0.8 % per year. This is 80-fold higher than mortality in the general population of children (Elenitoba-Johnson and Jaffe 1997). Primary immunodeficiency syndromes with a higher risk of lymphoma development are AT (10 %), WAS (7.6 %), and CVID (1.4 % to 7 %).

Pathogenesis

Before describing LPDs and lymphomas occurring in association with congenital immunodeficiencies, it is useful to summarize the pathogenesis of these lymphoid lesions (Elenitoba-Johnson and Jaffe 1997). There are three types of conditions which, regardless of the type of immunodeficiency, may play a role in the development of LPD and malignant lymphoma. In addition, the early type of immunodeficiency syndrome has additional, specific pathogenetic factors. The common conditions are the following:

1. Polyclonal activation of lymphoid proliferation, most frequently by viruses. Two types of viruses have been implicated:

1.1. EBV, particularly in X-linked immunoproliferative syndrome (Purtilo's syndrome) in which the origin of the LPD and malignant lymphoma is associated with a defective host-response to EBV (Okano et al. 1984, 1988).

1.2. Human herpes virus type 6 is also, but less frequently, associated with LPD and malignant lymphoma in such immunodeficiencies (Krueger and Sander 1989).

2. Dysregulation of lymphoid cell proliferation. The different types of immunodeficiencies have in common an abnormal regulation mostly of B-lymphoid cells. In WAS, there are also defects of the surface glycoprotein sialophorin/leukosialin (CD43), involved in T-cell proliferation (Mentzer et al. 1987). In adenosine deaminase (ADA)-deficient SCID, the lymphoproliferation is due to the selective sensitivity of EBV-reactive cytotoxic T-cells to the toxic conditions generated by the absence of ADA activity (Ratech et al. 1989). The high level of interleukin-6 (IL6) (Adelman et al. 1990) or the impaired NK-cell activity may be responsible for the lymphoproliferation occurring in other types of immunodeficiencies (Aparicio-Pafges et al. 1990).
3. Genetic abnormalities. Chromosomal abnormalities, mostly in AT and the chromosomal breakage syndrome may be responsible for lymphoproliferation. Development of several genetic and molecular aberrations may then lead to malignant lymphoma (Stern et al. 1989).

8.1.1 Ataxia-Telangiectasia

An increased incidence of the following lymphoid neoplasias have been observed in patients with AT. By contrast, there is an absence of myeloid tumors (Taylor et al. 1996).

1. *Acute lymphoblastic leukemia* often with mediastinal involvement almost always of T type (Toledano and Lange 1980).
2. *T-prolymphocytic leukemia* (T-PLL) occurs mostly in young adults with AT (Taylor et al. 1996). In some cases, T-PLL is preceded by a type of T-cell chronic lymphocyte leukemia (Foon and Gale 1992).
3. Other malignant lymphomas have also been reported: one case of *T-cell lymphoma* (Petkovic et al. 1992) and several *B-cell lymphomas*, either *diffuse large-B-cell lymphoma (centroblastic or immunoblastic type)* or *Burkitt's lymphoma* (Elenitoba-Johnson and Jaffe 1997).

Genetic Features

1. Rearrangement of genes coding for the T-cell receptor or for immunoglobulin heavy-chain (IgH) have been demonstrated.
2. EBV is not consistently present in B-cell lymphomas (Elenitoba-Johnson and Jaffe 1997).
3. Genetic abnormalities which characterize AT are present (Taylor et al. 1996):
   - Mutation of the ATM gene, which encodes a protein sharing the PI-3 kinase domain and which is involved in the detection and repair of DNA damage and the control of cell-cycle progression (Savitsky et al. 1995).
   - The presence in about 10% of T-lymphocytes of translocations and inversions. Chromosomes 7 and 14 are most often involved in defects of T-cell antigen-receptor genes (i.e. 14q11–12, 7q32–35, 7p15) and at the immunoglobulin gene loci (i.e. 2p11, 14q32.3, 22p11).
   - Other chromosomal rearrangements or translocations have been observed: inv(7)(p13q35), t(7;7)(p13;q35), t(7;14)(p13;q11), t(14;14)(q11;q32).

Occurrence

About 10% of individuals homozygous for AT develop a neoplasia, with a 70- to 250-fold higher incidence of leukemias and lymphomas, respectively (Morrell et al. 1986). There is a four- to five-fold increase in the frequency of T-cell neoplasias compared with B-cell neoplasias (Filipovich et al. 1992). Hodgkin's lymphoma, often with a pattern of lymphocyte depletion, represents approximately 10% of the malignancies developing in AT patients (Frizzera et al. 1980).

Non-lymphoid malignancies, mainly carcinomas, represent 13–22% of all neoplasias, particularly in older patients (median age: 17 years) (Morrell et al. 1986; Taylor et al. 1996).

Clinical Presentation

Patients present with cerebellar degeneration, progressive ataxia, oculocutaneous telangiectasia. Due to the immunodeficiency, most patients have sinopulmonary infections. Growth retardation, hypogonadism, and thymic hypoplasia are frequent. Biological abnormalities comprise elevated levels of α-fetoprotein, hypo-IgA sometimes with deficiency of IgG4 and IgG2 (Elenitoba-Johnson and Jaffe 1997). The lymphoid neoplasias are responsible for the development of adenopathies, mediastinal involvement (acute lymphoblastic leukemia), and peripheral blood modifications (leukemias). The prognosis is not very good. Acute lymphoblastic leukemia is frequently associated with an unusually high proportion of unfavorable prognostic signs.

8.1.2 Wiskott-Aldrich Syndrome

Morphology

In a group of 59 WAS patients, 75.6 % of the malignancies were non-Hodgkin's lymphoma (NHL); the incidence of Hodgkin's lymphoma was 3.8 % and of leukemia 9.0 %. In another series comprising 50 patients with WAS (Cotelingam et al. 1985), nine had lymphoma (18 %), eight with non-Hodgkin's type and one with Hodgkin's lymphoma (nodular sclerosing type). In seven patients, the NHL was of *immunoblastic type.* The majority of these NHLs developed at an extranodal site: brain (three patients), skin and subcutaneous tissue (two patients), small bowel (one patient), mediastinum (one patient). Elenitoba-Johnson and Jaffe (1997) described two patients: one with large-B-cell lymphoma of *immunoblastic type* of the tibia with cerebral and meningeal extension, and one with *lymphoplasmacytic lymphoma* secreting at one site IgM λ and at another IgD κ. Finally, there is an increased frequency of lymphomatoid granulomatosis in patients with WAS (Jaffe 2001).

Immunohistochemistry

In the study of Elenitoba-Johnson and Jaffe (1997), the majority of the lymphomas were of B-cell type. The absence of Burkitt's lymphoma and lymphoblastic acute leukemia/lymphoma should be stressed (Elenitoba-Johnson and Jaffe 1997; Cotelingam et al. 1985). Polyclonal B-lymphoproliferative diseases have also been reported. One T-cell lymphoma associated with a Kaposi's sarcoma was described (Meropol et al. 1992).

Molecular Biology

Only a few cases have been studied as far as we know. Some LPDs may be polyclonal. In situ hybridization for EBV demonstrated the presence of EBER-1 in 60 % of patients with LPD or NHL (Okano et al. 1984). Episomal EBV genome was demonstrated in the tumor cells.

Occurrence

Patients with WAS have a risk of malignancy that is 100 times greater than that of the age-matched normal population (Filipovich et al. 1992). Malignant lymphomas develop in about 10 – 20 % of WAS patients, mostly in children (Cotelingam et al. 1985). The number of malignant lymphomas increases with the age of the child (Perry et al. 1980).

The median age at time of diagnosis of malignant lymphoma in a group of 59 WAS patients was 6.2 years, and all patients were male, due to the fact that the disease has an X-linked (recessive) mode of inheritance (Cotelingam et al. 1985).

WAS has an incidence in the United States of 4.0 per one million male births.

Clinical Presentation

WAS patients have eczema and thrombocytopenia. During disease evolution, recurrent bacterial infections occur. In the serum, IgG is normal, IgM is reduced, and IgA and IgE are elevated, with defective antibody formation. T-lymphoid cells decrease and exhibit several functional and morphological abnormalities. The development of adenopathy is the first sign of a lymphoproliferative disease. Splenectomy and intravenous immunoglobulin therapy can prolong the life of WAS patients, Previously, patients died during the first decade of life from hemorrhage, infection, or lymphoid neoplasias (Elenitoba-Johnson and Jaffe 1997).

8.1.3 Common Variable Immunodeficiency Disorder

Morphology

Lymphoid hyperplasia and NHL develop in nodal and, more often, extranodal sites: gastrointestinal tract, skin, spleen, etc. (Sander et al. 1992).

A study of 30 biopsies (Sander et al. 1992) obtained from 17 patients with CVID revealed reactive lymphoid hyperplasia, including nodular lymphoid hyperplasia of the gastrointestinal tract, in 14 biopsies (47 %), atypical lymphoid hyperplasia in eight (27 %), chronic granulomatous inflammation in six (20 %), and malignant lymphoma in two (6.7%). Atypical lymphoid hyperplasia is defined as an infiltration effacing the architecture of the tissues or organs, mimicking lymphomas.

Most of the lymphoma seems to belong to the large-B-cell group (centroblastic or immunoblastic) and occur at an extranodal site (Sander et al. 1992). Reports of T-cell lymphoma remain rare (Sander et al. 1992).

Elenitoba-Johnson and Jaffe (1997) reported two cases of immunoblastic lymphoma, one associated with a Hodgkin's lymphoma, the other with a difficult to diagnose lesion between Hodgkin's lymphoma and T-cell-rich B-cell lymphoma. They also described a patient presenting with a follicular large-B-cell lymphoma at several sites and an immunoblastic lymphoma in the spleen.

Immunohistochemistry

Atypical lymphoid hyperplasia consists of a hyperplasia of both B- and T-cells, particularly immunoblasts and transformed cells. Immunohistochemistry demonstrates the B-cell origin of the majority of the lymphomas and the T-cell origin in a few cases.

Genetic Features

About 25% of patients with atypical lymphoid hyperplasia have positive in-situ hybridization for EBER-1. Clonal rearrangement in B- or T-lymphoid cells is absent. In some cases, clonal expansion of B- or T-lymphocytes occurs even in the absence of malignant histopathological changes and in patients with a long follow-up without lymphoid neoplasia. Some of the large-B-cell lymphomas are associated with an EBV infection.

In the cases reported by Elenitoba-Johnson and Jaffe (1992), IgH gene rearrangement as well as the presence of the EBV genome was demonstrated in the two patients with immunoblastic lymphomas. In the one patient with follicular large-cell lymphoma of different sites and immunoblastic lymphoma of the spleen, the clones were different in the two types of lymphoma.

Occurrence

An increase risk of neoplasias is well known in patients with CVID (Cunningham-Rundles et al. 1987). Malignant lymphomas occur in about 1–7% of the patients and 300 times more frequently in women (Cunningham-Rundles et al. 1987). These lymphomas develop mostly in patients in the fifth to seventh decade of life and not in children (Cunningham-Rundles et al. 1987).

Clinical Presentation

CVID comprises different types of dysimmune disorders affecting both sexes with several modes of inheritance and having in common a defect in the humoral immune response (Rosen et al. 1995). Patients present with hypogammaglobulinemia, discovered mostly during the second and third decades of life, which is responsible for recurrent opportunistic infections such as *Pneumocystis carinii, Giardia, mycobacteria, fungi, herpes simplex, and herpes zoster* (Elenitoba-Johnson and Jaffe 1997).

Various autoimmune diseases occur also with a high frequency: rheumatoid arthritis, pernicious anemia, hemolytic anemia, thrombocytopenia, and neutropenia (Rosen et al. 1995). Lymphoma develops in multiple sites, often extranodal. Other neoplasms can occur, for example gastric carcinoma. Acute myeloblastic leukemia is very rare. An insufficient number of T-cells which are thus unable to stimulate B-cells seems to be responsible for the immune deficiencies (Rosen et al. 1995).

8.1.4 Severe Combined Immunodeficiency

Morphology

Histology. A thymic involution is characteristic of many types of SCID, with atrophy of the lymph nodes, lymphoid tissue of the spleen, and digestive tract (Rosen 1990; Rosen et al. 1995; Huber et al. 1992).

Non-Hodgkin's lymphomas are the most frequent type of lymphoma, but Hodgkin's lymphoma can also occur. Multiple sites are involved in more than half of the patients, often with involvement of extranodal sites (Filipovich et al. 1992).

Immunohistochemistry and Genetic Features

Precise data are still lacking.

Occurrence

The incidence of malignancies is 1–5%. NHL accounts for almost 74% and Hodgkin's lymphoma for 9.5%.

At diagnosis, the median age of patients with NHL is 1.6 years and the male:female ratio is 3.3:1 (Elenitoba-Johnson and Jaffe 1997).

Clinical Presentation

SCID comprises diseases arising from a variety of genetic causes and resulting in combined T- and B-cell defects. All patients have in common the tendency to develop recurrent infections due to many different agents: *P. carinii*, *Candida albicans*, *Pseudomonas*, *cytomegalovirus*, *varicella* virus, *herpes* virus, and *adenovirus*, as well as giant-cell pneumonia resulting from measles infection and progressive vaccinia after smallpox vaccination. Many of these infections have a fatal outcome (Rosen et al. 1995). Some neonatal patients, have a syndrome resembling graft-versus-host disease, often referred to as Omenn's syndrome (WHO Scientific Group 1995).

Children with SCID have profound lymphopenia, with a normal or high number of NK cells (Rosen et al. 1995). Autosomal recessive forms are characterized by a severe deficiency of both T- and B-lymphocytes. Patients with the X-linked forms of SCID have, by contrast, a normal number of B-cells in the peripheral blood, and sometimes oligoclonal or polyclonal immunoglobulin in the blood. These latter forms of SCID are called Nezelof's syndrome.

NHL and Hodgkin's lymphoma can develop at any time during SCID evolution with a poor outcome.

8.1.5 X-linked Lymphoproliferative Disorder (Duncan's Disease/Purtilo Syndrome)

Morphology

Lymph nodes, tonsils, and spleen may be involved by infectious mononucleosis. Large transformed B-cells, immunoblasts, and numerous cells with plasma cell differentiation infiltrate these organs, obscuring the normal architecture. Reed-Sternberg-like cells may be present. Areas of necrosis are frequent. Often, hemophagocytic histiocytosis can be recognized. After 4 weeks of disease evolution, lymphoid depletion occurs. Diffuse large-B-cell lymphoma represents the most frequently occurring type of lymphoma. Extranodal sites are often involved. In a series of 100 patients published by Purtilo et al. (1982), 35 had a B-cell lymphoma and 26 of them were localized on the terminal ileum. In a series published by Harrington et al. (1987), comprising 17 patients, 41 % had Burkitt's lymphoma, 18 % immunoblastic, 12 % small-B-cell and 6 % were unclassifiable lymphomas.

Immunohistochemistry

Immunohistochemistry demonstrates the B-cell origin of the lymphomas and their monoclonality.

Genetic Features

EBER-1 is demonstrated in a high percentage of cells in the malignant lymphomas.

Occurrence

About 67 % of the patients develop severe or fatal infectious mononucleosis (Purtilo et al. 1982). Malignant lymphoma occurs in 25 % of the patients (Purtilo et al. 1982; Harrington et al. 1987).

Clinical Presentation

Duncan's disease is characterized by a familial lymphoid defect with a high susceptibility to diseases induced by EBV (Purtilo et al. 1982). The affected boys remain healthy during childhood and adolescence, until they have contact with EBV. These children have impairment of both humoral and cell-mediated immunity with an increased number of suppressor T-cells, a decrease of NK-cell function, and often an acquired hypogammaglobulinemia.

Approximately two thirds of the patients develop severe or fatal infectious mononucleosis. They often die from hemophagocytic histiocytosis with activated histiocyte (macrophage) syndrome. Development of malignant lymphoma represents the other cause of death.

8.1.6 Hyper-IgM Syndrome

Morphology

Lymph nodes and spleen show inactive germinal centers in the follicles (Rosen et al. 1995). Malignant lymphomas can occur. In a series of 16 tumors (Filipovich et al. 1992), nines were NHLs (56.3 %) and four Hodgkin's lymphomas (25 %), with mostly extranodal localizations (mainly gastrointestinal tract and brain).

These lymphomas should be distinguished from the extensive lymphoproliferation of IgM-secreting polyclonal plasma cells that can massively infiltrate the gastrointestinal tract, liver, and gall bladder, and which may have a fatal outcome (Rosen et al. 1995).

Immunohistochemistry

Demonstration of monotypic or polytypic secretion of immunoglobulins may be important to distinguish some types of malignant lymphoma from lymphoproliferations of polyclonal plasma cells.

Genetic Features

Precise data are lacking concerning lymphomas.

The genetic abnormality is a mutation in the gene, present on Xq26, coding for the CD40 ligand, which is normally expressed on activated T-cells and which reacts with the CD40 receptor expressed on B-cells for productive isotype switching in B-cells (WHO Scientific Group 1992).

Occurrence

The median age of patients who developed lymphomas was 7–8 years in the series of Filipovich et al. (1992) with a male:female ratio of 7:2.

Clinical Presentation

This syndrome comprises a group of entities having in common either a defective normal or an elevated IgM associated with diminished IgG and IgA levels. In the majority of patients, hyper-IgM syndrome is X-linked, in others it is autosomal recessive.

Patients with X-linked hyper-IgM syndrome present with recurrent pyogenic infections and/or *P. carinii* infection. They also have neutropenia, autoimmune hemolytic anemia, and thrombocytopenia with purpura. The peripheral blood B-lymphocytes are normal in number but bear only surface IgM and IgD.

Lymphomas of different types (non-Hodgkin's and Hodgkin's) occur at any time. Leukemia has never been observed, but other malignancies can develop (Filipovich et al. 1992).

8.1.7 JOB Syndrome

Morphology

Diffuse large-B-cell lymphoma, often disseminated, occurs in this syndrome (Elenitoba-Johnson and Jaffe 1997).

Immunohistochemistry

The lymphomas are of B-cell origin.

Genetic Features

Precise information concerning the lymphomas is lacking.

Clinical Presentation

Patients present with recurrent, often staphylococcal infections, a decreased total number of T-cells, and elevated IgE levels in the serum.

8.1.8 Nijmegen Breakage Syndrome

Morphology

Patients have thymic hypoplasia but lymph nodes and spleen are more or less normal.

In many patients, malignant lymphomas develop, often with multiple localizations mostly extranodal, particularly in the digestive tract. These lymphomas show a B-immunoblastic morphology (Chrzanowska et al. 1995).

Immunohistochemistry

The B-cell origin has been demonstrated in all cases, with λ-light-chain restriction (Chrzanowska et al. 1995).

Genetic Features

Neither EBV nor cytomegalovirus have been detected by PCR and in situ hybridization.

The disease is associated with chromosomal instability with multiple chromosome 7 or 14 rearrangements.

Occurrence

This autosomal recessive disorder was described in 1981 by Weemaes et al. Thirty patients were diagnosed in 21 families.

At present, in eight of the 30 patients a malignant lymphoma has occurred. The average age of the patients is 10.25 years, with a male:female ratio of 1:1 (Weemaes et al. 1994).

Clinical Features

Patients present with microcephaly, short stature, "bird-like" facies (Weemaes et al. 1994), with normal intelligence or mental retardation. They often suffer from recurrent infections (respiratory and urinary tract). The disease resemble AT but without cerebellar ataxia and telangiectasia. Hypogammaglobulinemia is frequent.

8.2 Lymphoma and Lymphoproliferative Disorders Associated with Acquired Immunodeficiency

Definition

The acquired immunodeficiencies that lead to lymphomas or LPDS include:

- Immunodeficiency associated with HIV infection
- Post-transplant lymphoproliferative disorders
- Liebow granulomatosis of the lung (see Chap. 6.7.1.4)
- Pyothorax-associated lymphoma (see Chap. 6.8.1.2)

8.2.1 HIV-Related Lymphoma

Definition

HIV-infected patients have a progressive severe immunodeficiency leading to a 60-fold higher overall incidence of NHL than in the general population (Beral et al. 1991). Lymphomas occur in 5–10% of HIV-infected patients either at presentation or during evolution of the disease (Raphael et al. 1991, 1994). Development of malignant lymphoma has been defined as a criteria for the diagnosis of AIDS. One of the most important factors for the occurrence of these lymphomas is a severe CD4-positive T-lymphocyte depletion.

Since the use of highly active antiretroviral therapy, there has been a decrease in the incidence of lymphoma in patients with AIDS. But more data are needed to confirm this finding (Grulich 1999).

Many of the lymphomas involve extranodal sites. The majority are diffuse large-B-cell lymphomas (DLBCLs). Only a few T-cell lymphomas have been reported. Some of these NHLs are similar to those observed in immunocompetent patients, others are specific to those with immunodeficiencies (Knowles 1999).

Morphology

1. *Diffuse large-B-cell lymphomas.* In the series of 448 cases published by the French Study Group, these lymphomas accounted for 53% of all lymphomas (Raphael et al. 1991, 1993a,b; Diebold et al. 1997). Their morphology resembles that of lymphomas described in immunocompetent patients (see Chap. 4.2.2).
   Centroblastic lymphoma. About 26% of the DLBCLs were centroblastic lymphoma, rarely monomorphic or multilobated, more often polymorphic (Diebold et al. 1997).
   Immunoblastic lymphoma. This type of lymphoma accounted for 23% of the series of the French Study Group. The majority had a plasmablastic differentiation.
   Anaplastic large-cell lymphoma B-cell type. This type of still controversial lymphoma was observed in about 4% of the patients of the French Study Group series.
   Plasmablastic lymphoma of the oral cavity. This type of lymphoma (see Chap. 8.2) was previously classified as immunoblastic lymphoma with plasmablastic differentiation (Fig. 8.1). Due to the localization, to the monotonous morphology – similar in all cases, their constant association with EBV infection, and their rapid growth it has been proposed to regard this type of large-B-cell lymphoma as a distinct entity (Delecluse et al. 1997; Porter et al. 1999) accepted by the WHO classification (Jaffe et al. 2001).
   Primary effusion lymphoma (PEL). This lymphoma is characterized by lymphomatous effusions in the serosa and was described in Chap. 6.8.1.1. It has been reported as a distinct entity due to its typical morphology, immunohistochemistry, and the presence in the lymphomatous cells of both Kaposi's sarcoma herpes virus (KSHV)/human herpes virus 8 (HHV8) and EBV. This type of lymphoma can be associated with Kaposi's sarcoma and multicentric Castleman's disease (Cesarman et al. 1995; Nador et al. 1996; Carbone and Gaidano 1997). The same type of lymphoma can present as a solid tumor mass, for example, in the gastrointestinal tract or soft tissue (DePond et al. 1997; Beaty et al. 1999)
2. *Burkitt's lymphoma.* These lymphomas resemble endemic and sporadic Burkitt's lymphoma in immunocompetent patients (see Chap. 4.2.3). In the French Study Group, they represent 38% of the cases (Davi et al. 1998). *Classical Burkitt's lymphoma* can be observed, but Burkitt's lymphoma *with plasmacytoid differentiation* and *atypical Burkitt's/Burkitt's-like* lymphoma are often observed (Fig. 8.2).
3. *Polymorphic B-cell lymphoproliferative disorders.* These lymphoproliferations resemble those observ-

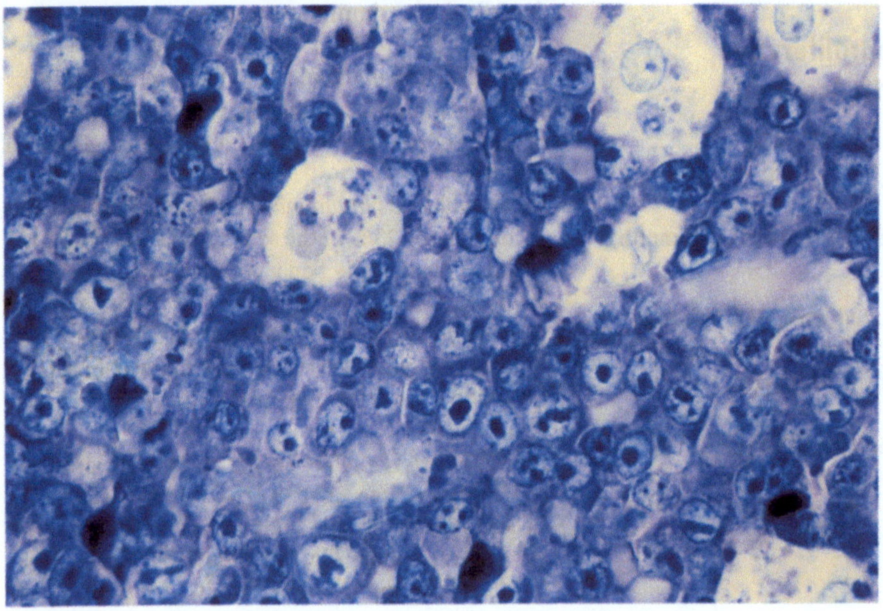

Fig. 8.1. Plasmablastic lymphoma of the gum. The cells produce a monoclonal intracytoplasmic IgA and are EBER-1-positive (not shown) (Giemsa stain)

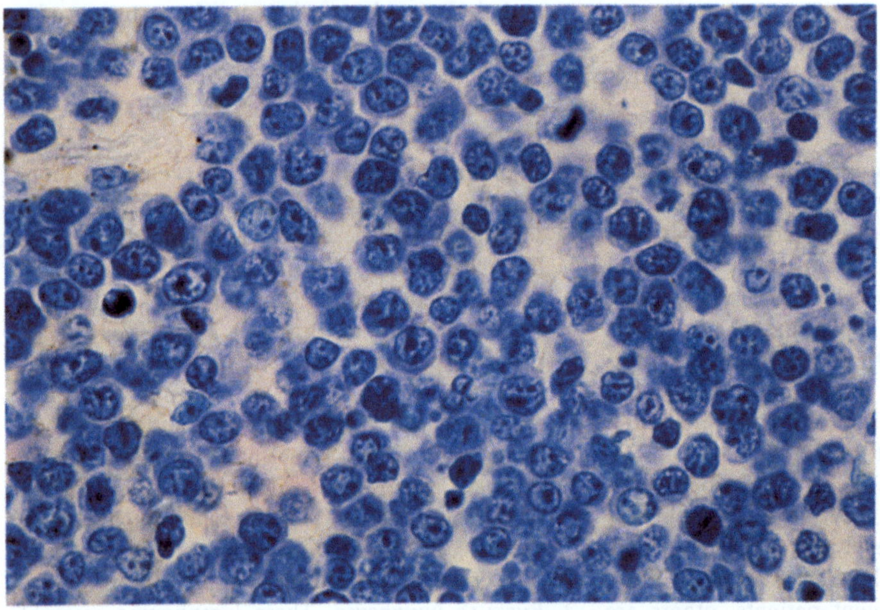

Fig. 8.2. Burkitt's lymphoma, atypical variant, featuring large cells and a plasmacytoid differentiation (Giemsa stain)

ed in post-transplant recipients but occur less frequently. In the French Study Group series, they represented 5% of the cases. The same criteria as for polymorphic B-cell post-transplant lymphoproliferative disorders (see Chap. 8.2.2) are used: a mixture of small cells, medium-sized cells, transformed cells, and immunoblasts (Fig. 8.3) with numerous cells showing a plasmacytoid differentiation. There are also mature plasma cells as well as some dispersed large-cells that are difficult to classify and which can resemble Reed-Sternberg cells (Raphael et al. 1994; Kaplan et al. 1995; Kingma et al. 1999; Martin et al. 1998).

4. *Plasmacytoma.* Rare extranodal plasmacytomas (Israel et al. 1983) and some cases of multiple myeloma (Ventura et al. 1995) have been reported in HIV-positive patients.

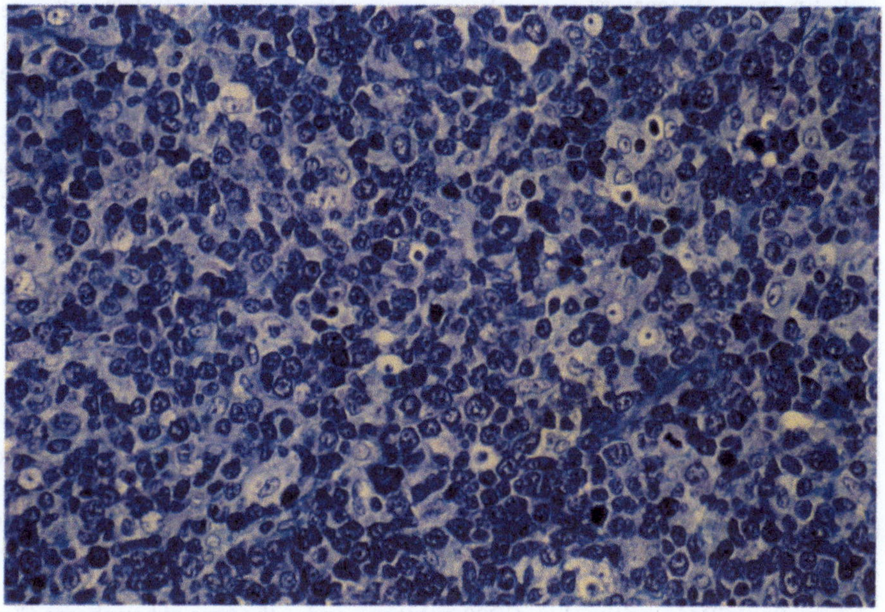

Fig. 8.3. Polymorphic B-cell lymphoproliferative disorder, Epstein-Barr virus (EBV)-associated. The nodal architecture is effaced by numerous immunoblasts and transformed lymphoid cells which are EBER-1-positive (not shown) (Giemsa stain)

5. *Small B-cell lymphoma*. Exceptional, probably incidental cases of *B-cell chronic lymphocytic leukemia* (B-CLL), *follicular lymphoma*, and *Waldenström's disease* have been observed in HIV-positive patients (Diebold et al. 1997). More interesting are the cases of *extranodal marginal zone lymphoma*, mostly of the digestive tracts (MALT), described in adults (Coker et al. 1992) and of the lung or parotid gland in children (Teruya-Feldstein et al. 1995; Chetty 1996). In addition, two cases of *nodal marginal zone lymphomas* with monocytoid B-cell component have been reported (Sheibani et al. 1990; Charton-Bain et al. 1997).
6. *T-cell lymphomas*. Very rare cases have been reported, mainly *peripheral T-cell lymphoma, unspecified* (Charton-Bain et al. 1997). They seem to occur fortuitously (Nasr et al. 1988; Herndier et al. 1993, 1994). Two cases of *angioimmunoblastic type* have also been published (Lust et al. 1989). An association of HIV with *adult T-cell leukemia lymphoma HTLV-1-positive* have been described and seems to also be an incidental association in patients living in areas of HTLV-1 endemic infection. *Anaplastic large-cell lymphoma of T type* have been published, for example with skin involvement and EBV expression (Filippa et al. 1996) or as a primary tumor in the liver (Baschinsky et al. 2001). *T-lymphoblastic leukemia and lymphoma* may also occur but are rare.

Immunophenotype

1. *Large-B-cell lymphomas*

Centroblastic lymphoma. On paraffin sections, these tumors can be shown to express B-cell markers (CD20, CD79α). Some express CD10 or CD5; bcl-2 protein can also be demonstrated. On frozen sections, monotypic surface immunoglobulin with a light-chain restriction and often a μ-heavy-chain restriction can be seen. Intracytoplasmic immunoglobulins are absent in the majority of the tumors, whereas EBV-LMP-1 is present in about 20–30% (Raphael et al. 1994). Latent EBV infection is very rare in monomorphic and multilobated centroblastic lymphomas but more frequent in polymorphic centroblastic lymphomas, which are positive in about 50% of the cases (Hamilton-Dutoit et al. 1993a,b; Raphael et al. 1994; Diebold et al. 1997).

Immunoblastic lymphoma. These tumors express CD20 and CD79α, often EMA, as well as CD138 due to plasmacytoid differentiation. Some immunoblastic lymphomas do not express CD20. Some are CD30-positive. Intracytoplasmic immunoglobulins with a light-chain restriction and expression of μ-, γ-, or α-heavy chains are disclosed. EBV-LMP-1 antigen is demonstrated in about 90% of the tumors (Knowles et al. 1988; Raphael et al. 1994). Bcl-2 is often expressed, particularly in LMP-1-positive tumors, mainly in primary CNS lymphoma (Camilleri-Broët et al. 1995). These results suggest a relationship between these two proteins in vivo as well as in vitro when transactivation of the bcl-2 gene by LMP-1 has been demonstrated. Thus, the oncoprotein bcl-2, which protects cells against apoptosis, might be part of the function of EBV in lymphomagenesis (Diebold et al. 1997).

Anaplastic large-cell lymphoma B type. In these lymphomas, CD45, CD30, and EMA are expressed as well as CD20 (Raphael et al. 1993a, b, 1994; Carbone et al. 1996).

Plasmablastic lymphoma of the oral cavity. These lymphomas are often CD20-negative, but CD79α- and CD30-positive. CD138 and VS38c are also positive. These tumors express monotypic IgA in the cytoplasm. EBV-LMP-1 is positive in more than 50 % of these *plasmablastic lymphomas.*

Primary effusion pleural lymphoma. As in plasmacytic lymphoma of the oral cavity, these lymphomas are often CD45-positive but CD20-negative, and even CD79α-negative. CD138 and VS38c are both positive. Primary effusion pleural lymphomas contain monotypic immunoglobulins often with an α-heavy-chain. EMA is expressed in more than 20 % of the tumors, as well as CD30. All of these tumors are EBV-LMP-1-positive (see Chap. 6.8.1.1).

2. *Burkitt's lymphoma.* These tumors have the same immunophenotype as Burkitt's lymphomas in immunocompetent patients (see Chap. 4.2.3). EBV-LMP-1 is positive in 30–50 % of the tumors.
3. *Polymorphic B-cell lymphoproliferative disorders.* The infiltrate consists of a mixture of B- and T-cells with a majority of cells expressing CD20 and CD79α. Some B-cell populations are polyclonal, some monoclonal, as determined by the expression of immunoglobulins. Some of these LPDs express EBV-LMP-1, others are negative.
4. *The small-B-*cell lymphocytes have a typical immunophenotype (see Chap. 4.2.1).
5. *Plasma cell neoplasias.* Different types have been reported (Diebold et al. 1997).

   Extranodal plasmacytoma. The neoplasias are made up of mature plasma cells, with only a few plasmablasts and/or immunoblasts, with monotypic intracytoplasmic immunoglobulin. Precise data concerning the outcome are lacking (Israel et al. 1983).

   Multiple myeloma. Reported cases are few. Ventura et al. found 23 cases in the literature in 1995. Clinical, radiographic, and morphological presentation are typical. Transformed myeloma may be difficult to differentiate from immunoblastic lymphoma with plasmacytoid differentiation or from plasmablastic lymphoma. Some myelomas can be EBV-positive (Ventura et al. 1995).
6. *T-cell lymphomas.* In these rarely occurring tumors, peripheral T-cell-associated antigens, with sometimes the loss of one or more antigens, are expressed. The rare anaplastic large-cell lymphomas express CD30, CD45, often EMA, as well as some T-cell markers.

Genetic Features

All B-cell lymphomas have in common a clonal rearrangement of the genes coding for IgH-chain immunoglobulin genes. T-cell lymphomas show a clonal rearrangement of T-cell receptor (TCR) genes. Demonstration of EBV genome by Southern blot or of EBER-1 by in situ hybridization gives various results according to the type of lymphoma (Knowles et al. 1989). Positivity was disclosed in 30 % of centroblastic lymphomas, 90 % of immunoblastic lymphomas, more than 50 % of plasmablastic lymphomas of the oral cavity (Delecluse et al. 1997), 100 % of PELs (Walts et al. 1990), 30 % of classic Burkitt's lymphomas (Raphael et al. 1994), 50–70 % of Burkitt's lymphomas with plasmacytoid differentiation (Davi et al. 1998), and 30–50 % in atypical Burkitt's/Burkitt's-like lymphomas. The presence of HIV in the lymphoma cells has never been demonstrated (Prévot et al. 1993).

Molecular genetic has shown that a very small number of high-grade lymphomas are bigenotypic (Samoszuk and Nguyen 1994; Diebold et al. 1997).

Polymorphic B-cell lymphoid proliferation can be positive or negative for EBV. In PEL and in a very few other B-cell lymphomas, HHV8/KSHV genomes are disclosed in the tumor cells (Cesarman et al. 1995; Carbone and Gaidano 1997; DePond et al. 1997; Beaty et al. 1999).

Several oncogenes and tumor suppressor genes have been studied. In Burkitt's lymphoma, the same type of genetic abnormalities affecting the c-myc locus have been disclosed in HIV-positive as in HIV-negative patients. Cytogenetic analysis has demonstrated the classic translocation t(8;14)(q24;q32) or one of the variants, as well as other abnormalities (DePond et al. 1997; Davi et al. 1998).c-myc gene rearrangements are observed not only in Burkitt's or Burkitt's-like lymphomas but also in some DLBCLs (Delecluse et al. 1993; Prévot et al. 1993).

Translocation involving the 8q24 band is detected in about 20% of DLBCLs but has never been found in PEL.

The proto-oncogene bcl-6 is rearranged in DLBCLs, mostly of centroblastic type, but not in Burkitt's lymphoma. Frequently, mutations of the 5'-non-coding region of the bcl-6 gene without bcl-6 rearrangement are observed in Burkitt's lymphomas and in some DLBCLs (Ballerini et al. 1993; Gaidano et al. 1994, 1997).

Mutations of the ras family of proto-oncogenes are present in about 15% of AIDS-associated lymphomas.

Abnormalities of the p53 tumor suppressor gene are detected in 50–60% of Burkitt's lymphomas and in 40% of DLBCLs. The gene is inactivated resulting in an overexpression of p53 (Martin et al. 1998).

Other tumor suppressor genes may be involved in other cytogenetic abnormalities, for example, deletions of the long arm of chromosome 6, which occurs in 25% of AIDS-related lymphomas (Gaidano and Carbone 1995).

Finally, DLBCLs in HIV-positive patients represent a distinct group of B-cell lymphomas showing more somatic IgH mutations in the CDRII and FWIII regions than DLBCLs developing in HIV-negative patients. In addition, a significant fraction of these lymphomas originate from EBV-driven lymphoproliferations and half of the lymphomas derive from pre-germinal-center B-cells (Delecluse et al. 1999).

Occurrence
The incidence of malignant lymphomas in HIV-positive is 60 to 200 times greater than in HIV-negative populations. Prior to the use of highly activated antiretroviral therapy, the incidence of primary central nervous system lymphoma and Burkitt's lymphoma was about 1,000-fold higher in HIV-positive patients than in the general population (Beral et al. 1991; Raphael et al. 2001). A decrease of the incidence of lymphoma following antiretroviral therapy has since been reported, but more information is needed to evaluate the effects of treatment (Grulich 1999).

Lymphoma represents the first lesion defining AIDS in about 3–5% of the patients.

Clinical Presentation
Clinical symptoms depend on the initial site of involvement, either nodal (presence of adenopathy in one or more sites in about 30% of the patients) or frequently extranodal (e.g. tumors of the central nervous system, gastrointestinal tract, oral cavity, liver, heart, serosa, and muscle). Often patients present with an advanced clinical-stage disease.

DLBCL develops mostly in patients with long-standing AIDS who present with one or more opportunistic infections. In these patients, the number of peripheral blood CD4-positive T-cells is very low (mean count less than 100×10^6/l). The level of LDH is high (Raphael et al. 1991; Diebold et al. 1997).

Burkitt's lymphoma occurs earlier during the evolution of HIV infection and the number of CD4-positive lymphocytes in the peripheral blood is higher (more than 200×10^6/l) (Raphael et al. 1991; Diebold et al. 1997; Davi et al. 1998). A few patients have Burkitt's leukemia.

The prognosis is not very good and depends on the histological subtype and the primary site of involvement. For example, PEL has a very poor prognosis with a very low complete remission rate. Complete remission was achieved in about 50% of the patients. The 2-year survival of patients with Burkitt's lymphoma is much better than that of patients with DLBCL.

The evolution of multiple myeloma is more aggressive in HIV-positive patients than in the HIV-negative population, and there is often multivisceral dissemination of the disease (Karnad et al. 1989).

8.2.2 Post-transplant Lymphoproliferative Disorders (ICD-O: 9970/1)

Definition
In the WHO classification (Jaffe 2001), these disorders are defined as "a lymphoid proliferation or lymphoma that develops as a consequence of immunosuppression in a recipient of a solid organ or bone marrow allograft. These disorders comprise a spectrum ranging from early Epstein-Barr Virus (EBV) driven polyclonal proliferations resembling infectious mononucleosis to EBV+ or EBV- lymphomas of predominantly B- or less often T-cell type" (Harris et al. 1997, 2001).

The frequency of post-transplant lymphoproliferative disorders (PTLDs) varies greatly, for example PTLDs are observed in about 1% of patients with renal allografts, 1–2% of patients with hepatic and cardiac allografts, and 5% of patients with heart-lung or liver-bowel allografts. Bone marrow allograft recipients have a low risk of PTLDs (1%), but for patients receiving HLA-mismatched or T-cell-depleted bone marrow or patients receiving immunosuppression for graft vs host disease, the risk is much more higher, up to 20% in patients with more than one of these risk factors (Curtis et al. 1999).

8.2.2.1 Plasmacytic Hyperplasia and Infectious-Mononucleosis-Like PTLD

Histology

Both of these conditions are characterized by a diffuse lymphoid hyperplasia with a more or less preserved architecture, i.e. the presence of sinuses in lymph nodes, epithelial crypts in tonsils, and even sometimes reactive follicles.

Plasmacytic hyperplasia consists of a diffuse infiltration of plasma cells with rare immunoblasts (Nalesnik et al. 1988). In infectious-mononucleosis-like PTLD, there is a diffuse infiltration, predominately of the paracortex, comprising immunoblasts, numerous lymphoid cells with plasmacytoid differentiation, and a large number of T-cells.

Immunophenotype

The plasma cells are polytypic, and in infectious-mononucleosis-like PTLD some of the immunoblasts are of the B type and polytypic, others are of the T type. The B-immunoblasts express EBV-LMP-1 (Lones et al. 1995).

Genetic Features

Rearrangements of immunoglobulin heavy-chain genes are polyclonal in both conditions. Some cases of plasmacytic hyperplasia are associated with EBV, some not and these negative cases should not be regarded as PTLD.

EBER-1 is positive in the B-immunoblasts of infectious-mononucleosis-like PTLD. Southern blotting with probes for episomal EBV may disclose small monoclonal or oligoclonal bands of unknown significance (Knowles et al. 1995; Wu et al. 1996).

Occurrence

Plasmacytic hyperplasia and infectious-mononucleosis-like PTLD are more frequent in younger patients (children, young adults) with solid organ transplantation and without prior EBV infection (Chadburn et al. 1998; Lones et al. 1995) They can occur at any time after transplantation, often during the first two years but sometimes later, until the fifth year (Nalesnik et al. 1988).

Clinical Presentation

Lymph nodes show mostly plasmacytic hyperplasia while infectious-mononucleosis-like PTLD more frequently involves Waldeyer's ring (particularly tonsils and adenoids). Other organs, such as the lung, can also be involved (Knowles et al. 1995).

Often, both types of lesions regress either spontaneously or after reduction of the immunosuppression and the prognosis can be good particularly in children (Lones et al. 1995). But infectious-mononucleosis-like PTLD can be more aggressive, sometimes fatal. In some cases, both types of lesions may be followed by the other types of PTLD (Nalesnik et al. 1988; Wu et al. 1996).

8.2.2.2 Polymorphic PTLD

The diffuse infiltration destroys the nodal architecture (Frizzera et al. 1981; Hanto et al. 1983) and consists of a very polymorphic cell population comprising small and medium-sized lymphocytes with round or irregular nuclei (centrocytic-like), transformed lymphoid cells, typical immunoblasts, and all the intermediate cells including plasma cells. Some large, difficult to classify, atypical cells are scattered through the infiltrate. Mitoses are numerous. Irregular areas of necrosis are often observed. According to the absence or presence of atypical large cells and necrosis, subdivision into a "polymorphic B-cell hyperplasia" and a "polymorphic B-cell lymphoma" has been proposed. This distinction has neither clinical nor practical value and should not be used (Knowles et al. 1995; Wu et al. 1996).

Immunophenotype

Many cells of the aggressive infiltrate are of B type, particularly many immunoblasts and the cells with plasmacytoid differentiation. The sIg and cIg are in some cases polytypic, in others monotypic (Frizerra et al. 1980; Wu et al. 1996). Many of these B-cells express EBNA2 and EBV-LMP-1. In addition, numerous cells, including immunoblasts, have a T-cell phenotype.

Genetic Features
PCR discloses clonal rearrangement of both immunoglobulin heavy-chain genes and EBV genome This monoclonality contrasts with the polymorphism of the cells.

In situ hybridization demonstrates the presence of EBER-1 in a large number of cells. The absence of EBER-1 or the finding of only a few positive cells rules out PTLD.

Occurrence
The reported frequency is variable, 20–80% in some series.

Clinical Features
Polymorphic PTLD usually develops during the first year after transplantation. Patients present with adenopathy, sometimes polyadenopathy and variable extranodal infiltrates. Regression can follow reduction of immunosuppression. Progression of the disease should be treated as lymphoma (Nalesnik et al. 1988; Knowles et al. 1995).

8.2.2.3 Monomorphic B-Cell PTLD

Morphology
The main characteristic of the infiltration is its aggressiveness, with destruction of the architecture of the nodal and extranodal organs.

The infiltrates consist of sheets of large transformed blastic cells. The polymorphism seen in polymorphic PTLD is lacking. Despite the monomorphic blastic background, some pleomorphism can still be observed due to the presence of a variable proportion of lymphoid cells with plasmacytoid differentiation as well as bizarre, sometimes multinucleated large cells. But the monomorphic pattern is still apparent due to the predominance of large transformed blastic cells.

The WHO classification (Harris et al. 2001) emphasizes that these monomorphic B-cell PTLDs should be classified according to the WHO classification scheme for DLBCL, adding the term PTLD. Four types of malignant lymphomas can be recognized and are discussed below.

8.2.2.3.1 Diffuse Large-B-Cell Lymphoma

The morphology of the majority of monomorphic B-cell PTLDs is that of DLBCL, mostly of the immunoblastic type, with a few being of centroblastic type. Rarely, B-cell PTLDs resemble anaplastic large-cell lymphoma (Kaplan et al. 1994).

8.2.2.3.2 Burkitt's Lymphoma

Only a few B-cell PTLDs have this morphology (Kaplan et al. 1994).

8.2.2.3.3 Plasma Cell Myeloma

This peculiar osseous lymphoma has been described in a very few transplant recipients.

8.2.2.3.4 Plasmacytoma-Like PTLD

Rare extramedullary plasmacytomas very similar to those seen in non-immunocompromised patients occur in different sites, nodal or extranodal, mainly in the gastrointestinal tract (Harris et al. 1997).

Immunophenotype
Whatever the subtype, monomorphic B-cell PTLDs express CD19, CD20, and CD79α. More than half show monotypic immunoglobulins, often with γ- or α-heavy-chain. In many cases CD30 is expressed even in the absence of a morphology of anaplastic large-cell lymphoma. In the majority of the cases, EBNA2 and EBV-LMP-1 are demonstrated in many cells.

Genetic Features
In almost all monomorphic B-cell PTLDs, it is possible to demonstrate clonal rearrangement of heavy-chain genes.

The majority of monomorphic B-cell PTLDs contain EBV genomes mostly in a clonal episomal form (Kaplan et al. 1994). Some plasma cell myelomas may be EBV negative.

Occurrence
Monomorphic B-cell PTLD occurs in the first year after transplantation.

Clinical Presentation
Patients present with lymphadenopathy in one or multiple sites, or extranodal localization (e.g. gastrointestinal tract for plasmacytoma-like lesions, or bone in plasma cell myeloma). Most of the cases should be treated as DLBCL or Burkitt's lymphoma. Decreased immunosuppression is not followed by regression in many patients.

8.2.2.4 Monomorphic T-Cell PTLD

Morphology
This term refers to lymphoproliferation consisting of T-cells and resembling certain T-cell lymphomas, but developing in transplant recipients. The following types have been described:

- Subcutaneous panniculitis-like lymphoma (Kaplan et al. 1993)
- Hepatosplenic γδ-T-cell lymphoma (Kraus et al. 1998; François et al. 1997)
- Aggressive NK-like T-cell or NK-cell lymphoma (Natkunam et al. 1999)
- T-cell large granular lymphocyte leukemia (Gentile et al. 1998)
- Peripheral T-cell lymphoma, unspecified (Van Gorp et al. 1994)

Immunophenotype
Their immunophenotype is identical to cases with the same histological subtype occurring in patients without immunosuppression. They have either αβ- or γδ-T-cell receptors. The phenotype of monomorphic T-cell PTLDs is often that of cytotoxic cells, NK-cells, or NK-like cells. In many cases, CD30 is expressed.

Genetic Features
T-cell-receptor genes are clonally rearranged. The presence of EBER-1-positive cells, as determined by in situ hybridization, is also variable. About 25% of monomorphic T-cell PTLDs have clonal episomal EBV genomes.

Clinical Presentation
Most patients present with adenopathy, either localized, multiple, or extranodal (skin, intestinal).

8.2.2.5 Hodgkin's-Like PTLD

Morphology
A small number of PTLDs resemble classic Hodgkin's lymphoma; they occur at nodal or extranodal sites (Nalesnik et al. 1993).

Immunophenotype
Reed-Sternberg-like cells express CD30 and CD15, and sometimes CD20. All Hodgkin's-like PTLDs are EBV-LMP-1-positive (Nalesnik et al. 1993; Harris et al. 1997).

Genetic Features
EBER-1 is positive by in situ hybridization in numerous cells in all Hodgkin's-like PTLDs.

Clinical Presentation
Development of either adenopathies or extranodal tumors occurs mostly during the first year after transplantation. Due to the small number of cases, the clinical behavior of Hodgkin's-like PTLDs is not well known. Some are clinically aggressive, others respond to classic Hodgkin's lymphoma treatment.

References

Adelman DC, Matsuda T, Hirano T, Kishimoto T, Saxon A (1990) Elevated serum interleukin-6 associated with a failure in B-cell differentiation in common variable immunodeficiency. J Allergy Clin Immunol 86:512–521

Aparicio-Pafges MN, Den Hartog G, Verspaget HW et al. (1990) Decreased natural killer cell activity in late-onset hypogammaglobulinaemia. Clin Sci 78:133–137

Ballerini P, Gaidano G, Gong JZ, Tassi V, Saglio G, Knowles DM, Dalla-Favera R (1993) Multiple genetic lesions in acquired immunodeficiency syndrome-related non-Hodgkin's lymphoma. Blood 81:166–176

Baschinsky DY, Weidner N, Baker PB, Frankel WL (2001) Primary hepatic anaplastic large-cell lymphoma of T-cell phenotype in acquired immunodeficiency syndrome: a report of an autopsy case and review of the literature. Am J Gastroenterol 96:227–232

Beaty MW, Kumar S, Sorbara L, Miller K, Raffeld M, Jaffe ES (1999) A biophenotypic human herpes virus 8-associated primary bowel lymphoma. Am J Surg Pathol 23:992–994

Beral V, Peterman T, Berkelman R, Jaffe H (1991) AIDS-associated non-Hodgkin's lymphoma. Lancet 337:805–809

Camilleri-Broët S, Davi F, Feuillard J et al (1995) High expression of latent membrane protein 1 (LMP1) of Epstein-Barr virus and bcl2 oncoprotein in AIDS-related primary brain lymphomas. Blood 86:432–435

Carbone A, Gaidano G (1997) HHV-8-positive body-cavity-based lymphoma: a novel lymphoma entity. Br J Haematol 97:515–522

Carbone A, Dolcetti R, Gloghini A et al (1996) Immunophenotypic and molecular analysis of AIDS-related and EBV-associated lymphomas: a comparative study. Human Pathol 27:133–146

Cesarman E, Chang Y, Moore PS, Said JW, Knowles DM (1995) Kaposi's sarcoma-associated herpesvirus-like DNA sequences in AIDS-related body-cavity-based lymphomas. N Engl J Med 332:1186–1191

Chadburn A, Chen JM, Hsu DT, Frizzera G, Cesarman E, Garrett TJ, Mears JG, Zangwill SD, Addonizion LJ, Michler RE, Knowles DM (1998) The morphologic and molecular genetic categories of posttransplantation lymphoproliferative disorders are clinically relevant. Cancer 82:1978–1987

Charton-Bain MC, Le Tourneau A, Weiss L, Bruneval P, Diebold J (1997) Lymphomes non hodgkiniens inhabituels au cours de l'infection par le VIH; 2 cas avec envahissement médullaire. Ann Pathol 17:38–40

Chetty R (1996) Parotid MALT lymphoma in an HIV positive child. Histopathology 29:195–196

Chrzanowska KH, Kleijer WJ, Krajewska Walasek M et al (1995) Eleven Polish patients with microcephaly, immunodeficiency and chromosomal instability: the Nijmegen breakage syndrome. Am J Med Genet 57:462–471

Coker RJ, Lau R, Isaacson PG, Kelly SA, Price P, Weber J (1992) Mucosa-associated gastric lymphoma occurring in an HIV-antibody-positive patient. AIDS 6:336–337

Cotelingam JD, Witebsky FG, Hsu SM et al (1985) Malignant lymphoma in patients with the Wiskott-Aldrich syndrome. Cancer Invest 3:515–522

Cunningham-Rundles C, Siegal FP, Cunningham-Rundles S et al (1987) Incidence of cancer in 98 patients with common varied immunodeficiency. J Clin Immunol 7:294–299

Curtis RE, Travis LB, Rowlings PA et al (1999) Risk of lymphoproliferative disorders after bone marrow transplantation: a multi-institutional study. Blood 94:2208–2216

Davi F, Delecluse HJ, Guiet P, Gabarre J, Fayon A, Gentilhomme O, Felman P, Bayle C, Berger F, Audouin J, Bryon PA, Diebold J, Raphael M (1998) Burkitt-like lymphomas in AIDS patients: characterization within a series of 103 human immunodeficiency virus-associated non-Hodgkin's lymphomas. Burkitt's Lymphoma Study Group. J Clin Oncol 16:3788–3795

Delecluse HJ, Raphael M, Magaud JP et al (1993) Variable morphology of human immunodeficiency virus-associated lymphomas with the c-myc rearrangement. Blood 82:552–563

Delecluse HJ, Anagnostopoulos I, Dallenbach F, Hummel M, Marafioti T, Schneider U, Huhn D, Schmidt-Westhausen A, Reichart PA, Gross U, Stein H (1997) Plasmablastic lymphomas of the oral cavity: a new entity associated with the human immunodeficiency virus infection. Blood 89:1413–1420

Delecluse HJ, Hummel M, Marafioti T, Anagnostopoulos I, Stein H (1999) Common and HIV-related diffuse large B-cell lymphomas differ in their immunoglobulin gene mutation pattern. J Pathol 188:133–138

DePond W, Said JW, Tasaka T, de Vos S, Kahn D, Cesarman E, Knowles DM, Koeffler HP (1997) Kaposi's sarcoma-associated herpesvirus and human herpesvirus 8(KSHV/HHV8)-associated lymphoma of the bowel. Report of two cases in HIV-positive men with secondary effusion lymphomas. Am J Surg Pathol 21:719–724

Diebold J, Raphael M, Prevot S, Audouin J (1997) Lymphomas associated with HIV infection. Cancer Surv 30:263–293

Elenitoba-Johnson KSJ, Jaffe ES (1997) Lymphoproliferative disorders associated with congenital immunodeficiencies. Semin Diagn Pathol 14:35–47

Filipovich AH, Mathur A, Kamat D, Shapiro RS (1992) Primary immunodeficiencies. Genetic risk factors for lymphoma. Cancer Res 52 [Suppl]:5465–5467

Filippa DA, Ladanyi M, Wollner N et al (1996) CD30 (Ki-1) positive malignant lymphomas: clinical, immunophenotypic, histologic and genetic characteristics and differences with Hodgkin's disease. Blood 87:2905–2917

Foon KA, Gale RP (1992) Is there a T-cell form of chronic lymphocytic leukaemia? Leukemia 6:867–868

François A, Lesesue JF, Stamatoullas A et al (1997) Hepatosplenic gamma/delta T-cell lymphoma: a report of two cases in immunocompromised patients, associated with isochromosome 7q. Am J Surg Pathol 21:781–790

Frizzera G, Rosai J, Dehner LP et al (1980) Lymphoreticular disorders in primary immunodeficiencies: new findings based on an up-to-date histologic classification of 35 cases. Cancer 46:692–699

Frizzera G, Hanto DW, Gajl-Peczalska KJ et al (1981) Polymorphic diffuse B-cell hyperplasias and lymphomas in renal transplant recipients. Cancer Res 41:4262–4279

Gaidano G, Carbone A (1995) AIDS-related lymphomas: from pathogenesis to pathology. Br J Haematol 90:235–243

Gaidano G, Lo CF, Ye BH, Shibata D, Levine AM, Knowles DM, Dalla-Favera R (1994) Rearrangements of the BCL-6 gene in acquired immunodeficiency syndrome-associated non-Hodgkin's lymphoma: association with diffuse large-cell subtype. Blood 84:397–402

Gaidano G, Carbone A, Pastore C, Capello D, Migliazza A, Gloghini A, Roncella S, Ferrarini M, Saglio G, Dalla-Favera R (1997) Frequent mutation of the 5'noncoding region of the BCL-6 gene in acquired immunodeficiency syndrome-related non-Hodgkin's lymphomas. Blood 89:3755–3762

Gentile TC, Hadlock KG, Uner AH et al (1998) Large granular lymphocyte leukaemia occurring after renal transplantation. Br J Haematol 101:507–512

Grulich AE (1999) AIDS-associated non-Hodgkin's lymphoma in the era of highly active antiretroviral therapy. J Acquir Immune Defic Syndr 21 [Suppl 1]:S27–S30

Hamilton-Dutoit SJ, Rea D, Raphael M et al (1993a) Epstein-Barr virus-latent gene expression and tumor cell phenotype in acquired immunodeficiency syndrome-related non-Hodgkin's lymphoma. Am J Pathol 143:1072–1085

Hamilton-Dutoit SJ, Raphael M, Audouin J et al (1993b) In situ demonstration of Epstein-Barr virus small RNAs (EBER 1) in acquired immunodeficiency syndrome-related lymphomas: correlation with tumor morphology and primary site. Blood 82:619–624

Hanto DW, Gajl-Peczalska KJ, Frizzerra G (1983) Epstein-Barr virus (EBV) induced polyclonal and monoclonal B-cell lymphoproliferative diseases occurring after renal transplantation. Clinical, pathologic and virologic findings and implications for therapy. Ann Surg 198:356–369

Harrington DS, Weisenburger DD, Purtilo DT (1987) Malignant lymphoma in the X-linked lymphoproliferative syndrome. Cancer 59:1419–1429

Harris NL, Ferry JA, Swerdlow SH (1997) Posttransplant lymphoproliferative disorders. Summary of the Society for Hematopathology workshop. Semin Diagn Pathol 14:8–14
Harris et al (2001) Post-transplant lymphoproliferative disorders. In: Jaffe ES, Harris NL, Stein H, Vardeman JW (eds) World Health Organization Classification of Tumours. Pathology and genetics of tumours of haematopoietic and lymphoid tissues. IARC, Lyon
Herndier BG, Sanchez HC, Chang KL, Chen YY, Weiss LM (1993) High prevalence of Epstein-Barr virus in the Reed-Sternberg cells of HIV-associated Hodgkin's disease. Am J Pathol 142:1073–1079
Herndier BG, Kaplan L, McGrath MS (1994) Pathogenesis of AIDS lymphomas. AIDS 8:1025–1049
Huber J, Zegers BJJM, Schuurman HJ (1992) Pathology of congenital immunodeficiencies. Semin Diagn Pathol 9:31–32
Israel AM, Koziner B, Strauss DJ (1983) Plasmacytoma and the AIDS. Ann Intern Med 99:635–636
Kaplan MA, Jacobson JO, Ferry JA, Harris NL (1993) T-cell lymphoma of the vulva in a renal allograft recipient with associated hemophagocytosis. Am J Surg Pathol 17:842–849
Kaplan MA, Ferry JA, Harris NL, Jacobson JO (1994) Post-transplant lymphoproliferative disorders episomal EBV in a more reliable marker of clonality than immunoglobulin gene rearrangement. Am J Clin Pathol 101:590–596
Kaplan LD, Shiramizu B, Herndier B et al (1995) Influence of molecular characteristics on clinical outcome in human immunodeficiency virus-associated non-Hodgkin's lymphoma: identification of a subgroup with favorable clinical outcome. Blood 85:1727–1735
Karnad AB, Martin AW, Koh HK, Brauer MJ, Novich M, Wright J (1989) Nonsecretory multiple myeloma in a 26-year-old man with acquired immunodeficiency syndrome, presenting with multiple extramedullary plasmacytoma and osteolytic bone disease. Am J Hematol 32:305–310
Kingma DW, Mueller BU, Frekko K, Sorbara LR, Wood LV, Katz D, Raffeld M, Jaffe ES (1999) Low-grade monoclonal Epstein-Barr virus-associated lymphoproliferative disorder of the brain presenting as human immunodeficiency virus-associated encephalopathy in a child with acquired immunodeficiency syndrome. Arch Pathol Lab Med 123:83–87
Knowles DM (1999) Morphologic, immunologic and genetic features of lymphoproliferative disorders associated with immunodeficiency. In: Mason DY, Harris NL (eds) Human lymphoma: clinical implications of the REAL classification. Springer, Berlin Heidelberg New York
Knowles DM, Chamulak GA, Subar M, Burke JS, Dugan M, Wernz J, Slywotzky C, Pelicci G, Dalla-Favera R, Raphael B (1988) Lymphoid neoplasia associated with the acquired immunodeficiency syndrome (AIDS). The New York University Medical Center experience with 105 patients (1981–1986). Ann Intern Med 108:744–753
Knowles DM, Inghirami G, Ubriaco A, Dalla-Favera R (1989) Molecular genetic analysis of three AIDS-associated neoplasms of uncertain lineage demonstrates their B-cell derivation and the possible pathogenetic role of the Epstein-Barr virus. Blood 73:792–799
Knowles DM, Cesarman E, Chadburn A et al (1995) Correlative morphologic and molecular genetic analysis demonstrates three distinct categories of post-transplantation lymphoproliferative disorders. Blood 85:552–565
Kraus MD, Crawford DF, Kaleem Z et al (1998) T gamma/delta hepatosplenic lymphoma in a heart transplant patient after an Epstein-Barr virus positive lymphoproliferative disorder: a case report. Cancer 82:983–992
Krueger GRF, Sander C (1989) What's new in human herpesvirus-6? Clinical immunopathology of the HHV-6 infection. Pathol Res Pract 185:915–929
Lones MA, Mishalani S, Shintaku IP et al (1995) Changes in tonsils and adenoids in children with post-transplant lymphoproliferative disorder: report of three cases with early involvement of Waldeyer's ring. Hum Pathol 26:525–530
Lust JA, Banks PM, Hooper WC et al (1989) T-cell non-Hodgkin lymphoma in human immunodeficiency virus-1-infected individuals. Am J Haematol 31:181–187
Martin A, Flaman JM, Frebourg T, Davi F, El Mansouri S, Amouroux J, Raphael M (1998) Functional analysis of the p53 protein in AIDS-related non-Hodgkin's lymphomas and polymorphic lymphoproliferations. Br J Haematol 101:311–317
Franklin EC, Kyle R, Seligmann M, Frangiona B (1979) Correlation of protein structure and immunoglobulin gene organization in the light of two new deleted heavy chain disease proteins. Mod Immunol 16 :919–921
Meropol NJ, Hicks D, Brooks JJ et al (1992) Coincident Kaposi's sarcoma and T-cell lymphoma in a patient with the Wiskott-Aldrich syndrome. Am J Hematol 40:126–134
Morrell D, Cromartie E, Swift M (1986) Mortality and cancer incidence in 263 patients with ataxia telangiectasia. J Natl Cancer Inst 77:89–92
Nador RG, Cesarman E, Chadburn A, Dawson DB, Ansari MQ, Sald J, Knowles DM (1996) Primary effusion lymphoma: a distinct clinicopathologic entity associated with the Kaposi's sarcoma-associated herpes virus. Blood 88:645–656
Nalesnik M, Jaffe E, Starzl T et al. (1988) The pathology of post-transplant lymphoproliferative disorders occurring in the setting of cyclosporin A-prednisone immunosuppression. Am J Pathol 133:173–192
Nalesnik MA, Randhawa P, Demetris AJ et al (1993) Lymphoma resembling Hodgkin disease after post-transplant lymphoproliferative disorder in a liver transplant recipient. Cancer 72:2568–2573
Nasr SA, Brynes RK, Garrison CP, Chan WC (1988) Peripheral T-cell lymphoma in a patient with AIDS. Cancer 61:947–951
Natkunam Y, Warnke RA, Zehnder JL, Cornbleet PJ (1999) Aggressive natural killer-like T-cell malignancy with leukemic presentation following solid organ transplantation. Am J Clin Pathol 111:663–671
Okano M, Mizumo F, Osato T et al (1984) Wiskott-Aldrich syndrome and Epstein-Barr virus-induced lymphoproliferation. Lancet 2:933–934
Okano M, Thiele GM, Davis JR (1988) Epstein-Barr and human diseases: recent advances in diagnosis. Clin Microbiol Rev 1:300–312
Perry GS, Spector BD, Schuman LM et al (1980) The Wiskott-Aldrich syndrome in the United States and Canada (1892–1979). J Pediatr 97:72–78
Petkovic I, Ligutic I, Dominis M et al (1992) Cytogenetic analysis in ataxia-telangiectasia with malignant lymphoma. Cancer Genet Cytogenet 60:158–163

Porter SR, Diz DP, Kumar N, Stock C, Barrett AW, Scully C (1999) Oral plasmablastic lymphoma in previously undiagnosed HIV disease. Oral Surg Oral Med Oral Pathol Oral Radiol Endod 87:730–734

Prévot S, Raphael M, Fournier JG, Diebold J (1993) Detection by in situ hybridization of HIV and c-myc RNA in tumour cells of AIDS-related B-cell lymphomas. Histopathology 22:151–156

Purtilo DT, Sakamoto K, Barnabei B et al (1982) Epstein-Barr virus-induced diseases in boy with the X-linked lymphoproliferaton syndrome (XLP): update on studies of the registry. Am J Med 73:49–56

Raphael M, Gentilhomme O, Tulliez M, Bryon PA, Diebold J (1991) Histopathologic features of high-grade non-Hodgkin's lymphomas in acquired immunodeficiency syndrome. The French Study Group of Pathology for Human Immunodeficiency Virus-Associated Tumors. Arch Pathol Lab Med 115:15–20

Raphael M, Audouin J, Tulliez M et al (1993a) Anatomic and histologic distribution of 448 cases of AIDS-related non Hodgkin's lymphomas. Blood 82:56a

Raphael M, Rea D, Hamilton-Dutoit S, Marelle L et al. and the French-Danish Study Group of Pathology of AIDS-Related Lymphoma (1993b) Expression of EBV latent antigens, activation and adhesion molecules in AIDS-related non-Hodgkin's lymphomas. Symposium on Epstein-Barr Virus, pp 649–656

Raphael M, Audouin J, Lamine M, Delecluse HJ, Vuillaume M, Lenoir GM, Gisselbrecht C, Lennert K, Diebold J (1994) Immunphenotypic and genotypic analysis of acquired immunodeficiency syndrome-related non-Hodgkin's lymphomas. Correlation with histologic features in 36 cases. French Study Group of Pathology for HIV-Associated Tumors. Am J Clin Pathol 101:773–782

Raphael M,Borisch B, Jaffe ES (2001) Lymphomas associated with infection by the human immune deficiency virus (HIV). In: Jaffe ES, Harris NL, Stein H, Vardeman JW (eds) World Health Organization Classification of tumours. Pathology and genetics of tumours of haematopoietic and lymphoid tissues? IARC, Lyon

Ratech H, Hirschhorn R, Greco MA (1989) Pathologic findings in adenosine deaminase deficient-severe combined immunodeficiency. II. Thymus, spleen, lymph node and gastrointestinal tract lymphoid tissue alterations. Am J Pathol 135:1145–1156

Report of a WHO Scientific Group (1995) Primary immunodeficiency diseases. Clin Exp Immunol Suppl 1:1–2

Rosen F (1990) Genetic deficiencies in specific immune responses. Semin Hematol 27:333–341

Rosen FS, Wedgwood RJ, Eibl M (1992) Primary immunodeficiency diseases: report of a World Health Organization Scientific Group. Immunodefic Rev 3:195–236

Rosen FS, Cooper MD, Wedgwood RJP (1995) The primary immunodeficiencies. N Engl J Med 333:431–440

Samoszuk M, Nguyen V (1994) Two cases of acquired immunodeficiency syndrome-related lymphomas with simultaneous clonal rearrangements of B-cell and T-cell genes. Blood 83:1444–1445

Sander CA, Medeiros LJ, Weiss LM et al (1992) Lymphoproliferative lesions in patients with common variable immunodeficiencies syndrome. Am J Surg Pathol 16:1170–1182

Savitsky K, Bar-Shira A, Gilad S et al (1995) A single ataxia-telangiectasia gene with a product similar to Pi-3 kinase. Science 268:1749–1753

Sheibani K, Ben Ezra I, Swartz WG, Rossi J, Kerizian J, Koo CH (1990) Monocytoid B-cell lymphoma in a patient with HIV infection. Arch Pathol Lab Med 114:1264–1267

Stern MH, Theodorou I, Aurias A et al (1989) T-cell nonmalignant clonal proliferation in ataxia-telangiectasia: a cytological immunological and molecular characterization. Blood 73:1285–1290

Taylor AMR, Metcalfe JA, Mak YF (1996) Leukemia and lymphoma in ataxia-telangiectasia. Blood 87:423–438

Teruya-Feldstein J, Temeck BK, Melisse Sloas M et al (1995) Pulmonary malignant lymphoma of mucosa-associated lymphoid tissue (MALT) arising in a pediatric HIV-positive patient. Am J Surg Pathol 19:357–363, 20:644

Toledano SR, Lange BJ (1980) Ataxia-telangiectasia and acute lymphoblastic leukemia. Cancer 45:1675–1678

Van Gorp J, Doornewaard H, Verdonck LF et al (1994) Post-transplant T-cell lymphoma. Report of 3 cases and a review of the literature. Cancer 73:3064–3072

Ventura G, Lucia MB, Damiano F, Cauda R, Larocca LM (1995) Multiple myeloma associated with EBV in an AIDS patient: a case report. Eur J Haematol 55:332–334

Walts AE, Shintaku IP, Said JW (1990) Diagnosis of malignant lymphoma in effusions from patients with AIDS by gene rearrangement. Am J Clin Pathol 94:170–175

Weemaes CMR, Smeets DFCM, Van Der Burgt CJAM (1994) Nijmegen breakage syndrome: a progress report. Int J Radiat Biol 66:185–188

Wu TT, Swerdlow SH, Locker J et al (1996) Recurrent Epstein-Barr virus-associated lesions in organ transplant recipients. Hum Pathol 27:157–164

9 Practical Guidelines for Lymphoma Diagnosis in Bone Marrow

Bone marrow is frequently involved in malignant lymphoma (ML). The frequency varies according to the histological type and the duration of evolution. Bone marrow biopsy (BMB) is now routinely performed for diagnosis and staging. The positivity or negativity of BMB is of prognostic value. BMB not only allows the presence of lymphomatous involvement to be recognized, but also gives important information concerning hematopoiesis and the presence of stromal modifications or granulomatous reactions. It can also be used to assess therapeutic responses and identify residual disease and/or relapse. Immunohistochemistry is very useful in the diagnosis of bone marrow involvement by ML and can be carried out on fixed tissue embedded in paraffin or in various plastic mediums.

9.1 Patterns of Involvement

Lymphomatous infiltrates of the bone marrow present as one of three main patterns according to the topography: paratrabecular, intertrabecular, and intravascular.

9.1.1 Paratrabecular Infiltrates

This type can be defined as a lymphomatous infiltrate along parts of bone trabeculae; it is always associated with localized myelofibrosis. Paratrabecular infiltrates may be discrete (Fig. 9.1) and demonstration of localized juxtatrabecular myelofibrosis by silver impregna-

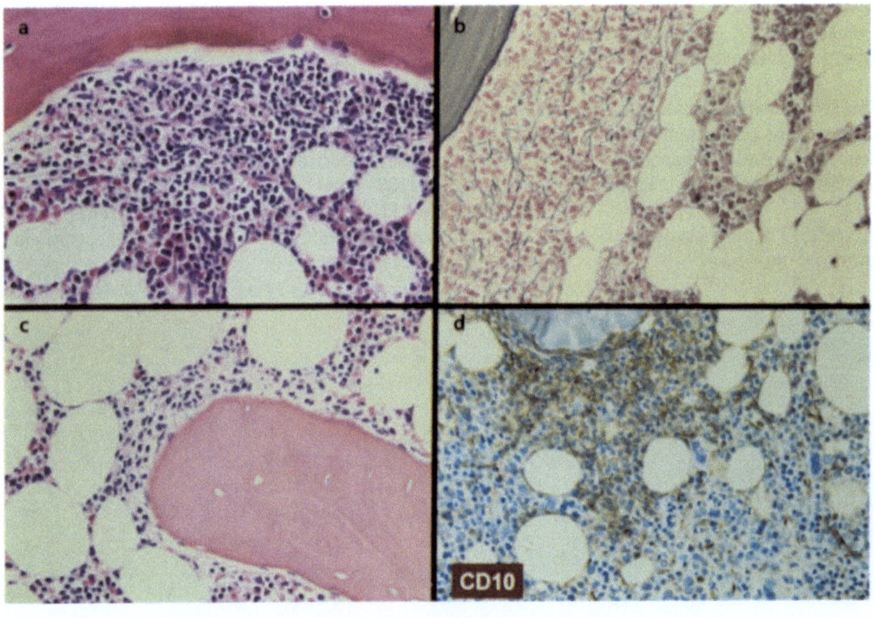

Fig. 9.1 a–d. Paratrabecular infiltrates. Several patterns are observed in follicular lymphomas: **a** typical infiltrate (H and E stain); **b** myelofibrosis underlined by silver impregnation in a paratrabecular infiltrate; **c** minimal paratrabecular infiltrate (H and E stain); **d** neoplastic centrofollicular cells expressing CD10 (immunoperoxide)

tion may be very useful (Fig. 9.1). Alternatively, these infiltrates may be more abundant, appearing either as a band-like infiltrate along trabeculae or as a nodule with a large base in direct contact with the bone trabeculae and a convexity compressing the hematopoietic tissue. Paratrabecular infiltrates are often multiple. They can be associated with intertrabecular infiltrates, either interstitial or nodular.

9.1.2 Intertrabecular Infiltrates

These lymphomatous infiltrates tend to develop at a distance from the bone trabeculae, in the center of the lacunae.

Three patterns can be distinguished.

9.1.2.1 Interstitial Infiltrate

This type can be defined as the presence of lymphoma cells between adipocytes with respect for the architecture of the bone marrow. Interstitial infiltrates can be *minimal* with persistence of normal hematopoietic cells, or *dense* with total replacement of the hematopoietic cell population (Fig. 9.2). The infiltrate can be *localized* or *diffuse* throughout the bone marrow lacunae, or associated with focal reinforcement forming lymphoid aggregates with an often irregular outline.

9.1.2.2 Nodular Infiltrate

This type of involvement can be defined as lymphoid nodules developing as reactive lymphoid nodules in the center of the bone marrow lacunae (Fig. 9.3), often near vessels (Fig. 9.4). Voluminous nodules may make contact with the bone trabeculae at their periphery, i.e. at the convexity of the nodule. This should not be interpreted as a paratrabecular nodule. The number of nodules is variable; there are often more than one or two in a BMB measuring 1 cm in length. A nodular infiltrate can be associated with an interstitial infiltrate and is then very similar to an interstitial infiltrate with nodular reinforcement.

In certain types of lymphoma, nodules with peculiar pattern can be observed.

Some nodules may show *marginal zone differentiation* (Fig. 9.5). The morphology of the cells, the pattern of the involvement, and the immunophenotype will allow follicular lymphoma with marginal zone differentiation to be distinguished from marginal zone lymphoma, mostly primary splenic type.

Rarely, nodules have a reactive germinal center. These nodules may also have marginal zone differenti-

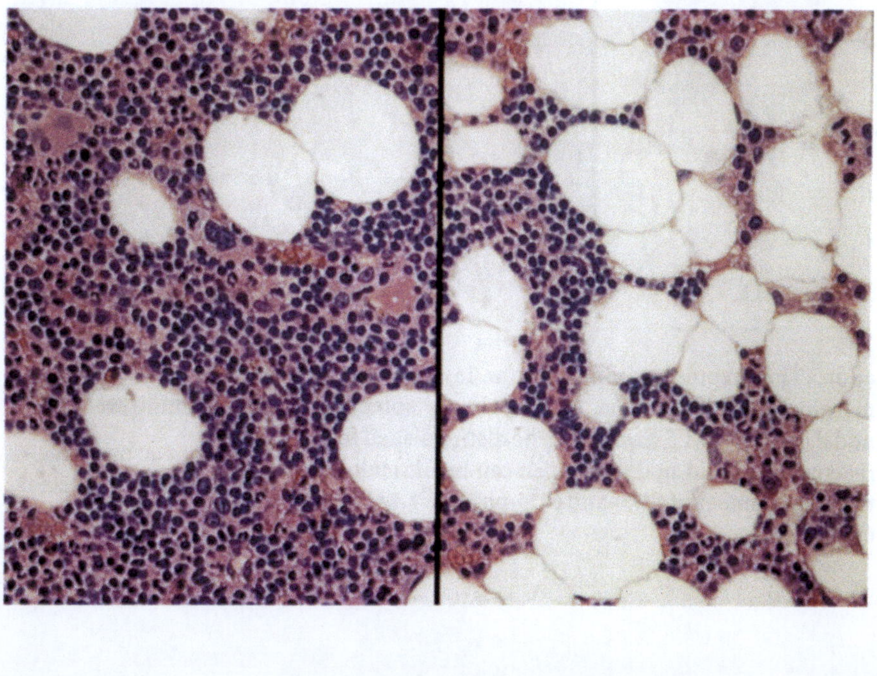

Fig. 9.2. Dense (*left*) and minimal (*right*) interstitial infiltrate in a mantle zone lymphoma (H and E stain)

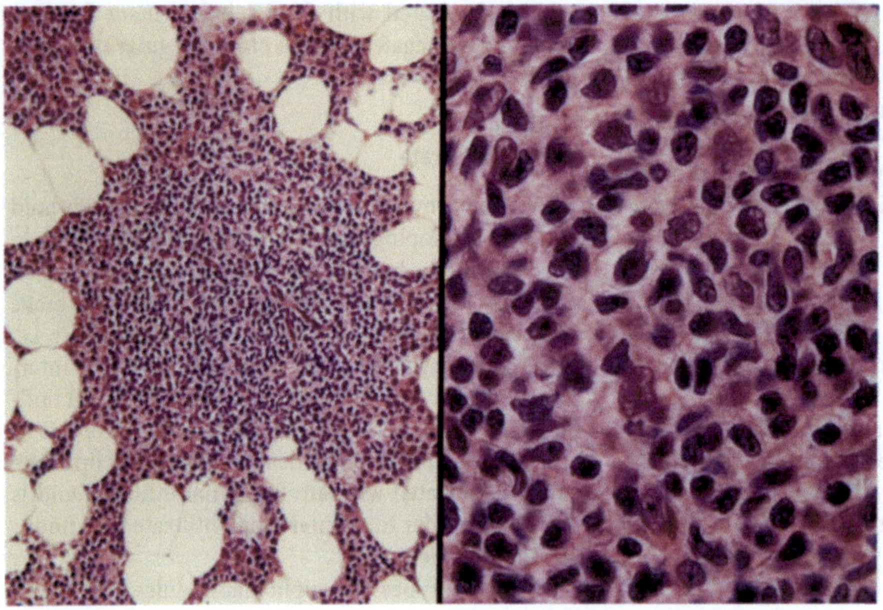

Fig. 9.3. Intertrabecular nodular infiltrate in follicular lymphoma (*left*), consisting mostly of centrocytes (*right*) (H and E stain)

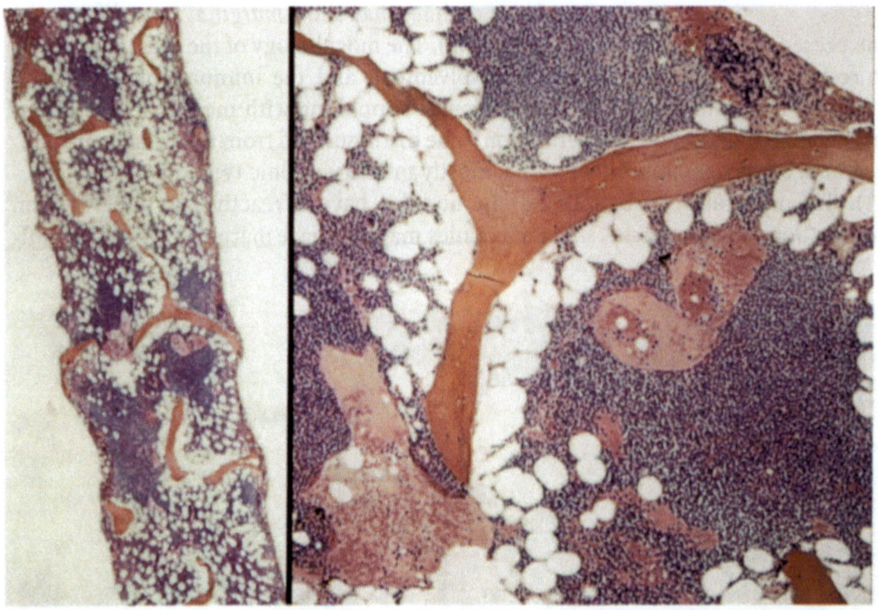

Fig. 9.4. Multiple intertrabecular nodular infiltrates in a mantle cell lymphoma (H and E stain)

ation. They represent bone marrow involvement by marginal zone lymphoma, either primary splenic or nodal or even MALT, and have to be distinguished from reactive lymphoid nodules, which can be difficult due to a large number of CD3- and CD5-positive T-lymphocytes.

9.1.2.3 Massive Infiltrate

This type can be defined as a diffuse, dense lymphomatous infiltrate. It destroys and replaces the bone marrow hematopoietic tissue either in one or two bone marrow lacunae or diffusely throughout all the lacunae, forming a densely packed infiltrate.

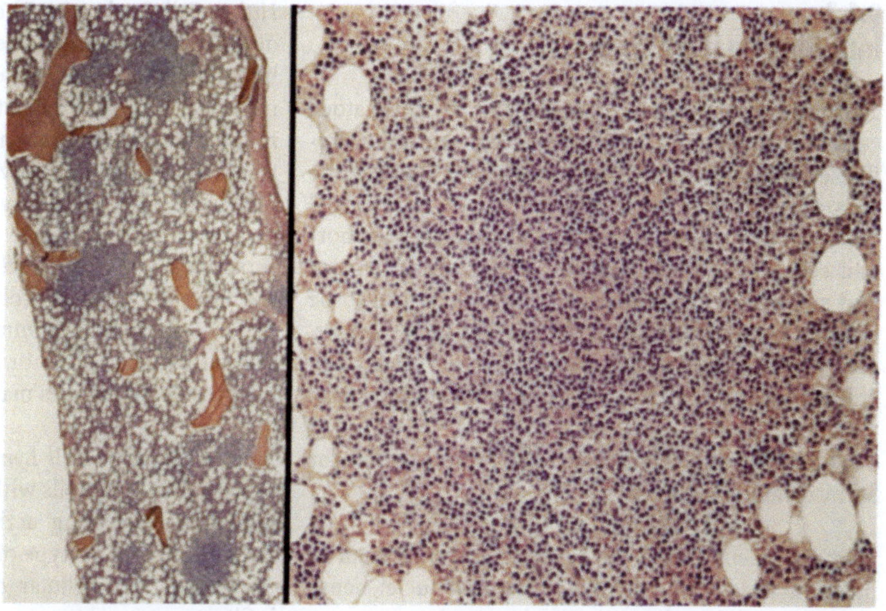

Fig. 9.5. Intertrabecular nodular infiltrates in splenic marginal zone lymphoma. Note the marginal zone at the periphery of the nodule (H and E stain)

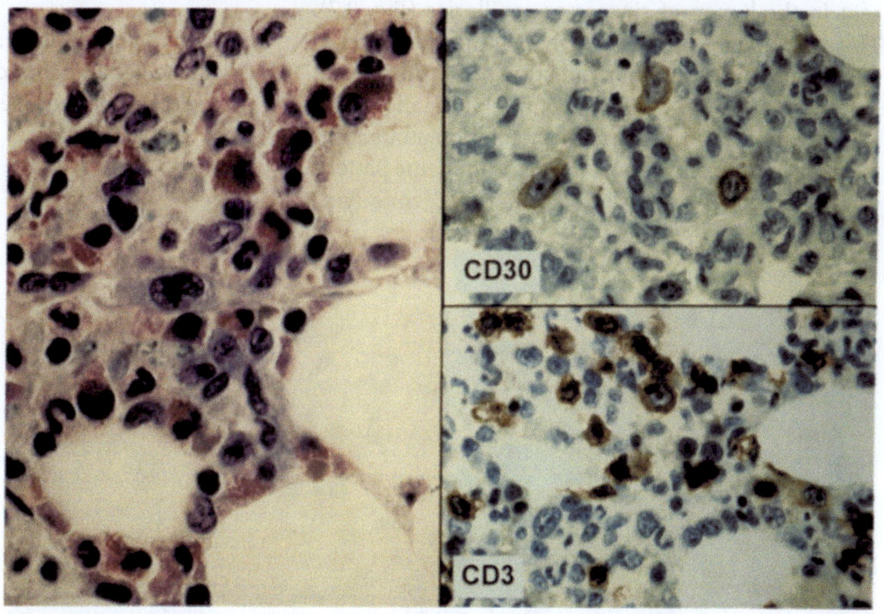

Fig. 9.6. Monocellular dispersion of large lymphoma cells (Giemsa stain), expressing CD30 and CD3, in an anaplastic large-cell lymphoma of NK/T type (both immunoperoxidase)

9.1.2.4
Monocellular Dispersion

This type of involvement can be defined as the presence of lymphomatous cells dispersed between normal hematopoietic cells without architectural modification and without myelofibrosis, representing a kind of minimal interstitial infiltrate. This pattern is very rarely observed, mostly in anaplastic large-cell lymphoma (Fig. 9.6) T/null type, or as residual disease in some lymphomas, e.g. hairy cell leukemia. Often, it is only recognized by immunohistochemistry.

9.1.3 Intrasinusoidal Infiltrate

This can be defined as the presence of lymphomatous cells in venous sinuses, often distended, and/or in capillaries. The number of cells is usually not high and the cells are separated from each other. An intrasinusal lymphomatous infiltrate may be associated with normal cells or erythrophagocytic histiocytes. A careful and systematic examination of the sinuses has to be done. When lymphoid cells are present in capillaries, they form an Indian-file pattern, which is often difficult to recognize and to distinguish from an interstitial infiltrate.

Different types of lymphoma can be responsible for an intrasinusal infiltrate.

Primary Splenic Marginal Zone Lymphoma. Small to medium-sized lymphoid cells with round nuclei, dense chromatin, and medium-sized pale cytoplasm are present in the lumen of sinuses or capillaries (Fig. 9.7). This type of intrasinusal involvement may be associated with nodules and/or an interstitial infiltrate or even a massive infiltrate. At the beginning of the disease or after treatment, an intravascular lymphomatous infiltrate may be the only lesion. Recently, the same pattern was observed in primary nodal-marginal zone lymphoma.

Hairy Cell Leukemia. The same vascular pattern as described for primary splenic or nodal marginal zone lymphoma has been observed; however, the typical infiltrate is mostly interstitial, associated with focal reinforcement. There are no nodules. In the past, when treatment was not effective, massive involvement was observed in advanced stages.

Intravascular Large-B-Cell Lymphoma. Large cells with the morphology of centroblast, immunoblast, anaplastic large-cells and a B immunophenotype. There is no interstitial or nodular or massive infiltrate. Erythrophagocytic histiocytes may be associated.

Anaplastic Large-Cell Lymphoma, T/Null Type. Large typical anaplastic cells with a T or null immunophenotype and expressing activated cell markers (CD30, EMA, ALK-1). This type of lymphoma can be associated with a monocellular dispersion or an interstitial infiltrate.

Hepatosplenic Lymphoma. Medium-sized cells with irregular nuclei and abundant pale cytoplasm, with a typical immunophenotype.

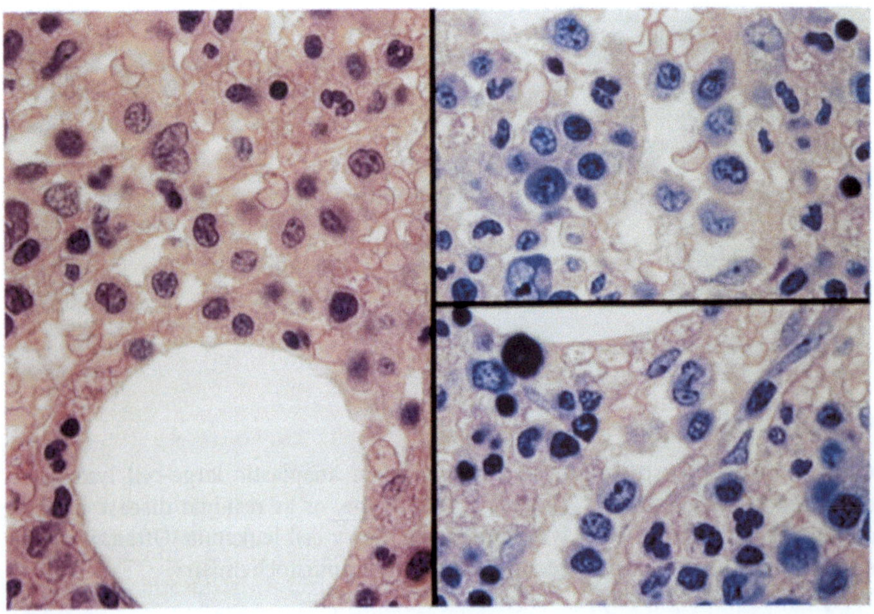

Fig. 9.7. Intrasinusal infiltrate in a splenic marginal zone lymphoma (left: H and E stain, right: Giemsa stain)

Table 9.1. Pattern of bone marrow involvement in the different types of malignant lymphoma. *ALC* Anaplastic large-cell, *AIBTCL* Angioimmunoblastic T-cell lymphoma, *NK* natural killer cell, *T-CLL* T-cell chronic lymphocytic leukemia with azurophilic granules, *B-CLL* B-cell chronic lymphocytic leukemia

Patterns	Paratrabecular infiltrate	Intertrabecular infiltrate	Interstitial localized	Interstitial diffuse	Nodular	Nodular plus interstitial	Nodular with marginal differentiation	Nodular with reactive germinal center	Monocellular dispersion	Massive localized	Massive diffuse	Intrasinusal
T-cell lymphomas												
ALC			+						+	+	+	+
Peripheral, unspecified			+	+						+	+	
AIBTCL			+	+						+	+	
Panniculitic			+	+						?	?	
Hepatosplenic			+	+						?	+	+
Intestinal			+	+						?	?	
Nasal			+	+						?	?	
Mycosis fungoides/ Sézary's syndrome			+	+						+	+	
Adult leukemia lymphoma			+	+		+				+	+	
Aggressive NK				+						+	+	
T-CLL			+	+								
T-prolymphocytic			+	+						+		
B-cell lymphomas												
Burkitt's										+	+	
Large-B-cell	+				+					+	+	(+)[a]
Hairy cell			+	+								+
Follicular	+				+		+			+	+	
Splenic marginal zone	+		+		+	+	+	+			+	+
Mantle-cell			+	+		+				+	+	
Lymphoplasmacytic			+	+						+	+	
B-CLL				+							+	
Hodgkin's lymphoma	+				+	+				+	+	

[a] Intravascular large B-cell lymphomas

9.2 Associated Lesions or Modifications

9.2.1 Reticulum Fibers Framework

An increase of collagen fibers or *myelofibrosis* is often observed in bone marrow localizations of ML. Myelofibrosis can be demonstrated by different techniques based on silver impregnation (Gomori, Gordon-Sweet, Goldner, etc.). The use of trichromic staining according to the method of Masson or Van Gieson is not really useful. Myelofibrosis may develop such that the architecture of the framework is preserved but the fibers are thickened and increased in number. Myelofibrosis can also be *mutilating, destroying* the normal architecture. It is usually present in areas involved by lymphoma and can be either *localized,* mainly when the lymphomatous infiltrate is patchy or nodular, or it can be *diffuse,* mainly when the lymphomatous infiltrate is also diffuse and often massive.

9.2.2 Vascular Modifications

Sinuses are often distended in patients with myelofibrosis. In some types of ML, arteriolocapillary hyperplasia can be observed, for example, in peripheral T-cell lymphoma of AILD (angioimmunoblastic lymphadenopathy with dysproteinemia) type. The lumen of the vessels should be studied carefully due to the possible presence of hemophagocytic (erythrophagocytic) histiocytes and, more importantly, of lymphomatous cells. (see Chap. 1.6).

9.2.3 Reactive Changes

9.2.3.1 Interstitial Edema

Interstitial edema with or without hemorrhages and/or fibrin deposits with a stellate pattern are more often seen in patients after treatment of lymphoma than in untreated patients.

9.2.3.2 Polyclonal Plasmacytosis

Polyclonal plasmacytosis is often observed associated or not with lymphomatous involvement. The mature plasma cells are mainly present around arterioles and capillaries.

9.2.3.3 Reactive Lymphoid Nodules

These nodules may be present in association with lymphomatous involvement or in the absence thereof and thus should not be confused with such an involvement. Reactive lymphoid nodules are always present in the center of bone marrow spaces, at a distance from bone trabeculae. Large nodules may develop contact with the bone trabeculae but only at their convexity. Such nodules are often associated with a sinus, a capillary, or a venule. They may present as a homogeneous pattern or show a marginal zone hyperplasia. Sometimes, a reactive germinal center can be recognized. This pattern is mostly regarded as reactive. But in a few patients with bone marrow involvement during the evolution of a primary splenic or nodal marginal zone lymphoma, a reactive germinal center surrounded by a neoplastic marginal zone can be observed.

These reactive lymphoid nodules should not exceed two or three on a BMB. Reactive lymphoid nodules are not associated with interstitial infiltrates. They consist of a mixture of B- and T-cells with a network of follicular dendritic cells.

9.2.3.4 Chronic Inflammation

Epithelioid cell clusters or *granulomas* with or without giant cells can be recognized in the bone marrow in patients with ML. They can be associated with typical ML involvement, but can also occur in the absence of neoplastic involvement. *Diffuse histiocytosis with hemophagocytosis (mostly erythrophagocytosis)* can be recognized, again even in the absence of ML. This pattern can be associated with an *activated histiocyte (macrophage) syndrome* which can have a fatal outcome.

9.2.3.5 Eosinophilic Necrosis

Eosinophilic necrosis, often of ischemic nature, destroys large areas of bone marrow tissue infiltrated by lymphoma. It occurs particularly in B- or T-cell lymphoblastic lymphoma and in acute leukemia as well as follicular or large-B-cell lymphoma.

9.2.3.6 Modifications of the Normal Hematopoietic Cell Lines

Hyperplasia of one, two, or three normal hematopoietic cell lines can be observed in patients with certain types of lymphoma with or without lymphomatous involvement of the bone marrow. Such hyperplasia, particularly of megakaryocytes, is frequently observed in patients with splenic lymphoma. There is often an associated reactive plasmacytosis as well as eosinophilia.

Hypoplasia of one, two, or three cell lines is observed mainly after treatment, with or without a myelodysplastic pattern.

Bone marrow modifications following treatment is a very important topic but is beyond the scope of this book. Four types of modifications are important to recognize: those due to the various types of bone marrow grafts, those due to the use of growth factors and/or multi-agent chemotherapy, and, finally, the difficult question of residual disease.

9.3 Diagnosis of Bone Marrow Involvement According to the Different Types of Lymphoma

The diagnosis is based on the pattern of the infiltration, on the morphology of the cells and on the presence or absence of myelofibrosis (Lambertenghi-Deliliers et al. 1992; McKenna 1992; Schmid and Isaacson 1992; Brunning and McKenna 1994).

9.3.1 Small B-Cell Lymphoma (Kroft et al. 1995)

9.3.1.1 B-Cell Chronic Lymphocytic Leukemia

- Pattern: About 50–95% of the bone marrow is involved either by an interstitial diffuse infiltrate without or with focal reinforcement, sometimes nodular, or a massive diffuse infiltrate. There is no paratrabecular infiltrate. Sometimes, proliferation centers are present. Patients with non-diffuse infiltrate have a better prognosis than those with a diffuse infiltrate (Rozman et al. 1984).
- Cell Morphology: Small lymphocytes with round nucleus, dense chromatin, and sometimes slight nuclear irregularities.
- Myelofibrosis: Absent.

9.3.1.2 B-Prolymphocytic Leukemia

- Pattern: Diffuse interstitial infiltrate with focal reinforcement (nodular) or a diffuse massive infiltrate.
- Cell morphology: Medium-sized lymphoid cells with large cytoplasm, round nucleus with dispersed chromatin, and a single, large, centrally situated nucleolus.

9.3.1.3 Lymphoplasmacytic Lymphoma

- Pattern: Interstitial localized or diffuse infiltrate with focal reinforcement, sometimes nodular. There is no paratrabecular infiltrate and no proliferative centers.
- Cell morphology: Plasma cells, lymphoplasmacytoid cells, less than 20% large cells (immunoblasts, plasmablasts); PAS positive intranuclear vacuoles (see Chap. 4.2.1.2).
- Myelofibrosis: Frequent, preservation of the normal architecture, localized or diffuse.

9.3.1.4 Follicular Lymphoma

- Pattern: Bone marrow replacement (25–50%), paratrabecular infiltrate (Fig. 9.1) either nodular or band-like along bone trabeculae in all the cases,

with in one third of the cases nodules in the bone marrow spaces (Fig. 9.4), but very rarely interstitial infiltrate.
- Cell morphology: Typical small and medium centrocytes sometimes large centrocytes (Fig. 9.4), often only a few centroblasts . Often the cell population is smaller than in the peripheral nodes. The presence of a follicular dendritic cell network and marginal zone differentiation can be observed (See Chap. 4.2.1.6).
- Myelofibrosis: Preservation of the normal architecture, localized around the lymphomatous cells, along the bone trabecular around or in the nodules.

9.3.1.5 Mantle Cell Lymphoma

- Pattern: Intertrabecular nodules replace 5–95 % of the bone marrow (Fig. 9.5) in about two thirds of the patients. There is often a paratrabecular infiltrate (about 50 % of the patients) and an interstitial infiltrate in more than two thirds of the patients (Fig. 9.3), but no proliferative center, no germinal center (Wasman et al. 1996; Pittaluga et al. 1996).
- Cell morphology: Mixture of small lymphocytes resembling the cells in B-cell chronic lymphocytic leukemia (B-CLL) and of small to medium-sized cells with an irregular nucleus, no large B-cells, occasionally presence of large clear histiocytes without tingible bodies.
- Myelofibrosis: Absent.

9.3.1.6 Primary Splenic and Nodal and Extranodal Marginal Zone Lymphoma

- Pattern: Pure intrasinusal infiltrate coinciding with early bone marrow involvement (Fig. 9.7), particularly in patients with peripheral blood villous lymphocytosis (Labouyrie et al. 1997; Franco et al. 1996). In more advanced disease, there is an interstitial infiltrate and nodules, either paratrabecular (Fig. 9.1) or intertrabecular (Fig. 9.6). Some of the nodules have a marginal zone (Fig. 9.6) and more rarely a reactive germinal center. A massive infiltrate can develop years after disease evolution.
- Cell morphology: Association of monocytoid B-cells and centrocytoid B-cells with more or less abundant clear cytoplasm. In about half of the patients (Duong et al. 2000) plasma cells with intracytoplasmic monotypic immunoglobulins are found (see Chap. 6.10.1.2).
- Myelofibrosis: Absent.

9.3.1.7 Hairy Cell Leukemia

- Pattern: Interstitial focal or diffuse infiltrate, rarely massive.
- Cell morphology: Medium-sized cells with ovoid, kidney-shaped nuclei and an abundant pale cytoplasm regularly disposed around the nucleus (Hounieu et al. 1992). There is a typical distribution of nuclei separated by identical clear spaces (see Chap. 6.10.1.1).
- Myelofibrosis: Constant only in the areas infiltrated by hairy cells. The normal framework architecture is preserved but thickened.

9.3.1.8 Myeloma

(See Chap. 7.1)

9.3.1.9 Differential Diagnosis

The difficulty in the differential diagnosis is to distinguish B-CLL from mantle cell lymphoma, due to the possible presence in B-CLL of some nuclear irregularities and in mantle cell lymphoma of the possible predominance of lymphoid cells with roundish nuclei. The discovery of proliferative centers is a good argument for B-CLL. Immunophenotyping is useful, particularly the expression of cyclin D1, which indicates a mantle cell lymphoma. In the absence of these morphologic and immunophenotypic criteria, demonstration of bcl-1 rearrangement by PCR and the presence of a t(11;14) by cytogenetics is needed.

Nodular patterns can be observed mainly in follicular, mantle cell, and marginal zone lymphomas. If the morphologic criteria are not clear enough to allow a diagnosis, then the immunophenotype, molecular genetic techniques, and cytogenetics are useful.

In the presence of plasmacytoid differentiation with intracytoplasmic monotypic immunoglobulins, the immunophenotype and the presence of proliferative centers are good arguments for diagnosing the lymphoplasmacytoid variant of B-CLL. In lymphoplasmacytic lymphoma, the pattern is not nodular and marginal zone differentiation with monocytoid B-cells is absent. Clinical data and the type of immunoglobulins secreted are useful in distinguishing some lymphoplasmacytic lymphomas from myeloma and marginal zone lymphoma.

9.3.2 Large-B-Cell Lymphoma

- Pattern: Patchy or massive infiltrate contacting the bone trabeculae .
- Cell morphology: All types of centroblastic and immunoblastic lymphoma (see Chap. 4.2.2.2). Remember that immunoblastic lymphoma with or without plasmablastic differentiation may represent a transformation from myeloma (hence the importance of clinical data).
- Myelofibrosis
- Variants: These are described below (Chap. 9.3.2.1 and 9.3.2.2).

9.3.2.1 T-Cell-Rich/Histiocyte-Rich Large-B-Cell Lymphoma

- Pattern: Patchy or massive infiltrate of small lymphoid cells with a variable number of histiocytes or epithelioid cells.
- Cell morphology: Large cells dispersed (see Chap. 4.2.2.2) in a sea of small or medium-sized T-lymphocytes.
- Myelofibrosis: Localized in the infiltrates. Immunohistochemistry is valuable in the diagnosis of this type of lymphoma (see Chap. 4.2.2.2).

9.3.2.2 Intravascular Large B-Cell Lymphoma

- Pattern: Accumulation of large-B-cells in the lumen of vessels mostly sinuses.
- Cell morphology: See Chap. 6.18. Possible association with erythrophagocytic histiocytosis (Dufau et al. 2000).
- Myelofibrosis: Absent.

9.3.3 Burkitt's Lymphoma

- Pattern: Patchy or massive infiltrate.
- Cell morphology: (see Chap. 4.2.3).
- Myelofibrosis: Localized, systematic in the infiltrates.

9.3.4 Precursor Cell Lymphoma (B- and T-Cell Lymphoblastic Lymphoma or Acute Leukemia)

- Pattern: Interstitial diffuse infiltrate, sometimes massive, with necrotic areas.
- Cell morphology: Medium-sized cells with pale or faintly stained cytoplasm, ovoid nuclei, sometimes convoluted, inconspicuous nucleoli (see Chaps. 4.1, 5.1). Immunophenotyping is necessary to distinguish B- and T-cell types.
- Myelofibrosis: Localized or diffuse, sometimes associated with a poor prognosis.

9.3.5 NK/T-Cell Lymphoma

As for B-cell lymphoma, the diagnosis of bone marrow involvement by NK/T-cell lymphoma is based on the pattern of infiltration, the cell morphology and the presence or absence of myelofibrosis (Caulet et al. 1990; Gaulard et al. 1991).

9.3.5.1 T-Prolymphocytic Leukemia

- Pattern: Diffuse interstitial infiltrate.
- Cell morphology: Medium-sized lymphoid cells with round nuclei and a central medium-sized nucleolus.
- Myelofibrosis: Absent.

9.3.5.2 T-Cell Large Granular Lymphocytic Leukemia

- Pattern: Interstitial infiltrate minimal and initially localized , then diffuse.
- Cell morphology: Lymphocytes with a large pale cytoplasm, but azurophilic granules are only seen on smears (see Chap. 6.10.1.8).
- Myelofibrosis: Absent.

9.3.5.3
Peripheral T-Cell Leukemia Lymphoma, Unspecified

- Pattern: Interstitial infiltrate localized or with focal enlargement (patchy), sometimes paratrabecular infiltrate.
- Cell morphology: Small, medium-sized or large lymphoid cells with irregular nuclei and large pale cytoplasm (see Chap. 5.2.2.2).
- Myelofibrosis: Localized around the neoplastic cell infiltrates.
- Variants:
  - *Adult T-cell leukemia lymphoma*: Same pattern and cell population as in peripheral T-cell leukemia lymphoma, unspecified.
  - *Lymphoepithelioid T-cell lymphoma* : Same pattern as in peripheral T-cell leukemia lymphoma, unspecified; presence of nests of epithelioid cells.
  - *Mycosis fungoides/Sézary's syndrome* : Same pattern as in peripheral T-cell leukemia lymphoma, unspecified; presence of lymphoid cells with cerebriform nuclei (Salhany et al. 1989).

9.3.5.4
Peripheral T-Cell Lymphoma, Angioimmunoblastic

- Pattern: Patchy with localized interstitial infiltrate, sometimes paratrabecular, vascular hyperplasia in the infiltrated areas.
- Cell morphology: Medium-sized and large lymphoid cells with pale cytoplasm in reactive cells (plasma cells, eosinophils, histiocytes, epithelioid cells and B-immunoblasts).
- Myelofibrosis: Localized in the infiltrated areas.

9.3.5.5
Anaplastic Large-Cell Lymphoma

- Pattern: Intravascular or interstitial monocellular infiltrate (Fig.) can be seen or sometimes massive dense localized infiltrate (Fraga et al. 1995; Wong et al. 1991).
- Cell morphology: Large anaplastic cells and Reed-Sternberg giant cells (see Chap. 5.2.2.4).
- Myelofibrosis: Localized in patchy or massive infiltrate.

9.3.5.6
Hepatosplenic T-Cell Lymphoma

- Pattern: Intrasinusal accumulation of neoplastic lymphoid cells.
- Cell morphology: Medium-sized cells with ovoid nuclei (see Chap. 6.10.1.7) and sometimes erythrophagocytic histiocytosis.
- Myelofibrosis: Absent.

9.3.5.7
General Comments

Immunohistochemistry is mandatory for the diagnosis of all types of NK/T-cell lymphoma and particularly of anaplastic large-cell lymphoma.

9.4
Differential Diagnosis

The following lesions or diseases should be distinguished from bone marrow lymphoma involvement.

9.4.1
Reactive Lymphoid Nodules

These are normally observed in elderly patients and are often present in patients with dysimmune disorders; they may be seen in patients with lymphomas even in the absence of bone marrow involvement. Other characteristics are:

- Less than three nodules in one bone marrow trephine biopsy.
- No paratrabecular localization.
- No interstitial infiltrate. No myelofibrosis. Sometimes reactive germinal centers.
- Mixture of B- and T-lymphoid cells.

Reactive lymphoid nodules are sometimes very difficult to distinguish from lymphoma. Clinical data and evaluation of immunoglobulin gene rearrangement are important for the diagnosis.

9.4.2 Reactive Intravascular Lymphocytosis

Small lymphoid cells, sometimes binucleated, expressing B-cell markers have been observed in female patients with peripheral-blood B lymphocytosis who are heavy smokers (Labouyrie et al. 1997).

9.4.3 Hodgkin's Lymphoma

The involvement may be patchy or massive and consists of collagenous fibrosis infiltrated by reactive lymphoid cells, plasma cells, and eosinophils surrounding typical Reed-Sternberg cells.

9.4.4 Non-lymphoid Acute Leukemia

Interstitial infiltrate with focal reinforcement or massive infiltrate. Cytological evaluation of imprints, immunohistochemistry, etc., are of diagnostic value.

9.4.5 Systemic Mastocytosis

There is an interstitial localized or massive infiltrate with collagenous fibrosis. Medium-sized cells with ovoid or kidney-shaped nuclei and a large cytoplasm containing numerous basophilic granules make up the infiltrate. Cytological evaluation of smears, the use of Giemsa staining, and tryptase demonstration by immunohistochemistry on histological sections are of diagnostic value.

9.4.6 Undifferentiated Carcinoma

This should be discussed only when considering a diagnosis of large B-cell or anaplastic large-cell lymphoma T/null-cell type. Immunohistochemistry and analysis of the expression of cytokeratin as well as CD45 negativity are useful.

References

Bartl R, Frisch B, Fateh-Moghadam A, Kettner G, Jaeger K, Sommerfeld W (1987) Histologic classification and staging of multiple myeloma. A retrospective and prospective study of 674 cases. Am J Clin Pathol 87:342–355

Brunning RD, McKenna RD (1994) Tumors of the bone marrow. Armed Forces Institute of Pathology, Washington DC

Caulet S, Delmer A, Audouin J, Le Tourneau A, Bernadou A, Zittoun R, Diebold J (1990) Histopathological study of bone marrow biopsies in 30 cases of T-cell lymphoma with clinical, biological and survival correlations. Hematol Oncol 8:155–168

Dufau JP, Le Tourneau A, Molina T, Le Houcq M, Claessens YE, Rio B, Delmer A, Diebold J (2000) Intravascular large B-cell lymphoma with bone marrow involvement at presentation and haemophagocytic syndrome: two western cases in favour of a specific variant. Histopathology 37:509–512

Duong Van Huyen JP, Molina T, Delmer A, Audouin J, Le Tourneau A, Zittoun R, Bernadou A, Diebold J (2000) Splenic marginal zone lymphoma with or without plasmacytic differentiation. Am J Surg Pathol 24:1581–1592

Fraga M, Brousset P, Schlaifer D, Payen C, Robert A, Rubie H, Huguet-Rigal F, Delsol G (1995) Bone marrow involvement in anaplastic large cell lymphoma. Am J Clin Pathol 103:82–89

Franco V, Florena AM, Campesi G (1996) Intrasinusoidal bone marrow infiltration: a possible hallmark of splenic lymphoma. Histopathology 29:571–575

Gaulard P, Kanavarros P, Farcet JP, Rocha FD, Haioun C, Divine M, Reyes F, Zafrani ES (1991) Bone marrow histologic and immunohistochemical findings in peripheral T-cell lymphoma: a study of 38 cases. Hum Pathol 22:331–338

Hounieu H, Chittal SM, Al Saati T, de Mascarel A, Sabattini E, Pileri S, Falini B, Ralfkiaer E, Le Tourneau A, Selves J, Voigt JJ, Laurent G, Diebold J, Delsol G (1992) Hairy cell leukemia. Diagnosis of bone marrow involvement in paraffin-embedded sections with monoclonal antibody DBA-44. Am J Clin Pathol 98:26–33

Kroft SH, Finn WG, Peterson LC (1995) The pathology of the chronic lymphoid leukaemias. Blood 9:234–250

Labouyrie F, Marit G, Vial JP, Lacombe F, Fialon P, Bernard P, Mascarel A de, Merlio JP (1997) Intrasinusoidal bone marrow involvement by splenic lymphoma with villous lymphocytes: a helpful immunohistologic feature. Mod Pathol 10:1015–1020

Lambertenghi-Deliliers G, Annaloro C, Soligo D, Oriani A, Pozzoli E, Quirica N, Luksca R, Polli EE (1992) Incidence and histological features of bone marrow involvement in malignant lymphomas. Ann Hematol 65:61–65

McKenna RW (1992) The bone marrow manifestations of Hodgkin's disease, non-Hodgkin's lymphomas and lymphoma-like disorders. In: Knowles DB (ed) Neoplastic hematopathology. Williams and Wilkins, New York, pp 1135–1180

Pittaluga S, Verhoef G, Criel A, Maes A, Nuyts J, Bougaerts M, De Wolf-Peeters C (1996) Prognostic significance of bone marrow trephine and peripheral blood smears in 55 patients with mantle cell lymphoma. Leuk Lymph 21:115–125

Rozman C, Montserrat E, Rodriguez-Fernandez JM et al (1984) Bone marrow histologic pattern: the best single prognostic parameter in chronic lymphocytic leukemia. A multivariate survival analysis of 329 cases. Blood 64:642–648

Salhany KE, Greer JP, Cousar JB et al (1989) Marrow involvement in cutaneous T-cell lymphoma. A clinicopathologic study of 60 cases. Am J Clin Pathol 92:747–754

Schmid C, Isaacson PG (1992) Bone marrow trephine biopsy in lymphoproliferative disease. J Clin Pathol 45:745–750

Wasman J, Rosenthal NS, Fahri DC (1996) Mantle cell lymphoma. Morphologic findings in bone marrow involvement. Am J Clin Pathol 106:196–200

Wong KF, Chang JKC, Ng CS, Chu YC, Lam PWWY, Yen HL (1991) Anaplastic large cell Ki-1 lymphoma involving bone marrow: marrow findings and association with reactive hemophatocytosis. Am J Hematol 37:112–119

Chapter 10

Practical Advice: Methods for the Diagnosis of Malignant Lymphoma

10.1 The Diagnosis of Malignant Lymphoma

10.1.1 Practical Tips

1. The diagnosis of lymphoma begins with the biopsy excision. The surgeon must avoid squeezing the tissue and must obtain a specimen of adequate size. If possible, imprints from the freshly cut surface of the node should be prepared by carefully touching it on well-degreased glass slides. If adequate material is available, one piece should be shock-frozen immediately (best within 10 min after excision in order to also preserve RNA). A representative part of the tissue should then be immediately placed in fixative.
2. As a rule, fixation for 6 – 12 h in diluted (4 – 6 %) *buffered formalin* is sufficient. Tissue pieces should be not larger than 1.5 cm at their largest diameter. Sections of especially high cytological quality are obtained from tissue fixed in special solutions, such as one consisting of 750 ml absolute alcohol, 200 ml undiluted formalin, and 50 ml acetic acid. Bouin's fixative is not recommended. Moreover, proper dehydration with high-quality alcohol is of major importance.
3. The most common faults in the processing of lymph nodes are *embedding* the tissue improperly and inadequate *sectioning and stretching* of sections. Embedding in paraffin (Paraplast) is sufficient for routine diagnoses. To analyze cytological details, lymph nodes must be embedded more carefully than other specimens. Hence it is essential to separately embed lymph nodes. The improvement in quality is often so dramatic that it is hard to believe that one is looking at the same tissue (Fig. 10.1a and b).
4. When the lymph node has been properly embedded, it is easy to prepare 4-μm thick sections. Stretching or drying of the sections at too high temperatures (> 45 °C; see Table 10.1) must be avoided. Figure 10.2 shows examples of poorly (Fig. 10.2a) and well-cut (Fig. 10.2b) sections from the same paraffin block.
5. In the diagnosis of lymph node lesions, *Giemsa staining* is the most useful (Fig. 10.3). It is the only method that allows a precise cytological diagnosis according to the rules of hematology. The staining must be of high quality (Table 10.2). A poor Giemsa stain is worse than none at all. The stock solutions

Table 10.1. Preparation of high-quality sections

Fixation (4 – 6 % buffered formalin)
Tissue processing:

Step	Solution	Hours
1	70 % alcohol	1
2	96 % alcohol	1
3	96 % alcohol	1
4	100 % alcohol	1
5	100 % alcohol	1
6	100 % alcohol	1.5
7	Xylene	1
8	Xylene	1
9	Xylene	1.5
10	Paraplast+	1
11	Paraplast+	2
12	Paraplast+	2

Embedding: Paraplast or Paraplast+ in an embedding mould

Cutting: Cut sections. Use a Feather knife holder and disposable blades (S35). Remove four or five sections and dispose of them so as to avoid holes and cracks.
Float the sections on warm water (40 – 42 °C). Remove wrinkles and bubbles.

Drying: 2 h at 42 °C or 5 min at 45 – 50 °C and 5 min at 80 °C.

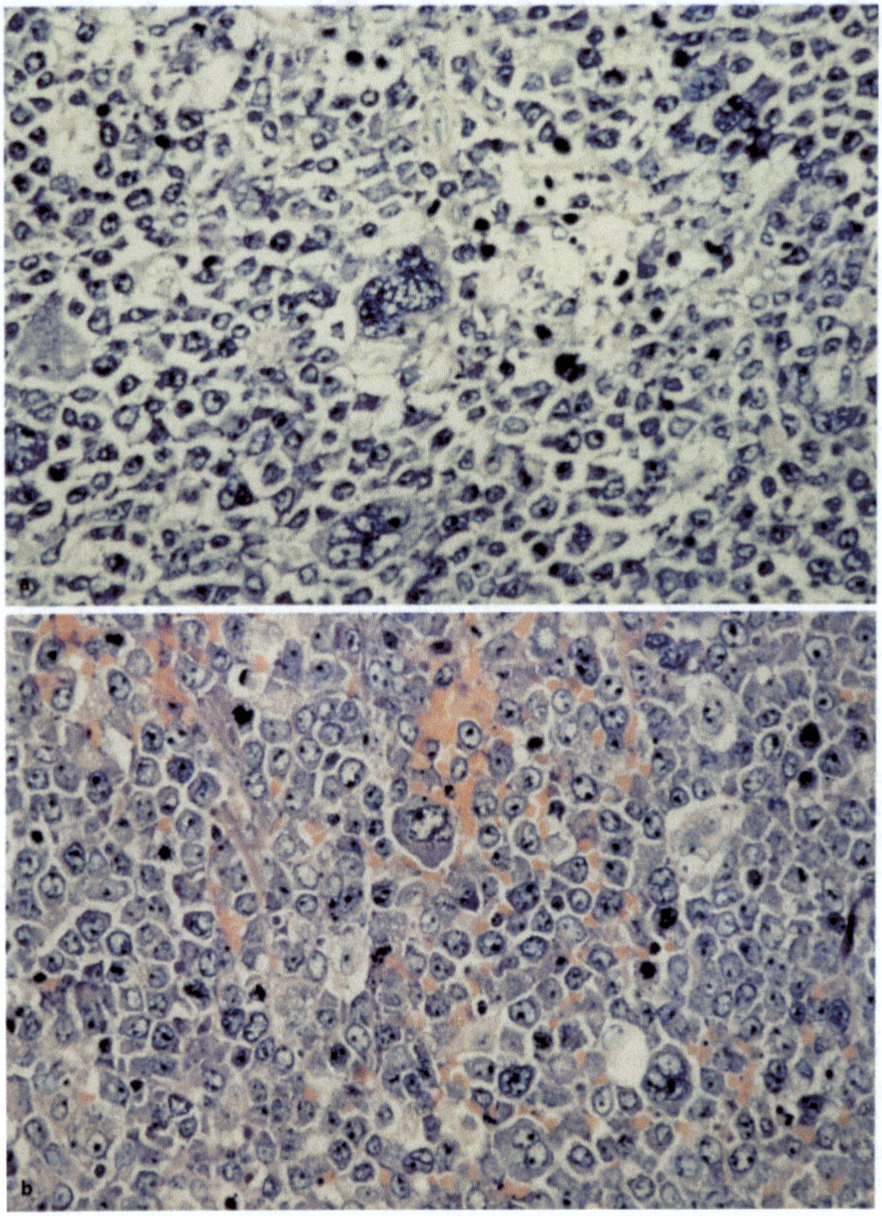

Fig. 10.1. a Original Giemsa-stained section of a lymph node with a blastic lymphoma. **b** Re-embedding of the material and new section also in Giemsa stain shows a typical Burkitt's morphology

should be purchased from Merck (Darmstadt, Germany); the results obtained with other Giemsa solutions are, as a rule, poor and often worthless. In addition to the Giemsa-stained slides, one should always examine sections stained by silver impregnation (e.g. Gomori's method), with periodic acid-Schiff (PAS) and with hematoxylin and eosin (H and E)

6. Imprints are very useful in cytological analysis. For this purpose, we stain them with Pappenheim (May-Grünwald-Giemsa) no earlier and, if possible, not much later than 1 day after biopsy.
7. One should examine lymph node sections (and imprints) *before* looking at the clinical data. Not until a preliminary diagnosis has been made should the clinical data be checked to see whether they

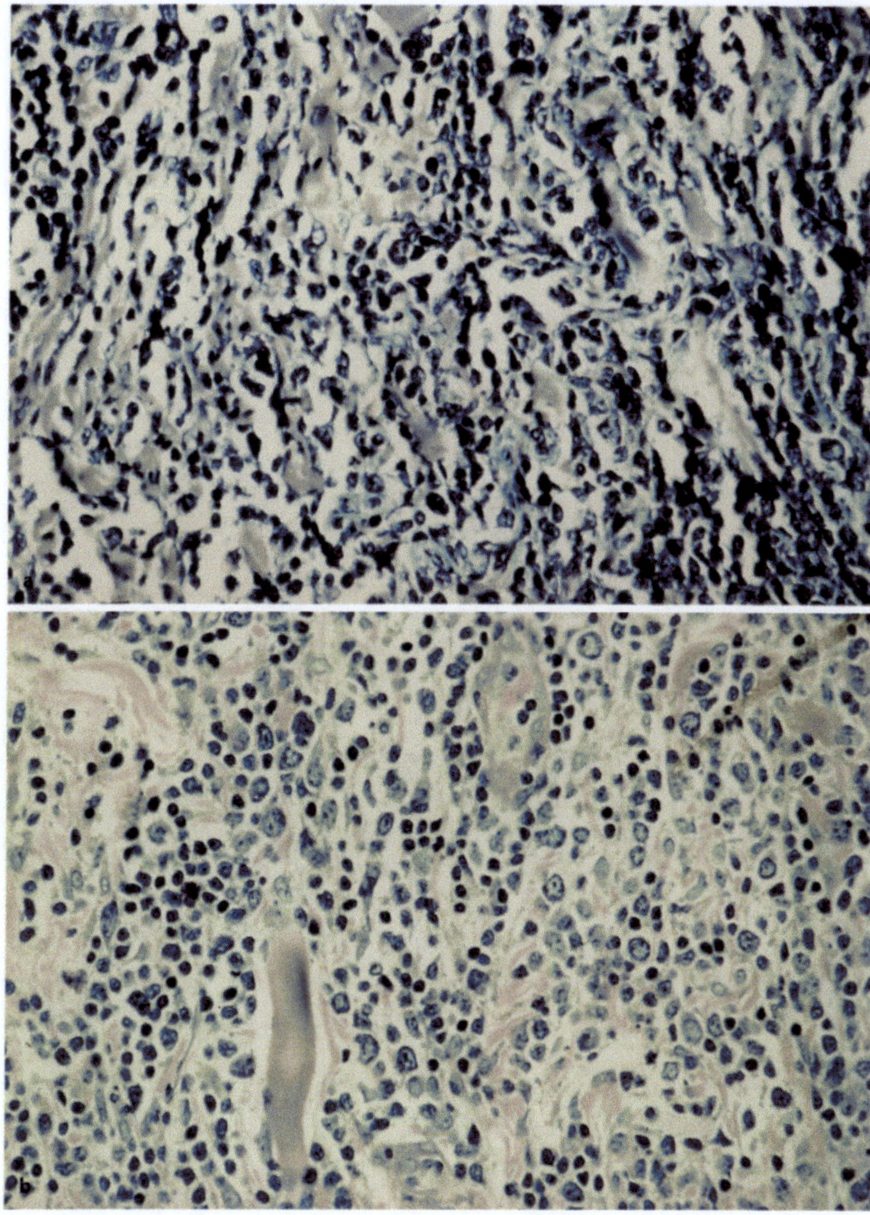

Fig. 10.2. a Giemsa-stained original section; note the poor morphology of the infiltrate and shrinking artifacts. **b** New, well performed section from the same paraffin block with standardized Giemsa stain reveals a diffuse follicular lymphoma in the skin

agree with the morphological picture. The reverse procedure often puts the pathologist on the wrong track, or at least precludes an objective, independent evaluation. The most important clinical information is the age of the patient.

8. Every histological examination of a lymph node begins with microscopy at low magnification in order to determine whether the lymph node architecture is effaced or intact. It is generally effaced in malignant neoplasms. One should be cautious, however, because it may also be effaced in reactive processes (viral infections such as Epstein-Barr virus) and at least partially intact in partial infiltrations of malignant neoplasms. At low magnification, it is also possible to recognize focal lesions (e.g. small areas of necrosis), metastatic tumors, and lesions in

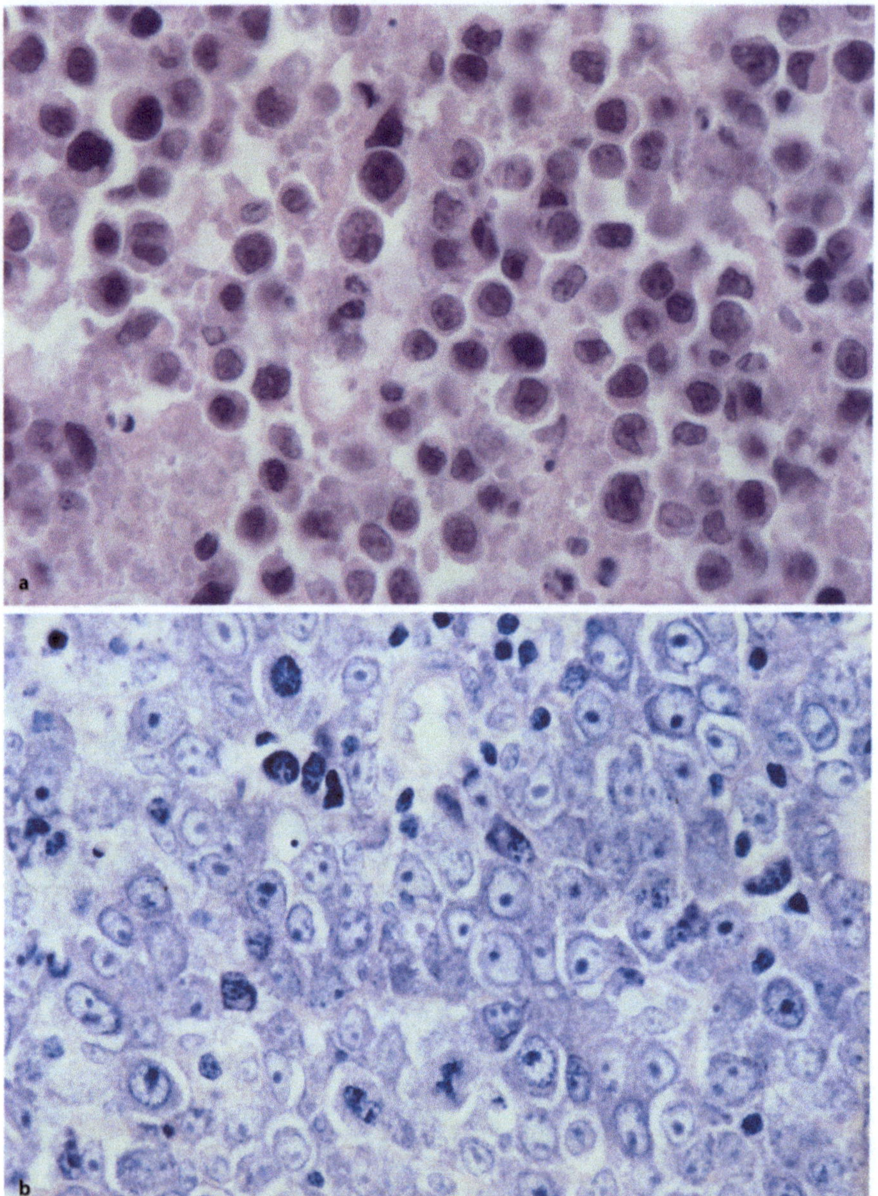

Fig. 10.3. a Original section (H and E) stain of a diffuse large-B-cell lymphoma. **b** Re-sectioning the same block and staining for Giemsa perfectly reveals the morphology of a B-immunoblastic lymphoma. The chromatin and the cytoplasm are well-stained with Giemsa

the tissue surrounding the lymph node. A nodular pattern is of particular diagnostic significance. This approach is also valuable for extranodal lymphoproliferations.

9. When the lymph node architecture is effaced, i.e. when follicles or sinuses are not recognizable, cytological analysis at a higher, or the highest magnification must be performed to determine the nature of the malignant process. First, Giemsa-stained sections are examined to see whether there is a "monotonous" (uniform) or of a mixed population of cells. If the process is monotonous looking, one then determines whether the cells are small, medium-sized, or large. Other criteria for defining the type of cell are: nuclear shape; number, size and location of the nucleoli; and amount and staining of the cyto-

Table 10.2. Giemsa staining of paraffin sections (modified from Lennert 1952, 1961)

1. The de-waxed sections are removed from distilled water and put into the following solution for 1 h:
   80 ml distilled water
   20 ml Giemsa solution (Merck, Darmstadt, Germany)
2. The sections are removed from the Giemsa solution and put into 100 ml distilled water, to which 3–4 drops of undiluted glacial acetic acid have been added. The sections are agitated gently in this solution for a few seconds, slightly differentiated and then immediately put into:
3. 96% ethyl alcohol, in which they are differentiated further until the desired staining is achieved (microscopic control).
4. Differentiation is stopped and, at the same time, dehydration is achieved by dipping in 3 changes of isopropanol for 2 min each and
5. in 3 changes of xylene for 2 min each.
6. Mount with Eukitt (Kindler, Freiburg, Germany).
7. Results:

7a RNA, DNA: blue ("basophilic")
7b Acidophilic substances: pink or reddish orange
7c Acid mucopolysaccharides: reddish violet

plasm. Imprints are examined to find out more about chromatin structure; they also reveal the staining properties and the presence or absence of granules in the cytoplasm.

10. With silver impregnation it is particularly easy to survey the lymph node architecture and to recognize a nodular or follicular growth pattern. Moreover, the number and arrangement of small vessels (capillaries and venules) can be more clearly determined with silver impregnation than with any other stain. This is of minor importance in extranodal localizations. An increase in the number of capillaries may be indicative of a myelomonocytic neoplasm; an increase in the number of epithelioid venules may represent a T-cell neoplasm. The *density* of reticulin fibers is not, in general, a useful criterion. The fiber *pattern* also helps in making a distinction between tumor metastases and malignant lymphomas. Finally, silver impregnation of sections of totally necrotic lymph nodes makes the underlying architecture and, in many cases, even the tumor cells visible; this prevents a false diagnosis of a lymph node infarction and sometimes even makes it possible to determine the nature of a tumor (e.g. follicular lymphoma!).
11. When Giemsa staining reveals a monotonous looking proliferation of medium-sized cells ("lymphoblastic" proliferation), chloroacetate esterase staining or detection of myelomonocytic antigens, including CD34 and myeloperoxidase, to exclude the possibility of a myeloid neoplasm should be applied. When the blood picture is leukemic, blood smears may also be used.
12. Electron microscopy hardly provides more diagnostic information than does a technically good, light microscopic preparation. It is thus no more helpful in lymphoma diagnosis.
13. *Overall in 20–30% of* malignant lymphomas, it is necessary to apply immunohistochemical methods to make a distinct diagnosis. As a rule, these methods can be used in ambiguous cases to distinguish between T-cell and B-cell lymphomas and between lymphomas and non-lymphoid undifferentiated tumors. Today, most diagnostic immunohistochemical stainings can be done on paraffin sections.
    However, it is still a matter of discussion whether the diagnosis of a malignant lymphoma has to be proven in each case by immunohistochemistry. Working in a reference center for lymphoma diagnosis, we employ at least a basic panel of antibodies to each case to substantiate the diagnosis even if it is already clear on a purely morphological basis.
    – Even though one may have high expectations of immunohistochemistry, it is still possible to misinterpret the results. Consistent, useful results can be obtained only by regular application of the methods. An antibody may show a considerable number of cross-reactions; these must always be taken into consideration, especially when interpreting the expression of a single antigen. In a few cases, it is impossible to reconcile the immunohistochemical and morphological findings. When the actively proliferating cells are labeled clearly, we favor the immunohistochemical results. In all other discrepancies, one has to increase the number of immunohistochemical stains.
    – If even this approach does not achieve a consensus result, the discrepancy has to be reported and possibly discussed with the clinician.
14. When the morphological and immunohistochemical results are contradictory and the clonality of a

T-cell proliferation has to be proven, it is sensible to perform a molecular genetic analysis to determine the rearrangement of characteristic gene segments of the T-cell receptor (TCR). So far, this is the only method available for identifying the clonality of a T-cell lymphoproliferation. The method can also be used to determine the clonality of a B-cell proliferation, in which clonal Ig light-chain expression is not detectable. By applying molecular genetic techniques, it is possible to clarify the vast majority of doubtful cases, at least with respect to the clonality and cellular origin of the tumor. Again, a consensus between morphology, results of immunohistochemistry, and results of PCR analysis is essential, as it has become clear that the detection of clonality does not by itself indicate malignancy. This aspect has to be taken into particular account in skin biopsies.

15. The diagnostic report should be clear. If it was not possible to determine the exact type of lymphoma, proper treatment can still often be chosen if the pathologist states whether the lymphoma is a small-cell (so-called low-grade) or blastic/large-cell (so-called high-grade) malignancy. The pathologist should endeavor to provide this information in all cases, even if it means obtaining another biopsy.

10.2 Immunohistochemistry and Molecular Clonality Analysis in the Diagnosis of Lymphoma

An immunohistochemical analysis has four major aims:

1. Determining the cellular origin and distinguishing a lymphoma from non-lymphomatous neoplasms
2. Classification of the malignant lymphoma
3. Demonstration of the clonality of a lymphoproliferative process
4. Substantiation and objectification of the morphological diagnosis

To 1: A large number of antibodies that react with formalin-resistant antigens and which can be applied to *paraffin* sections is available. Using these antibodies, it is possible to determine in almost all of the ambiguous cases whether a neoplasm is a T-cell or B-cell lymphoma. Moreover, non-lymphoid tumors can also be recognized. This is especially important in the distinction of large-cell undifferentiated tumors. About 60–80% of those cases in which it is impossible to decide between an undifferentiated carcinoma and a lymphoma by morphology alone can be classified immunohistochemically as malignant lymphoma, most often as anaplastic large-cell lymphoma or diffuse large-B-cell lymphoma. Only a few antibodies are of high specificity, however. Hence several antibodies have to be used to draw up an antigen profile. Table 10.3 and 10.4 list the major antibodies that are suitable for diagnosis of a lymphoproliferation on formalin-fixed tissue. Systematic analysis of monoclonal and polyclonal antibodies on formalin-fixed tissue has resulted in a steadily growing number of useful reagents. Antibodies which can be used as first-line antibodies for confirming a lymphoma diagnosis are indicated in the table.

The antibodies in Table 10.3 are listed in defined clusters, allowing a comparative analysis when various antibodies are used. The clusters are defined by the antigens whose molecular weight has been determined.

The benign or malignant nature and the cellular origin of only a small number (about 5%) of lymphoproliferative processes cannot be clarified by examining paraffin sections stained by immunohistochemical methods.

An antigen profile of an infiltrate showing partial antigen loss compared to normal lymphoid cells is indicative of a neoplastic, non-reactive proliferation. This is especially helpful in the diagnosis of T-cell lymphomas. Viral infections in lymph nodes, however, may also result in partial antigen loss in blast cells.

To 2: The antigen profiles given in Tables 10.5–7 are characteristic immunohistochemical reaction patterns of malignant lymphoma. One must bear in mind, however, that there are no absolute criteria. Hence, a deviation from the characteristic antigen profile must be considered possible in each case (CD23-negative lymphocytic lymphomas, CD23-positive mantle lymphoma, etc.). Only the use of a combination of antibodies makes it possible to classify a lymphoma as a defined entity with a degree of certainty. It is not permissible to interpret the expression of a single antigen by itself.

To 3: The clonality of a lymphoproliferative process still serves as an important criterion for determining its benign or malignant nature. Although biclonal B-cell lymphomas, polyclonal Epstein-Barr virus (EBV)-induced B-cell lymphomas, and monoclonal benign

Table 10.3. Antigens listed according to their cluster of differentiation (CD). For these antigens, antibodies that react in formalin-fixed material are available. *FDC* Follicular dendritic cells, *ALCL* anaplastic large-cell lymphoma, *LGL* large granular lymphocytic leukemia

Cluster	Specifications: expression on normal lymphoid and hematopoietic cells	Neoplasia: expression on lymphoid and hematopoietic malignancies
CD1a	Cortical thymocytes, Langerhans' cells interdigitating cells	T-lymphoblastic, Langerhans cell histiocytosis
CD2	Immature and mature T-cells	T-cell lymphomas
CD3	Immature and mature T-cells	T-cell lymphomas
CD4	Helper/inducer T-cells	Most T-cell lymphomas
CD5	Most immature and mature T-cells	Most T-cell lymphomas+B-CLL+MCL
CD7	Cortical thymocytes, most peripheral T-cells	T-LB; most peripheral T-cell lymphomas
CD8	Suppressor/cytotoxic T-cells	Some T-cell lymphomas including NK/T
CD10	Cortical thymocytes	Lymphoblastic lymphomas; DLBCL-centroblastic, follicular lymphomas
CD13	Myelomonocytic cells; NK cells	Myelomonocytic neoplasms; some NK-cell neoplasms
CD14	Myelomonocytic cells	Myelomonocytic neoplasms
CD15	Granulocytes	Hodgkin and Reed-Sternberg cells
CD20	Most B-cells	Most B-cell lymphomas
CD21	B-cell subpopulation; FDC	Some B-cell lymphomas
CD23	Follicular mantle cells; FDC	B-cell lymphocytic lymphomas
CD25	Activated T-cells	Some T-cell lymphomas (HTLV-1+), HCL
CD30	Activated T- and B-cells	Hodgkin and Reed-Sternberg cells, ALCL
CD33	Immature myelomonocytic cells	Myelomonocytic neoplasms
CD34	Hematopoietic progenitor cells	Acute myelomonocytic leukemias
CD35	Myelomonocytic cells, B-lymphocytes, 10% T-cells; FDC	Myelomonocytic, B-cell and some T-cell neoplasms
CD38	Plasma cells	Plasmacytomas
CD45	All leukocytes	All lymphomas (exception 40% of ALCL are negative)
CD45RA	Many leukocytes, predominantly B-cells	Most B-cell lymphomas (not lineage specific)
CD45RB	Many leukocytes, predominantly B-cells	Most B-cell lymphomas (not lineage specific)
CD45R0	Many leukocytes-predominantly B-cells	Most B-cell lymphomas (not lineage specific)
CD56	NK/T-cells	NK/T-cells neoplasms
CD57	NK cells, LGL	LGL
CD68	Myelomonocytic cells	Myelomonocytic leukemias
CD72	B-cell subpopulation	Some B-cell lymphomas
CD79α	B-cell subpopulation; plasma cells	Some B-cell lymphomas, especially plasmacytomas, plasmablastic lymphomas
CD117	Hematopoietic stem cells; most cells	Acute myeloid leukemias

tumors (e.g. meningioma) have been described, in ambiguous cases clonality is still the most important diagnostic criterion of malignancy in addition to the histological and clinical pictures.

DNA extraction and subsequent PCR analysis for Ig heavy-chain genes as well as for TCR genes allows reliable demonstration of clonality in both the B-cell and the T-cell system. Depending on the use of different primers and the preceding method of formalin fixation, 70–80% of the clonal tumors can be detected.

During the differentiation of a cell in the B-cell or T-cell system, various segments of the genes coding for the TCR- and for Ig are rearranged. This means that gene segments located on different parts of a chromosome are first rearranged in order to form a functional gene that can then be transcribed. The rearranged gene segments or those that have remained in the germline can be fragmented by restriction enzymes and then electrophoretically separated. In a *polyclonal* lymphoproliferative process, this results in fragments of multiple sizes and thus a smear in PCR electrophoresis. In contrast, a monoclonal lymphoproliferative process is characterized by identical rearrangements of the gene segments of one cell clone. Hence fragments of the same size migrate on electrophoresis to the same position, forming a distinct band. This type of molecular genetic analysis makes it possible to recognize monoclonal proliferations that make up at least even 1% of a

Table 10.4. Antigens for lymphoma diagnosis, which are not yet clustered as those in table 10.3. The antibodies react in formalin-fixed material

Antigen/Antibody	Expression on normal lymphoid and hematopoietic cells	Expression on lymphoid and hematopoietic malignancies
ALK	Not expressed	T-anaplastic large cell lymphoma, rare B-immunoblastic/plasmablastic lymphoma
bcl-2	Follicular mantle cells, marginal zone cells T-cells	Nodal follicular lymphoma, many other lymphomas
bcl-6	Follicular center cells, some CD4+ T-cells thymic cortex cells	Follicular lymphoma, Burkitt's lymphoma, 70% DLBCL
CNA 42	Follicular dendritic cells	Follicular dendritic cells
Cyclin D1	Not expressed	Mantle cell lymphoma, plasmacytoma, hairy cell leukemia
EMA	Plasma cells	Anaplastic large cell lymphoma, plasmacytoma, some DLBCL
Immunoglobulins: IgG, A, M, Kappa; Lambda	B-cells	B-cell lymphomas
Granzyme B	Cytotoxic T-cells	NK/T-cell lymphomas, anaplastic large cell lymphoma
MUM 1	Plasma cells, some GC cells, some T-cells	Lymphoplasmacytic lymphoma, DLBCL, plasmacytoma
OCT 2	B-cells	Most B-cell lymphomas
Pax 5	B-cells	Most B-cell lymphomas, L + H cells
TdT	Thymic cortex cells	Lymphoblastic lymphoma/leukemia
TIA 1	Cytotoxic T-cells	NK/T-cell lymphomas, anaplastic large cell lymphoma

Table 10.5. Immunophenotypes of small B-cell lymphomas. *B-CLL* Chronic lymphocytic leukemia, *B-PLL* Prolymphocytic leukemia, *HCL* hairy cell leukemia, *MZBCL* marginal zone B-cell lymphoma

	CD20	CD5	CD10	CD23	bcl-2	Cyclin D1	CD 38
B-CLL	+	+	–	+	+	–	–
B-PLL	+	+	–	–	+	–	–
HCL	+	–	–	–	+/–	–	–
LP-cytic lymphoma	+	–/+	–	–	+	–	–
Mantle cell lymphoma	+	+	–	–	+	+	–/+
Follicular lymphoma	+	–	+	–	+	–	–
MZBCL	+	–	–	–	+	–	–
Plasmocytoma	–/(+)	–	–	–	–	+/–	+

Table 10.6. Immunophenotypes of precursor B-lymphoblastic leukemia/lymphoma. *ALL* Acute lymphoblastic leukemia

	CD19	CD20	CD79a	cμ	CD10	TdT
Precursor B-ALL	+	–	–/+	–	–	+
Common B-ALL	+	–/+	+	–	+	+
Pre-B-ALL	+	+	+	+	+	–/+

Table 10.7. Immunophenotypes of mature NK/T-cell neoplasms

	CD2	CD3	CD4	CD5	CD8	CD30	CD56	TIA-1
Angioimmunoblastic T-cell lymphoma	+	+	+/–	+	–/+	–/+	–	–
Peripheral T-cell lymphoma, unspecified	+	+/–	+/–	+	–/+	–/+	–/+	+/–
Anaplastic large-cell lymphoma (primary systemic)	+/–	–/+	+/–	–	–	+	–/	+/–
Adult T-cell lymphoma/leukemia (HGLV1+)	+	+	+/–	+	–/+	+/–	–	–
Mycosis fungoides; Sézary syndrome	+	+	+	+	–/+	–	–	–
Extranodal NK/T-cell lymphoma, nasal type	+/–	–/+	–	+	–	–/+	+	+
Subcutaneous panniculitis-like T-cell lymphoma	+	+/–	–	+	+	–	–/+	+
Enteropathy-type T-cell lymphoma	+	+	–	–	–/+	–/+	–/+	+
Hepatosplenic T-cell lymphoma	+	+	–	–	–/+	–	+/–	+

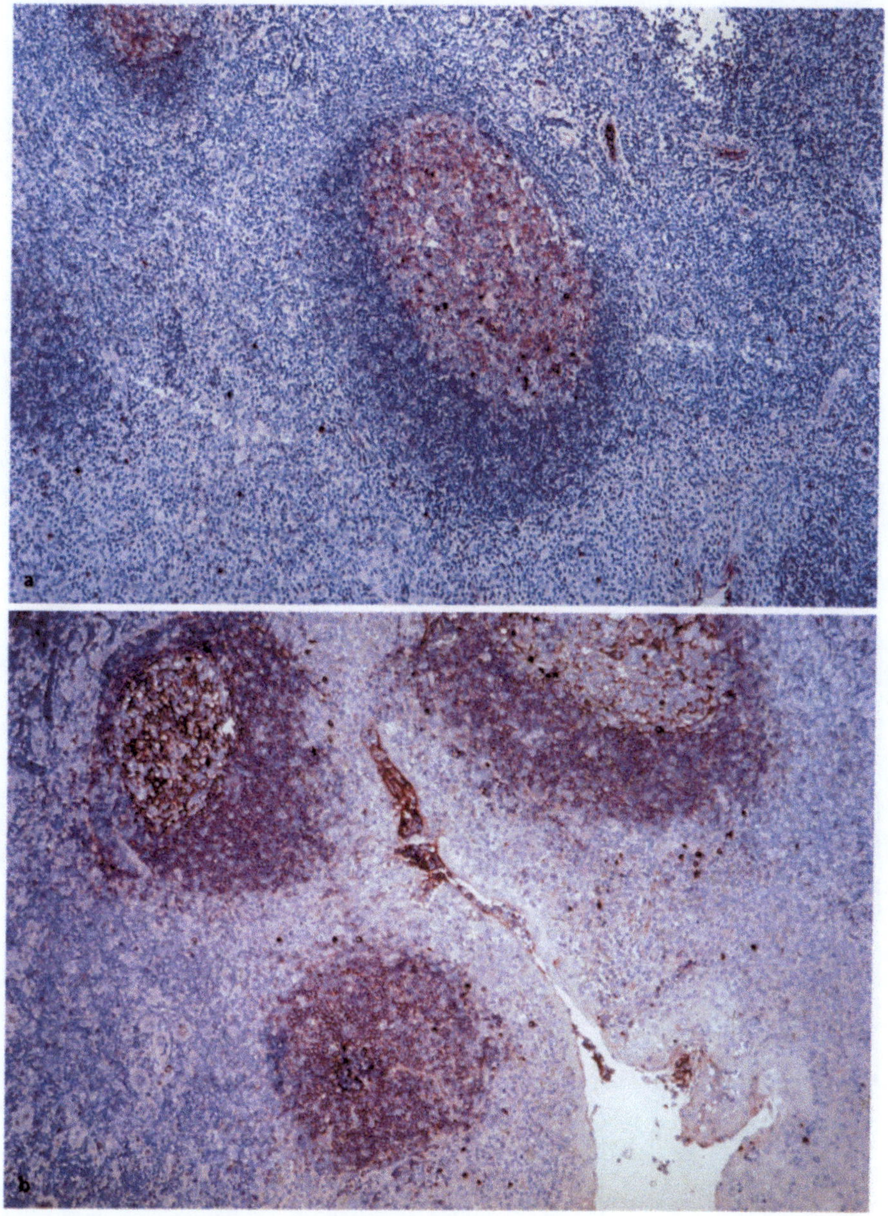

Fig. 10.4 a, b. IgM staining of a tonsilar section. **a** Conventional APAAP staining without pretreatment. Positive germinal center and faint staining of the follicular mantle. b Same staining method but with microwave pretreatment. The staining, especially in the follicular mantle, is clearly intensified

cell population. However, the high sensitivity also leads to the problem that even in some inflammatory processes monoclonal or oligoclonal B- or T-cell proliferations can be detected. Thus clonality is not by itself a sign of definite malignancy.

Immunophenotyping and molecular genetic rearrangement studies allow practically all lymphomas to be classified in the B-cell or T-cell system (Pelicci et al. 1985). So-called null-cell lymphomas are probably extremely rare exceptions. In such cases, true NK cell neoplasms as well as myelomonocytic neoplasias have to considered.

To 4: Although immunohistochemistry is necessary only in the minority of cases for correctly diagnosing a malignant lymphoma, it is still a matter of debate whether every lymphoma should be analyzed by this

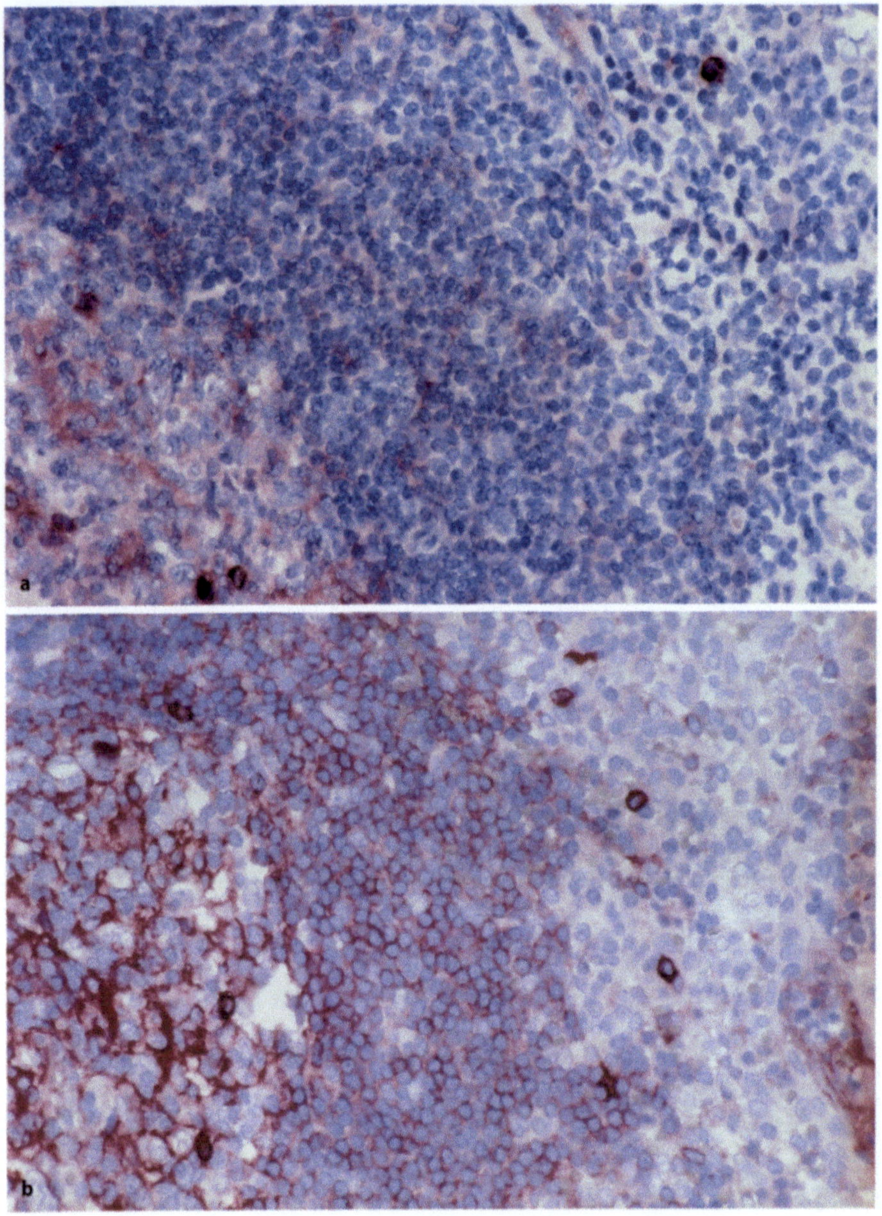

Fig. 10.5 a, b. High-power view of Fig. 10.4. Note the intensively stained follicular mantle cells in **b**. This staining pattern, with detection of surface Ig, can only be produced with the additional use of antigen retrieval techniques

technique or whether it should be limited to morphologically doubtful cases.

In our reference center for hematopathology, we apply a basic panel of immunohistochemistry assays to all malignant and benign lymphoproliferations. However, application of this basic panel is decided upon only after a primary morphological diagnosis has been made. This procedure is followed for two reasons.

A. Morphology should still lead the lymphoma diagnosis as it indicates the general direction of the diagnosis, Hodgkin's vs. non-Hodgkin's, small lymphocytic vs large-cell lymphoma, lymphoma vs carcinoma, T-cell vs B-cell, etc. The morphological evaluation is less objective if it is influenced from the beginning by immunohistochemistry.

Thus, for routine purposes the antibody panel can

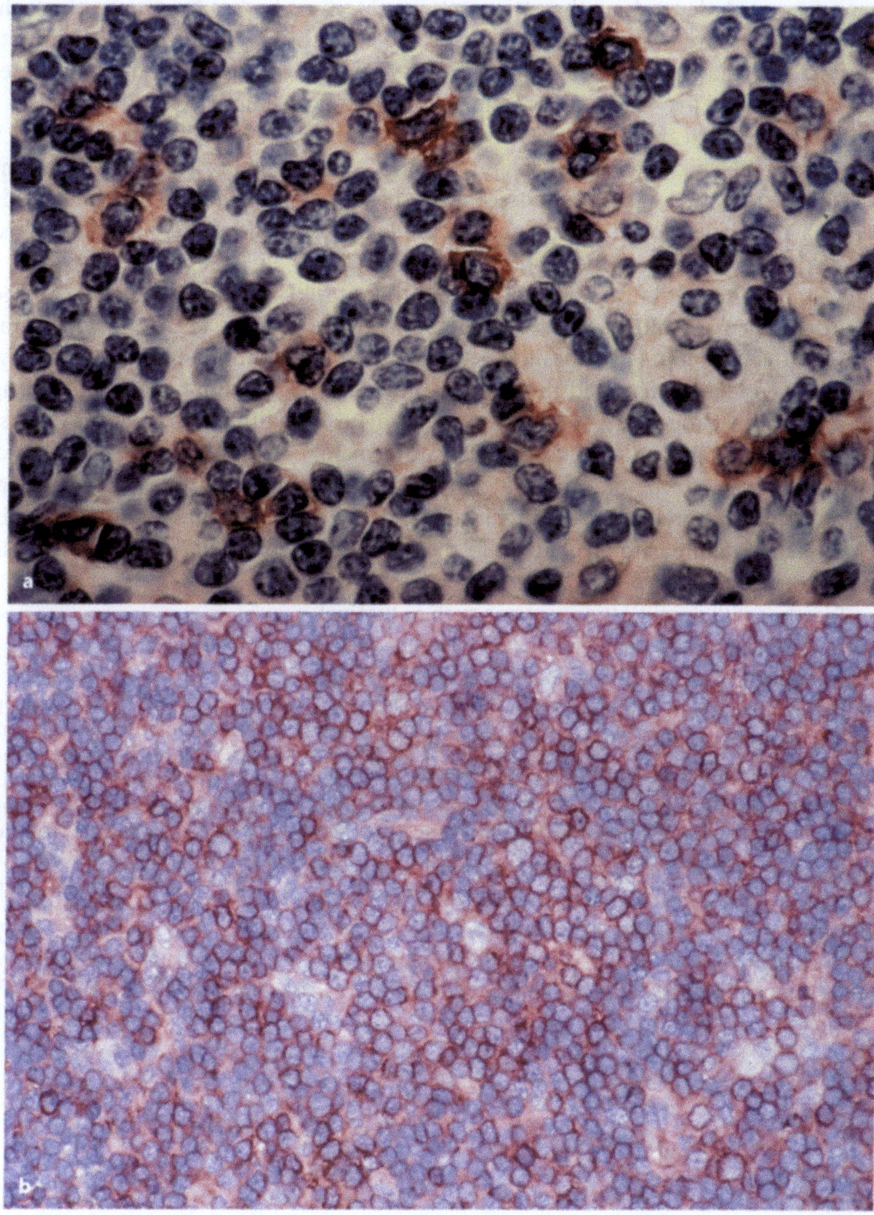

Fig. 10.6. a Staining for CD5 in a follicular mantle of a normal lymph node. Both strongly and lightly stained CD5-positive cells are visible after staining following the use of an antigen retrieval technique. The lightly stained cells may be the CD5-positive B-cells, which are the reactive counterparts of CD5-positive lymphocytic lymphomas. **b** Intensive surface staining for IgM in a lymphocytic lymphoma using an antigen retrieval technique (microwave). If the retrieval step is omitted, surface IgM is difficult to detect in lymphocytic lymphomas

be limited if the overall direction of the morphological diagnosis is fixed.

B. Immunohistochemistry allows for an objective morphological diagnosis, which by definition is a subjective one in the latter case.

Therefore, we recommend, at least for those who have limited experience in lymphoma diagnosis, the application of a basic panel of antibodies in order to determine preservation or destruction of the lymph node architecture, the B- or T-cell components, and the proliferative activity. Details for further analysis and subtyping lymphomas are given in Tables 10.4 – 10.6.

An increasing number of monoclonal antibodies suitable for formalin-fixed material has become available. However, the detection quality for different antigens very much depends on the antigen retrieval technique (for an overview see Shi et al. 2000). It has become clear that proteins react with aldehydes such as formaldehyde. This leads to protein modification, although it is unclear what kind of cross-linking actually occur and which are irreversible.

For this reason, a number of different retrieval systems have been developed in order to increase sensitivity. In principle, these systems may lead to antigen demasking or to amplification of antigen binding sites. In order to demask antigens, heating together with the use of different buffers provides the best results. Both microwave enhancement and the use of a household pressure cooker together with citrate buffer (pH 6.0) are widely used techniques (Figs. 10.4, 10.5). The major mistakes which can be made are due to the fact that temperature and pressure are difficult to standardize. Thus each system has to be adapted to the individual laboratory system.

Together with amplification systems such as biotinyl-thyramin-based enhancement, excellent results can be achieved with the use of highly diluted primary antibodies. Even antigens expressed at low levels can be made visible using an amplification system (Fig. 10.6a, b).

It is clear that tissue processing, antigen retrieval, and subsequent immunohistochemistry techniques have to be standardized not only alone but also with respect to each other. Fixation time has to be limited when buffered paraformaldehyde is used. The use of antigen retrieval systems such as microwave ovens or pressure cookers has to balance achieving maximum effect while still preserving cellular morphology. Antibodies for immunohistochemistry have to be adapted to minimize background staining. Without such a standardization, the results are not completely reliable and thus may lead to pitfalls.

It is also of importance to recognize that systematic quality control for immunohistochemistry, except the internal controls of individual laboratories, is not available. Different immunohistochemistry techniques are in use that, in part, lead to slightly different results, which, however, can be decisive in the final diagnosis. It has to be considered that pretreatment of paraffin sections may dramatically increase the sensitivity of immunohistochemistry, again making it sometimes difficult to compare results between different laboratories. Therefore, at least a constant, well-defined internal control has to be established in each laboratory using immunohistochemistry. The same is true for molecular clonality analysis.

References

Lennert K (1952) Zur histologischen Diagnose der Lymphogranulomatose. Habilitationsschrift, Frankfurt/Main

Lennert K (1961) Lymphknoten. Diagnostik in Schnitt und Ausstrich. Cytologie und Lymphadenitis. Springer, Berlin Göttingen Heidelberg (Handbuch der speziellen pathologischen Anatomie und Histologie, vol 1, part 3A)

Pelicci P-G, Knowles II DM, Dalla Favera R (1985) Lymphoid tumors displaying rearrangements of both immunoglobulin and T-cell receptor genes. J Exp Med 162:1015–1020

Shi SR, Gu J, Táylor CR (eds) (2000) Antigen retrieval techniques: immunohistochemistry and molecular morphology. Eaton, Natick, Massachusetts

Subject Index

MIX
Papier aus verantwortungsvollen Quellen
Paper from responsible sources
FSC® C105338

If you have any concerns about our products,
you can contact us on
ProductSafety@springernature.com

In case Publisher is established outside the EU,
the EU authorized representative is:
Springer Nature Customer Service Center GmbH
Europaplatz 3, 69115 Heidelberg, Germany

Printed by Libri Plureos GmbH
in Hamburg, Germany